# Iserson's
# Getting Into
# A Residency

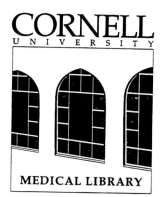

# Iserson's Getting Into A Residency

## A Guide for Medical Students

### Fifth Edition

**Kenneth V. Iserson**
**M.D., MBA, FACEP**

Galen Press, Ltd. • Tucson, Arizona

First Published 1988
Second Edition 1990
Third Edition 1993
Fourth Edition 1996
Fifth Edition 2000

Kenneth V. Iserson, M.D., MBA, FACEP
Professor of Surgery, Section of Emergency Medicine
University of Arizona College of Medicine
1501 N. Campbell Avenue
Tucson, AZ 85724 USA

AMA-FREIDA and FREIDA are registered trademarks of the American Medical Association. Windows is a registered trademark of Microsoft, Inc.

**Library of Congress Cataloging-in-Publication Data**
Iserson, Kenneth V.
  Iserson's getting into a residency : a guide for medical students / Kenneth V. Iserson. – 5th ed.
    p. ; cm.
  Rev. ed. of: Getting into a residency / Kenneth V. Iserson. 4th ed. 1996.
  Includes bibliographical references and index.
  ISBN 1-883620-27-9 (pbk.)
    1. Residents (Medicine)–Selection and appointment–United States. 2. Medical education–United States. I. Title: Getting into a residency. II. Iserson, Kenneth V. Getting into a residency. III. Title.
    [DNLM: 1. Internship and Residency–United States. 2. Education, Medical, Graduate–United States. W 20 I78i 2000]
  RA972 .I74 2000
  610'.71"550973–dc21                                                          00-025401

**Galen Press, Ltd.**
P.O. Box 64400 • Tucson, AZ 85728-4400
Phone (520) 577-8363 • FAX (520) 529-6459
Orders (U.S. & Canada) 1-800-442-5369
Special bulk purchase terms are available. Please contact our special sales department.

Printed in the United States of America
10  9  8  7  6  5  4  3  2  1

# Contents

# List of Figures

# Acknowledgments

*Those having torches will pass them on to others.*
— Plato, *The Republic*

*Of the making of books, there is no end.*
— Ecclesiastes, 12

This book would not exist but for the significant help I received from others. First and foremost is the fantastic assistance and support from my wife, Mary Lou Iserson, C.P.A. Acting as both a skilled and persistent editor, and the resident computer whiz, she midwifed every edition.

I greatly appreciate the help of the many students and physicians who took time to add to the book's content by using the Feedback Form, letters, and E-mail to send me comments (some of which are quoted in this edition).

Special thanks also goes to Donald Witzke, Ph.D., now at the University of Kentucky Medical Center, Lexington, who has strongly supported this book's concept and has acted as a superb content reviewer for every edition.

As always, I owe a debt of gratitude to my friends at the University of Arizona Health Sciences Library, who find sources of information in inscrutable ways. I am especially grateful to Nga T. Nguyen, B.A., B.S., Senior Library Specialist; Ms. Hannah Fisher, R.N., M.L.S., AHIP; and Mary L. Riordan, Research Librarian, who helped to update important details, such as organization addresses and bibliographic references. Also thanks to an ingenious and always reliable researcher, Robert Fisher, M.L.S, Tucson, AZ.

Other reviewers added to the text's completeness, including Harry Jonas, M.D., Director, Division of Undergraduate Medical Education, American Medical Association; Kenneth Ryan, M.D., Interim Dean, University of Arizona College of Medicine; and Sam Keim, M.D., President, Emergency Medicine Council of Residency Directors and Associate Professor, University of Arizona.

A variety of people at the organizations helped supply valuable and updated information for this edition. These include Verna Bronersky, Graduate Education Division, American Osteopathic Association; Waldo

Wentz, National Residency Matching Program; Douglas Perry, Executive Director, San Francisco Matching Program; Regina Damon, Fifth-Pathway Program Coordinator, New York Medical College; Katalin Scherer, M.D., Tucson, AZ; Russell B. Rayman, M.D., Executive Director, Aerospace Medical Association; David Reiley, medical student, University of Arizona College of Medicine; Sarah Brotherton, Ph.D., Director, Dept. of Research & Data Analysis, American Medical Association; Phil Kletke, Ph.D., Center for Health Policy Research, American Medical Association; Pamela Ingham, American Geriatrics Society; and Gerald Whelan, M.D., FACEP, Vice President, ECFMG.

Not only I, but also the medical students at the University of Arizona, express our gratitude to the Arizona Medical Association, to its Executive Director Chic Older, and to the Mallory Trust, who believe that this book is so essential to medical students' careers that they supply each student with a copy.

My special appreciation goes to George H. Zimny, Ph.D., for graciously allowing a markedly abbreviated version of his Medical Specialty Preference Inventory to be included in this text.

I would be remiss if I did not also thank the people at Galen Press: Mary Lou Sherk and Jennifer Gilbert, who have been wonderful in supporting this project and helping make it the success it has been. Part of that success is due to Lynn Bishop, who produced the new cover and Anne Olson, who gave the book its newly designed interior.

Finally, I wish to thank Dr. Louis Olsen, M.D., of Baltimore, Maryland. One of the few ideal physicians I know, this Family Physician suffered the strain of acting as my mentor throughout medical school—for which I will be ever grateful. It is to him that I owe much of what I am as a clinician and teacher.

# A Personal Note

*To cure sometimes, to relieve often, to comfort always.*
– Anonymous, 15th C. or earlier

I wrote this book primarily for my students who, not knowing the complex and changing systems, often got lost in the morass of details as they progressed through medical school, searched for the "right" specialty, and applied for residency positions. Many told me that they were just happy to survive the process, not knowing that they often missed options that would have saved them time, money, and grief.

I began the first edition of this book in January 1987, after I counseled several students during the same week about the specialty selection and residency application processes. None were going into my specialty of Emergency Medicine. All were desperate for this information and told me that they could not find it easily. Talk about a wake-up call!

Since the first edition came out, I have had the opportunity to speak with many medical students throughout the country when I spoke to their classes about how they could best find and achieve the exciting career opportunities that medicine has to offer. Their positive response to this book is heartwarming. I have also spoken to many student advisers and residency directors who have found that this book supplies them with some of the information they need to best counsel students and select residents for their programs.

As the new millennium dawns, I continue to have a marvelous career in clinical medicine, education, research, public policy development and, of course, writing. My hope is that this book will, in some measure, help others to achieve the same joy in their life that the medical profession has brought to mine. As Dr. Mark Siegler, one of my teachers and friends, tells students, "Medicine is a wonderful profession—ancient, noble, and surprisingly unchanging in its focus. It is a great way of life."

Kenneth V. Iserson, M.D., 2000

# Preface to the First Edition

*Knowing how to get a job is as important as knowing how to do a job.*
– Robert Half

Over the years, many students have come to me seeking career advice. In some cases, the advice was about my own specialty. But often it concerned the mechanics of finding a personal niche in medicine and assuring that the individual was able to get a training position in his or her area of interest. Sadly, most of these medical students had not spent enough time investigating all the choices available. Many believed that since they had chosen medicine as a career, and since they had achieved the long-sought-after goal of entering medical school, the significant choices were behind them. Nothing could be further from the truth.

Medicine is a diverse and complicated profession. The physician practicing Pathology is in a different world from the Family Practitioner or Physiatrist. The Radiologist's practice has little in common with that of the Anesthesiologist. Unfortunately, these differences are not as obvious as they might be in many medical school settings.

While they know, or will know, something about the practices of the Internist, Family Physician, General Surgeon, Pediatrician, Obstetrician, and Psychiatrist from their required third-year rotations, even here their knowledge may be skewed toward picturing the individuals only in the hospital setting. Rarely does this setting constitute the majority of the clinician's practice. This is insufficient knowledge upon which to base a career. In addition, most medical students are unaware of their many training options. (Many haven't even heard the term "Physiatrist" before. This is a specialist in Physical and Rehabilitation Medicine.)

The first part of this book briefly describes the specialty choices available to you. It also provides you with a method of analyzing your own interests to compare them with those of physicians practicing in various medical fields.

Even if you do make a career decision, how do you use your medical school experience to optimize your chances of getting into the specialty and program that you finally decide upon? The basic medical school wisdom is that an industrious student will get his or her just rewards. Not necessarily!

There is so much to do and so little time in which to accomplish it. You need to know how to maximize your efforts. The second part of the book encompasses this.

And then, how do you know where to interview, how to get an interview, and how to interview? Although students in other professions are given basic information on how to get their first job, this information is not generally passed on to medical students. You need this knowledge as you prepare to get your first job in medicine. You will find it in the third part of the book.

Finally, how to best utilize the Matching systems? What pitfalls must you avoid? What opportunities can you take advantage of? The last part of the book deals with these questions.

This text, in concert with your mentor and Dean of Students, is designed to guide you through the process of selecting a specialty field, helping you to maximize your efforts toward getting into your chosen specialty and program, selecting programs that meet your personal needs, getting interviews at these programs, doing well at the interviews and ultimately matching with these programs.

This book is intended to serve as a guide for the student who wants to be a winner—who is actively participating in taking those steps necessary to get into the residency he or she wants. Different parts of the book will be relevant to different students with diverse goals in mind. To make this book work for you, you should read it all, charting the course to your goal. This can be done by checking or flagging those items relevant to your goal and what you must do to achieve it. After you have charted your course, you can then use this as a plan for action. As you complete each activity, check it off. Write in the book, highlight what is relevant, and make it work for you.

If you are reading this book, it means that you are willing to put forth a little effort in preparing for your upcoming major career step. Just owning the book will not be sufficient. You must read it and apply the information diligently. Success can be yours if you expend the energy.

If any part of this book particularly helps you, or you find errors or omissions, please let me know. You can be assured that any insights you share will be considered for the future editions of this book.

Best of luck in your exciting life in medicine!

K.V. Iserson, M.D.
December, 1987

# 1

# Overview–The Problem

*Luck is a crossroad where preparation and opportunity meet.*

– Anonymous

If your rich relative just donated $3 million to endow a desperately needed chair of advanced biohypergraphics at the institution you would like to attend, you may not have much of a problem securing a residency slot there. Unfortunately, most of us are not in this position. And, with the rapidly decreasing number of quality residency positions, even the rich-relative ploy may not guarantee you entrance.

In recent years, more than 7% of the U.S. medical students attempting to find a residency position through the National Residents Matching Program (NRMP) did not match. Not exactly the kind of odds you would choose! And the odds are even worse in some of the specialties that do not go through the NRMP.

Getting a residency in the specialty you desire, at the institution you crave, is a **COMPETITION**. It has **RULES**, which you may not know unless you have been out in the working world as a professional before entering medical school. These rules correspond in many ways to those used to get executive positions in the business world. They even more closely approximate the rules you will follow to get a job after residency—assuming that you, like more than half of your colleagues, join a group practice of some type.

In many ways, however, resident-selection rules are arcane—having been derived from the ancient art of choosing an apprentice. One thing is certain: just as in the days of our ancestors, choice apprenticeship positions are few and far between.

A physician from the Philippines related a horrifying story of his experiences not many years ago. As now, the Philippines had very good quality medical schools. They taught from American texts and utilized the curriculum that is so near and dear to our hearts. But they produced more medical graduates than there were spaces available for residency training. And, since physicians were required to have advanced training to get a medical license, many medical school graduates ended up driving taxicabs and doing other odd jobs until they could get residency positions in the United States.

These events happened when we still had a doctor shortage in this country. At that time, physicians graduating from U.S. medical schools could get into almost any specialty that they desired. The only real question was where.

Today's graduating medical students are part of an ever-worsening doctor glut. While there were 142 physicians per 100,000 population in 1960 (1 physician per 703 persons), by 1998 there were 238 per 100,000 (1 physician per 420 persons). This represents a 168% growth in the number of physicians while the population increased by only 46%. Yet, while it's suggested that the physician supply in the United States will exceed the need, it may be instructive to look at the supply of physicians in some other countries (Figure 1.1).

Most of the U.S. physician surplus seems to be in the non-primary care areas (although the definition of "primary care" remains unclear). While primary care providers may be in short supply, specialists and subspecialists

FIGURE 1.1

### Physicians Per Capita in Various Countries
*(Number of persons per each physician)*

| | | | | | |
|---|---|---|---|---|---|
| Georgia | 170 | Netherlands | 410 | Philippines | 1,016 |
| Latvia | 200 | **United States** | **420** | Egypt | 1,320 |
| Italy | 210 | Australia | 438 | South Korea | 1,370 |
| Russia | 210 | Canada | 450 | South Africa | 1,750 |
| Kazakhstan | 250 | Japan | 610 | Algeria | 2,330 |
| Norway | 309 | Britain | 611 | India | 2,460 |
| Uruguay | 341 | China | 724 | Honduras | 3,090 |
| France | 350 | Ecuador | 980 | Iran | 3,140 |

Source: World Bank; Asiaweek, 1998.

abound. Therefore, the federal government is targeting many of these non-primary care training programs for destruction. Positions in most of these specialties, already difficult to obtain, will become extremely competitive.

In 1998-99, there was a total of 97,383 ACGME-approved residency positions. This was essentially the same number as in 1993-94, although there had been a marginal increase in the intervening years. But some training programs exist in name only. Among subspecialty training programs, 677 had no residents in 1998-99; 122 specialty programs had no residents. While the number of residents and fellows has increased 95% since 1970, their percentage in relation to the total U.S. physician population has decreased from 15.3% (1970) to 13.2% (1997).

In 1999, international medical graduates (IMGs) (26.1%) and Osteopathic Physicians (D.O.s) (3.7%) comprised a steadily increasing percentage of all residents, while Canadians remained constant (0.6%) and the percentage of U.S. medical graduates decreased (68.9%). There were 21,732 GY-1 positions available to students. This is more than 100 positions fewer than there were in 1994. The number of programs, however, increased from 7,435 in 1994 to 7,892 in 1999.

Applicants already overwhelm the most sought-after residency programs and institutions. But don't despair. This book will show you how to get the residency that you long for. Basically, success comes from applying the **three golden rules**:

**1. Be Assertive!** No one can look out for your best interests better than you. Don't be a wimp! Determine what you want and need, then go after it. This means that you should get yourself a mentor/adviser, research opportunities, special externships or rotations, or additional career counseling and information. Remember—the course of *your entire professional life* depends on whether or not you get a good residency in your chosen field!

**2. Time It Right!** Nothing is worse than doing all the right things—but at the wrong time. This includes getting started. As you will learn from this book, if you are a senior medical student, you are probably already behind the eight ball. The wolves howl at your door and you risk losing your desired career to unpreparedness. If you are a third-year student, you have a little more time to get your act together—but you had better work fast. The essence of timing is to *start early, apply early, and interview late.* While "the early bird gets the worm" is a rather trite expression, it is worth heeding—at least until you schedule your interviews. (See Chapter 15 for more information.)

**3. Go for the Gold!** Most medical students I know tend to "put down" both themselves and the training they received from their medical school. "It's only a state school," they say. "I wasn't AOA," they moan. This negative attitude makes them aim much lower than they should, both in the specialty they seek and in the institutional slots they pursue. My father was a professional salesman. His advice for success was, *"Sell yourself—no one will do it for you."* While you compete for your goal, keep these words close to your heart. Remember, it's your life and your career!

# 2

# The Specialties

*If you don't know where you are going,*
*you won't know when you get there.*

– Anonymous

## The Choices

In going through the process of tentatively selecting a specialty—because a tentative selection is all you should make if you are reading this during your preclinical or early clinical years—*make sure to choose for yourself.* Don't select a specialty based on:

- **What your parents want you to do.** "You're going to be a Surgeon, just like your old man," your father has said since you were knee-high to a grasshopper.
- **What your spouse wants you to do.** "Make sure that you go into something where you will be home nights and weekends—and, of course, make a lot of money."
- **What your lab partner is going into.** Did you forget that while your partner was dissecting those tiny little nerves in Anatomy you had trouble finding the biceps muscle?
- **Images from those trashy books and television shows** which first attracted you to medicine. Do you really think *any* Emergency Physician sees only crises interspersed with sexual escapades as *ER* depicts?

### "Knowing" The Specialty You Will Enter

Many students enter medical school "knowing" the specialty they will follow as their career. Most of them are wrong. Studies suggest that more than one-third of medical students make a specialty selection before medical school (although it often subsequently changes), about the same number decide during their third-year clerkships, and fewer decide either during their basic science years or after their basic clerkships.

Overall, only 20% of students who "know" what field they want to practice upon entering medical school actually pursue that field for residency training. For those with a specific specialty in mind upon entering medical school, more than one-third of those interested in Obstetrics/ Gynecology, Psychiatry, Family Practice, and Emergency Medicine ultimately pursue those fields. Even with these specialties, however, the likelihood is that you will change your mind as you experience new and exciting adventures in your route through medical school. Some people, of course, are the exception to the rule.

Even in my student days, we knew that our specialty choices would probably not last out the first year. My anatomy partner, for example, foolishly blurted out during our first day of medical school that he would be a Pediatric Surgeon. Okay, so he was good at dissection, but no one believed that he would really follow through with that goal. We now send mail to him care of the Section of Pediatric Surgery.

In general, older students are more likely to commit to a career path early in medical school.

## A Medical Career?
An uncomfortable question needs to be raised early in your considerations about selecting a career path in medicine. That is, do you really want to be a physician? Of course you have already spent a great deal of time ardently pursuing this goal. But is it still what you want? You now know a lot more about medicine and, hopefully, about yourself than when you entered upon this trek towards a medical career. Perhaps now is the time to reflect upon whether the career path you have chosen is still right for you.

An American Medical Association survey yielded disturbing results— *39% of practicing physicians probably or definitely would not go to medical school,* if they had known as much about a career in medicine when entering as they know now. If you also feel that way, now would be an appropriate time to consider jumping ship. Yes, this could deal a large blow to your self-esteem. And you might feel that you have failed the relatives and friends who have been cheering you on. But the bottom line is to do a personal assessment to determine whether your goals and desires will still be met by a medical career.

## Medicine's Opportunities

Before you do anything too hastily, however, consider that medicine has more options for its practitioners than any other profession (Figures 2.8, 2.9, and 2.10). Many of those who say that they are not happy in medicine may only be dissatisfied with their specialty. If you choose your specialty wisely, you stand the best chance of being fulfilled by your medical career (Figure 2.1).

Choose a specialty that fits your own needs, wants, and interests (Figure 2.2). Medical students considering which specialty to enter say that they give consideration to: the time they will have for their family and personal life (81%); their professional autonomy within the specialty (53%); potential income (29%); risk of malpractice (29%); and risk of contracting AIDS (10%). In assessing your own needs, you may need to consider the presence of a family in your future. You may also realize that given the increase in managed care organizations, professional autonomy is an illusion for many physicians. The debt you owe, however, is real and current.

Don't let your financial burden unduly influence your decision. Don't choose a specialty just for the big bucks. Unfortunately, that is how some of your classmates may decide upon their future direction (Figures 5.1 and 5.2). But forty or more years of being miserable in a specialty that does not really interest you is not worth it. The happiest physicians are those who

### FIGURE 2.1

### *Essentials for Specialty Selection*

1. Keep an open mind about your career direction in medicine. Many exciting career possibilities exist in medicine. Most students enter medical school with a limited view of the range of career opportunities in medicine, even (or especially) if their parents are physicians.

2. Be open to the many new possibilities and experiences that medical school offers.

3. Know that even the largest medical centers and extensive medical school curricula do not expose students to the entire scope of available medical careers.

4. Aggressively seek new, interesting career opportunities—wherever you find them.

5. Remember what excites you about a medical career.

really enjoy their work. Between 60% and 75% of medical students change their specialty choice during medical school; 20% of residents in training switch to unrelated areas; and 16% of physicians in practice change their specialty identification. Try to figure out which area of medicine you will enjoy for your entire professional life. It will be worth the time you spend doing it.

## Specialty Choice

The process of choosing a specialty is complex (Figure 2.4). It involves multiple steps. Initially, you must assess your own strengths and weaknesses, and likes and dislikes. The process has been described as "trying on possible selves" (i.e., projecting oneself into hypothetical career and personal roles). Medical students must make specialty choices that fit with their own personalities, so that they are compatible with other practitioners in the specialty, and with their comfort and ability to master the specialty's content and skills. They make these choices as they go through medical school in three ways:

1. They confirm that a pre-existing specialty choice does meet their needs.

2. They select a specialty that includes many of the areas they find interesting.

3. They eliminate specialties as they discover things about themselves and various specialties that are not compatible.

The biggest decision point for most students in their specialty selection is whether to enter a surgical or a non-surgical specialty. Those entering a surgical area want a high level of control when practicing medicine, while those entering non-surgical specialties are especially interested in a manageable caseload (Figure 2.2).

After looking over the available specialties, you can make a tentative choice. Then you must gather enough information, both by reading and through experience, to confirm that you have made the correct personal selection of a specialty. With this commitment you will experience some relief and stability. But this decision can also lead to anxiety. Such anxiety is a normal part of making a major decision and is termed "post-purchase dissonance." If your anxiety is more severe than this (more than the feeling that you get after you have signed the papers on a new car or expensive sound system), your career decision should be investigated further—and perhaps changed.

---

## FIGURE 2.2

### *Factors Important to Students When Selecting a Residency Program*

**Very Important**

- House officer satisfaction
- General impression at the interview
- Diversity of training experience
- Geographic location

**Important**

- Conference/didactic teaching
- High level of management responsibility
- Opportunities for post-residency training
- High patient volume
- Program's prestige
- Proportion of IMGs in program

**Not Very Important**

- Department's and faculty's prestige
- Extent of staff supervision
- Manageable case load
- Call schedules
- Electives availability
- Support services
- Physical plant
- Opportunity to conduct research
- Benefits
- Salary

**Not Important**

- Opportunity to treat AIDS patients
- Absence of AIDS from patient population
- Training in one hospital

Adapted from: Simmonds AC, Robbins JM, Brinker MR, Rice JC, Kerstein MD: Factors important to students in selecting a residency program. *Acad Med.* 1990;65(10):640-43 and Riley JD, Hannis M, Rice KG: Are international medical graduates a factor in residency program selection? A survey of fourth-year medical students. *Acad Med.* 1996;71(4):381-6.

---

Once you make a career decision, expect to hear negative comments about other specialties as you rotate through clerkships. This behavior is typical of medical practitioners. Physicians, as well as other professionals, often believe that the "holy grail" is whatever professional area they chose, and everyone else does less important work, simply works less hard, makes too much money for what they do, or is incompetent. Whether this is a way to bolster their self-esteem, reinforce their career choice, or results from their interactions with other practitioners and their patients is uncertain. However, just as professional baseball pitchers cannot allow themselves to be affected by catcalls from the stands, medical students allow these comments to influence their career decisions only at their own peril.

## Jobs—The Ultimate Goal

Completing medical school and residency seems pointless if you cannot ultimately get a position in your specialty. You will have to take a realistic look at the specialties. Some fields are already crowded; others, according to the best estimates, soon will be. Some recent graduates, especially in Anesthesiology, Plastic Surgery, and Pathology are having trouble finding jobs (Figure 2.5). In response, many residency programs are planning to reduce the number of training positions over the next few years.

Those programs in which the most positions have been lost include Anesthesiology, Radiation Oncology, and Pathology. Anesthesiology, Radiation Oncology, Radiology, and Pathology expect additional decreases. Twice as many residency directors in university-based programs anticipate losing positions as do those in university-affiliated and community-based programs. This will dramatically increase the competition for university-based positions.

However, positions have been recently added at many residencies in Family Medicine, Emergency Medicine, Pediatrics, and Internal Medicine, with all but Pediatrics anticipating additional increases. Residency directors expect increased competition for all training positions in Pediatrics, Internal Medicine, Emergency Medicine, General Surgery, Family Medicine, and Anesthesiology.

Residency directors foresee an increase in job opportunities for residency graduates in Anesthesiology (due to decreasing numbers of grad- uates to fill the positions opened by retiring anesthesiologists), Family Medicine, Internal Medicine, and Pediatrics. They believe fewer jobs will be available for new Radiation Oncologists, Ophthalmologists, Orthopedic Surgeons, Radiologists, and Pathologists.

Despite these predictions, any specialty that you find that you really like, whether it is likely to be populated by a horde of other physicians or not, will most likely suit you the best.

So where are these physicians practicing? The U.S. regions with the most physicians per population are New England (CT, ME, MA, NH, RI, VT) with one physician for every 265 people and the Middle Atlantic (PA, NJ, NY) with one physician for every 282 people. The regions with the fewest physicians per capita are the West South Central (AR, LA, OK, TX) with only one physician per 466 people and the Mountain (AZ, CO, ID, MT, NV, NM, UT, WY) with one physician per 437 people.

The states with the highest physician-to-population ratios are listed in Figure 2.3.

FIGURE 2.3

**U.S. States with the Highest Number of Physicians per Capita**
*(Number of persons per each physician)*

| | | | |
|---|---|---|---|
| District of Columbia | 131 | Rhode Island | 283 |
| Massachusetts | 230 | Vermont | 300 |
| New York | 248 | New Jersey | 320 |
| Maryland | 251 | Pennsylvania | 324 |
| Connecticut | 263 | Hawaii | 336 |

Adapted from Table 7, *Physician Characteristics and Distribution in the U.S., 1999.* Chicago, IL: American Medical Association, 1999, p. 17.

## Medicine's Future

I hope you will have a long career in medicine. This means that you will see many changes, not only in the science and art of medicine but also in health care delivery systems. Your choice of specialty will, in part, determine how well you weather these changes. At present, three important factors appear to be influencing the course of health care delivery: the role of primary care versus specialist physicians, the role of managed care delivery systems, and the number of physicians in each specialty compared to those that are needed to provide adequate care for the population. While these factors are clearly interrelated, I will attempt to provide you with a brief overview of the individual elements.

FIGURE 2.4

**Process of Choosing a Specialty**

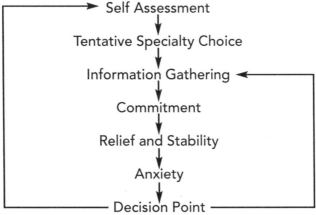

Adapted from: *New Physician.* July-August 1986, p. 19.

FIGURE 2.5

## Will There be Jobs in the Specialty?

| Specialty | Employed When Completing Residency* | Difficulty Finding Preferred Position# | Work in Closed-Panel HMO | % of Training in Managed Care Setting |
|---|---|---|---|---|
| Vascular Surgery | 100.0% | 0.0% | 5.3% | 7.3% |
| Neurological Surgery | 100.0 | 3.8 | 0.0 | 12.4 |
| Orthopedic Surgery | 100.0 | 9.5 | 11.4 | 9.0 |
| Hand Surgery (Orth) | 100.0 | 10.7 | 11.1 | 9.5 |
| Colon & Rectal Surgery | 100.0 | 33.3 | 0.0 | 18.8 |
| Urology | 98.3 | 15.0 | 10.0 | 12.0 |
| Otolaryngology | 98.1 | 20.5 | 9.9 | 10.8 |
| Emergency Medicine | 97.8 | 11.4 | 6.8 | 17.7 |
| Obstetrics & Gynecology | 97.7 | 15.0 | 10.5 | 16.7 |
| Neonatology | 97.5 | 35.3 | 18.8 | 6.8 |
| Dermatology | 96.4 | 11.8 | 14.1 | 16.4 |
| Thoracic Surgery | 96.3 | 22.9 | 3.0 | 9.3 |
| Cardiology | 95.3 | 15.4 | 3.2 | 11.5 |
| Plastic Surgery | 94.9 | 37.7 | 9.8 | 11.6 |
| Nephrology | 94.7 | 13.6 | — | — |
| Family Practice | 94.5 | 8.2 | 9.7 | 12.5 |
| Child Psychiatry | 93.6 | 4.5 | 14.0 | 12.2 |
| Oncology | 93.1 | 22.2 | 11.1 | 13.6 |
| Pediatric Surgery | 92.9 | 0.0 | 16.7 | 0.1 |
| Pain Management | 92.9 | 17.1 | 5.0 | 14.7 |
| Neurology | 92.7 | 19.7 | 11.9 | 7.3 |
| Radiation Oncology | 92.5 | 45.0 | 10.0 | 10.3 |
| Diagnostic Radiology | 92.0 | 32.7 | 6.3 | 8.6 |
| General Surgery | 91.8 | 21.3 | 6.7 | 13.0 |
| Physical Medicine/Rehab | 91.7 | 29.0 | 9.1 | 8.7 |
| Anesthesiology | 91.5 | 28.1 | 4.7 | 13.0 |
| Gastroenterology | 91.4 | 41.0 | 7.4 | 15.4 |
| Allergy/Immunology | 90.7 | 41.7 | 4.2 | 17.0 |
| Hematology/Oncology | 90.3 | 34.5 | 7.4 | 5.8 |
| Geriatrics (IM) | 90.2 | 45.0 | 15.8 | 5.5 |
| Psychiatry | 90.0 | 21.6 | 10.7 | 9.2 |
| Infectious Diseases | 89.8 | 30.8 | 7.9 | 8.4 |
| Pediatrics | 89.2 | 21.2 | 9.1 | 15.4 |
| Ophthalmology | 87.7 | 32.4 | 16.3 | 8.9 |
| Endocrinology | 87.1 | 31.4 | 11.4 | 13.8 |

FIGURE 2.5 (continued)

| Specialty | Employed When Completing Residency* | Difficulty Finding Preferred Position# | Work in Closed-Panel HMO | % of Training in Managed Care Setting |
|---|---|---|---|---|
| Rheumatology | 86.0% | 26.7% | 0.0% | 7.5% |
| Critical Care (IM) | 84.6 | 30.8 | 15.4 | 1.8 |
| Nephrology | 84.4 | 15.6 | 4.8 | 11.4 |
| Internal Medicine | 83.9 | 27.1 | 13.5 | 10.6 |
| Child Neurology | 83.3 | 27.3 | 9.1 | 9.9 |
| Pulmonary Disease (IM) | 83.3 | 44.4 | 5.6 | 12.2 |
| Pathology (Anat & Clinical) | 81.3 | 44.6 | 1.9 | 4.5 |
| Preventive Medicine (All) | 79.5 | 20.0 | 16.7 | 11.4 |
| Nuclear Medicine | 76.5 | 50.0 | 11.1 | 8.9 |
| Hematology | 73.3 | 0.0 | 0.0 | 3.5 |

#Osteopathic training programs may not exist in all approved specialties and subspecialties.
*Also available to diplomates of other AOA Boards.

Adapted from AMA statistics, 1999. (To order specialties, numbers were not rounded, as they were in the specialty descriptions.)

## Primary Care

Before looking at individual specialties, you should know what is meant by the term "primary care"—a hot topic among health planners, politicians, and medical school deans.

What is primary care? Primary care is ideally the point at which patients enter the health treatment system. Primary care practitioners, now also referred to as "Generalists," should be able to diagnose and treat 80% or more of the patients that present themselves, oversee the activities of any specialists involved in their patient's care, and provide continuity of care. Whether many practitioners actually do all these is questionable. It is often especially difficult to provide continuity of care, since patients frequently switch their managed care plans (HMOs, PPOs, IPAs, etc.).

What specialties are considered "primary care"? Certainly the term encompasses General Internal Medicine, Family Practice, and General Pediatrics. Does it also include Obstetrics and Gynecology, Emergency Medicine, Psychiatry, Internal Medicine subspecialties, Dermatology, and Neurology? All have been proposed as being "primary care." In some cases their practitioners do exactly what the definition implies—sometimes better than those in the three generalist specialties. Most Physician Assistants and Nurse Practitioners also fall into this category. But why all this fuss?

The answer is, for money and survival. Over the past several decades, the federal government's regulatory and funding arms have attempted to limit the number of non-primary care residency and fellowship (except Geriatrics) positions. Multiple groups continue to advocate increasing primary care residency positions, although it has become clear that there are enough, if not too many, primary care practitioners—they just are not distributed where they are most needed.

A key national policy question is what percentage of graduates practice medicine in a rural or underserved urban environment? While we produce many primary care practitioners, they don't seem to go where they are needed. About 88% of all primary care physicians practice in metropolitan areas, compared with nearly 90% of all U.S. physicians. Among primary care physicians, about 70% are office-based. General Practice and Obstetricians and Gynecologists (76%) most commonly have office-based practices. Internists are the least commonly office based (63%).

A primary care designation has, therefore, been politically important for survival. What does this mean to you? The relevant question is, what will "primary care" include?

You may have noticed that many senior faculty extol the virtues of primary care. Perhaps this is because national groups and legislators have recently been reviewing medical schools based on the percentage of their graduates that go into primary care specialties. With more than one-third of U.S. medical schools having an explicit mission to produce primary care physicians, the folks who control the purse strings are carefully reviewing whether they are meeting this goal. Medical schools have been successful in promoting primary care specialties, with the number of graduates planning a career in Family Practice, General Internal Medicine, or General Pediatrics growing from 14.6% of 1992's graduating class to 35.6% in 1999. (Although, for the fourth straight year, more than 50% of the 1999 class took residencies in Family Practice, Internal Medicine, or Pediatrics, many are expected to subspecialize.) Family Practice gained the most, with 9% of 1992's class entering the field but with 14.6% of 1999's class choosing this specialty.

At most U.S. medical schools, about 50% of each graduating class enters a primary care residency—although many subsequently enter subspecialties. Among M.D.-granting schools, this percentage ranges from about 75% at Morehouse School of Medicine and the University of Minnesota-Duluth to about 33% at the Universidad Central del Caribe. Osteopathic medical schools have a much firmer primary care orientation, with more than two-thirds of all students entering primary care. This ranges from about 70% at the Chicago and the Texas Colleges of Osteopathic Medicine to about 97% at Michigan State University. Of those D.O.s entering primary care, nearly all go into Family Practice.

According to many state government descriptions, "Primary Care" includes Family Practice, General Practice, Internal Medicine, Obstetrics and Gynecology, and Pediatrics, excluding the subspecialties in these areas. Over the past three decades, the number of physicians in primary care specialties more than doubled, as did the total number of U.S. physicians. Among them, Internists comprise 38.7% of all primary care physicians; Family Practitioners, 26.3%; Obstetrician/Gynecologists, 12.4%; Pediatricians, 17.3%; and General Practitioners, 5.3%. (General Practitioners are usually physicians who practice general medicine and do not hold board certification; nearly half are at least 65 years old.) The subspecialties in these fields also increased, with the largest increase occurring in Pediatric subspecialties.

States with the highest ratio of primary care physicians to all physicians are Illinois (38%), New Jersey and Michigan (36%), Ohio and New York (35%), and Texas (34%). More than 39% of all international medical graduates practice in primary care, as do 33% of U.S. medical graduates and 27% of Canadian medical graduates practicing in the United States.

While about 63% of all U.S. physicians are Board certified, only about 56% of primary care physicians have their Boards. The highest percentage of those with primary care Board certification is in Family Practice (68%), while the lowest (excluding General Practice) is in Internal Medicine (49%). About 83% of primary care subspecialists have their Boards.

Why do students choose to enter primary care, especially Family Practice? Studies suggest that students are strongly influenced by: coming from a rural background; having low income expectations and little debt; being Hispanic, a woman, married, or older; not being concerned about control of one's work hours; and perhaps most important, whether they entered medical school thinking that they would be a Family Practitioner. (Other factors are listed in Figure 2.6.) One study also suggested that students who were less Machiavellian tended to go into primary care. (Heh! Heh! Heh! Were you saying you wanted to subspecialize?)

No one really knows how many primary care practitioners we need. Some studies now suggest that the United States has adequate generalist physicians to meet current needs. As an AAMC spokesman said, "In recent years, there has been no insufficiency in primary care doctors. We were giving people the wrong message." The real problem seems to be an overabundance of specialists. Plans were afoot to retrain specialists into

---

**FIGURE 2.6**

*Reasons Why Students Choose Primary Care/*
*Non-Primary Care Specialties*

**Factors important when selecting a primary care specialty:**

1. Continuity of care.

2. Preventive interventions.

3. Diverse patient populations.

4. Enhanced patient interactions.

5. Breadth of clinical activities and content.

6. Influence of role models and mentors.

**Factors important when selecting a non-primary care specialty:**

1. Physician lifestyle and quality of life.

2. Seeing immediate results of interventions.

3. Doing procedures and having technical skills.

4. Intellectual challenge.

5. Pace of practice.

6. Specific setting: ED, OR, ICU.

Adapted from: Burack JH, Irby DM, Carline JD, et al.: A study of medical students' specialty-choice pathways: trying on possible selves. *Acad Med.* 1997;72(6):534-41.

---

primary care (a fruitless endeavor that has now been all but abandoned). Specialists, rather than primary care physicians, provide most care for one in five Americans, with most of these patients being elderly.

As alternative practitioners (Physician Assistants and Nurse Practitioners) assume many duties formerly performed by primary care physicians, the era of the primary care practitioner may have passed. Yet bureaucrats with little grasp of the big picture will probably determine the balance of training positions. As with their response to the "physician shortage" only a few years ago, they are certain to overreact.

At the present time, residency graduates intending to practice primary care are doing very well; they report that they get more than fifty recruitment offers during their residency (IMGs get fewer). Their salary expectations are also rising, although whether they will get what they hope for still remains to be seen.

## The Managed Care Environment

Health care delivery is changing and managed care organizations are taking the lead in that change. "Managed care" includes a wide variety of structures, from large group practices relying on salaried physicians and their own hospitals to every other imaginable permutation of physicians, insurance companies, and hospitals. What they have in common is that, rather than emphasizing quality medical care or the physician-patient relationship (some may still have these), they emphasize cost-effectiveness. With the runaway cost of medical care and the increasing availability of high-technology, high-cost diagnostic and treatment modalities, such a change was inevitable.

A wag once commented that if we treated medicine like agriculture and paid every unneeded licensed physician $100,000 to not practice medicine, we could balance the federal budget. Indeed, the more physicians we have, the more medical tests and procedures are ordered and the more costs increase. Specialists do far more tests and procedures than primary care practitioners; hospitalized patients get the most tests and the most procedures. Managed care organizations, therefore, profit by keeping as many patients as possible away from specialists and hospitals. They have been very successful at doing this in many parts of the country. You can see the effect of this in the many hospitals that have closed or been forced to merge, the specialists who wish to retrain into primary care, the new specialty graduates who cannot get jobs in locales they desire, and the specialty societies that plan to close residency and fellowship programs.

Among the key skills needed to be a successful practitioner within the managed care environment are the ability to diagnose and treat a wide variety of common illnesses, the ability to recognize when you are beyond your depth clinically, an ability and willingness to see many patients quickly, an ability to work with many other physicians and non-physician health care providers, an understanding of how to effectively use information systems (computers), and a willingness to tolerate the unwieldy clinical and financial maze of managed care organizations.

These are skills that, for the most part, can and should be learned during medical school and residency. An optimal place to learn such skills is to work within a managed care framework, gaining experience by either dealing with such organizations from the outside or, better yet, spending some time working in managed care groups. Unfortunately, only 20% of teaching hospitals use such facilities for residency training, and the amount of education in managed care settings varies by specialty (Figure 2.5).

As can be seen in Figure 2.7, it is now common for physicians to participate in managed care. Soon the full impact of managed care will be felt throughout the country. Making money (for owners and insurance companies) and saving money (by employers and government) are strong incentives. It would be wise for you to consider the impact of managed care systems on medical practice in the United States as you make your career decisions.

While managed care is the current buzzword in health care delivery, the caveat when charting your future career is to always plan for the next system—and perhaps for the system after that.

## The "Right" Number of Physicians

Medicine and medical care delivery systems are changing so fast that no one can predict exactly how many physicians we will need or what will be the optimal balance of specialties over the course of your career—or even for the next ten years. An educated guess of how many physicians will be in the various specialties can be found in Figure 5.4. Whether these numbers represent too many or too few physicians is, at present, unclear. Some pessimistic studies suggest that about 40% of all medical specialists could be unnecessary by the end of this decade.

FIGURE 2.7
### *Percentage of Specialty Physicians in Practices with Managed Care Contracts*

| Specialty | Any Managed Care Contract | Private | Medicare | Medicaid |
|---|---|---|---|---|
| Obstetrics/Gynecology | 98% | 96% | 83% | 70% |
| Radiology | 98 | 98 | 73 | 74 |
| Anesthesiology | 98 | 96 | 82 | 77 |
| Surgical Subspecialty | 98 | 96 | 72 | 66 |
| General Surgery | 98 | 95 | 72 | 73 |
| Int Med Subspecialty | 97 | 95 | 72 | 67 |
| Pediatrics | 97 | 95 | 17 | 80 |
| **ALL PHYSICIANS** | **94** | **91** | **67** | **67** |
| Emergency Med | 93 | 90 | 73 | 75 |
| Gen Internal Med | 92 | 89 | 71 | 65 |
| Family Practice | 91 | 86 | 64 | 62 |
| Pathology | 86 | 82 | 64 | 59 |
| Other Specialties | 86 | 81 | 56 | 56 |
| Psychiatry | 84 | 77 | 56 | 50 |

Adapted from: American Medical Association. *Physician Socioeconomic Statistics 1999-2000.* Chicago, IL: AMA, 1999, pp. 106-7.

Economic necessity is pushing the health care system to encourage more non-physicians to practice medicine; including Nurse Practitioners, Nurse-Anesthetists, Nurse- and lay-midwives, Physician Assistants, and others. In some cases, they are decreasing the need for specialist physicians (Anesthesiologists, Ophthalmologists) while in other cases, such as primary care specialties, their numbers have hardly dented the need for practitioners.

When considering what specialty to enter, you will hear conflicting opinions about the future need for physicians in various specialties. As the truism goes, "There are liars, damn liars, and statisticians." Worse yet are those who interpret those statistics, often incompletely or incorrectly, to make their points. Take all these prognostications with a grain of salt.

Your best course of action is to use all the factors you believe, including the potential job markets. Next, assess which specialty best fits your needs, your interests, and your personality. Then pursue it with all of your determination.

The future will come, no matter what you do. Therefore, your best strategy is to prepare yourself to *enjoy* your medical career.

FIGURE 2.8

### American Board of Medical Specialties (M.D.)-Approved Specialty Boards, Certifications, and Special Qualification Categories

| American Board | Certification | Subspecialty |
|---|---|---|
| Allergy & Immunology | Allergy & Immunology | Clinical & Lab Immun |
| Anesthesiology | Anesthesiology | Critical Care Medicine<br>Pain Management |
| Colon & Rectal Surgery | Colon & Rectal Surgery | |
| Dermatology | Dermatology | Dermatopathology<br>Clinical & Lab Derm Immun |
| Emergency Medicine | Emergency Medicine | Medical Toxicology<br>Pediatric Emergency Med<br>Sports Medicine |
| Family Practice | Family Practice | Geriatric Medicine<br>Sports Medicine |
| Internal Medicine | Internal Medicine | Adolescent Medicine<br>Cardiovascular Disease<br>Clin Cardiac Electrophysiology<br>Clinical & Lab Immun<br>Critical Care Medicine |

FIGURE 2.8 (continued)

| American Board | Certification | Subspecialty |
|---|---|---|
| Internal Medicine (continued) | | Endocrin, Diabetes & Met |
| | | Gastroenterology |
| | | Geriatric Medicine |
| | | Hematology |
| | | Infectious Diseases |
| | | Interventional Cardiology |
| | | Medical Oncology |
| | | Nephrology |
| | | Pulmonary Disease |
| | | Rheumatology |
| | | Sports Medicine |
| Medical Genetics | Clinical Biochemical Genetics | Molecular Genetic Pathology |
| | Clinical Cytogenetics | |
| | Clinical Genetics (M.D. only) | |
| | Clinical Molecular Genetics | |
| | Medical Genetics (Ph.D. only) | |
| Neurological Surgery | Neurological Surgery | |
| Nuclear Medicine | Nuclear Medicine | |
| Obstetrics & Gynecology | Obstetrics & Gynecology | Critical Care Medicine |
| | | Gynecologic Oncology |
| | | Maternal & Fetal Med |
| | | Reproductive Endocrinology |
| | | Urogynecology/Reconstructive Pelvic Surgery |
| Ophthalmology | Ophthalmology | |
| Orthopedic Surgery | Orthopedic Surgery | Hand Surgery |
| Otolaryngology | Otolaryngology | Otology/Neurotology |
| | | Pediatric Otolaryngology |
| Pathology | Anatomic & Clinical Pathology | Blood Bank/Transfus Med |
| | Anatomic Pathology | Chemical Pathology |
| | Clinical Pathology | Cytopathology |
| | | Dermatopathology |
| | | Forensic Pathology |
| | | Hematology |
| | | Immunopathology |
| | | Medical Microbiology |
| | | Neuropathology |
| | | Pediatric Pathology |

FIGURE 2.8 (continued)

| American Board | Certification | Subspecialty |
|---|---|---|
| Pediatrics | Pediatrics | Adolescent Medicine |
| | | Clinical & Lab Immunology |
| | | Developmental-Behavioral Peds |
| | | Medical Toxicology |
| | | Neonatai-Perinatal Med |
| | | Pediatric Cardiology |
| | | Ped Critical Care Med |
| | | Ped Emergency Med |
| | | Ped Endocrinology |
| | | Ped Gastroenterology |
| | | Ped Hematology-Oncology |
| | | Ped Infectious Diseases |
| | | Pediatric Nephrology |
| | | Pediatric Pulmonology |
| | | Pediatric Rheumatology |
| | | Sports Medicine |
| Physical Medicine & Rehabilitation | Physical Medicine & Rehabilitation | Pain Management |
| | | Pediatric Rehabilitation Med |
| | | Spinal Cord Injury Medicine |
| Plastic Surgery | Plastic Surgery | Hand Surgery |
| Preventive Medicine | Aerospace Medicine | Medical Toxicology |
| | Occupational Medicine | Underseas Med |
| | Public Health & General Preventive Medicine | |
| Psychiatry & Neurology | Psychiatry | Addiction Psychiatry |
| | Neurology | Child & Adolescent Psych |
| | Neurology with Special Qualifications in Child Neurology | Clinical Neurophysiology |
| | | Forensic Psychiatry |
| | | Geriatric Psychiatry |
| | | Neurodevelopmental Disabilities |
| | | Pain Management |
| Radiology | Diagnostic Radiology | Neuroradiology |
| | Radiation Oncology | Nuclear Radiology |
| | Radiological Physics | Pediatric Radiology |
| | Radiology | Vascular/Interventional Rad |
| Surgery | Surgery | General Vascular Surgery |
| | | Pediatric Surgery |
| | | Surgery of the Hand |
| | | Surgical Critical Care |
| Thoracic Surgery | Thoracic Surgery | |
| Urology | Urology | |

Adapted from: American Board of Medical Specialties. *1999 Annual Report & Reference Handbook*. Atlanta, GA:ABMS, 1999.

FIGURE 2.9

## Approved Specialty Boards, Certification, and Special Qualification Categories (D.O.)#

| American Osteopathic Board | General Certification | Certification of Special Qualifications† | Certification of Added Qualifications†† |
|---|---|---|---|
| Anesthesiology | Anesthesiology | | Addiction Medicine<br>Critical Care Medicine<br>Pain Management |
| Dermatology | Dermatology | | Dermatopathology<br>Micrographic Surgery |
| Emergency Medicine | Emergency Medicine | | Emergency Med Services<br>Medical Toxicology*<br>Sports Medicine |
| Family Physicians | Family Practice | | Addiction Medicine<br>Adolescent & Young<br>  Adult Medicine<br>Geriatric Medicine<br>Sports Medicine |
| Internal Medicine | Internal Medicine | Allergy & Immunology<br>Cardiology<br>Endocrinology<br>Gastroenterology<br>Hematology<br>Hematology/Oncology<br>Infectious Disease<br>Pulmonary Diseases<br>Nephrology<br>Oncology<br>Rheumatology | Addiction Medicine<br>Critical Care Medicine<br>Clin Card Electrophysiology<br>Geriatric Medicine<br>Sports Medicine |
| Neurology & Psychiatry | Neurology<br>Psychiatry | | Child Neurology<br>Child Psychiatry |
| Nuclear Medicine | Nuclear Medicine | | Nuclear Cardiology<br>Nuclear Imaging & Therapy<br>In Vivo & In Vitro Nuclear Med |
| Obstetrics & Gynecology | Obstetrics & Gynecology | | Gynecologic Oncology<br>Maternal & Fetal Medicine<br>Reproductive Endocrinology |
| Ophthalmology & Otolaryngology– Head & Neck Surg | Ophthalmology<br>Otolaryngology<br>Facial Plastic Surg<br>Otolaryngology & Facial Plastic Surg | | |
| Orthopedic Surg | Orthopedic Surg | | |
| Pathology | Anatomic Pathology<br>Anatomic Pathology & Lab Med<br><br>Laboratory Med | Forensic Pathology | Blood Bank/Transfus Med<br>Chemical Pathology<br><br>Cytopathology<br>Dermatopathology<br>Hematology<br>Immunopathology<br>Medical Microbiology<br>Neuropathology |

FIGURE 2.9 (continued)

| American Osteopathic Board | General Certification | Certification of Special Qualifications[†] | Certification of Added Qualifications[††] |
|---|---|---|---|
| Pediatrics | Pediatrics | Adolescent & Young Adult Medicine<br>Neonatology<br>Ped Allergy/Immunology<br>Ped Cardiology<br>Ped Endocrinology<br>Ped Hematology-Oncology<br>Ped Infectious Diseases<br>Ped Intensive Care<br>Ped Nephrology<br>Ped Pulmonary | Sports Medicine |
| Preventive Medicine | Preventive Med/ Aerospace Med<br>Preventive Med/ Occupational-Environmental Med<br>Preventive Med/ Public Health | | Occupational/Environmental Medicine** |
| Proctology | Proctology | | |
| Radiology | Diagnostic Radiology | | Angiography & Interventional Radiology |
| | Radiation Oncology | | Body Imaging<br>Diagnostic Ultrasound<br>Neuroradiology<br>Nuclear Radiology<br>Pediatric Radiology |
| Rehabilitation Med | Rehabilitation Med | | Sports Medicine |
| Special Proficiency in Osteopathic Manipulative Med | Special Proficiency in Osteopathic Manipulative Med | | Sports Medicine |
| Surgery | Gen Vascular Surgery<br>Neurological Surgery<br>Plastic & Reconstructive Surgery<br>Surgery (General)<br>Thoracic Surgery<br>Urological Surgery | Gen Vascular Surgery | Surgical Critical Care |

[#]Osteopathic training programs may not exist in all approved specialties and subspecialties.
*Also available to diplomates of other AOA Boards.
**Available only to diplomates from other AOA Boards.
[†]Requires General Certification—Equivalent to "Subspecialty."
[††]Requires General Certification or Certification of Special Qualifications—Equivalent to "Subspecialty."

Adapted from: American Osteopathic Association: *1999 Yearbook and Directory of Osteopathic Physicians*, 90th ed. Chicago, IL: AOA, 1999.

FIGURE 2.10

## M.D. and D.O. Physicians in Practice by Specialty

| Specialty | Total Physicians | Osteopathic Physicians | % That Practice This Specialty |
|---|---|---|---|
| Aerospace Medicine | 586 | 112 | 0.1 |
| Allergy & Immunology | 3,772 | 77 | 0.5 |
| Anesthesiology | 33,730 | 1,448 | 4.4 |
| Cardiovascular Disease | 19,287 | 573 | 2.5 |
| Child Psychiatry | 5,620 | 115 | 0.7 |
| Colon & Rectal Surgery | 1,033 | 1 | 0.1 |
| Dermatology | 9,062 | 305 | 1.2 |
| Emergency Medicine | 20,605 | 2,669 | 2.7 |
| Family Practice | 64,611 | 19,656 | 8.5 |
| Forensic Pathology | 514 | na | 0.1 |
| Gastroenterology | 9,728 | 285 | 1.3 |
| General Practice | 16,835 | 65 | 2.2 |
| General Preventive Medicine | 1,550 | 302 | 0.2 |
| General Surgery | 40,935 | 922 | 5.4 |
| Internal Medicine | 128,435 | 3,244 | 17.0 |
| Medical Genetics | 250 | na | <0.1 |
| Neurological Surgery | 4,913 | 78 | 0.6 |
| Neurology | 11,714 | 397 | 1.5 |
| Nuclear Medicine | 1,434 | 22 | 0.2 |
| Obstetrics & Gynecology | 39,257 | 1,369 | 5.2 |
| Occupational Medicine | 3,049 | na | 2.3 |
| Ophthalmology | 17,822 | 349 | 2.3 |
| Orthopedic Surgery | 22,888 | 972 | 3.0 |
| Osteo. Manipulative Medicine | na | 418 | <0.1 |
| Otolaryngology | 9,096 | 392 | 1.2 |
| Pathology-Anat/Clin | 18,236 | 279 | 2.4 |
| Pediatrics | 55,427 | 1,020 | 7.3 |
| Pediatric Cardiology | 1,362 | na | 0.2 |
| Physical Med & Rehab | 5,850 | 456 | 0.8 |
| Plastic Surgery | 5,981 | 65 | 0.8 |
| Psychiatry | 39,064 | 966 | 5.2 |
| Public Health | 1,670 | na | 0.2 |
| Pulmonary Diseases | 6,759 | 254 | 0.9 |
| Radiation Oncology | 3,697 | 56 | 0.5 |
| Radiology (All) | 28,259 | 940 | 2.3 |
| Thoracic Surgery | 2,269 | 80 | 0.3 |
| Urology | 10,028 | 194 | 1.3 |
| Other Specialties | 6,168 | 1,090 | 0.8 |
| Others in Practice | 15,060 | na | 2.0 |

Adapted from: American Medical Association. *Physician Characteristics & Distribution in the U.S., 1999.* Chicago, IL: AMA, 1999, pp. 20-21, and American Osteopathic Association. *1999 Yearbook and Directory of Osteopathic Physicians,* 90th ed. Chicago, IL: AOA, 1999, pp. 630-1.

na = Information not available.

# 3

# Specialty Descriptions

First, take a look at the wide range of medical specialties that are available. You will probably be surprised at the diversity within the house of medicine. There are probably many specialties listed here that you have never heard of; there definitely are many that you will have no contact with during your training. You may have encountered others only peripherally. But they all are options for you. Most of the specialties listed below provide certification—either primarily, such as Internal Medicine and Surgery, or as a subspecialty, such as Forensic Pathology and Child Psychiatry. Some, however, such as Trauma Surgery, Hospitalists, and Medical Informatics, while gradually being accepted as distinct subspecialties by the medical community, do not yet have individual subspecialty examinations or certifications.

More than half of all U.S. physicians hold specialty or subspecialty board certification. Overall, the vast majority of physicians who do get board certified have done better in medical school and residency than their counterparts who don't. (Currently, physicians passing an initial exam to become certified, with periodic recertification in some cases. Pressed by an AMA-sponsored certification program and public demand for more physician accountability, the American Board of Medical Specialties is working on a plan to continually assess specialists. Your future will include continual performance assessment, not just an evaluation of your knowledge.)

Read through these descriptions to open your mind to the scope of career choices you have. There is no point in leaping ahead until you know what lies before you.

The ease of acquiring a residency position in each specialty varies. This can be expressed by assigning each specialty a relative difficulty factor, just as in competitive diving. While it is impossible to give exact numbers, it is possible to approximate this difficulty. Beside each specialty's name in the descriptions below, I have indicated this factor by using a one (*) to five (*****) asterisk scale. *In specialties with one asterisk, you should have the least difficulty getting a residency position (or, if there is no residency, into the field); and in those with five asterisks, the most difficulty.* Remember, though, that even the easiest specialties to enter have some very competitive programs, and even the most difficult to enter have some less competitive programs. So, only use the asterisk system as *a general guide, not as an absolute truth.*

Some specialties are entered by completing Fellowship training after finishing training in a prerequisite residency. These specialties are designated by "(F)." The terminology PGY-1, PGY-2, etc. (or occasionally R-1, R-2, etc. for Osteopaths) equates to the specified "postgraduate year."

Some specialties have programs that accept new residents other than in July. The number of programs offering these slots is listed. The specific programs, as well as those that offer part-time (shared-schedule) positions, are listed in the American Medical Association's *Graduate Medical Education Directory—Supplement* for the current year.

The figures in Chapter 22 contain additional information that may guide you when making a decision. This includes the prerequisites for training in the various specialties, the total number of programs in each specialty, and the approximate number of entry-level positions open each year. Figure 2.10 lists the total number of physicians currently practicing in each specialty. A visual description of the length of specialty training for both M.D. and Osteopathic (D.O.) physicians can be found in Figures 3.1 and 3.2, following the verbal descriptions of the specialties. Figure 3.3 ranks most specialties and subspecialties by how well they meet current practitioners' expectations of what they were seeking when they entered the specialty.

After you have looked through this chapter, you will have an opportunity (in Chapter 4) to assess your likes and dislikes in medical practice, as well as your own perceived aptitudes. Then you can compare them to those of practitioners in a few of the major specialties.

For clarification, "ACGME" stands for the Accreditation Council for Graduate Medical Education, the body that approves M.D. residencies. "AOA" in "AOA-Approved Programs" stands for the American Osteopathic Association, the body that approves D.O. residencies. For M.D.s, "AOA" also stands for a prestigious medical school honorary society.

"NRMP" stands for the National Residency Matching Program. This is the method most medical students use to obtain a residency position. It is described in detail in Chapter 22.

## Legend for Specialty Descriptions

\*   Entry into a training program is **Very Easy**
\*\*   Entry into a training program is **Easy**
\*\*\*  Entry into a training program is **Difficult**
\*\*\*\*  Entry into a training program is **Very Difficult**
\*\*\*\*\* Entry into a training program is **Extremely Difficult**

(**F**) **Fellowship** training following completion of an initial residency.

The Osteopathic listings are for funded programs and positions only.

In the boxes listing the positions for each specialty, the terms mean:

"ACGME-Approved Programs"—Programs approved for M.D.s
"AOA-Approved Programs"—Programs approved for D.O.s
"1st-Yr Positions"—Beginning positions in specialty training
"PGY-1 Positions"—Positions available at the intern level
"Part-Time Programs"—Shared-schedule positions
"Positions through NRMP Specialties Matching Services"—Positions listed in the NRMP's Specialty Matches outside the normal Match. Contact: the NRMP, 2501 M Street N.W., Suite 1, Washington, DC 20037-1307.

## Aerospace Medicine \*\*\*\*

**Specialty Overview:** Aerospace Medicine is a specialty within Preventive Medicine. Practitioners are responsible for the medical care and safety of individuals involved in military and civilian aviation and space travel. This includes crew members and ground personnel. The Federal Aviation Administration, NASA, the military, or the aerospace industry employs most flight surgeons or aviation medical examiners. They are usually engaged in clinical medicine, research and development, or administration. Medical certification of pilots for flight duty often constitutes a large part of their clinical practice, and most physicians in this field are pilots themselves. Note: for information in *FREIDA* (see Chapter 9), look under Preventive Medicine.

**Training:** Two years of residency training are required after internship. One of these years must be spent obtaining an advanced degree in a relevant area, usually a master's degree in Public Health. The second residency year has more time devoted to clinical Aerospace Medicine. A fourth year of training, teaching, practice, and/or research is required to take the Board examination. There are two military Aerospace Medicine programs (Brooks

Air Force Base, Texas, and Pensacola Naval Air Station, Florida) and one civilian program (Wright State University, Ohio).

**Match:** To be eligible for the military programs, an individual must already be in the military and practicing as a Flight Surgeon.

| AEROSPACE MEDICINE | | | |
|---|---|---|---|
| ACGME-Approved Programs | 4 | 1st-Yr Positions (M.D.) | 42 |
| AOA-Approved Programs | 0 | 1st-Yr Positions (D.O.) | 0 |
| PGY-1 Positions | 0 | Part-Time Programs | 0 |

*For more information, contact:*

- Aerospace Medical Association, 320 S. Henry Street, Alexandria, VA 22314-3524; www.asma.org.
- American College of Preventive Medicine, 1660 L Street N.W., Suite 206, Washington, DC 20036; www.acpm.org.
- American Osteopathic College of Occupational and Preventive Medicine, 5405 Alton Parkway, Suite 5A-246, Irvine, CA 92604; www.aocopm.org.

# Allergy and Immunology (F) *

**Specialty Overview:** Allergy and Immunology is a subspecialty of both Internal Medicine and Pediatrics devoted to the diagnosis and treatment of allergic, asthmatic, and immunologic diseases. There is a great deal of art, as well as science, in the practice of the Allergist-Immunologist. The patients seen most frequently have asthma and chronic or seasonal allergies. Practitioners get most of their patients through referrals. There is usually very little emergency or night call. Practice opportunities are more restricted than in the past, due to an increasing number of physicians, both in this field and in other fields, who do allergy testing and treatment. Allergist-Immunologists are mainly office-based and are concentrated in metropolitan areas. Research opportunities in this field are increasing dramatically because of the increasing recognition of the role of immunologic factors in diseases.

**Specialists' View:** According to recent AMA surveys, 60% of Allergists-Immunologists in academic and clinical positions felt that their practice activities met their expectations. On a scale of 1=very unsatisfied with their current practice position to 5=very satisfied, those surveyed averaged 3.4. They average 42 hours per week doing patient care. Among new residency graduates, 42% had difficulty finding a job they preferred; 9% were unemployed at graduation. The numbers for Clinical & Laboratory Immunologists were too small to interpret.

**Training:** Training is two years after completing either a Pediatric or an Internal Medicine residency. It includes experiences in both pediatric and adult diseases. A special qualification in Clinical & Laboratory Immunology requires an extra year of training.

**Match:** Applicants should contact programs directly.

### ALLERGY AND IMMUNOLOGY

| | | | |
|---|---|---|---|
| ACGME-Approved Programs | 79 | 1st-Yr Positions (M.D.) | 127 |
| AOA-Approved Programs | 0 | 1st-Yr Positions (D.O.) | 0 |
| PGY-1 Positions | 0 | Part-Time Programs | 14 |
| % Women Residents | 40 | % IMG Residents | 48 |
| Avg. Res. Work Hours/Week | 42.6 | Avg. Days Off Per Month | 7.0 |
| % Pursuing Additional Specialty Training | 10 | Programs Offering Multiple Start Dates | 13 |
| Positions through NRMP Specialties Matching Services | 0 | | |

### CLINICAL AND LABORATORY IMMUNOLOGY

| | | | |
|---|---|---|---|
| ACGME-Approved Programs | 12 | 1st-Yr Positions (M.D.) | 12 |
| AOA-Approved Programs | 0 | 1st-Yr Positions (D.O.) | 0 |
| PGY-1 Positions | 0 | Part-Time Programs | 1 |
| % Women Residents | 25 | % IMG Residents | 50 |
| Avg. Res. Work Hours/Week | 47.8 | Avg. Days Off Per Month | 6.7 |
| Positions through NRMP Specialties Matching Services | 0 | | |

### For more information, contact:

- American Academy of Allergy, Asthma, & Immunology, 611 E. Wells Street, Milwaukee, WI 53202; www.aaaai.org.
- American College of Allergy, Asthma, & Immunology, 85 W. Algonquin Road, Suite 550, Arlington Heights, IL 60005; www.allergy.mcg.edu.
- American Osteopathic College of Allergy and Immunology, 3030 North Hayden Road, #26, Scottsdale, AZ 85251.

# Anesthesiology *

**Specialty Overview:** Anesthesiologists give general and regional anesthesia during surgical, obstetric, diagnostic, and therapeutic procedures; function as Critical Care physicians; and give anesthetic blocks in conjunction with pain clinics. They often specialize in Pediatric, Neurosurgical, Obstetric, Cardiothoracic, or Ambulatory Anesthesia, although Critical Care (see Critical Care) and Pain Management (see Pain Management) are the only formal subspecialties. Anesthesiology is a hospital-based specialty with frequent night call for most practitioners. Research is continuing to push the practice of Anesthesiology into an ever more elegant and scientific realm. The growing use of less-expensive Nurse-Anesthetists and a declining number of surgeries has decreased the need for Anesthesiologists; this trend is expected to continue. Yet, the markedly decreased number of Anesthesiology residents in recent years has led to increased job opportunities for the positions that Anesthesiologists continue to fill.

**Specialists' View:** According to recent AMA surveys, 62% of Anesthesiologists in academic and clinical positions felt that their practice activities met their expectations. On a scale of 1=very unsatisfied with their current practice position to 5=very satisfied, those surveyed averaged 3.3. They average 54 hours per week doing patient care. Among new residency graduates, 28% had difficulty finding a job they preferred; 9% were unemployed at graduation.

**Training:** Training consists of a "base" year, essentially a Transitional, Preliminary, or Categorical internship in a clinical specialty, followed by three years of training in Clinical Anesthesiology and Critical Care. Residency programs in Anesthesiology start at either the first (PGY-1) or the second (PGY-2) postgraduate year. The training is essentially the same for Osteopathic physicians. Anesthesiology residents spend about 65 (15) hours per week in the hospital. Training in the subspecialties of Anesthesia Critical Care Medicine (103 positions) or Anesthesia Pain Management (146 positions) takes a minimum of one year after completing an Anesthesiology residency. No programs are currently available in Pediatric Anesthesiology.

**Match:** In recent years, about 37% of the available PGY-1 positions filled through the NRMP Match and 54% of the positions were subsequently filled. Of the PGY-2 positions available through the NRMP Match, about 37% filled in the Match and about 44% subsequently filled. Some PGY-4 positions are available in specialty areas (Pediatric, Neurosurgical, etc.) and can be applied for separately from normal Anesthesiology programs.

**Other Useful Information:** Anesthesiology residencies tend to look both for good performance in preclinical Physiology and Pharmacology courses and for how well students have done in their Internal Medicine and Anesthesiology clerkships. Since working with a team is vital, great importance is given to the applicant's interview.

| ANESTHESIOLOGY | | | |
|---|---|---|---|
| ACGME-Approved Programs | 147 | 1st-Yr Positions (M.D.) | 1,075 |
| AOA-Approved Programs | 13 | 1st-Yr Positions (D.O.) | 10 |
| PGY-1 Positions | 381 | Part-Time Programs | 19 |
| % Women Residents | 27 | % IMG Residents | 44 |
| Avg. Res. Work Hours/Week | 60.9 | Avg. Days Off Per Month | 7.2 |
| % Pursuing Additional Specialty Training | 27 | Programs Offering Multiple Start Dates | 61 |

### For more information, contact:

- American Academy of Pain Management, 4700 W. Lake Avenue, Glenview, IL 60025-1485; www.painmed.org.
- American Osteopathic College of Anesthesiologists, 17201 E. Highway 40, Suite 204, Independence, MO 64055-6427.
- American Society of Anesthesiologists, 520 N. Northwest Highway, Park Ridge, IL 60068-2573; www.asahq.org.

# Cardiology (F) *

**Specialty Overview:** Cardiologists, who practice the specialty officially known as "Cardiovascular Disease," primarily deal with adult patients who have diseases of the heart and circulatory system. They are involved in both the diagnosis and the medical treatment of these diseases. The core of the specialty is the medical history and physical diagnosis, frequently augmented by the latest medical technology and medications. Recently, Cardiologists have become involved with the angiographic (catheters in arteries) treatment of obstructions of vessels, primarily the coronary arteries. This will be a rapidly expanding area of practice for those in the specialty. Practicing Cardiologists can now be divided by the nature of their practices into invasive and non-invasive specialists. Cardiologists are generally office-based, but spend about one-third of their professional time in hospitals. This frequently includes long hours and significant night call.

Between 1965 and 2000, there was more than an eight-fold increase in the number of Cardiologists; at this rate, the number will nearly double again by 2010. However, since Cardiology has been targeted as a specialty with too many practitioners, especially in the highly paid area of invasive Cardiology, the number of available positions will decrease in the future.

**Specialists' View:** According to recent AMA surveys, 75% of Cardiologists in academic and clinical positions felt that their practice activities met their expectations. On a scale of 1=very unsatisfied with their current practice position to 5=very satisfied, those surveyed averaged 3.7. They average 60 hours per week doing patient care. Among new residency graduates, 27% had difficulty finding a job they preferred; 5% were unemployed at graduation.

Among Pediatric Cardiologists in academic and clinical positions, 77% felt that their practice activities met their expectations. On a scale of 1=very unsatisfied with their current practice position to 5=very satisfied, those surveyed averaged 3.2. They average 50 hours per week doing patient care. Among new residency graduates, 60% had difficulty finding a job they preferred; 8% were unemployed at graduation.

**Training:** Training is currently a three-year fellowship following completion of an Internal Medicine or Pediatric residency. One year (or in a few 4-year programs, two years) is devoted to research. Specialty certification in Cardiology is time-limited, requiring periodic recertification. Additional training is necessary for certification in Electrophysiology. Post-fellowship training is also available in Nuclear Cardiology and Cardiac Catheterization. For Osteopathic physicians, training follows internship and two years of Internal Medicine residency.

**Match:** About 70% of ACGME-approved programs and positions in adult Cardiology are available through the NRMP Specialty Match. Match results are announced in June, one year before the applicant starts specialty training. (Applicants must contact Pediatric Cardiology programs individually.) In recent years, about 63% of all enrolled applicants found a position through the Match, while 97% of available positions filled in the Match.

### CARDIOLOGY (INTERNAL MEDICINE)

| | | | |
|---|---|---|---|
| ACGME-Approved Programs | 199 | 1st-Yr Positions (M.D.) | 656 |
| AOA-Approved Programs | 7 | 1st-Yr Positions (D.O.) | 15 |
| PGY-1 Positions | 0 | Part-Time Programs | 16 |
| % Women Residents | 15 | % IMG Residents | 40 |
| Avg. Res. Work Hours/Week | 55.0 | Avg. Days Off Per Month | 6.2 |
| Positions through NRMP Specialties Matching Services | 463 | Programs Offering Multiple Start Dates | 7 |

### CARDIOLOGY (PEDIATRICS)

| | | | |
|---|---|---|---|
| ACGME-Approved Programs | 48 | 1st-Yr Positions (M.D.) | 101 |
| AOA-Approved Programs | 0 | 1st-Yr Positions (D.O.) | 0 |
| PGY-1 Positions | 0 | Part-Time Programs | 8 |
| % Women Residents | 33 | % IMG Residents | 35 |
| Avg. Res. Work Hours/Week | 50.4 | Avg. Days Off Per Month | 7.4 |
| Positions through NRMP Specialties Matching Services | 0 | Programs Offering Multiple Start Dates | 3 |

*For more information, contact:*
- American College of Cardiology, 9111 Old Georgetown Road, Bethesda, MD 20814-1699; www.acc.org.
- American College of Osteopathic Internists, 3 Bethesda Metro Center, Suite 508, Bethesda, MD 20814; www.acoi.org.
- American Academy of Pediatrics, 141 Northwest Point Boulevard, Elk Grove Village, IL 60007; www.aap.org.

## Child and Adolescent Psychiatry (F) *

**Specialty Overview:** Child and Adolescent Psychiatrists diagnose and treat mental, emotional, and behavioral disorders in children, adolescents, and their families. Child Psychiatrists work with Pediatricians, courts, schools, and social service agencies. They often have both inpatient and outpatient practices, and frequently work as part of a multidisciplinary team.

**Specialists' View:** According to recent AMA surveys, 58% of Child Psychiatrists in academic and clinical positions felt that their practice activities met their expectations. On a scale of 1=very unsatisfied with their current practice position to 5=very satisfied, those surveyed averaged 3.4. They average 45 hours per week doing patient care. Among new residency graduates, 5% had difficulty finding a job they preferred; 6% were unemployed at graduation.

**Training:** Fellowships in for both M.D.s and D.O.s, consist of two years of Child and Adolescent Psychiatry in addition to at least two years (following internship) of General Psychiatry. Child and Adolescent Psychiatry training can start any time after the internship year, but generally begins after the PGY-2 year in Psychiatry. There are also ten programs with five years of training combining Pediatrics, Psychiatry, and Child and Adolescent Psychiatry. These programs consist of two years of Pediatrics, one-and-a-half years of adult Psychiatry, and one-and-a-half years of Child and Adolescent Psychiatry, making trainees eligible for Board certification in all three specialties. For information about these programs, contact both the Pediatrics-Psychiatry Joint Training Committee and the individual programs. These programs are more difficult to match with than programs in either Pediatrics or Psychiatry.

**Match:** No straight Child and Adolescent Psychiatry programs are in the NRMP Match, but the programs have agreed to announce their decisions about residents for the next academic year on the second Monday in November (the National Uniform Entry Plan). There are 21 positions combining Pediatrics, Psychiatry, and Child and Adolescent Psychiatry available to medical students through the NRMP PGY-1 Match.

| CHILD AND ADOLESCENT PSYCHIATRY | | | |
|---|---|---|---|
| ACGME-Approved Programs | 116 | 1st-Yr Positions (M.D.) | 387 |
| AOA-Approved Programs | 1 | 1st-Yr Positions (D.O.) | 0 |
| PGY-1 Positions | 0 | Part-Time Programs | 74 |
| % Women Residents | 55 | % IMG Residents | 33 |
| Avg. Res. Work Hours/Week | 42.7 | Avg. Days Off Per Month | 8.3 |
| Positions through NRMP Specialties Matching Services | 0 | Programs Offering Multiple Start Dates | 28 |

## For more information, contact:

- American Academy of Child & Adolescent Psychiatry, 3615 Wisconsin Avenue, N.W., Washington, DC 20016; www.aacap.org.
- American College of (Osteopathic) Neuropsychiatry, 28595 Orchard Lake Road, Suite 200, Farmington Hills, MI 48334-2979.
- Pediatrics-Psychiatry Joint Training Committee, 111 Silver Cedar Ct., Chapel Hill, NC 27514-1651.

# Child Neurology (F) *

**Specialty Overview:** Child Neurologists diagnose and manage neurological disorders of the infant, child, and adolescent. They treat diseases of the brain, spinal cord, and neuromuscular system. Many such problems are congenital or developmental in nature. Practitioners, most often based at academic medical centers, usually see patients in consultation for primary care physicians.

**Specialists' View:** According to recent AMA surveys, 75% of Child Neurologists in academic and clinical positions felt that their practice activities met their expectations. On a scale of 1=very unsatisfied with their current practice position to 5=very satisfied, those surveyed averaged 3.4. They average 64 hours per week doing patient care. Among new residency graduates, 27% had difficulty finding a job they preferred; 17% were unemployed at graduation.

**Training:** Applicants must have completed at least two years of an approved Pediatric residency before entering the program. Training in Child Neurology is an additional three years: one year in clinical adult Neurology and one year in clinical Child Neurology. The third year is devoted to studying Electrodiagnostic Neurology, Neuropathology, Neuroradiology, Neuro-Ophthalmology, Child Psychiatry, and the basic neurosciences. Trainees are eligible to take the American Board of Pediatrics examination after their second year of Child Neurology training.

**Match:** Applicants should contact individual training programs, since this specialty has no match.

| CHILD NEUROLOGY (F) | | | |
|---|---|---|---|
| ACGME-Approved Programs | 71 | 1st-Yr Positions (M.D.) | 84 |
| AOA-Approved Programs | 0 | 1st-Yr Positions (D.O.) | 0 |
| PGY-1 Positions | 0 | Part-Time Programs | 14 |
| % Women Residents | 51 | % IMG Residents | 48 |
| Avg. Res. Work Hours/Week | 61.7 | Avg. Days Off Per Month | 5.9 |
| Programs Offering Multiple Start Dates | 14 | | |

## For more information, contact:

- American Academy of Neurology, 1080 Montreal Street, St. Paul, MN 55116-2325; www.aan.com.
- American College of (Osteopathic) Neuropsychiatry, 28595 Orchard Lake Road, Suite 200, Farmington Hills, MI 48334-2979.
- Child Neurology Society, 3900 Northwoods Drive, Suite 175, St. Paul, MN 55112.

# Colon and Rectal Surgery (F) ***

**Specialty Overview:** Colon and Rectal Surgeons diagnose and treat disorders of the intestinal tract, rectum, anal canal, and perianal areas that are amenable to surgical treatment. They are involved not only in operative treatment but also in diagnostic procedures, including colonoscopy. Other physicians refer most patients. Most practitioners in this specialty are located in medium to large cities.

**Specialists' View:** According to recent AMA surveys, 61% of Colon and Rectal Surgeons in academic and clinical positions felt that their practice activities met their expectations. On a scale of 1=very unsatisfied with their current practice position to 5=very satisfied, those surveyed averaged 3.5. They average 60 hours per week doing patient care. Among new residency graduates, 33% had difficulty finding a job they preferred; 29% were unemployed at graduation.

**Training:** The training consists of a complete residency in General Surgery followed by a one-year fellowship in Colon and Rectal Surgery. While there are no Osteopathic training programs in this specialty, the more limited specialty of Proctology, consisting of two years of training after internship, is available.

**Match:** Most positions are listed through the NRMP Specialties Matching Services. Results of the Match for positions beginning in July are released in December of the prior year. The ratio of applicants to available positions is approximately 1.5:1. In recent years, 71% of applicants matched and 96% of available positions filled in the NRMP Specialty Match.

### COLON AND RECTAL SURGERY

| | | | |
|---|---|---|---|
| ACGME-Approved Programs | 30 | 1st-Yr Positions (M.D.) | 55 |
| AOA-Approved Programs | 0 | 1st-Yr Positions (D.O.) | 0 |
| PGY-1 Positions | 0 | Part-Time Programs | 3 |
| % Women Residents | 20 | % IMG Residents | 14 |
| Avg. Res. Work Hours/Week | 56.2 | Avg. Days Off Per Month | 4.6 |
| Positions through NRMP Specialties Matching Services | 53 | % Pursuing Additional Specialty Training | 3 |

### PROCTOLOGY (OSTEOPATHIC ONLY)

| | | | |
|---|---|---|---|
| AOA-Approved Programs | 1 | 1st-Yr Positions (D.O.) | 1 |

*For more information, contact:*
- American Osteopathic College of Proctology, 2721 Derby Road, Toledo, OH 43615.
- American Society of Colon & Rectal Surgeons, 85 Algonquin Road, Suite 550, Arlington Heights, IL 60005; www.fascrs.org.

# Critical Care (F) *

**Specialty Overview:** Critical Care physicians work in hospital intensive care units managing the overall care of critically ill medical and surgical patients. The practice requires both a broad knowledge of the medical and surgical conditions that cause patients to be in the intensive care unit, and a specialized knowledge of the respiratory, fluid, and cardiovascular management needed to maintain these patients.

Many Critical Care physicians alternate their duties in the critical care unit with practice in their primary specialty. The majority of Critical Care physicians in adult units are Internists, most commonly specialists in Pulmonary Diseases. Night call or night duty in the intensive care unit is common. Most individuals in this specialty are located in large cities.

**Specialists' View:** According to recent AMA surveys, 56% of Anesthesiologist Critical Care physicians in academic and clinical positions felt that their practice activities met their expectations. On a scale of 1=very unsatisfied with their current practice position to 5=very satisfied, those surveyed averaged 3.1. They average 49 hours per week doing patient care. Among new residency graduates, 40% had difficulty finding a job they preferred; 12% were unemployed at graduation.

Among Internist Critical Care physicians in academic and clinical positions, 55% felt that their practice activities met their expectations. On a scale of 1=very unsatisfied with their current practice position to 5=very satisfied, those surveyed averaged 3.2. They average 55 hours per week doing patient care. Among new residency graduates, 31% had difficulty finding a job they preferred; 15% were unemployed at graduation.

Among Surgeon Critical Care physicians in academic and clinical positions, 44% felt that their practice activities met their expectations. On a scale of 1=very unsatisfied with their current practice position to 5=very satisfied, those surveyed averaged 3.1. They average 58 hours per week doing patient care. Among new residency graduates, 33% had difficulty finding a job they preferred; all were employed at graduation.

Among Pediatric Critical Care physicians in academic and clinical positions, 50% felt that their practice activities met their expectations. On a scale of 1=very unsatisfied with their current practice position to 5=very satisfied, those surveyed averaged 3.2. They average 58 hours per week doing patient care. Among new residency graduates, 20% had difficulty finding a job they preferred; 4% were unemployed at graduation.

**Training:** At present, positions leading to certificates of special competence are offered in Critical Care from the American Boards of Internal Medicine (1 to 3 years after residency), Anesthesiology (1 year), and Surgery (1 year). Pediatrics offers Critical Care as a subspecialty (3 years after residency). Other Boards may offer a similar certification in the future. Internal Medicine offers two routes to certification: either a one-year fellowship following completion of subspecialty training, or a two-year fellowship following residency. A common program design is to incorporate Critical Care into a three-year Pulmonary Diseases fellowship leading to dual subspecialty certification (see Pulmonary Diseases).

**Match:** Virtually all adult Critical Care programs combined with Pulmonary Disease training are in the NRMP Medical Specialties Matching Programs. Applicants for other Critical Care training should contact individual programs. A list of programs is published early each year in *Critical Care Medicine*.

### ADULT CRITICAL CARE (ANESTHESIOLOGY)

| | | | |
|---|---|---|---|
| ACGME-Approved Programs | 57 | 1st-Yr Positions (M.D.) | 136 |
| AOA-Approved Programs | 0 | 1st-Yr Positions (D.O.) | 0 |
| PGY-1 Positions | 0 | Part-Time Programs | 8 |
| % Women Residents | 25 | % IMG Residents | 30 |
| Avg. Res. Work Hours/Week | 59.1 | Avg. Days Off Per Month | 6.9 |
| Positions through NRMP Specialties Matching Services | 0 | Programs Offering Multiple Start Dates | 19 |

### ADULT CRITICAL CARE (INTERNAL MEDICINE)

| | | | |
|---|---|---|---|
| ACGME-Approved Programs | 50 | 1st-Yr Positions (M.D.) | 145 |
| AOA-Approved Programs | 4 | 1st-Yr Positions (D.O.) | 1 |
| PGY-1 Positions | 0 | Part-Time Programs | 2 |
| % Women Residents | 24 | % IMG Residents | 54 |
| Avg. Res. Work Hours/Week | 56.1 | Avg. Days Off Per Month | 6.4 |
| Positions through NRMP Specialties Matching Services (Pulmonary) | 268 | Programs Offering Multiple Start Dates | 3 |

### ADULT CRITICAL CARE (SURGERY)

| | | | |
|---|---|---|---|
| ACGME-Approved Programs | 57 | 1st-Yr Positions (M.D.) | 111 |
| AOA-Approved Programs | 0 | 1st-Yr Positions (D.O.) | 0 |
| PGY-1 Positions | 0 | Part-Time Programs | 4 |
| % Women Residents | 21 | % IMG Residents | 13 |
| Avg. Res. Work Hours/Week | 60.5 | Avg. Days Off Per Month | 6.1 |
| Positions through NRMP Specialties Matching Services (Pulmonary) | 0 | Programs Offering Multiple Start Dates | 2 |

### PEDIATRIC CRITICAL CARE

| | | | |
|---|---|---|---|
| ACGME-Approved Programs | 63 | 1st-Yr Positions (M.D.) | 94 |
| AOA-Approved Programs | 0 | 1st-Yr Positions (D.O.) | 0 |
| PGY-1 Positions | 0 | Part-Time Programs | 9 |
| % Women Residents | 39 | % IMG Residents | 33 |
| Avg. Res. Work Hours/Week | 58.9 | Avg. Days Off Per Month | 8.0 |
| Positions through NRMP Specialties Matching Services | 0 | Programs Offering Multiple Start Dates | 14 |

## For more information, contact:

- American College of Osteopathic Internists, 3 Bethesda Metro Center, Suite 508, Bethesda, MD 20814; www.acoi.org.
- Society of Critical Care Medicine, 8101 E. Kaiser Boulevard, Suite 300, Anaheim Hills, CA 92808-2259; www.sccm.org.

# Dermatology *****

**Specialty Overview:** Dermatologists deal with patients who have both acute and chronic disorders of the skin. They diagnose skin lesions and use both chemotherapeutic agents and surgery to effect cures. Dermatologists get referrals from other physicians and from patients who refer themselves. There is little night call and very rarely an inpatient service associated with a Dermatology practice. With the increase in managed care, many patients who once would have been referred to Dermatologists are now being treated by primary care practitioners, decreasing the need for Dermatologists.

Following Dermatology training, fellowships are available in Clinical & Laboratory Dermatological Immunology and in Dermatopathology. Dermatopathology is a subspecialty of both Pathology and Dermatology. Emphasis is placed on the diagnosis of skin disorders using appropriate microscopic techniques including light and electron microscopy, immuno-pathology, histochemistry, and aspects of cutaneous mycology, bacteriology, and entomology. At least six months of the training must be in either clinical Dermatology for those trained in Pathology, or Anatomic Pathology for those trained in Dermatology.

**Specialists' View:** According to recent AMA surveys, 71% of Derma-tologists in academic and clinical positions felt that their practice activities met their expectations. On a scale of 1=very unsatisfied with their current practice position to 5=very satisfied, those surveyed averaged 3.8. They average 40 hours per week doing patient care. Among new residency graduates, 12% had difficulty finding a job they preferred; 4% were unemployed at graduation.

Among Dermatopathologists in academic and clinical positions, 70% felt that their practice activities met their expectations. On a scale of 1=very unsatisfied with their current practice position to 5=very satisfied, those surveyed averaged 3.9. They average 37 hours per week doing patient care. Among new residency graduates, 10% had difficulty finding a job they preferred; all were employed at graduation.

**Training:** Dermatology residencies are three years following initial training. There are approximately 20 PGY-1 positions in 4-year programs. Dermatopathology training consists of a one-year fellowship. It is designed for either a research or a clinical practice. At least six months of the training must be in either clinical Dermatology for those trained in Pathology, or Anatomic Pathology for those trained in Dermatology.

**Match:** Nearly all positions beginning at the PGY-2 level are available to medical students through the NRMP Match. Most applicants must arrange their own internship. Several programs require the prior completion of a residency in another specialty. Entrance to the specialty is very competitive. In recent years, only about 66% of applicants found a position through the Match, while 93% of positions filled through the Match.

### DERMATOLOGY

| | | | |
|---|---|---|---|
| ACGME-Approved Programs | 101 | 1st-Yr Positions (M.D.) | 291 |
| AOA-Approved Programs | 11 | 1st-Yr Positions (D.O.) | 8 |
| PGY-1 Positions | 41 | Part-Time Programs | 4 |
| % Women Residents | 50 | % IMG Residents | 6 |
| Avg. Res. Work Hours/Week | 42.8 | Avg. Days Off Per Month | 6.8 |
| % Pursuing Additional Specialty Training | 16 | Programs Offering Multiple Start Dates | 3 |

### DERMATOPATHOLOGY (F)

| | | | |
|---|---|---|---|
| ACGME-Approved Programs | 41 | 1st-Yr Positions (M.D.) | 50 |
| AOA-Approved Programs | 0 | 1st-Yr Positions (D.O.) | 0 |
| PGY-1 Positions | 0 | Part-Time Programs | 3 |
| % Women Residents | 31 | % IMG Residents | 29 |
| Avg. Res. Work Hours/Week | 44.7 | Avg. Days Off Per Month | 7.2 |
| Positions through NRMP Specialties Matching Services | 0 | | |

*For more information, contact:*

- American Academy of Dermatology, 930 N. Meacham Road, Schaumburg, IL 60173; www.aad.org.
- American Osteopathic College of Dermatology, 800 W. Jefferson, P.O. Box 7525, Kirksville, MO 63501.

## Emergency Medicine *****

**Specialty Overview:** Emergency Physicians deal with the entire spectrum of acute illness and injury in all age groups. Hands-on physical diagnosis and the use of both medical and surgical therapeutic modalities are an integral part of the specialty. Emergency Physicians are trained to stabilize patients with acute injuries and deal with life-threatening conditions. Hours are long, but schedules are fixed in advance. There is rarely a call schedule outside of assigned working hours in this specialty.

Emergency Physicians are mainly hospital-based. Most practitioners in the specialty work in medium to large cities. Many new Emergency Medicine opportunities are available at academic centers and in research. All sources agree that there will still be a shortage of Emergency Physicians in the year 2025. Less than 1% of Emergency Physicians leave the field each year.

**Specialists' View:** According to recent AMA surveys, 87% of Emergency Physicians in academic and clinical positions felt that their practice activities met their expectations. On a scale of 1=very unsatisfied with their current practice position to 5=very satisfied, those surveyed averaged 3.8. They average 39 hours per week doing patient care. Among new residency graduates, 11% had difficulty finding a job they preferred; 2% were unemployed at graduation. The numbers for Emergency Physician-Internists and Emergency Physician-Pediatricians were too small to interpret.

**Training:** Training is three to four years in length. Programs also exist combining Emergency Medicine with either Internal Medicine or Pediatrics. These are five years long and lead to dual certification. Osteopathic physicians have the option of combining Emergency Medicine with training in Family Practice.

Fellowships following residency leading to subspecialty certification are offered in Medical Toxicology, Pediatric Emergency Medicine, and Sports Medicine. Some Critical Care programs accept Emergency Medicine residency graduates. Fellowships are also available in Research, Hyperbaric Medicine, Medical Education, Medical Information Services, and Emergency Medical Service Administration.

**Match:** Most programs begin in the first year and are available through the NRMP PGY-1 Match or the Advanced Match. Those that begin at the PGY-2 level require at least one year of prior training in a Transitional internship or an Internal Medicine, Surgery, or Family Practice residency. Students can also enter the five-year combined programs in Emergency Medicine-Internal Medicine and Emergency Medicine-Pediatrics. A Pediatric Emergency Medicine (fellowship) Match is run by the NRMP Specialties Matching Services. In recent years, 68% of enrolled applicants found positions through this Match and 80% of available positions filled.

**Other Useful Information:** Emergency Medicine has become extremely competitive. Programs look for high United States Medical Licensing Examination (USMLE) scores, research experience, election to AOA (honorary), and outstanding performance on Emergency Medicine clerkships. In recent years, about 79% of the available PGY-1 positions filled through the NRMP Match and 100% of these positions were subsequently filled. Of the PGY-2 positions available through the NRMP Match, about 84% filled in the Match and about 99% subsequently filled.

### EMERGENCY MEDICINE

| | | | |
|---|---|---|---|
| ACGME-Approved Programs | 119 | 1st-Yr Positions (M.D.) | 1,131 |
| AOA-Approved Programs | 28 | 1st-Yr Positions (D.O.) | 96 |
| PGY-1 Positions | 967 | Part-Time Programs | 12 |
| % Women Residents | 27 | % IMG Residents | 2 |
| Avg. Res. Work Hours/Week | 56.0 | Avg. Days Off Per Month | 6.9 |
| % Pursuing Additional Specialty Training | 5 | Programs Offering Multiple Start Dates | 3 |

### EMERGENCY MEDICINE–PEDIATRICS **

| | | | |
|---|---|---|---|
| ACGME-Approved Programs | 4 | 1st-Yr Positions (M.D.) | 7 |
| AOA-Approved Programs | 1 | 1st-Yr Positions (D.O.) | 1 |
| PGY-1 Positions | 7 | Part-Time Programs | 1 |
| % Women Residents | 30 | % IMG Residents | 0 |
| Avg. Res. Work Hours/Week | 63.3 | Avg. Days Off Per Month | 5.3 |

### PEDIATRIC EMERGENCY MEDICINE (F) **

| | | | |
|---|---|---|---|
| ACGME-Approved Programs | 59 | 1st-Yr Positions (M.D.) | 88 |
| AOA-Approved Programs | 0 | 1st-Yr Positions (D.O.) | 0 |
| PGY-1 Positions | 7 | Part-Time Programs | 0 |
| Positions through NRMP Specialties Matching Services | 0 | | |

### EMERGENCY MEDICINE–INTERNAL MEDICINE *****

| | | | |
|---|---|---|---|
| ACGME-Approved Programs | 11 | 1st-Yr Positions (M.D.) | 21 |
| AOA-Approved Programs | 12 | 1st-Yr Positions (D.O.) | 17 |
| PGY-1 Positions | 21 | Part-Time Programs | 2 |
| % Women Residents | 23 | % IMG Residents | 3 |
| Avg. Res. Work Hours/Week | 58.8 | Avg. Days Off Per Month | 6.0 |

### EMERGENCY MEDICINE–FAMILY PRACTICE (OSTEOPATHS ONLY)

| | | | |
|---|---|---|---|
| AOA-Approved Programs | 4 | 1st-Yr Positions (D.O.) | 4 |

## For more information, contact:

- American College of Emergency Physicians, P.O. Box 619911, Dallas, TX 75261-9911; www.acep.org.
- American College of Osteopathic Emergency Physicians, 142 E. Ontario Street, Suite 550, Chicago, IL 60611; www.acoep.org.
- Society for Academic Emergency Medicine, 901 N. Washington, Lansing, MI 48906; www.saem.org.

# Endocrinology, Diabetes, and Metabolism (F) *

**Specialty Overview:** Endocrinologists treat patients with diseases of the endocrine (glandular) system and with a wide variety of hormonal abnormalities. The most common endocrine diseases include diabetes mellitus, high lipid (blood fats or cholesterol) levels, and thyroid disorders. Patients are often referred to Endocrinologists for failure to grow, early or late puberty, excess hair growth, high calcium levels, osteoporosis, pituitary tumors, or reproductive problems. Endocrinologists also consult in the rapidly growing areas of Nutrition and Metabolism. This includes helping with postoperative and chronic-disease patients needing extra nutritional support. Many Endocrinologists also participate in clinical or basic-science research.

**Specialists' View:** According to recent AMA surveys, 57% of Endocrinologists in academic and clinical positions felt that their practice activities met their expectations. On a scale of 1=very unsatisfied with their current practice position to 5=very satisfied, those surveyed averaged 3.2. They average 44 hours per week doing patient care. Among new residency graduates, 31% had difficulty finding a job they preferred; 13% were unemployed at graduation.

Among Pediatric Endocrinologists in academic and clinical positions, 43% felt that their practice activities met their expectations. On a scale of 1=very unsatisfied with their current practice position to 5=very satisfied, those surveyed averaged 3.1. They average 36 hours per week doing patient care. Among new residency graduates, none had difficulty finding a job they preferred, although 22% were unemployed at graduation.

**Training:** Training is two years following an Internal Medicine residency or three years following a Pediatric residency. For Osteopathic physicians, training follows internship and two years of Internal Medicine residency.

**Match:** Applicants should contact individual training programs, since this specialty has no match.

### ENDOCRINOLOGY (INTERNAL MEDICINE)

| | | | |
|---|---|---|---|
| ACGME-Approved Programs | 130 | 1st-Yr Positions (M.D.) | 213 |
| AOA-Approved Programs | 0 | 1st-Yr Positions (D.O.) | 0 |
| PGY-1 Positions | 0 | Part-Time Programs | 24 |
| % Women Residents | 49 | % IMG Residents | 58 |
| Avg. Res. Work Hours/Week | 43.2 | Avg. Days Off Per Month | 7.4 |
| Positions through NRMP Specialties Matching Services | 0 | Programs Offering Multiple Start Dates | 17 |

| ENDOCRINOLOGY (PEDIATRICS) | | | |
|---|---|---|---|
| ACGME-Approved Programs | 63 | 1st-Yr Positions (M.D.) | 67 |
| AOA-Approved Programs | 0 | 1st-Yr Positions (D.O.) | 0 |
| PGY-1 Positions | 0 | Part-Time Programs | 10 |
| % Women Residents | 59 | % IMG Residents | 54 |
| Avg. Res. Work Hours/Week | 43.5 | Avg. Days Off Per Month | 7.7 |
| Positions through NRMP Specialties Matching Services | 0 | Programs Offering Multiple Start Dates | 7 |

### For more information, contact:

- American College of Osteopathic Internists, 3 Bethesda Metro Center, Suite 508, Bethesda, MD 20814; www.acoi.org.
- Endocrine Society, 4350 East-West Highway, Suite 500, Bethesda, MD 20814; www.endo-society.org.
- American Academy of Pediatrics, 141 Northwest Point Boulevard, Elk Grove Village, IL 60007; www.aap.org.

# Family Practice ***

**Specialty Overview:** Family Physicians treat entire families, as did the General Practitioners of the past. They spend more than 90% of their time in direct patient care. The spectrum of their practice varies with the extent of their training, their interests, the area of the country, the number of other medical practitioners in the local area, and the rules of their local hospitals. Family Physicians practice medicine mostly in an outpatient setting. They provide primary care to a diverse population, unlimited by the patient's age, sex, organ system affected, or disease. They usually have a significant number of pediatric and geriatric patients.

Delivering babies, although always a part of the training, is not always a part of the practice. Due to the rising cost of professional liability insurance and the irregular hours involved, and other factors, many Family Physicians now severely limit this aspect of their practices. Dealing with the behavioral aspects of medicine, including family life-cycle events (birth, stress, grief), and delivering other psychological services also are a large part of Family Practice.

Most Family Physicians enter group practices, and nearly 75% participate in some type of managed health care delivery system (HMO, PPO, IPA). Many have assumed the often-uncomfortable role of "gatekeeper" or "case manager" within these systems and end up allocating services to patients. The average Family Physician works 57 hours per week, with 69% of the time spent on office visits, 13% on hospital rounds, 14% on other patient visits, and 4% doing surgical/manipulative procedures.

There is a shortage of Family Physicians, aggravated by an increased demand in managed care systems and rural areas. Part of the reason for this shortage is that the specialty suffers from a lack of recognition, both publicly and professionally, which discourages new physicians from entering this field. And, while many Family Physicians work longer hours than their colleagues and often must know how to treat a broader range of medical problems, their remuneration is lower. Physicians in this field get satisfaction from providing continuity of care to patients, in the context of their entire family, throughout the various stages of life.

**Specialists' View:** According to recent AMA surveys, 77% of Family Physicians in academic and clinical positions felt that their practice activities met their expectations. On a scale of 1=very unsatisfied with their current practice position to 5=very satisfied, those surveyed averaged 3.6. They average 46 hours per week doing patient care. Among new residency graduates, 8% had difficulty finding a job they preferred; 6% were unemployed at graduation. The numbers for Family Physician-Internists and Family Physician-Psychiatrists were too small to interpret.

**Training:** Training is three years in length. Residencies combining Family Practice and Internal Medicine last four years; those combining Family Practice and Psychiatry are five years long. Osteopathic residencies are generally two years in length following internship and one program exists combining Family Practice with Osteopathic Manipulative Medicine. Family Practice faculty rely heavily on applicant interviews and performance on clinical rotations to select residents. About 10% of Family Practitioners specialize. Family Practice graduates (M.D.s) can take Geriatric Medicine or Sports Medicine fellowships following initial residency training. Osteopathic graduates can take a two-year Geriatrics fellowship after their first year of Family Practice residency, or a two-year Osteopathic Manipulative Medicine fellowship after completing residency.

**Match:** In recent years, about 71% of the available PGY-1 positions filled through the NRMP Match and 87% of these positions were subsequently filled.

| FAMILY PRACTICE | | | |
|---|---|---|---|
| ACGME-Approved Programs | 489 | 1st-Yr Positions (M.D.) | 3,365 |
| AOA-Approved Programs | 117 | 1st-Yr Positions (D.O.) | 373 |
| PGY-1 Positions | 3,365 | Part-Time Programs | 109 |
| % Women Residents | 45 | % IMG Residents | 13 |
| Avg. Res. Work Hours/Week | 64.9 | Avg. Days Off Per Month | 5.2 |
| % Pursuing Additional Specialty Training | 3 | Programs Offering Multiple Start Dates | 65 |

### FAMILY PRACTICE–INTERNAL MEDICINE *

| | | | |
|---|---|---|---|
| ACGME-Approved Programs | 3 | 1st-Yr Positions (M.D.) | 11 |
| AOA-Approved Programs | 0 | 1st-Yr Positions (D.O.) | 0 |
| PGY-1 Positions | 11 | Part-Time Programs | 2 |
| % Women Residents | 48 | % IMG Residents | 5 |
| Avg. Res. Work Hours/Week | 66.7 | Avg. Days Off Per Month | 4.3 |

### FAMILY PRACTICE–PSYCHIATRY ***

| | | | |
|---|---|---|---|
| ACGME-Approved Programs | 12 | 1st-Yr Positions (M.D.) | 23 |
| AOA-Approved Programs | 0 | 1st-Yr Positions (D.O.) | 0 |
| PGY-1 Positions | 23 | Part-Time Programs | 6 |
| % Women Residents | 40 | % IMG Residents | 0 |
| Avg. Res. Work Hours/Week | 65.4 | Avg. Days Off Per Month | 7.0 |
| Programs Offering Multiple Start Dates | 1 | | |

### FAMILY PRACTICE–OSTEOPATHIC MANIPULATIVE MEDICINE (D.O.s ONLY)

| | | | |
|---|---|---|---|
| AOA-Approved Programs | 4 | 1st-Yr Positions (D.O.) | 2 |

### For more information, contact:

- American Academy of Family Physicians, 8880 Ward Parkway, Kansas City, MO 64114; www.aafp.org.
- American College of Osteopathic Family Physicians, 330 E. Algonquin Road, Arlington Heights, IL 60005; www.acofp.org.

# Gastroenterology (F) *

**Specialty Overview:** Gastroenterologists are Internists and Pediatricians who specifically deal with diseases of the esophagus, stomach, small and large intestines, liver, pancreas, and gallbladder. A large number of their patients have ulcer disease or chronic diseases of the liver, intestinal tract, or pancreas. Recent advances in endoscopy (esophagogastroduodenoscopy, colonoscopy, and endoscopic retrograde cholangiopancreatography) have increased the number of procedures that Gastroenterologists perform.

Gastroenterologists are predominantly office-based. They do take some night call and many have active inpatient services. The field of Gastroenterology grew about twelve-fold between 1965 and 2000; it is still growing rapidly and has been targeted as an over-populated specialty. The specialty's leaders are considering a 50% decrease in available training positions.

**Specialists' View:** According to recent AMA surveys, 69% of Gastroenterologists in academic and clinical positions felt that their practice activities met their expectations. On a scale of 1=very unsatisfied with their current practice position to 5=very satisfied, those surveyed averaged 3.7. They average 54 hours per week doing patient care. Among new residency graduates, 41% had difficulty finding a job they preferred; 9% were unemployed at graduation.

Among Pediatric Gastroenterologists in academic and clinical positions, 67% felt that their practice activities met their expectations. On a scale of 1=very unsatisfied with their current practice position to 5=very satisfied, those surveyed averaged 3.5. They average 45 hours per week doing patient care. Among new residency graduates, none had difficulty finding a job they preferred although 17% were unemployed at graduation.

**Training:** As a subspecialty of Internal Medicine, training consists of a two-year fellowship following completion of an Internal Medicine residency. Pediatric Gastroenterology fellowships last three years after a Pediatric residency. For Osteopathic physicians, training follows internship and two years of Internal Medicine residency.

**Match:** Very few Gastroenterology positions fill through the NRMP Medical Specialties Match. For most positions, including all Pediatric Gastroenterology positions, contact the programs directly.

### GASTROENTEROLOGY (INTERNAL MEDICINE)

| | | | |
|---|---|---|---|
| ACGME-Approved Programs | 170 | 1st-Yr Positions (M.D.) | 329 |
| AOA-Approved Programs | 5 | 1st-Yr Positions (D.O.) | 3 |
| PGY-1 Positions | 0 | Part-Time Programs | 15 |
| % Women Residents | 15 | % IMG Residents | 46 |
| Avg. Res. Work Hours/Week | 50.7 | Avg. Days Off Per Month | 6.3 |
| Positions through NRMP Specialties Matching Services | 100 | Programs Offering Multiple Start Dates | 6 |

### GASTROENTEROLOGY (PEDIATRICS)

| | | | |
|---|---|---|---|
| ACGME-Approved Programs | 46 | 1st-Yr Positions (M.D.) | 47 |
| AOA-Approved Programs | 0 | 1st-Yr Positions (D.O.) | 0 |
| PGY-1 Positions | 0 | Part-Time Programs | 3 |
| % Women Residents | 47 | % IMG Residents | 53 |
| Avg. Res. Work Hours/Week | 47.5 | Avg. Days Off Per Month | 5.8 |
| Positions through NRMP Specialties Matching Services | 0 | Programs Offering Multiple Start Dates | 8 |

*For more information, contact:*

- American College of Gastroenterology, 4900-B S. 31st Street, Arlington, VA 22206-1656; www.acg.gi.org.
- American College of Osteopathic Internists, 3 Bethesda Metro Center, Suite 508, Bethesda, MD 20814; www.acoi.org.
- American Gastroenterological Association, 7910 Woodmont Avenue, Suite 700, Bethesda, MD 20814, www.gastro.org.
- American Academy of Pediatrics, 141 Northwest Point Boulevard, Elk Grove Village, IL 60007; www.aap.org.

## Geriatric Medicine (F) *

**Specialty Overview:** Geriatric Medicine is a primary-care subspecialty that deals with the complex medical and psychosocial problems of older adults. Due to the significant growth of the elderly population, the demand for physicians with special skills in Geriatric Medicine is rapidly increasing. With almost 13% of Americans now older than 65, about 20,000 Geriatric clinicians are currently needed to treat the elderly. However, only 6,011 Internists (M.D.), 2,809 Family Physicians (M.D.), and 172 Osteopathic Internists and Family Physicians have been certified in Geriatric Medicine

By 2030, 20% of all Americans will be older than 65 and the U.S. will need more than 36,000 Geriatricians. Obviously, there are far fewer Geriatricians than are needed currently and the demand is expected to vastly increase.While one-third of all patients seen by Internists are over 65 years old, nearly half of Geriatricians' patients are over 75 years old.

Opportunities exist in academic medicine and research, corporate (HMO) medicine, community medicine, long-term care, and private practice. At present, most graduates of Geriatric Medicine and Geriatric Psychiatry fellowships hold academic faculty appointments, although relatively few do research or publish. Geriatricians must be able to work within a multispecialty team of both medical and non-medical personnel.

**Specialists' View:** According to recent AMA surveys, 60% of Family Physician-Geriatricians in academic and clinical positions felt that their practice activities met their expectations. On a scale of 1=very unsatisfied with their current practice position to 5=very satisfied, those surveyed averaged 4.0. They average 36 hours per week doing patient care. Among new residency graduates, none had difficulty finding a job they preferred; 11% were unemployed at graduation.

Among Internist-Geriatricians in academic and clinical positions, 70% felt that their practice activities met their expectations. On a scale of 1=very unsatisfied with their current practice position to 5=very satisfied, those surveyed averaged 3.4. They average 40 hours per week doing patient care. Among new residency graduates, 45% had difficulty finding a job they preferred; 10% were unemployed at graduation.

Among Geriatric Psychiatrists in academic and clinical positions, 88% felt that their practice activities met their expectations. On a scale of 1=very unsatisfied with their current practice position to 5=very satisfied, those surveyed averaged 4.4. They average 41 hours per week doing patient care. Among new residency graduates, 36% had difficulty finding a job they preferred; 9% were unemployed at graduation.

**Training:** Most specialists begin from a base of training in Family Practice, Internal Medicine, or Psychiatry. Some of the programs operate jointly, with both the Internal Medicine and Family Practice programs participating. A directory of fellowships in Geriatrics is available from the American Geriatric Society. Fellowships of varying lengths, either in Geriatric Medicine (programs accredited by the ACGME must currently be two years in length) or in Geriatric Psychiatry (one year) are now being offered at many sites. The American Psychiatric Association's *Directory of Psychiatry Residency Training Programs* has a list of available Geriatric Psychiatry fellowships. Osteopathic fellowships are available for those completing one or two years of any other residency.

**Match:** Applicants should apply directly to the programs.

### GERIATRIC MEDICINE (FAMILY PRACTICE)

| | | | |
|---|---|---|---|
| ACGME-Approved Programs | 17 | 1st-Yr Positions (M.D.) | 30 |
| AOA-Approved Programs | 4 | 1st-Yr Positions (D.O.) | 4 |
| PGY-1 Positions | 0 | Part-Time Programs | 10 |
| % Women Residents | 41 | % IMG Residents | 38 |
| Avg. Res. Work Hours/Week | 45.1 | Avg. Days Off Per Month | 7.2 |
| Positions through NRMP Specialties Matching Services | 0 | Programs Offering Multiple Start Dates | 7 |

### GERIATRIC MEDICINE (INTERNAL MEDICINE)

| | | | |
|---|---|---|---|
| ACGME-Approved Programs | 90 | 1st-Yr Positions (M.D.) | 232 |
| AOA-Approved Programs | 2 | 1st-Yr Positions (D.O.) | 2 |
| PGY-1 Positions | 0 | Part-Time Programs | 19 |
| % Women Residents | 42 | % IMG Residents | 58 |
| Avg. Res. Work Hours/Week | 43.7 | Avg. Days Off Per Month | 7.2 |
| Positions through NRMP Specialties Matching Services | 0 | Programs Offering Multiple Start Dates | 31 |

### GERIATRIC PSYCHIATRY

| | | | |
|---|---|---|---|
| ACGME-Approved Programs | 47 | 1st-Yr Positions (M.D.) | 107 |
| AOA-Approved Programs | 0 | 1st-Yr Positions (D.O.) | 0 |
| PGY-1 Positions | 0 | Part-Time Programs | 15 |
| % Women Residents | 36 | % IMG Residents | 56 |
| Avg. Res. Work Hours/Week | 42.1 | Avg. Days Off Per Month | 7.5 |
| Positions through NRMP Specialties Matching Services | 0 | Programs Offering Multiple Start Dates | 5 |

## For more information, contact:

- American Academy of Family Physicians, 8880 Ward Parkway, Kansas City, MO 64114.
- American College of Osteopathic Internists, 3 Bethesda Metro Center, Suite 508, Bethesda, MD 20814; www.acoi.org.
- American Geriatric Society, 770 Lexington Avenue, Suite 300, New York, NY 10021; www.americangeriatrics.org.
- American Association for Geriatric Psychiatry, 7910 Woodmont Avenue, Suite 1350, Bethesda, MD 20814; www.aagpgpa.org.

# Hand Surgery (F) *****

**Specialty Overview:** Hand surgeons primarily treat diseases of and injuries to the hand and forearm. Nearly all have training in either Orthopedic Surgery or Plastic Surgery. Advances in the specialty have come with development of new microsurgical techniques. Some Hand Surgeons do reimplantation surgery after traumatic amputations. This surgery normally requires a specialized center. One benefit to Hand Surgery is that it is usually done sitting down. Much of the surgery is now done on outpatients.

**Specialists' View:** According to recent AMA surveys, 33% of General Surgery-trained Hand Surgeons in academic and clinical positions felt that their practice activities met their expectations. On a scale of 1=very unsatisfied with their current practice position to 5=very satisfied, those surveyed averaged 3.3. They average 74 hours per week doing patient care. Among new residency graduates, none had difficulty finding a job they preferred; 13% were unemployed at graduation.

Among Orthopedic Surgery-trained Hand Surgeons in academic and clinical positions, 76% felt that their practice activities met their expectations. On a scale of 1=very unsatisfied with their current practice position to 5=very satisfied, those surveyed averaged 3.5. They average 58 hours per week doing patient care. Among new residency graduates, 11% had difficulty finding a job they preferred; all were employed at graduation.

Among Plastic Surgery-trained Hand Surgeons in academic and clinical positions, 57% felt that their practice activities met their expectations. On a scale of 1=very unsatisfied with their current practice position to 5=very satisfied, those surveyed averaged 3.1. They average 56 hours per week doing patient care. Among new residency graduates, 17% had difficulty finding a job they preferred; 11% were unemployed at graduation.

**Training:** Fellowship training in Hand Surgery lasts one year after a residency in Orthopedic Surgery, Plastic Surgery, or General Surgery.

**Match:** Most Hand Surgery positions fill through the Specialty Match run by the NRMP Specialties Matching Services. In recent years, about 73% of enrolled applicants found a position through the Match and about 74% of all available Hand Surgery positions filled through the Match.

### HAND SURGERY (ORTHOPEDIC SURGERY)

| | | | |
|---|---|---|---|
| ACGME-Approved Programs | 53 | 1st-Yr Positions (M.D.) | 100 |
| AOA-Approved Programs | 0 | 1st-Yr Positions (D.O.) | 0 |
| PGY-1 Positions | 0 | Part-Time Programs | 4 |
| % Women Residents | 7 | % IMG Residents | 0 |
| Avg. Res. Work Hours/Week | 59.2 | Avg. Days Off Per Month | 6.6 |
| Positions through NRMP Combined Musculoskeletal Match | 114 | Programs Offering Multiple Start Dates | 6 |

### HAND SURGERY (PLASTIC SURGERY)

| | | | |
|---|---|---|---|
| ACGME-Approved Programs | 17 | 1st-Yr Positions (M.D.) | 24 |
| AOA-Approved Programs | 0 | 1st-Yr Positions (D.O.) | 0 |
| PGY-1 Positions | 0 | Part-Time Programs | 1 |
| % Women Residents | 16 | % IMG Residents | 0 |
| Avg. Res. Work Hours/Week | 57.4 | Avg. Days Off Per Month | 6.9 |
| Positions through NRMP Specialties Matching Services | 0 | | |

### HAND SURGERY (GENERAL SURGERY)

| | | | |
|---|---|---|---|
| ACGME-Approved Programs | 2 | 1st-Yr Positions (M.D.) | 11 |
| AOA-Approved Programs | 0 | 1st-Yr Positions (D.O.) | 0 |
| PGY-1 Positions | 0 | Part-Time Programs | 0 |
| % Women Residents | 19 | % IMG Residents | 48 |
| Avg. Res. Work Hours/Week | 45.0 | Avg. Days Off Per Month | 6.5 |
| Positions through NRMP Specialties Matching Services | 0 | Programs Offering Multiple Start Dates | ·1 |

*For more information, contact:*
- American Academy of Orthopaedic Surgeons, 6300 N. River Road, Rosemont, IL 60018-4262; www.aaos.org.
- American Osteopathic Academy of Orthopedics, Box 291690, Davie, FL 33329-1690; www.aaos.org.
- American Association for Hand Surgery, 444 E. Algonquin Road, Suite 120, Arlington Heights, IL 60005; www.handsurgery.org.
- American Society for Surgery of the Hand, 6060 Greenwood Plaza Boulevard, Suite 100, Englewood, CO 80111-4801; www.hand-surg.org.

# Hematology-Oncology (F) *

**Specialty Overview:** Although separate specialties, Hematology (the diagnosis and treatment of diseases of the blood) and Oncology (the diagnosis and treatment of patients with cancer) are often combined in both training and practice. This specialty's patients, once seen as victims of hopeless diseases, frequently can now be offered significant life-extending treatments.

The specialty is predominantly office-based, but practitioners often have a large primary or consultative inpatient service. Night call and emergencies can be frequent. Most specialists in this field work in medium to large cities. Hematologists and Oncologists are drawn from the specialties of Pediatrics and Internal Medicine.

**Specialists' View:** According to recent AMA surveys, 61% of Hematologist-Oncologist Internists in academic and clinical positions felt that their practice activities met their expectations. On a scale of 1=very unsatisfied with their current practice position to 5=very satisfied, those surveyed averaged 3.5. They average 55 hours per week doing patient care. Among new residency graduates, 35% had difficulty finding a job they preferred; 10% were unemployed at graduation.

Of Pediatric Hematologist-Oncologists in academic and clinical positions, 44% felt that their practice activities met their expectations. On a scale of 1=very unsatisfied with their current practice position to 5=very satisfied, those surveyed averaged 3.6. They average 36 hours per week doing patient care. Among new residency graduates, 67% had difficulty finding a job they preferred; 8% were unemployed at graduation.

Among Hematologist Internists in academic and clinical positions, 75% felt that their practice activities met their expectations. On a scale of 1=very unsatisfied with their current practice position to 5=very satisfied, those surveyed averaged 3.5. They average 47 hours per week doing patient care. Among new residency graduates, none reported difficulty finding a job they preferred although 27% were unemployed at graduation.

Among Hematologist Pathologists in academic and clinical positions, 86% felt that their practice activities met their expectations. On a scale of 1=very unsatisfied with their current practice position to 5=very satisfied, those surveyed averaged 3.6. They average 45 hours per week doing patient care. Among new residency graduates, 67% had difficulty finding a job they preferred; 7% were unemployed at graduation.

Among Oncologist Internists in academic and clinical positions, 69% felt that their practice activities met their expectations. On a scale of 1=very unsatisfied with their current practice position to 5=very satisfied, those surveyed averaged 3.1. They average 49 hours per week doing patient care. Among new residency graduates, 22% had difficulty finding a job they preferred; 7% were unemployed at graduation.

**Training:** Training in either Hematology or Oncology is usually a two-year fellowship, but many programs combine the two specialties into three-year fellowships. Training in these specialties follows completion of an Internal Medicine or Pediatric residency or three years of a Pathology residency for a one-year fellowship in Hematology. For Osteopathic physicians, training follows internship and two years of Internal Medicine residency.

**Match:** Applicants should contact programs directly.

### HEMATOLOGY (INTERNAL MEDICINE)

| | | | |
|---|---|---|---|
| ACGME-Approved Programs | 38 | 1st-Yr Positions (M.D.) | 79 |
| AOA-Approved Programs | 0 | 1st-Yr Positions (D.O.) | 0 |
| PGY-1 Positions | 0 | Part-Time Programs | 2 |
| % Women Residents | 35 | % IMG Residents | 55 |
| Avg. Res. Work Hours/Week | 50.2 | Avg. Days Off Per Month | 5.7 |
| Positions through NRMP Specialties Matching Services | 0 | Programs Offering Multiple Start Dates | 4 |

### HEMATOLOGY (PATHOLOGY)

| | | | |
|---|---|---|---|
| ACGME-Approved Programs | 60 | 1st-Yr Positions (M.D.) | 68 |
| AOA-Approved Programs | 0 | 1st-Yr Positions (D.O.) | 0 |
| PGY-1 Positions | 0 | Part-Time Programs | 6 |
| % Women Residents | 38 | % IMG Residents | 36 |
| Avg. Res. Work Hours/Week | 49.3 | Avg. Days Off Per Month | 7.3 |
| Positions through NRMP Specialties Matching Services | 0 | Programs Offering Multiple Start Dates | 4 |

### ONCOLOGY (INTERNAL MEDICINE)

| | | | |
|---|---|---|---|
| ACGME-Approved Programs | 45 | 1st-Yr Positions (M.D.) | 133 |
| AOA-Approved Programs | 0 | 1st-Yr Positions (D.O.) | 0 |
| PGY-1 Positions | 0 | Part-Time Programs | 3 |
| % Women Residents | 25 | % IMG Residents | 51 |
| Avg. Res. Work Hours/Week | 51.0 | Avg. Days Off Per Month | 6.0 |
| Positions through NRMP Specialties Matching Services | 0 | Programs Offering Multiple Start Dates | 6 |

### HEMATOLOGY–ONCOLOGY (INTERNAL MEDICINE)

| | | | |
|---|---|---|---|
| ACGME-Approved Programs | 105 | 1st-Yr Positions (M.D.) | 289 |
| AOA-Approved Programs | 1 | 1st-Yr Positions (D.O.) | 1 |
| PGY-1 Positions | 0 | Part-Time Programs | 8 |
| % Women Residents | 28 | % IMG Residents | 47 |
| Avg. Res. Work Hours/Week | 49.4 | Avg. Days Off Per Month | 4.9 |
| Positions through NRMP Specialties Matching Services | 0 | Programs Offering Multiple Start Dates | 20 |

### HEMATOLOGY–ONCOLOGY (PEDIATRICS)

| | | | |
|---|---|---|---|
| ACGME-Approved Programs | 65 | 1st-Yr Positions (M.D.) | 99 |
| AOA-Approved Programs | 0 | 1st-Yr Positions (D.O.) | 0 |
| PGY-1 Positions | 0 | Part-Time Programs | 13 |
| % Women Residents | 46 | % IMG Residents | 40 |
| Avg. Res. Work Hours/Week | 52.0 | Avg. Days Off Per Month | 6.6 |
| Positions through NRMP Specialties Matching Services | 0 | Programs Offering Multiple Start Dates | 9 |

## *For more information, contact:*

- American College of Osteopathic Internists, 3 Bethesda Metro Center, Suite 508, Bethesda, MD 20814; www.acoi.org.
- American Society of Clinical Oncology, 435 N. Michigan Avenue, Suite 1717, Chicago, IL 60611; www.asco.org.
- American Society of Hematology, 1200 19th Street N.W., Suite 300, Washington, DC 20036-2412; www.hematology.org.

# Hospitalists *

**Specialty Overview:** Hospitalists care for inpatients. Under current definitions, physicians are hospitalists if they spend 25% or more of their time caring for patients admitted or transferred to the hospital by their primary doctors. Their practice has been described as caring for horizontal patients; when patients are discharged, office-based physicians assume take over their care. This specialty's growth has been encouraged by managed care organizations that want their office-based physicians to primarily see outpatients while streamlining the treatment given to inpatients, i.e., reduce lengths of stay and reduce costs. Having Hospitalists see all inpatients saves the time required for the rest of the physicians to do rounds. In some cases, Hospitalists also compensate for the reduction in resident physicians some hospitals have experienced by doing the work they used to do.

About 90% of Hospitalists are Internists, about 5% are Pediatricians, and 5% are Family Physicians. At some academic centers, Hospitalists do most of the inpatient teaching to residents and students. However, some managed care organizations require the use of their Hospitalist, rather than allowing the primary physician to provide patient care. This has raised serious and organized opposition to their presence.

The original article describing Hospitalists raised a known concern: Burnout. Similar to other hospital-based inpatient specialties, few physicians can withstand the pressures of constantly attending on the wards. Hospitalists also must balance the demands of patients, families, primary physicians, hospitals, and insurers. How (and how well) Hospitalist groups will handle this aspect of their work remains to be seen. Yet one benefit of being a Hospitalist is having set hours to work. The pay is 20% higher than what General Internists receive.

**Training:** Currently, training generally consists of completing an Internal Medicine or Family Practice residency. In mid-1998, the University of California-San Francisco slightly modified their Internal Medicine residency to accommodate those who wished to become Hospitalists. They also began a one-year fellowship for those who wished to pursue the field in an academic setting.

Special training will be added in end-of-life care, interacting with other specialists, dealing with managed care, and improving business and communication skills.

### For more information, contact:

- National Association of Inpatient Physicians, 190 N. Independence Mall West, Philadelphia, PA 19106; www.naiponline.org.

# Infectious Diseases (F) *

**Specialty Overview:** Infectious Disease specialists deal with the diagnosis and treatment of contagious diseases. At the onset of the antibiotic era, the specialty was thought to be on the edge of extinction. It is now making a large comeback due to the great diversity of drug-resistant bacteria and the AIDS epidemic. Some people have even suggested starting an HIV specialty akin to the "syphilologists" at the beginning of the twentieth century. Infectious Disease specialists act as consultants to other physicians. Many are also involved in research and most work in major medical centers. With the increased importance of nosocomial infections, many Infectious Disease specialists work part-time as hospital infection control officers. Physicians in this subspecialty generally receive lower salaries than those specialists who are more procedure-oriented. Many Infectious Disease specialists also practice General Internal Medicine.

**Specialists' View:** According to recent AMA surveys, 69% of Infectious Disease Internists in academic and clinical positions felt that their practice activities met their expectations. On a scale of 1=very unsatisfied with their current practice position to 5=very satisfied, those surveyed averaged 3.5. They average 46 hours per week doing patient care. Among new residency graduates, 31% had difficulty finding a job they preferred; 10% were unemployed at graduation.

**Training:** Training consists of either a two-year fellowship following completion of an Internal Medicine residency or a three-year fellowship after a Pediatric residency. (At present, no active Pediatric programs exist.) For Osteopathic physicians, training follows internship and two years of an Internal Medicine residency.

**Match:** Applicants match with Infectious Diseases fellowships by using the NRMP Specialties Matching Services. In recent years, 83% of enrolled applicants found a position through the Match, while 74% of available positions filled through the Match.

### INFECTIOUS DISEASE (INTERNAL MEDICINE)

| | | | |
|---|---|---|---|
| ACGME-Approved Programs | 142 | 1st-Yr Positions (M.D.) | 307 |
| AOA-Approved Programs | 2 | 1st-Yr Positions (D.O.) | 2 |
| PGY-1 Positions | 0 | Part-Time Programs | 23 |
| % Women Residents | 36 | % IMG Residents | 41 |
| Avg. Res. Work Hours/Week | 50.7 | Avg. Days Off Per Month | 5.6 |
| Positions through NRMP Specialties Matching Services | 230 | Programs Offering Multiple Start Dates | 17 |

## For more information, contact:

- American College of Osteopathic Internists, 3 Bethesda Metro Center, Suite 508, Bethesda, MD 20814; www.acoi.org.
- Infectious Diseases Society of America, 1200 19th Street N.W., Suite 300, Washington, DC 20036-2401; www.idsociety.org.

# Internal Medicine *

**Specialty Overview:** Internists (specialists in Internal Medicine, not to be confused with "interns") are divided into General Internists and subspecialists in Internal Medicine (see the subspecialties listed under "Internal Medicine" in Figure 2.8). The General Internist provides longitudinal care to adult patients with both acute and chronic diseases. In rural areas, the General Internist often acts as a consultant to other practitioners on complex medical cases. In suburban and urban areas, however, other primary care practitioners usually consult with Internal Medicine subspecialists; surgical specialists consult with both General and subspecialty Internists. Urban General Internists provide primary health care and treat non-surgical diseases such as diabetes, hypertension, and congestive heart failure on both an inpatient and an outpatient basis. They are also very active in managed care plans such as HMOs.

Students attracted to General Internal Medicine seek an intellectual challenge, have an interest in primary care, and often had a positive experience during their third-year Internal Medicine rotation. The field of General Internal Medicine, however, has been less popular among students and housestaff in recent years. This trend may be due to several factors, including: the Internist's income being lower than that of either the average physician or the Internal Medicine subspecialist, General Internal Medicine's relatively low prestige, the perception that caring for chronically ill patients is burdensome, and the increasing hassles of practice. Many students avoid Internal Medicine because they perceive that the housestaff and attendings they work with are overworked, unhappy, and under-rewarded. However, the growth of managed care plans and societal pressure to enhance primary care have led to increased job opportunities for General Internists.

Internal Medicine is often described as "less procedural and more cerebral" than other specialties. While this may be true for General Internists, it is not true of the procedurally oriented subspecialists in Gastroenterology, Critical Care, Pulmonary Diseases, and Cardiology. The average Internist (General and subspecialists) has a 63-hour work week, with 49% of the time spent in office visits, 27% spent on hospital rounds, 21% on other patient care activities, and 3% spent doing surgical/manipulative procedures. In some areas of the country, the amount of hospital time is decreasing as Hospitalists assume inpatient tasks.

**Specialists' View:** According to recent AMA surveys, 63% of Internists in academic and clinical positions felt that their practice activities met their expectations. On a scale of 1=very unsatisfied with their current practice position to 5=very satisfied, those surveyed averaged 3.3. They average 49 hours per week doing patient care. Among new residency graduates, 27% had difficulty finding a job they preferred; 16% were unemployed at graduation.

**Training:** Training in Internal Medicine is three years in length. Programs that combine Internal Medicine with Family Practice (see Family Practice-Internal Medicine), Pediatrics (see below), or Preventive Medicine are four years. Programs combining Internal Medicine with Emergency Medicine (see Emergency Medicine-Internal Medicine), Neurology, Physical Medicine and Rehabilitation, or Psychiatry last five years. These combined programs qualify graduates for board examinations in both specialties. If an Osteopathic graduate enters an Internal Medicine "specialty-track" internship, the Internal Medicine training time is shortened by one year. Approximately 100 trainees enter this type of internship each year.

One of the advantages of Internal Medicine training is the number of options available following residency. About 58% of all Internal Medicine residency graduates go on to subspecialize. However, residents completing Internal Medicine residencies in markets with high managed care penetration are less likely to subspecialize than are Internal Medicine residents training in areas with less managed care impact. Many physicians do not finalize their decision to practice as either General Internists or subspecialists until well into their residency.

Following residency, fellowships are available in: Adolescent Medicine; Cardiovascular Disease; Clinical Cardiac Electrophysiology; Critical Care Medicine; Clinical & Laboratory Immunology; Endocrinology, Diabetes & Metabolism; Gastroenterology; Geriatric Medicine; Hematology; Infectious Diseases; Medical Oncology; Nephrology; Pulmonary Diseases; Rheumatology; and Sports Medicine.

The *NRMP Directory* lists some positions as "Internal Medicine" and some as "Medicine-Primary." The difference between the two types of programs is that there is more, but often only slightly more, time spent in an ambulatory clinic and a continuity clinic in the latter type. Graduates of both programs take the same Board examination. Some programs, labeled "Primary Care Internal Medicine," emphasize outpatient clinic training, although they seldom have more clinic hours than inpatient training. These come closer than the usual residency programs to mimicking the actual practice of a General Internist, although all Internal Medicine programs have increased the amount of time spent in ambulatory settings over the past few years.

**Match:** Virtually all ACGME-approved positions in Internal Medicine are listed in the NRMP PGY-1 Match. Just over one thousand of these positions, though, are for only one year of training (preliminary positions) and are designed for those continuing their training in other specialties. In recent years, about 58% of the available PGY-1 positions filled through the NRMP Match and 92% of these positions were subsequently filled. Only about 73% of the Preliminary Internal Medicine positions filled.

**Other Useful Information:** Internal Medicine leads the way in the reform of postgraduate education. All Internal Medicine training programs must limit the number of hours residents work to 80 hours per week, averaged over four weeks. Residents at all levels of training are to have, on average, at least one day per week free of hospital duties. They also must spend at least 25% of their three-year training in ambulatory settings. Not all programs, though, are complying with these requirements.

### INTERNAL MEDICINE

| | | | |
|---|---|---|---|
| ACGME-Approved Programs | 415 | 1st-Yr Positions (M.D.) | 7,556 |
| AOA-Approved Programs | 50 | 1st-Yr Positions (D.O.) | 198 |
| PGY-1 Positions | 6,868 | Part-Time Programs | 94 |
| % Women Residents | 37 | % IMG Residents | 40 |
| Avg. Res. Work Hours/Week | 66.4 | Avg. Days Off Per Month | 4.6 |
| % Pursuing Additional Specialty Training | 41 | Programs Offering Multiple Start Dates | 49 |

### INTERNAL MEDICINE–NEUROLOGY *

| | | | |
|---|---|---|---|
| ACGME-Approved Programs | 16 | 1st-Yr Positions (M.D.) | 19 |
| AOA-Approved Programs | 0 | 1st-Yr Positions (D.O.) | 0 |
| PGY-1 Positions | 19 | Part-Time Programs | 5 |
| % Women Residents | 33 | % IMG Residents | 38 |
| Avg. Res. Work Hours/Week | 61.7 | Avg. Days Off Per Month | 4.5 |
| Programs Offering Multiple Start Dates | 2 | | |

### INTERNAL MEDICINE–PHYSICAL MEDICINE/REHABILITATION ***

| | | | |
|---|---|---|---|
| ACGME-Approved Programs | 15 | 1st-Yr Positions (M.D.) | 16 |
| AOA-Approved Programs | 0 | 1st-Yr Positions (D.O.) | 0 |
| PGY-1 Positions | 16 | Part-Time Programs | 5 |
| % Women Residents | 24 | % IMG Residents | 10 |
| Avg. Res. Work Hours/Week | 59.0 | Avg. Days Off Per Month | 5.1 |
| Programs Offering Multiple Start Dates | 1 | | |

### INTERNAL MEDICINE–PREVENTIVE MEDICINE *

| | | | |
|---|---|---|---|
| ACGME-Approved Programs | 3 | 1st-Yr Positions (M.D.) | 3 |
| AOA-Approved Programs | 0 | 1st-Yr Positions (D.O.) | 0 |
| PGY-1 Positions | 3 | Part-Time Programs | 2 |
| % Women Residents | 100 | % IMG Residents | 0 |
| Avg. Res. Work Hours/Week | 71.0 | Avg. Days Off Per Month | 4.0 |

### INTERNAL MEDICINE–PSYCHIATRY **

| | | | |
|---|---|---|---|
| ACGME-Approved Programs | 28 | 1st-Yr Positions (M.D.) | 49 |
| AOA-Approved Programs | 0 | 1st-Yr Positions (D.O.) | 0 |
| PGY-1 Positions | 49 | Part-Time Programs | 10 |
| % Women Residents | 44 | % IMG Residents | 25 |
| Avg. Res. Work Hours/Week | 64.0 | Avg. Days Off Per Month | 4.7 |
| Programs Offering Multiple Start Dates | 2 | | |

### INTERNAL MEDICINE–PRIMARY

| | | | |
|---|---|---|---|
| ACGME-Approved Programs | 95 | 1st-Yr Positions (M.D.) | 707 |
| AOA-Approved Programs | 0 | 1st-Yr Positions (D.O.) | 0 |
| PGY-1 Positions | 649 | Part-Time Programs | 29 |
| % Women Residents | 37 | % IMG Residents | 40 |
| Avg. Res. Work Hours/Week | 66.4 | Avg. Days Off Per Month | 4.6 |

### For more information, contact:

- American College of Osteopathic Internists, 3 Bethesda Metro Center, Suite 508, Bethesda, MD 20814; www.acoi.org.
- American College of Physicians–American Society of Internal Medicine, 190 Independence Mall West, Philadelphia, PA 19106-1572; www.acponline.org.
- Society of General Internal Medicine, 2501 M Street N.W., Suite 575, Washington, DC 20037; www.sgim.org.

## Internal Medicine–Pediatrics ****

**Specialty Overview:** Combined Internal Medicine–Pediatrics training programs are designed for the individual who wishes to have a primary care practice for families without offering obstetric and surgical services.

Graduates of these combined training programs report that they feel as comfortable as other Pediatricians handling infant, child, and adolescent cases, but less comfortable than Family Practitioners treating adolescent health problems. Although they are more comfortable than Family Practitioners dealing with complex Internal Medicine patients, they report being less comfortable than other Internists treating intensive care and geriatric patients.

Completion of combined programs makes the individual eligible to take the specialty Board examination in both Pediatrics and Internal Medicine. The combined programs are not reviewed by the certifying bodies (Residency Review Committees) as a whole program. Rather, the Internal Medicine and Pediatrics programs are each reviewed and approved separately. The number of programs is growing. A listing of the combined programs can be found in the "Green Book's" Appendices.

**Specialists' View:** According to recent AMA surveys, 77% of Internist-Pediatricians in academic and clinical positions felt that their practice activities met their expectations. On a scale of 1=very unsatisfied with their current practice position to 5=very satisfied, those surveyed averaged 3.5. They average 49 hours per week doing patient care. Among new residency graduates, 5% had difficulty finding a job they preferred; 14% were unemployed at graduation.

**Training:** Training is four years in length, with a minimum of twenty months of Internal Medicine. The programs are, for the most part, integrated. Trainees take blocks of Internal Medicine and then blocks of Pediatrics. This often leads to spending nearly two years at the intern level of training.

**Match:** In recent years, about 77% of the available PGY-1 positions filled through the NRMP Match and 87% of these positions were subsequently filled.

### INTERNAL MEDICINE–PEDIATRICS

| | | | |
|---|---|---|---|
| ACGME-Approved Programs | 108 | 1st-Yr Positions (M.D.) | 463 |
| AOA-Approved Programs | 0 | 1st-Yr Positions (D.O.) | 0 |
| PGY-1 Positions | 454 | Part-Time Programs | 32 |
| % Women Residents | 45 | % IMG Residents | 11 |
| Avg. Res. Work Hours/Week | 69.9 | Avg. Days Off Per Month | 4.5 |
| Programs Offering Multiple Start Dates | 10 | | |

## For more information, contact:

- American College of Physicians–American Society of Internal Medicine, 190 Independence Mall West, Philadelphia, PA 19106-1572; www.acponline.org.
- American Academy of Pediatrics, 141 Northwest Point Boulevard, Elk Grove Village, IL 60007; www.aap.org.

# Medical Genetics *

**Specialty Overview:** Medical Genetics is the newest medical specialty. Currently, more than 650 physicians have been certified in Clinical Genetics or a laboratory subspecialty (Clinical Biochemical Genetics, Clinical Molecular Genetics, Clinical Cytogenetics, and M.D. Clinical Genetics). Most of them come from the specialties of Pediatrics, Obstetrics and Gynecology, or Internal Medicine. While the field is still quite small, the rapid changes occurring in clinical genetics suggest that there may be a much greater need in the future for practitioners in the specialty for both diagnosis and treatment.

**Training:** Training in the specialty requires two years in another medical specialty before admission for two or more additional years of Medical Genetics. Some programs offer all four years of training. Two programs combine training in Medical Genetics with Pediatrics.

**Match:** The only way to get a list of programs is through the American Society for Human Genetics in their *Guide to North American Postgraduate Training Programs in Human Genetics.* This book lists the available programs; their areas of concentration; the type of individuals (masters, M.D., Ph.D.) currently enrolled, graduated, and on faculty; the contact person; their application deadline; and a narrative about each program.

**MEDICAL GENETICS**

| | | | |
|---|---|---|---|
| ACGME-Approved Programs– M.D. Clinical Genetics | 45 | Programs in Clinical Biochemical Genetics* | 38 |
| Programs in Clinical Cytogenetics* | 58 | Programs in Clinical Molecular Genetics* | 49 |
| AOA-Approved Programs | 0 | 1st-Yr Positions (M.D.)# | 70 |
| PGY-1 Positions | 0 | 1st-Yr Positions (D.O.) | 0 |
| % Women Residents | 48 | % IMG Residents | 42 |
| Avg. Res. Work Hours/Week | 47.5 | Avg. Days Off Per Month | 6.2 |
| % Pursuing Additional Specialty Training | 18 | | |

*Programs approved by the American Board of Medical Genetics.
#Funded positions for M.D. Clinical Genetics.

## For more information, contact:

- American College of Medical Genetics–American Society for Human Genetics, 9650 Rockville Pike, Bethesda, MD 20814-3998; www.faseb.org/genetics.

# Medical Management *

**Specialty Overview:** Medical managers have existed almost as long as the profession. (As soon as there were two physicians, one was assuredly the administrator.) Recently, medical management has come into its own with the increasing complexity of Byzantine government rules, the web of managed care organizations, and the constantly changing patient and payer demands. Also called "Medical Administration," this specialty competes with non-physicians who also try to manage health care systems.

Since managing physicians is somewhat like herding cats, it is often a thankless job. Yet many physicians try it at various stages of their careers—especially in the decade before retirement. Many such positions are available in hospitals, group practices, clinics, insurance companies, and corporations.

Closely linked to Medical Management is "Managed Care Medicine." Those taking courses in this area also intend to manage other physicians, but often with the more defined goal of working within managed care. According to the *New England Journal of Medicine* (1999 Dec 16;341(25): 1945-8), the inherent conflicts in the medical directors' role are "satisfying the desires of patients and physicians, on the one hand, and the financial profit or survival of the organization, on the other, and between the unlimited demands of individual patients and the limited resources of society."

**Training:** Courses are available through the American College of Physician Executives, the American College of Managed Care Medicine, and through various MBA and MPH programs.

### For more information, contact:

- American College of Managed Care Medicine, 4435 Waterfront Drive, Suite 101, Glen Allen, VA 23060; www.acmcm.org.
- American College of Physician Executives, 4890 W. Kennedy Boulevard, Suite 200, Tampa, FL 33609; www.acpe.org.
- American Medical Directors Association, 10480 Little Patuxent Parkway, Suite 760, Columbia, MD 21044; www.amda.com.

# Medical Toxicology (F) *

**Specialty Overview:** Medical Toxicologists diagnose, treat, and consult on a wide variety of intentional, accidental, and industrial poisonings. While the specialists in this field have been practicing and fellowships have been available for some time, the subspecialty was approved by the American Board of Medical Specialties only in 1992. It is sponsored by Emergency Medicine, Pediatrics, and Preventive Medicine.

**Training:** Programs are usually two years following the primary residency. A list of current training programs and their contact information is available through the American College of Medical Toxicology, www.acmt.net.

**Match:** Fellowships, usually within Emergency Medicine or Pediatrics departments, are obtained by contacting each program directly.

### MEDICAL TOXICOLOGY (F)

| | | | |
|---|---|---|---|
| ACGME-Approved Programs | 28 | 1st-Yr Positions (M.D.) | 42 |
| AOA-Approved Programs | 0 | 1st-Yr Positions (D.O.) | 0 |
| PGY-1 Positions | 0 | | |

*For more information, contact:*
- American Academy of Pediatrics, 141 Northwest Point Boulevard, Elk Grove Village, IL 60007; www.aap.org.
- American College of Emergency Physicians, P.O. Box 619911, Dallas, TX 75261-9911; www.acep.org.
- American College of Occupational and Environmental Medicine, 1114 N. Arlington Heights Road, Arlington Heights, IL 60004-4770; www.acoem.org.
- Society for Academic Emergency Medicine, 901 N. Washington, Lansing, MI 48906; www.saem.org.
- Society of Toxicology, 1767 Business Center Drive, Suite 302, Reston, VA 22190; www.toxicology.org.

## Neonatal–Perinatal Medicine (F) *

**Specialty Overview:** Neonatologists treat the problems associated with premature births. Their practice centers on the neonatal intensive care unit. They are Pediatricians who do critical care on those neonates who do not yet have the capacity to live without medical assistance.

As with other critical care specialists, they must be able to skillfully perform procedures—but they must work on *very* small babies. The size of the infants they work with has progressively decreased. Neonatologists work closely with a specialized team of nurses, social workers, and respiratory therapists. They also work closely with families to sort out both medical and ethical issues of care.

**Specialists' View:** According to recent AMA surveys, 71% of Neonatologists in academic and clinical positions felt that their practice activities met their expectations. On a scale of 1=very unsatisfied with their current practice position to 5=very satisfied, those surveyed averaged 3.5. They average 45 hours per week doing patient care. Among new residency graduates, 35% had difficulty finding a job they preferred; 3% were unemployed at graduation.

**Training:** These fellowships are two years in length following a Pediatric residency.

**Match:** Applicants should contact individual training programs, since this specialty has no match.

| NEONATAL–PERINATAL MEDICINE (F) | | | |
|---|---|---|---|
| ACGME-Approved Programs | 100 | 1st-Yr Positions (M.D.) | 181 |
| AOA-Approved Programs | 0 | 1st-Yr Positions (D.O.) | 0 |
| PGY-1 Positions | 0 | Part-Time Programs | 25 |
| % Women Residents | 48 | % IMG Residents | 55 |
| Avg. Res. Work Hours/Week | 52.7 | Avg. Days Off Per Month | 8.0 |
| Programs Offering Multiple Start Dates | 25 | | |

### For more information, contact:

- American Academy of Pediatrics, P.O. Box 927, 141 Northwest Point Road, Elk Grove Village, IL 60007; www.aap.org.
- American College of Osteopathic Pediatricians, 5550 Friendship Boulevard, Suite 300, Chevy Chase, MD 20815-7201.

# Nephrology (F) *

**Specialty Overview:** Nephrologists diagnose and treat diseases of the kidney and the urinary system. Most patients cared for by these specialists have chronic diseases requiring long-term care. Managing dialysis and the treatment of dialysis and renal transplant patients are large parts of most Nephrologists' practices. The specialty is predominantly office-based. However, practitioners may have large primary or consultative inpatient services. Night call can be frequent.

**Specialists' View:** According to recent AMA surveys, 61% of Nephrologists in academic and clinical positions felt that their practice activities met their expectations. On a scale of 1=very unsatisfied with their current practice position to 5=very satisfied, those surveyed averaged 3.4.

They average 55 hours per week doing patient care. Among new residency graduates, 16% had difficulty finding a job they preferred; 16% were unemployed at graduation.

Among Pediatric Nephrologists in academic and clinical positions, 57% felt that their practice activities met their expectations. On a scale of 1=very unsatisfied with their current practice position to 5=very satisfied, those surveyed averaged 3.6. They average 44 hours per week doing patient care. Among new residency graduates, all had difficulty finding a job they preferred, yet all were employed at graduation.

**Training:** Training is generally a two-year fellowship following the completion of an Internal Medicine residency or three years after a Pediatric residency. For Osteopathic physicians, training follows internship and two years of an Internal Medicine residency.

**Match:** Applicants should contact programs directly.

### NEPHROLOGY (INTERNAL MEDICINE)

| | | | |
|---|---|---|---|
| ACGME-Approved Programs | 135 | 1st-Yr Positions (M.D.) | 321 |
| AOA-Approved Programs | 2 | 1st-Yr Positions (D.O.) | 2 |
| PGY-1 Positions | 0 | Part-Time Programs | 16 |
| % Women Residents | 26 | % IMG Residents | 60 |
| Avg. Res. Work Hours/Week | 51.8 | Avg. Days Off Per Month | 6.7 |
| Programs Offering Multiple Start Dates | 19 | | |

### NEPHROLOGY (PEDIATRICS)

| | | | |
|---|---|---|---|
| ACGME-Approved Programs | 45 | 1st-Yr Positions (M.D.) | 46 |
| AOA-Approved Programs | 0 | 1st-Yr Positions (D.O.) | 0 |
| PGY-1 Positions | 0 | Part-Time Programs | 4 |
| % Women Residents | 49 | % IMG Residents | 63 |
| Avg. Res. Work Hours/Week | 46.5 | Avg. Days Off Per Month | 7.3 |
| Programs Offering Multiple Start Dates | 5 | | |

## For more information, contact:

- American College of Osteopathic Internists, 3 Bethesda Metro Center, Suite 508, Bethesda, MD 20814; www.acoi.org.
- American Society of Nephrology, 1200 19th Street N.W., Suite 300, Washington, DC 20036; www.asn-online.com.
- Renal Physicians Association, 2011 Pennsylvania Avenue, N.W., Suite 800, Washington, DC 20006-1808; www.kdp-baptist.louisville.edu/rpa/.

# Neurological Surgery ****

**Specialty Overview:** Neurosurgeons provide operative and non-operative management of lesions of the brain, spinal cord, peripheral nerves, and their supporting structures (skull, spine, meninges, CNS blood supply). Many are also involved in pain management. This requires much manual dexterity and a willingness to accept both dramatic successes and long-term failures in patient care. New developments in autologous and fetal tissue transplantation and in stereotactic surgery for epilepsy, Parkinson's Disease, and tumors may increase the need for Neurosurgeons during the next decade. Patients range in age from neonates to the elderly. Night call and emergency surgery are frequent parts of Neurosurgical practice.

**Specialists' View:** According to recent AMA surveys, 63% of Neurosurgeons in academic and clinical positions felt that their practice activities met their expectations. On a scale of 1=very unsatisfied with their current practice position to 5=very satisfied, those surveyed averaged 3.5. They average 63 hours per week doing patient care. Among new residency graduates, 4% had difficulty finding a job they preferred; all were employed at graduation.

**Training:** Residency training lasts five years following one year of General Surgery. A minimum of 36 months must be spent in clinical Neurosurgery and three months in clinical Neurology. The balance of time can be spent in the study of relevant basic sciences, such as Neuropathology and Neuroradiology, or other related fields, such as Pediatric Neurosurgery or Spinal Surgery. The areas covered during these extra months are the key differences among this specialty's training programs.

**Match:** All civilian Neurosurgery residency programs are in the Neurological Surgery Matching Program, sponsored by the Society of Neurological Surgeons, P.O. Box 7584, San Francisco, CA 94120-7584. About 34 ACGME-approved positions are listed at 24 programs in the *NRMP Directory*, but these are probably all "prematched" in the specialty Match. The Matching Program suggests that applications be submitted to the Centralized Application Service by late August. Rank-Order Lists are due in late-January and results are distributed in early February. Students in the Neurosurgery Match should also sign up with the NRMP PGY-1 Match for an internship position. (Although some programs have associated internships, applicants need to be in the NRMP PGY-1 Match to get a position.) Participants in the Neurosurgery Match get their results before they must submit their NRMP Rank-Order Lists.

**Other Useful Information:** The average applicant to a Neurosurgery residency submits 32 applications and interviews at 10 programs. All application materials (except the Dean's letter) must be at residency programs before November 1, and program directors notify applicants whether they have been invited for an interview by November 15.

In recent years, U.S. medical students matched with a Neurosurgery program about 85% of the time, U.S. medical school graduates matched 31% of the time, and IMGs matched 25% of the time. In most years, 95% of available positions fill in the specialty's Match.

### NEUROLOGICAL SURGERY

| | | | |
|---|---|---|---|
| ACGME-Approved Programs | 99 | 1st-Yr Positions (M.D.) | 136 |
| AOA-Approved Programs | 6 | 1st-Yr Positions (D.O.) | 4 |
| PGY-1 Positions | 34 | Part-Time Programs | 3 |
| % Women Residents | 10 | % IMG Residents | 8 |
| Avg. Res. Work Hours/Week | 75.9 | Avg. Days Off Per Month | 5.2 |
| % Pursuing Additional Specialty Training | 15 | Programs Offering Multiple Start Dates | 3 |

### For more information, contact:

- American Association of Neurological Surgeons, 22 S. Washington Street, Suite 100, Park Ridge, IL 60068; www.aans.org.
- American College of Osteopathic Surgeons, 123 N. Henry Street, Alexandria, VA 22314-2903.
- Society of Neurological Surgeons, 750 Washington Street, NEMC Suite 178, Boston, MA 02111; www.aans.org.

# Neurology *

**Specialty Overview:** Neurologists diagnose and treat patients with diseases of the brain, spinal cord, peripheral nerves, and neuromuscular system. Much of the practice deals with the diagnosis and, more and more often, the treatment of patients seen in consultation. Many of these patients have headaches, strokes, or seizure disorders. Neurologists follow not only these patients but also those with chronic neuromuscular diseases. It is anticipated that the need for Neurologists will increase as the population ages. The specialty is predominantly office-based. Neurologists may, however, have large primary or consultative inpatient services. Night call can be frequent, especially in solo or small group practices.

**Specialists' View:** According to recent AMA surveys, 65% of Neurologists in academic and clinical positions felt that their practice activities met their expectations. On a scale of 1=very unsatisfied with their current practice position to 5=very satisfied, those surveyed averaged 3.6. They average 49 hours per week doing patient care. Among new residency graduates, 20% had difficulty finding a job they preferred; 7% were unemployed at graduation.

**Training:** Training is three years after a general first-year residency, most often in Internal Medicine, Pediatrics, Family Practice, or a Transitional program. Some Neurology programs have their own PGY-1 year, and so are four years long. Combined programs, which take five years to complete, exist in Internal Medicine-Neurology (see Internal Medicine) and Neurology-Physical Medicine & Rehabilitation (two programs). Four programs, which are seven years long, combine Neurology, Diagnostic Radiology, and Neuroradiology. Nine programs also exist combining Neurology and Psychiatry. Basic Neurology training programs are similar for Osteopathic physicians.

**Match:** ACGME-approved programs generally match through the Neurology Matching Program, sponsored by the Association of University Professors of Neurology, P.O. Box 7584, San Francisco, CA 94120-7584. Most positions are filled a year ahead of time (matching for the year after internship). However, positions not previously filled are offered for the same year to those who have finished at least an internship. This Match requires that Rank-Order Lists be submitted in mid-January and releases results in late January. ACGME-approved programs that offer a first-year position integrated into the Neurology residency, in most cases, also go through the regular NRMP PGY-1 Match. Positions in programs combining Neurology with another specialty, such as Psychiatry or Internal Medicine, generally must be obtained through the NRMP Match or negotiated directly with the program.

**Other Useful Information:** The average applicant to a Neurology residency submits 19 applications and interviews at five programs. In recent years, U.S. medical students matched with a Neurology program 97% of the time, U.S. medical school graduates matched 81% of the time, and IMGs matched 36% of the time. Overall, only 86% of Neurology positions fill through the Match. Many positions not originally filled in the specialty Match are available again the next year (five months before the start of the program) to those already in internship. Applicants also go through the Neurology Matching Program for these positions.

| NEUROLOGY | | | |
|---|---|---|---|
| ACGME-Approved Programs | 122 | 1st-Yr Positions (M.D.) | 432 |
| AOA-Approved Programs | 4 | 1st-Yr Positions (D.O.) | 6 |
| PGY-1 Positions | 56 | Part-Time Programs | 16 |
| % Women Residents | 33 | % IMG Residents | 48 |
| Avg. Res. Work Hours/Week | 62.4 | Avg. Days Off Per Month | 5.4 |
| % Pursuing Additional Specialty Training | 54 | Programs Offering Multiple Start Dates | 13 |

*For more information, contact:*

- American Academy of Neurology, 1080 Montreal Street, St. Paul, MN 55116-2325; www.aan.com.
- American Association of Electrodiagnostic Medicine, 421 First Avenue, S.W., Suite 300E, Rochester, MN 55902; www.aaem.net.
- American College of (Osteopathic) Neuropsychiatry, 28595 Orchard Lake Road, Suite 200, Farmington Hills, MI 48334-2979.
- American Neurological Association, 5841 Cedar Lake Road, Suite 204, Minneapolis, MN 55416; www.aneuroa.org.

# Nuclear Medicine *

**Specialty Overview:** Specialists in Nuclear Medicine use radioactive materials both to diagnose and to treat diseases by imaging the body's physiologic function. The field combines medical practice with certain aspects of the physical sciences, including physics, mathematics, statistics, computer science, chemistry, and radiation biology. Specialists in Nuclear Medicine, unlike those in Radiation Oncology, use radioactive materials that are "unsealed," i.e., free in the bloodstream, for their diagnostic studies and treatments. At some institutions, they are also responsible for performing radioimmunoassay tests.

Practitioners in the specialty have no primary patient-care responsibility and little night call. Many individuals who are currently practicing Nuclear Medicine have been neither formally trained nor certified in the specialty. However, anyone entering the field now is expected to have been fully trained. The future of the specialty may either be very dynamic or rather static, depending upon how rapidly some currently innovative techniques become available to the specialty.

**Specialists' View:** According to recent AMA surveys, 55% of Nuclear Medicine physicians in academic and clinical positions felt that their practice activities met their expectations. On a scale of 1=very unsatisfied with their current practice position to 5=very satisfied, those surveyed averaged 3.2. They average 47 hours per week doing patient care. Among new residency graduates, 50% had difficulty finding a job they preferred; 24% were unemployed at graduation.

**Training:** Training consists of two years of Nuclear Medicine following, interspersed with, or, in a few cases, preceding two years of initial training in a clinical specialty. These clinical specialties are most commonly Radiology, Internal Medicine, or Pathology. Other fields of clinical training have also been rather freely accepted. Nearly all positions are obtained by negotiating with individual programs. Osteopathic programs also accept two years of initial training in Family Practice. Radiology residents doing a year of training in Nuclear Radiology occupy some of the positions that exist for training in Nuclear Medicine. Note, however, that Nuclear Medicine is a specialty distinct from Nuclear Radiology.

**Match:** Except for the few programs in the NRMP Match, contact the programs directly.

### NUCLEAR MEDICINE

| | | | |
|---|---|---|---|
| ACGME-Approved Programs | 76 | 1st-Yr Positions (M.D.) | 113 |
| AOA-Approved Programs | 0 | 1st-Yr Positions (D.O.) | 0 |
| PGY-1 Positions | 5 | Part-Time Programs | 4 |
| % Women Residents | 27 | % IMG Residents | 48 |
| Avg. Res. Work Hours/Week | 45.5 | Avg. Days Off Per Month | 7.1 |
| % Pursuing Additional Specialty Training | 33 | Programs Offering Multiple Start Dates | 10 |

### For more information, contact:

- American College of Nuclear Medicine, P.O. Box 175, Landisville, PA 17538; www.acnucmed.org.
- American Osteopathic Board of Nuclear Medicine, 1000 E. 53rd Street, Chicago, IL 60615.
- Society of Nuclear Medicine, 1850 Samuel Morse Drive, Reston, VA 20190; www.snm.org.

## Obstetrics and Gynecology ★★★★

**Specialty Overview:** Obstetrician-Gynecologists manage pregnancies and treat disorders of the female reproductive tract. Obstetricians deal with pregnancy in women. Gynecologists deal with medical and surgical diseases of the female reproductive tract and infertility. While some specialists in this field work primarily in one or the other area, most work in both Obstetrics and Gynecology. This is the only surgical specialty that is considered

"Primary Care." Obstetrics has been greatly affected by the rising cost of medical liability insurance and the increasing propensity to sue physicians. Due to this risk of being sued, Obstetricians are, in increasing numbers, eliminating deliveries from their practice or reducing the provision of care to patients who have or are likely to have high-risk pregnancies.

As the population ages and there is a greater awareness of women's health care needs, there will be a need for more Gynecologists. The specialty combines both surgical and non-surgical approaches to disease, and is increasingly using endoscopic surgical techniques (minimally invasive surgery).

The average Obstetrician-Gynecologist, in a 50-hour work week, spends 53% of the time seeing patients in the office, 30% in surgery or deliveries, 10% on hospital rounds, and 7% on other patient visits. The field of Obstetrics and Gynecology is primarily office-based, but frequently has a sizable inpatient service load. A busy Obstetric practice consists of considerable emergency and night call. An increasing number of women are entering this field. In general, the smaller the program and the fewer patients they see, the less competitive it is.

**Specialists' View:** According to recent AMA surveys, 76% of Obstetrician-Gynecologists in academic and clinical positions felt that their practice activities met their expectations. On a scale of 1=very unsatisfied with their current practice position to 5=very satisfied, those surveyed averaged 3.6. They average 50 hours per week doing patient care. Among new residency graduates, 15% had difficulty finding a job they preferred; 2% were unemployed at graduation.

**Training:** The basic training program in Obstetrics and Gynecology consists of four years of training following medical school. If Osteopathic graduates enter an Obstetrics/Gynecology "specialty-track" internship, their Obstetrics and Gynecology training time is shortened by one year. The malpractice climate has had an adverse effect on some training programs, leading to Obstetrics residents not being given an opportunity to exercise a level of responsibility appropriate to their training level.

Following residency, physicians can take subspecialty fellowships in Reproductive Endocrinology (more commonly known as Infertility) or Gynecologic Oncology, which requires extra surgical training. The two newest subspecialties are Maternal and Fetal Medicine in which physicians treat the developing child *in utero* and Urogynecology/Reconstructive Pelvic Surgery.

**Match:** In recent years, about 85% of the available PGY-1 positions filled through the NRMP Match and 97% of these positions were subsequently filled.

| OBSTETRICS AND GYNECOLOGY | | | |
|---|---|---|---|
| ACGME-Approved Programs | 264 | 1st-Yr Positions (M.D.) | 1,246 |
| AOA-Approved Programs | 37 | 1st-Yr Positions (D.O.) | 55 |
| PGY-1 Positions | 1,135 | Part-Time Programs | 8 |
| % Women Residents | 63 | % IMG Residents | 6 |
| Avg. Res. Work Hours/Week | 75.1 | Avg. Days Off Per Month | 5.6 |
| % Pursuing Additional Specialty Training | 7 | Programs Offering Multiple Start Dates | 3 |

### For more information, contact:

- American College of Obstetricians & Gynecologists, 409 12th Street S.W., Washington, DC 20024-2188; www.acog.org.
- American College of Osteopathic Obstetricians & Gynecologists, 900 Auburn Road, Pontiac, MI 48342-3365; www.acoog.com.
- American Society for Reproductive Medicine, 1209 Montgomery Highway, Birmingham, AL 35216-2809; www.asrm.org.

# Occupational Medicine **

**Specialty Overview:** Occupational Medicine is one of the specialties of Preventive Medicine. It focuses on the effects of specific occupations on health. Occupational physicians work in industry, teaching hospitals, government, or occupational health clinics. As the positions in industry decrease, private practice within occupational health clinics has become a burgeoning area for those trained or interested in Occupational Medicine. Specialists rarely take night call or have inpatient responsibilities. Note: for information in *FREIDA* (see Chapter 9), look under Preventive Medicine.

**Training:** Training consists of two or three years following internship. Part of the time is used to get a graduate degree in an appropriate area, usually a Master of Public Health. A fourth year of training, teaching, practice, and/or research is required to take the Board examination.

**Match:** Contact individual programs directly.

| OCCUPATIONAL MEDICINE | | | |
|---|---|---|---|
| ACGME-Approved Programs | 29 | 1st-Yr Positions (M.D.) | 78 |
| AOA-Approved Programs | 1 | 1st-Yr Positions (D.O.) | 1 |
| PGY-1 Positions | 16 | | |

*For more information, contact:*

- American College of Occupational and Environmental Medicine, 1114 N. Arlington Heights Road, Arlington Heights, IL 60004-4770; www.acoem.org.
- American College of Preventive Medicine, 1660 L Street N.W., Suite 206, Washington, DC 20036; www.acpm.org.
- American Osteopathic College of Occupational and Preventive Medicine, 5405 Alton Parkway, Suite 5A-246, Irvine, CA 92604; www.aocopm.org.

# Ophthalmology ***

**Specialty Overview:** Ophthalmologists prevent, diagnose, and treat the diseases and abnormalities of the eye and periocular structures. A combination of office-based medical practice and surgical treatment of eye diseases makes this one of the most popular and competitive of specialties. Ophthalmologists treat patients of all ages, often using high-technology equipment in both diagnosis and therapy. Patients are usually seen as outpatients. Many Ophthalmologists take some night call, but they rarely have to go into the hospital after-hours. Inpatient services represent a small proportion of the care they deliver. With Optometrists performing many of the functions once reserved for Ophthalmologists, the field is rapidly becoming over-staffed.

**Specialists' View:** According to recent AMA surveys, 66% of Ophthalmologists in academic and clinical positions felt that their practice activities met their expectations. On a scale of 1=very unsatisfied with their current practice position to 5=very satisfied, those surveyed averaged 3.5. They average 46 hours per week doing patient care. Among new residency graduates, 32% had difficulty finding a job they preferred; 12% were unemployed at graduation.

**Training:** The training consists of three years following an internship. Residency programs place great emphasis on high class-standing and research experience. They try to officially limit each student to one "audition elective," but this has had varying success. The average Ophthalmology program applicant submits about 30 applications and has 7 residency interviews. In recent years, 98% of residency positions filled in the Match. U.S. medical students matched with an Ophthalmology program 83% of the time; about half of U.S. medical school graduates and fewer than one-fifth of IMG applicants matched. Over the past decade, entering Ophthalmology has become slightly less difficult, although it retains its reputation as a "difficult-to-enter" specialty.

**Match:** Matching is through the Ophthalmology Matching Program, sponsored by the Association of University Professors of Ophthalmology, and run by the San Francisco Matching Programs, P.O. Box 7584, San Francisco, CA 94120-7584; www.sfmatch.org. They also run the Central Application Service for all civilian Ophthalmology applicants. You should get this information when you request information from the Ophthalmology Matching Program. They suggest that applications be submitted to the Centralized Application Service by late August. Rank-Order Lists must be submitted by mid-January and Match results are announced in late January, so applicants have their results before they must submit their NRMP Rank-Order Lists for PGY-1 positions. Individuals usually arrange their own internships through the NRMP PGY-1 Match. The Matching Program also runs a Vacancy Information System, available through their Web address or at (415) 561-8535.

Fellowship positions are offered through the Ophthalmology Fellowship Match in Anterior Segment Surgery, External Disease/Cornea, Glaucoma, Histopathology, Neuro-Ophthalmology, Pediatric Ophthalmology, Retina-Vitreous, and Uveitis/Immunology, among others. The Fellowship Match is in mid-December. Unlike the others, most Oculoplastic fellowships go through the NRMP Match.

| OPHTHALMOLOGY | | | |
|---|---|---|---|
| ACGME-Approved Programs | 132 | 1st-Yr Positions (M.D.) | 467 |
| AOA-Approved Programs | 10 | 1st-Yr Positions (D.O.) | 11 |
| PGY-1 Positions | 9 | Part-Time Programs | 8 |
| % Women Residents | 29 | % IMG Residents | 9 |
| Avg. Res. Work Hours/Week | 52.1 | Avg. Days Off Per Month | 6.4 |
| % Pursuing Additional Specialty Training | 42 | Programs Offering Multiple Start Dates | 2 |

### For more information, contact:

- American Academy of Ophthalmology, 655 Beach Street, San Francisco, CA 94109; www.eyenet.org.
- American Osteopathic Colleges of Ophthalmology, Otorhinolaryngology, and Head & Neck Surgery, 3 Mackoil Avenue, Dayton, OH 45403.

# Orthopedic Surgery *****

**Specialty Overview:** Orthopedic Surgeons treat diseases and injuries of the spine and the extremities. Using surgery, medications, and physical therapy, their goal is to preserve maximal function of the musculoskeletal system.

Much Orthopedic Surgery that was once done on an inpatient basis is now done as ambulatory surgery. Individuals who go into this specialty like to work with their hands. Many have hobbies such as woodworking that emphasize this, and the majority are sports-oriented. Many Orthopedic Surgeons continue to take night and emergency call during their entire career.

**Specialists' View:** According to recent AMA surveys, 77% of Orthopedic Surgeons in academic and clinical positions felt that their practice activities met their expectations. On a scale of 1=very unsatisfied with their current practice position to 5=very satisfied, those surveyed averaged 3.8. They average 61 hours per week doing patient care. Among new residency graduates, 10% had difficulty finding a job they preferred; all were employed at graduation.

Among Adult Reconstructive Orthopedic Surgeons in academic and clinical positions, 60% felt that their practice activities met their expectations. On a scale of 1=very unsatisfied with their current practice position to 5=very satisfied, those surveyed averaged 3.4. They average 49 hours per week doing patient care. Among new residency graduates, 50% had difficulty finding a job they preferred; 13% were unemployed at graduation.

The numbers for Musculoskeletal Oncology were too small to interpret.

Among Orthopedic Spinal Surgeons in academic and clinical positions, 44% felt that their practice activities met their expectations. On a scale of 1=very unsatisfied with their current practice position to 5=very satisfied, those surveyed averaged 2.6. They average 51 hours per week doing patient care. Among new residency graduates, 33% had difficulty finding a job they preferred; all were employed at graduation.

Among Pediatric Orthopedic Surgeons in academic and clinical positions, 60% felt that their practice activities met their expectations. On a scale of 1=very unsatisfied with their current practice position to 5=very satisfied, those surveyed averaged 3.6. They average 53 hours per week doing patient care. Among new residency graduates, 50% had difficulty finding a job they preferred; all were employed at graduation.

**Training:** Training consists of one year in a broad medical specialty followed by four years of Orthopedics. Orthopedic Surgery is one of the most competitive specialties. Programs look for high USMLE scores, research experience, election to AOA (honorary), and successful "audition clerkships." Both subspecialty training and certification are available in Hand Surgery (see Hand Surgery). One-year fellowship positions also exist in Musculoskeletal Oncology, Adult Reconstructive Orthopedics, Foot and Ankle Surgery (22 programs), Orthopedic Sports Medicine (see Sports

Medicine), Pediatric Orthopedics, Orthopedic Trauma (4 programs), and Surgery of the Spine.

**Match:** In recent years, about 89% of the available PGY-1 positions filled through the NRMP Match and 100% of these positions were subsequently filled. Of the relatively few PGY-2 positions available through the NRMP Match, about 72% filled in the Match and 100% subsequently filled. Virtually all positions in Foot and Ankle Surgery, Orthopedic Hand Surgery, Pediatric Orthopedics, and Orthopedic Sports Medicine go through the NRMP's Combined Musculoskeletal Match.

### ORTHOPEDIC SURGERY

| | | | |
|---|---|---|---|
| ACGME-Approved Programs | 157 | 1st-Yr Positions (M.D.) | 601 |
| AOA-Approved Programs | 28 | 1st-Yr Positions (D.O.) | 49 |
| PGY-1 Positions | 560 | Part-Time Programs | 5 |
| % Women Residents | 7 | % IMG Residents | 2 |
| Avg. Res. Work Hours/Week | 68.7 | Avg. Days Off Per Month | 5.4 |
| % Pursuing Additional Specialty Training | 57 | Programs Offering Multiple Start Dates | 2 |

### ADULT RECONSTRUCTIVE ORTHOPEDICS (F)

| | | | |
|---|---|---|---|
| ACGME-Approved Programs | 12 | 1st-Yr Positions (M.D.) | 18 |
| AOA-Approved Programs | 0 | 1st-Yr Positions (D.O.) | 0 |
| PGY-1 Positions | 0 | Part-Time Programs | 0 |
| % Women Residents | 0 | % IMG Residents | 50 |
| Avg. Res. Work Hours/Week | 50.6 | Avg. Days Off Per Month | 7.9 |
| Programs Offering Multiple Start Dates | 1 | | |

### MUSCULOSKELETAL ONCOLOGY (F)

| | | | |
|---|---|---|---|
| ACGME-Approved Programs | 8 | 1st-Yr Positions (M.D.) | 9 |
| AOA-Approved Programs | 0 | 1st-Yr Positions (D.O.) | 0 |
| PGY-1 Positions | 0 | Part-Time Programs | 0 |
| % Women Residents | 57 | % IMG Residents | 14 |
| Avg. Res. Work Hours/Week | 51.8 | Avg. Days Off Per Month | 8.1 |

### ORTHOPEDIC SURGERY OF THE SPINE (F)

| | | | |
|---|---|---|---|
| ACGME-Approved Programs | 14 | 1st-Yr Positions (M.D.) | 21 |
| AOA-Approved Programs | 0 | 1st-Yr Positions (D.O.) | 0 |
| PGY-1 Positions | 0 | Part-Time Programs | 1 |
| % Women Residents | 0 | % IMG Residents | 14 |
| Avg. Res. Work Hours/Week | 53.0 | Avg. Days Off Per Month | 6.4 |
| Programs Offering Multiple Start Dates | 1 | | |

| PEDIATRIC ORTHOPEDIC SURGERY (F) | | | |
|---|---|---|---|
| ACGME-Approved Programs | 27 | 1st-Yr Positions (M.D.) | 43 |
| AOA-Approved Programs | 0 | 1st-Yr Positions (D.O.) | 0 |
| PGY-1 Positions | 0 | Part-Time Programs | 1 |
| % Women Residents | 14 | % IMG Residents | 24 |
| Avg. Res. Work Hours/Week | 51.5 | Avg. Days Off Per Month | 8.4 |
| Positions Available through the NRMP Combined Musculoskeletal Match | 24 | Programs Offering Multiple Start Dates | 4 |

*For more information, contact:*

- American Academy of Orthopaedic Surgeons, 6300 N. River Road, Rosemont, IL 60018-4226; www.aaos.org.
- American Osteopathic Academy of Orthopedics, Box 291690, Davie, FL 33329-1690; www.aoao.org.

# Otolaryngology *****

**Specialty Overview:** Otolaryngologists, or Head and Neck Surgeons, specialize in the evaluation and treatment of medical and surgical problems of the head and neck region, including disorders of the ears, upper respiratory tract, and upper GI tract. The specialty is frequently referred to as ENT (Ear, Nose, & Throat). Physicians in this specialty have a substantial office practice with varying amounts of surgery. The majority of head and neck surgery is now performed in an ambulatory setting and most practitioners have few inpatients. Since managed care organizations have targeted some of this specialty's common procedures, such as tympanotomies, for decreased use, this field may quickly become over-staffed.

**Specialists' View:** According to recent AMA surveys, 71% of Otolaryngologists in academic and clinical positions felt that their practice activities met their expectations. On a scale of 1=very unsatisfied with their current practice position to 5=very satisfied, those surveyed averaged 3.7. They average 53 hours per week doing patient care. Among new residency graduates, 21% had difficulty finding a job they preferred; 2% were unemployed at graduation.

**Training:** Training consists of one or two years of General Surgery followed by three or four years of ENT training. Fellowships and certification are available in Otology/Neurotology (two programs, an additional two years) and Pediatric Otolaryngology (no programs currently exist). Additional fellowships are available in Facial Plastic & Reconstructive Surgery and in Head & Neck Cancer Surgery. About 25% of all residency graduates take additional fellowship training. Most Osteopathic programs combine Otolaryngology with Facial Plastic Surgery. Osteopathic residents who take a "specialty-track" internship in the specialty can shorten their training by one year.

**Match:** Virtually all civilian ENT programs go through the Otolaryngology Matching Program, sponsored by the Association of Academic Departments of Otolaryngology-Head & Neck Surgery, P.O. Box 7584, San Francisco, CA 94120-7584. They also run the Central Application Service (CAS) for all civilian Otolaryngology applicants and many subspecialty fellowship matches. You should get this information when you request information from the Otolaryngology Matching Program. They suggest that applications be submitted to the CAS by mid-August. This Match requires the Rank-Order List to be submitted in early January, with Match results announced in mid-January. Internship positions are obtained through the NRMP PGY-1 Match.

**Other Useful Information:** The average applicant to an Otolaryngology program submits 36 applications and has 8 residency interviews. About 98% of residency positions fill in the Match. U.S. medical students matched with Otolaryngology programs 75% of the time, U.S. medical school graduates matched 23% of the time, and IMGs matched 10% of the time.

### OTOLARYNGOLOGY

| | | | |
|---|---|---|---|
| ACGME-Approved Programs | 105 | 1st-Yr Positions (M.D.) | 277 |
| AOA-Approved Programs | 2 | 1st-Yr Positions (D.O.) | 2 |
| PGY-1 Positions | 44 | Part-Time Programs | 5 |
| % Women Residents | 18 | % IMG Residents | 3 |
| Avg. Res. Work Hours/Week | 68.0 | Avg. Days Off Per Month | 5.8 |
| % Pursuing Additional Specialty Training | 24 | Programs Offering Multiple Start Dates | 2 |

### OTOLARYNGOLOGY/FACIAL PLASTIC SURGERY (OSTEOPATHS ONLY)

| | | | |
|---|---|---|---|
| AOA-Approved Programs | 19 | 1st-Yr Positions (D.O.) | 12 |

### For more information, contact:

- American Academy of Otolaryngology–Head & Neck Surgery, 1 Prince Street, Alexandria, VA 22314; www.entnet.org.
- American Osteopathic Colleges of Ophthalmology, Otorhinolaryngology, and Head & Neck Surgery, 3 Mackoil Avenue, Dayton, OH 45403.

# Pain Management (F) *

**Specialty Overview:** Pain Medicine is concerned with the study of pain, prevention of pain, and the evaluation, treatment, and rehabilitation of persons in pain. A Pain Medicine physician serves as a consultant to other physicians but is often the principal treating physician and may provide care at various levels. A relatively new subspecialty of Anesthesiology, Neurology, Physical Medicine & Rehabilitation, and Psychiatry, it has expanded rapidly with the recognition that chronic pain control has often been poorly managed in the past. Specialists work in both hospitals and independent pain control clinics, employing a variety of pain management techniques.

**Specialists' View:** According to recent AMA surveys, 50% of Pain Management physicians in academic and clinical positions felt that their practice activities met their expectations. On a scale of 1=very unsatisfied with their current practice position to 5=very satisfied, those surveyed averaged 3.1. They average 54 hours per week doing patient care. Among new residency graduates, 17% had difficulty finding a job they preferred; 7% were unemployed at graduation.

**Training:** Pain Management fellowships are one year following completion of a core residency in one of the sponsoring specialties.

**Match:** Contact programs directly.

### PAIN MANAGEMENT (F)

| | | | |
|---|---|---|---|
| ACGME-Approved Programs | 95 | 1st-Yr Positions (M.D.) | 250 |
| AOA-Approved Programs | 0 | 1st-Yr Positions (D.O.) | 0 |
| PGY-1 Positions | 0 | Part-Time Programs | 12 |
| % Women Residents | 20 | % IMG Residents | 34 |
| Avg. Res. Work Hours/Week | 49.2 | Avg. Days Off Per Month | 7.1 |
| Programs Offering Multiple Start Dates | 25 | | |

*For more information, contact:*

- American Academy of Pain Medicine, 4700 W. Lake Avenue, Glenview, IL 60025; www.painmed.org.

# Pathology *

**Specialty Overview:** Pathologists are laboratory-based physicians who are often said to be the "doctor's doctor." They act as consultants for other physicians, helping them to determine the nature of disease in tissue, body fluids, or the entire organism. They apply the methods of the basic sciences to the detection of disease, but generally have little or no direct contact with (live) patients. Their interactions are with other physicians. Pathologists' lives are generally low-key and there is little or no in-hospital nightcall.

The field is divided into the areas of *Anatomic Pathology*, i.e., autopsies, Cytopathology, Surgical Pathology (gross and microscopic pathology); and *Clinical Pathology*, i.e., Hematology, Microbiology, Clinical Chemistry, and Blood Banking/Transfusion Medicine. Most Pathologists, especially the Anatomic Pathologists, are hospital-based. Many Pathologists also function as researchers and teachers in university medical centers/medical schools—frequently while also maintaining an active Pathology practice. In the past, the income has been very generous—especially for Clinical Pathology. However, changes in reimbursement have decreased Pathologists' income. Many recent Pathology residency graduates have had difficulty finding desirable positions.

**Specialists' View:** According to recent AMA surveys, 76% of Pathologists in academic and clinical positions felt that their practice activities met their expectations. On a scale of 1=very unsatisfied with their current practice position to 5=very satisfied, those surveyed averaged 3.5. They average 45 hours per week doing clinical work. Among new residency graduates, 45% had difficulty finding a job they preferred; 19% were unemployed at graduation.

Among Blood Banking/Transfusion Pathologists in academic and clinical positions, 38% felt that their practice activities met their expectations. On a scale of 1=very unsatisfied with their current practice position to 5=very satisfied, those surveyed averaged 2.6. They average 41 hours per week doing clinical work. Among new residency graduates, 100% had difficulty finding a job they preferred; 50% were unemployed at graduation.

Among Cytopathologists in academic and clinical positions, 74% felt that their practice activities met their expectations. On a scale of 1=very unsatisfied with their current practice position to 5=very satisfied, those surveyed averaged 3.7. They average 50 hours per week doing clinical work. Among new residency graduates, 33% had difficulty finding a job they preferred; 4% were unemployed at graduation.

Among Forensic Pathologists in academic and clinical positions, 67% felt that their practice activities met their expectations. On a scale of 1=very unsatisfied with their current practice position to 5=very satisfied, those surveyed averaged 4.0. They average 32 hours per week doing clinical work. Among new residency graduates, 46% had difficulty finding a job they preferred; 25% were unemployed at graduation.

The numbers for all other pathology subspecialties were too small to interpret.

**Training:** A residency can be taken separately in either Clinical Pathology or Anatomic Pathology (three years), or the two can be combined (four years). A "credentialing year" is required prior to taking the Board examination. This is usually taken before beginning a Pathology residency. It can consist of a clinical year, clinical experience, or clinically related research. Positions available for subspecialty training following the initial residency include: Neuropathology, requiring two years; Immunopathology (9 programs), requiring one or two years; Forensic Pathology, Dermato-pathology (see Dermatopathology), Blood Banking/Transfusion Medicine, Chemical Pathology (5 programs), Pediatric Pathology, Hematology (see Hematology), Selective Pathology (9 programs), Cytopathology, and Medical Microbiology (9 programs), all requiring one year.

**Match:** Many Pathology programs are pressuring students to contract for a position outside of the NRMP Match (during the interview), even though both the student and the program are contracted to participate in the Match. In recent years, about 61% of the available PGY-1 positions filled through the NRMP Match and 84% of these positions were subsequently filled.

### PATHOLOGY, ANATOMIC AND CLINICAL

| | | | |
|---|---|---|---|
| ACGME-Approved Programs | 174 | 1st-Yr Positions (M.D.) | 549 |
| AOA-Approved Programs | 1 | 1st-Yr Positions (D.O.) | 1 |
| PGY-1 Positions | 452 | Part-Time Programs | 21 |
| % Women Residents | 43 | % IMG Residents | 40 |
| Avg. Res. Work Hours/Week | 47.6 | Avg. Days Off Per Month | 7.0 |
| % Pursuing Additional Specialty Training | 53 | Programs Offering Multiple Start Dates | 32 |

### BLOOD BANKING/TRANSFUSION MEDICINE (F)

| | | | |
|---|---|---|---|
| ACGME-Approved Programs | 48 | 1st-Yr Positions (M.D.) | 56 |
| AOA-Approved Programs | 0 | 1st-Yr Positions (D.O.) | 0 |
| PGY-1 Positions | 0 | Part-Time Programs | 8 |
| % Women Residents | 53 | % IMG Residents | 38 |
| Avg. Res. Work Hours/Week | 42.4 | Avg. Days Off Per Month | 7.6 |
| Programs Offering Multiple Start Dates | 9 | | |

### CYTOPATHOLOGY (F)

| | | | |
|---|---|---|---|
| ACGME-Approved Programs | 70 | 1st-Yr Positions (M.D.) | 100 |
| AOA-Approved Programs | 0 | 1st-Yr Positions (D.O.) | 0 |
| PGY-1 Positions | 0 | Part-Time Programs | 3 |
| % Women Residents | 51 | % IMG Residents | 40 |
| Avg. Res. Work Hours/Week | 45.4 | Avg. Days Off Per Month | 7.8 |
| Programs Offering Multiple Start Dates | 5 | | |

### FORENSIC PATHOLOGY (F)

| | | | |
|---|---|---|---|
| ACGME-Approved Programs | 42 | 1st-Yr Positions (M.D.) | 72 |
| AOA-Approved Programs | 0 | 1st-Yr Positions (D.O.) | 0 |
| PGY-1 Positions | 0 | Part-Time Programs | 5 |
| % Women Residents | 37 | % IMG Residents | 15 |
| Avg. Res. Work Hours/Week | 42.4 | Avg. Days Off Per Month | 6.6 |
| Programs Offering Multiple Start Dates | 3 | | |

### NEUROPATHOLOGY (F)

| | | | |
|---|---|---|---|
| ACGME-Approved Programs | 46 | 1st-Yr Positions (M.D.) | 39 |
| AOA-Approved Programs | 0 | 1st-Yr Positions (D.O.) | 0 |
| PGY-1 Positions | 0 | Part-Time Programs | 6 |
| % Women Residents | 47 | % IMG Residents | 34 |
| Avg. Res. Work Hours/Week | 47.2 | Avg. Days Off Per Month | 7.5 |
| Programs Offering Multiple Start Dates | 7 | | |

### PEDIATRIC PATHOLOGY (F)

| | | | |
|---|---|---|---|
| ACGME-Approved Programs | 25 | 1st-Yr Positions (M.D.) | 28 |
| AOA-Approved Programs | 0 | 1st-Yr Positions (D.O.) | 0 |
| PGY-1 Positions | 0 | Part-Time Programs | 3 |
| % Women Residents | 65 | % IMG Residents | 57 |
| Avg. Res. Work Hours/Week | 43.3 | Avg. Days Off Per Month | 6.5 |
| Programs Offering Multiple Start Dates | 5 | | |

## For more information, contact:

- American Osteopathic College of Pathologists, 12368 N.W. 13th Court, Pembroke Pines, FL 33026.
- American Society of Clinical Pathologists, 2100 W. Harrison Street, Chicago, IL 60612; www.ascp.org.
- College of American Pathologists, 325 Waukegan Road, Northfield, IL 60093-2750; www.cap.org.

# Pediatric Surgery (F) ****

**Specialty Overview:** Pediatric Surgeons diagnose and treat surgical diseases in children. Depending upon their training, they deal with abdominal, urologic, and thoracic problems, as well as multiple trauma. Because of the volume of patients that is needed to support such a specialized practice, most Pediatric Surgeons live in moderate- or large-size cities, and are associated with major medical centers. Since this is a subspecialty of General Surgery, applicants for training must first complete a General Surgery residency.

**Specialists' View:** According to recent AMA surveys, 80% of Pediatric Surgeons in academic and clinical positions felt that their practice activities met their expectations. On a scale of 1=very unsatisfied with their current practice position to 5=very satisfied, those surveyed averaged 3.9. They average 62 hours per week doing patient care. Among new residency graduates, none had difficulty finding a job they preferred; 7% were unemployed at graduation.

**Training:** The training in Pediatric Surgery is two years in length.

**Match:** Applications must be submitted for positions that begin 18 months after appointment. Applicants should contact the programs directly. A list can be found on the American Pediatric Surgical Association's website. Generally, 100% of the available positions fill.

**Other Useful Information:** Fellowship directors look for individuals who work well with others, do well in interviews, and who have been favorably recommended during phone calls by practicing Pediatric Surgeons whom the directors know.

### PEDIATRIC SURGERY (F)

| | | | |
|---|---|---|---|
| ACGME-Approved Programs | 32 | 1st-Yr Positions (M.D.) | 28 |
| AOA-Approved Programs | 0 | 1st-Yr Positions (D.O.) | 0 |
| PGY-1 Positions | 0 | Part-Time Programs | 4 |
| % Women Residents | 24 | % IMG Residents | 7 |
| Avg. Res. Work Hours/Week | 74.3 | Avg. Days Off Per Month | 4.1 |
| Positions through NRMP Specialties Matching Services | 0 | | |

*For more information, contact:*

- American Pediatric Surgical Association, 13 Elm Street, Manchester, MA 01944; www.ped-surg.org.

# Pediatrics **

**Specialty Overview:** Pediatricians take care of pediatric patients. While that may sound circular, it is the only way to describe many Pediatric practices. Pediatricians may at one time have dealt primarily with children, but they have now expanded the scope of their practice to include adolescents and young adults. Patients from 12 to 21 years old make up 22% of the average Pediatrician's practice. In some cases, Pediatricians continue to care for patients with illnesses, such as cystic fibrosis, that were in the past uniformly fatal during childhood. With the shrinking pediatric population, this specialty may become over-staffed. Pediatricians do a great deal of well-child and preventive care. More recently, they are being asked to fill the often-uncomfortable role of "gatekeeper" or "case manager" for prepaid health plans. In this position, they determine their patients' access to care.

Progressively fewer Pediatricians are opting for private practice, with two-thirds working in group practices. Much of the intensive exposure to ill children seen by residents and medical students during their training does not exist for the practicing Pediatrician. Office-based for the most part, Pediatricians rarely utilize surgical techniques such as suturing or fracture reduction. The average Pediatrician, in a 43-hour work week, spends 55% of the time on office visits, 21% on non-clinical care activities, 16% on hospital rounds, 6% on other patient visits, and 2% doing surgical/manipulative procedures. Pediatrics is one of the lowest paying medical specialties, averaging about $143,000 per year before taxes. Most Pediatricians choose this field, nevertheless, because they love working with children.

**Specialists' View:** According to recent AMA surveys, 74% of Pediatricians in academic and clinical positions felt that their practice activities met their expectations. On a scale of 1=very unsatisfied with their current practice position to 5=very satisfied, those surveyed averaged 3.5. They average 43 hours per week doing patient care. Among new residency graduates, 21% had difficulty finding a job they preferred; 11% were unemployed at graduation.

**Training:** Initial Pediatric residency training is three years. The *NRMP Directory* lists 116 positions as "Pediatrics-Primary." These positions are integrated into normal Pediatric programs, but offer slightly more outpatient and continuity clinic experience. Graduates of both types of programs take the same Board examination. There are also residencies combining Pediatrics with Internal Medicine, with Emergency Medicine, with Psychiatry/Child Psychiatry, with Medical Genetics, and with Physical Medicine & Rehabilitation. (See listings under Internal Medicine, Emergency Medicine, and Child and Adolescent Psychiatry for additional information.) Osteopathic residents who take a "specialty-track" internship in Pediatrics can shorten their training by one year.

Following initial Pediatric residency training, about 38% of all graduates go on to specialize. White male Pediatricians are more likely to specialize than others. Positions available for subspecialty training (each two to three years long) following the initial residency include: Medical Toxicology, Neonatal-Perinatal Medicine, Pediatric Cardiology, Pediatric Critical Care, Pediatric Emergency Medicine, Pediatric Endocrinology, Pediatric Gastroenterology, Pediatric Hematology-Oncology, Pediatric Nephrology, Neurodevelopmental Disabilities, Pediatric Pulmonology, and Sports Medicine. Fellowships are also possible in Adolescent Medicine, Allergy-Immunology, Pediatric Infectious Diseases, and Pediatric Rheumatology. Pediatric Neurology training can be started after two years of Pediatrics residency.

**Match:** In recent years, about 73% of the available PGY-1 positions filled through the NRMP Match and 96% of these positions were subsequently filled.

PEDIATRICS

| | | | |
|---|---|---|---|
| ACGME-Approved Programs | 216 | 1st-Yr Positions (M.D.) | 2,515 |
| AOA-Approved Programs | 12 | 1st-Yr Positions (D.O.) | 65 |
| PGY-1 Positions | 2,314 | Part-Time Programs | 70 |
| % Women Residents | 64 | % IMG Residents | 26 |
| Avg. Res. Work Hours/Week | 71.8 | Avg. Days Off Per Month | 5.1 |
| % Pursuing Additional Specialty Training | 24 | Programs Offering Multiple Start Dates | 19 |

*For more information, contact:*
- American Academy of Pediatrics, 141 Northwest Point Road, Elk Grove Village, IL 60007; www.aap.org.
- American College of Osteopathic Pediatricians, 5550 Friendship Boulevard, Suite 300, Chevy Chase, MD 20815-7201.

# Physical Medicine and Rehabilitation *

**Specialty Overview:** Physiatrists (specialists in Physical Medicine and Rehabilitation, or PM & R) deal with the diagnosis, evaluation, and treatment of patients with impairments or disabilities which involve musculoskeletal, neurologic, cardiovascular, or other body systems. Physiatrists diagnose and treat patients of all ages with: (1) musculoskeletal pain syndromes, industrial and sports injuries, degenerative arthritis, or lower back pain; (2) severe impairments amenable to rehabilitation, from strokes, spinal cord and brain injuries, amputations, and multiple trauma; and (3) electrodiagnosis (i.e., EMG, nerve conduction, somatosensory evoked potentials). The physiatrist's goal is to maximize the patient's physical, psychosocial, and job-related recovery, as well as to alleviate pain. Depending upon their practice, they may have frequent or no night call.

**Specialists' View:** According to recent AMA surveys, 66% of Physiatrists in academic and clinical positions felt that their practice activities met their expectations. On a scale of 1=very unsatisfied with their current practice position to 5=very satisfied, those surveyed averaged 3.5. They average 47 hours per week doing patient care. Among new residency graduates, 29% had difficulty finding a job they preferred; 8% were unemployed at graduation.

**Training:** Residency training is four years. This can either be three years following at least one year of prior training or a straight four-year program. For a directory of the ACGME-approved programs, contact the Association of Academic Physiatrists. There are combined programs in

Internal Medicine-PM & R (36 entry-level positions at 17 programs), Pediatrics-PM & R (13 positions at 17 programs), and Neurology-PM & R (1 program). Following residency, fellowship training is available in Pain Management, Pediatric Rehabilitation Medicine, and Spinal Cord Injury Medicine.

Osteopathic physicians can also take training in Osteopathic Manipulative Medicine (sometimes called Osteopathic Principles and Practice or Osteopathic Manipulative Treatment [OMT]). Many D.O.s with advanced training in these techniques have the "problem" of having too many patients seeking their services. Training lasts two years after internship or one year following completion of a primary care specialty. Some programs allow M.D.s to apply.

**Match:** In recent years, about 54% of the available PGY-1 positions filled through the NRMP Match and 72% of these positions were subsequently filled. Of the PGY-2 positions available through the NRMP Match, about 44% filled in the Match and about 70% subsequently filled.

**Other Useful Information:** There are many more positions available for graduates of Physiatry residency training programs than there are graduates to fill them. The average residency candidate applies to 14 programs and spends 20 days interviewing.

| PHYSICAL MEDICINE AND REHABILITATION | | | |
|---|---|---|---|
| ACGME-Approved Programs | 81 | 1st-Yr Positions (M.D.) | 330 |
| AOA-Approved Programs | 1 | 1st-Yr Positions (D.O.) | 3 |
| PGY-1 Positions | 76 | Part-Time Programs | 5 |
| % Women Residents | 35 | % IMG Residents | 26 |
| Avg. Res. Work Hours/Week | 51.1 | Avg. Days Off Per Month | 6.8 |
| % Pursuing Additional Specialty | | Programs Offering | |
| Training | 14 | Multiple Start Dates | 15 |

| OSTEOPATHIC MANIPULATIVE MEDICINE | | | |
|---|---|---|---|
| AOA-Approved Program | 9 | 1st-Yr Positions (D.O.) | 24 |

## For more information, contact:

- American Academy of Physical Medicine & Rehabilitation, One IBM Plaza, Suite 2500, Chicago, IL 60611-3604; www.aapmr.org.
- American Congress of Rehabilitation Medicine, 4700 W. Lake Avenue, Glenview, IL 60025; www.acrm.org.
- American Osteopathic College of Rehabilitation Medicine, 2214 Elmira, Des Plaines, IL 60016.
- Association of Academic Physiatrists, 5987 E. 71st Street, Suite 112, Indianapolis, IN 46220; www. physiatry.org

# Plastic Surgery (F) ****

**Specialty Overview:** Plastic Surgeons operatively treat disfigurements of the body, whether they are congenitally or traumatically induced, or are caused by aging. This area of Surgery is as much an art as a science, and an artist's vision is said to be necessary to excel in the field. Microsurgery and liposuction are two of the newer techniques being used both in reconstructive and cosmetic surgery. The practice consists of a large amount of night call to the emergency room, especially early in a practitioner's career. Much of Plastic Surgery is done on an ambulatory basis. While the field is quite lucrative at present, the area of Plastic Surgery is expected to have many more practitioners than necessary in the near future.

**Specialists' View:** According to recent AMA surveys, 65% of Plastic Surgeons in academic and clinical positions felt that their practice activities met their expectations. On a scale of 1=very unsatisfied with their current practice position to 5=very satisfied, those surveyed averaged 3.7. They average 59 hours per week doing patient care. Among new residency graduates, 38% had difficulty finding a job they preferred; 5% were unemployed at graduation.

**Training:** Training in Plastic Surgery lasts at least two, and often three, years after completing at least three years of General Surgery or an entire Otolaryngology or Orthopedic Surgery residency. Individual programs vary in their preferences regarding previous training. All programs accept applicants who have completed General Surgery training, and most accept those who have completed Otolaryngology or Orthopedic residencies. Many programs will consider candidates with four years of General Surgery; some, mainly those programs of three years duration, accept applicants with only three years of General Surgery. Some programs accept medical students into five- or six-year Plastic Surgery programs.

Applicants must ascertain the minimum requirements by contacting each program and obtain the "Preliminary Evaluation of Training" form from the American Board of Plastic Surgery. This form must be completed prior to applying for residencies. Individuals with more training have a better chance of getting a position. Postgraduate fellowships and certification are available in Hand Surgery. Additional training in Plastic Surgery, and fellowships in Craniofacial Surgery, Microsurgery, and Burn Surgery are also available following completion of the primary residency.

**Match:** Relatively few positions are available to graduating medical students through the NRMP Match. The other positions are available through the Plastic Surgery Matching Program, P.O. Box 7584, San

Francisco, CA 94120-7584. Rank Order Lists are due at the Matching Program by mid-May and the results are announced in late May.

**Other Useful Information:** In recent years, 97% of all positions filled through the Match. The average applicant applies to 22 programs and interviews at 7 programs.

| PLASTIC SURGERY (F) | | | |
|---|---|---|---|
| ACGME-Approved Programs | 98 | 1st-Yr Positions (M.D.) | 195 |
| AOA-Approved Programs | 3 | 1st-Yr Positions (D.O.) | 5 |
| PGY-1 Positions | 49 | Part-Time Programs | 4 |
| % Women Residents | 17 | % IMG Residents | 5 |
| Avg. Res. Work Hours/Week | 65.1 | Avg. Days Off Per Month | 5.6 |
| % Pursuing Additional Specialty Training | 28 | | |

### For more information, contact:

- American Academy of Facial & Reconstructive Surgery, 310 S. Henry Street, Alexandria, VA 22314; www.aafprs.org.
- American Association of Plastic Surgeons, 4900 B South 31st Street, Arlington, VA 22206; www.aaps1921.org.
- American College of Osteopathic Surgeons, 123 N. Henry Street, Alexandria, VA 22314-2903.
- American Society of Plastic & Reconstructive Surgeons, 444 E. Algonquin Road, Arlington Heights, IL 60005; www.plasticsurgery.org.

## Preventive Medicine * to ****
### (see individual areas)

**Specialty Overview:** Preventive Medicine, unlike most other primary specialties, requires that those entering the field do so through one of three specialty areas: Public Health and General Preventive Medicine, Occupational Medicine, or Aerospace Medicine. Each of these is covered more fully in this chapter in its own section.

A list of programs and positions is available from the American College of Preventive Medicine, (202) 466-2044. In some cases, Family Practice programs have made arrangements so that training in both specialties can take place concurrently. Two subspecialty certifications are now available in Preventive Medicine: Medical Toxicology and Undersea & Hyperbaric Medicine. Note: for information in *FREIDA* (see Chapter 9) for the specialty areas, look under Preventive Medicine.

**Specialists' View:** According to recent AMA surveys, 60% of all Preventive Medicine specialists in academic and clinical positions felt that their practice activities met their expectations. On a scale of 1=very unsatisfied with their current practice position to 5=very satisfied, those surveyed averaged 3.3. They average 33 hours per week doing patient care. Among new residency graduates, 20% had difficulty finding a job they preferred; 21% were unemployed at graduation.

**Training:** All three specialty areas require that a Master of Public Health or equivalent degree be obtained for completion of the program.

**Match:** There are no matches in the Preventive Medicine specialties, other than those included under the military matching program. A few ACGME-approved programs are listed in the NRMP PGY-1 Match, but these positions are often prearranged with the programs. Applicants can usually make arrangements with individual programs to begin at the PGY-2 level. The intern year is obtained through the NRMP PGY-1 Match.

| PREVENTIVE MEDICINE (GEN PREV MED, OCC MED, AER MED, AND PUB HLTH) | | | |
|---|---|---|---|
| ACGME-Approved Programs | 89 | 1st-Yr Positions (M.D.) | 299 |
| AOA-Approved Programs | 0 | 1st-Yr Positions (D.O.) | 0 |
| PGY-1 Positions | 15 | Part-Time Programs | 45 |
| % Women Residents | 34 | % IMG Residents | 13 |
| Avg. Res. Work Hours/Week | 41.9 | Avg. Days Off Per Month | 8.4 |
| % Pursuing Additional Specialty Training | 4 | Programs Offering Multiple Start Dates | 24 |

## *For more information, contact:*

- American College of Preventive Medicine, 1660 L Street N.W., Suite 206, Washington, DC 20036; www.acpm.org.
- American Osteopathic College of Occupational and Preventive Medicine, 5405 Alton Parkway, Suite 5A-246, Irvine, CA 92604; www.aocopm.org.

# Psychiatry *

**Specialty Overview:** Psychiatrists diagnose and treat disorders of the mind. They deal with the entire spectrum of mental illness, from mild situational problems to severe, incapacitating psychotic illnesses. Psychiatrists practice in a variety of settings, including private offices, community mental health centers, psychiatric hospitals, prisons, and substance abuse programs. The majority, though, are office- rather than hospital-based. While there may be night call, it is easier than it might otherwise be, since many Psychiatrists use other health care workers to screen their calls for them.

The wide diversity of potent psychotropic medications has given the Psychiatrist a powerful pharmacological armamentarium. Treatment results can often be obtained that would have been unbelievable a few years ago. Many more disease-specific drugs are anticipated in the future. This may increase the ties between Psychiatry and other types of clinical practice. There are many job openings for Psychiatry residency graduates.

Students choose to specialize in Psychiatry because they seek an intellectual challenge, want to return to a humanities/social science background, want novel and unique problems, or want to treat the "whole person."

**Specialists' View:** According to recent AMA surveys, 66% of Psychiatrists in academic and clinical positions felt that their practice activities met their expectations. On a scale of 1=very unsatisfied with their current practice position to 5=very satisfied, those surveyed averaged 3.5. They average 44 hours per week doing patient care. Among new residency graduates, 22% had difficulty finding a job they preferred; 10% were unemployed at graduation.

**Training:** Training is three years following a clinical internship that is usually very similar in structure to a Transitional year. The residency consists of not only training in Psychiatry, but also includes a significant amount of Neurology training. Subspecialty fellowships and certification are available in Addiction Psychiatry, Clinical Neurophysiology, Child & Adolescent Psychiatry, Forensic Psychiatry, Geriatric Psychiatry, Neurodevelopmental Disabilities, and Pain Management. Twenty-seven programs exist combining Psychiatry with Internal Medicine, 13 combine Psychiatry with Family Practice, and 9 combine Neurology and Psychiatry.

Fellowships in Child and Adolescent Psychiatry, for both M.D.s and D.O.s, consist of a minimum of two years of Child and Adolescent Psychiatry in addition to at least two years (following internship) of general Psychiatry. The Child Psychiatry training can start any time after the internship year. There are also 6 programs with 5 years of training combining Pediatrics, Psychiatry, and Child Psychiatry. All Psychiatry, Child and Adolescent Psychiatry, and other subspecialty programs are listed in the *Directory of Psychiatry Residency Training Programs*, available from the American Psychiatric Association.

**Match:** In recent years, about 50% of the available PGY-1 positions filled through the NRMP Match and 78% of these positions were subsequently filled. There are 17 ACGME-approved programs in Internal Medicine-Psychiatry offering 36 positions through the NRMP PGY-1 Match.

| PSYCHIATRY | | | |
|---|---|---|---|
| ACGME-Approved Programs | 192 | 1st-Yr Positions (M.D.) | 1,179 |
| AOA-Approved Programs | 5 | 1st-Yr Positions (D.O.) | 17 |
| PGY-1 Positions | 1,080 | Part-Time Programs | 90 |
| % Women Residents | 45 | % IMG Residents | 43 |
| Avg. Res. Work Hours/Week | 53.9 | Avg. Days Off Per Month | 6.0 |
| % Pursuing Additional Specialty Training | 30 | Programs Offering Multiple Start Dates | 46 |

*For more information, contact:*

- American College of (Osteopathic) Neuropsychiatry, 28595 Orchard Lake Road, Suite 200, Farmington Hills, MI 48334-2979.
- American Psychiatric Association, 1400 K Street N.W., Washington, DC 20005; www.psych.org.
- American Society of Addiction Medicine, Upper Arcade Suite 101, 4601 N. Park Avenue, Chevy Chase, MD 20815-4520; www.asam.org.

# Public Health and General Preventive Medicine *

**Specialty Overview:** Specialists in Public Health and General Preventive Medicine deal with health promotion and disease prevention. They work in governmental and private health agencies, academic institutions, and health service research organizations. They deal with the health problems of entire communities and countries, as well as with those of individual patients.

Their goals are to promote health and to understand the risks of disease, injury, disability, and death. Their roles are to (1) assess information about the community's health, (2) develop comprehensive public health policies, and (3) assure the provision of services necessary to achieve the public health goals. This frequently involves dealing with the administrative and political sides of medicine.

This specialty usually has no night call and very low (usually government) pay. Preventive Medicine practitioners allocate their time among administrative duties (32%), patient care (29%), research (20%), teaching (8%), consulting (8%), and other activities (3%). The dearth of residency programs (a number have closed in the past few years due to lack of funding) has made these specialists some of the most sought-after in medicine (although still one of the worst paid). Note: for information in *FREIDA* (see Chapter 9) and program numbers, look under Preventive Medicine.

**Specialists' View:** See Preventive Medicine

Training: Training in General Preventive Medicine consists of two years following a clinical internship. One of these years is spent obtaining an advanced degree, usually a Master of Public Health. There are also eleven institutions offering one- or two-year appointments in Public Health. A fourth year of training, teaching, practice, and/or research is required to take the Board examination. Some programs in Family Practice, Internal Medicine, and Pediatrics have dual training with Preventive Medicine.

Match: For the most part, there is no matching program in Preventive Medicine. Applications must be made to the individual programs. Students can arrange to begin a program following a clinical year which should be obtained through the NRMP PGY-1 Match.

### For more information, contact:

- American Association of Public Health Physicians, 777 S. Mills Street, Madison, WI 53715; www.aaphp.org.
- American College of Preventive Medicine, 1660 L Street, N.W., Suite 206, Washington, DC 20036; www.acpm.org.
- American Osteopathic College of Occupational and Preventive Medicine, 5405 Alton Parkway, Suite 5A-246, Irvine, CA 92604; www.aocopm.org.

# Pulmonary Diseases (F) *

Specialty Overview: Pulmonologists diagnose and treat patients with diseases of the lungs in both the inpatient and outpatient setting. They deal most often with patients having lung cancer, asthma, and many types of chronic lung disease. In many cases, Pulmonologists, because of their background, act as full- or part-time Critical Care physicians. The specialty combines patient care and manipulative procedures with a strong underlying base of physiology. The major manipulative procedures performed by Pulmonologists are bronchoscopy, endotracheal intubation, management of mechanical ventilators, and placement of pulmonary artery catheters. Night call depends upon the type of practice.

Specialists' View: According to recent AMA surveys, 64% of adult Pulmonologists in academic and clinical positions felt that their practice activities met their expectations. On a scale of 1=very unsatisfied with their current practice position to 5=very satisfied, those surveyed averaged 3.3. They average 52 hours per week doing patient care. Among new residency graduates, 44% had difficulty finding a job they preferred; 17% were unemployed at graduation.

Among Pediatric Pulmonologists in academic and clinical positions, 50% felt that their practice activities met their expectations. On a scale of 1=very unsatisfied with their current practice position to 5=very satisfied, those surveyed averaged 3.0. They average 48 hours per week doing patient care. There was insufficient data on new residency graduates' employment.

Among Pulmonologists-Critical Care physicians in academic and clinical positions, 67% felt that their practice activities met their expectations. On a scale of 1=very unsatisfied with their current practice position to 5=very satisfied, those surveyed averaged 3.6. They average 56 hours per week doing patient care. Among new residency graduates, 21% had difficulty finding a job they preferred; 4% were unemployed at graduation.

**Training:** Training consists of a two- or three-year fellowship following completion of an Internal Medicine residency or three years following a Pediatric residency. Many adult programs that are three years in length fulfill the requirements for certification in Critical Care as well as Pulmonary Diseases. For Osteopathic physicians, training follows internship and two years of an Internal Medicine residency.

**Match:** Fellowship applications are available between November and May from the NRMP Specialties Matching Services. Virtually all programs and positions are in the Match. In recent years, about 67% of enrolled applicants found a position through the NRMP Specialty Match and about 92% of the available positions filled in the Match. Results of the Match are released in June one year prior to the start of the program. Applicants should contact Pediatric Pulmonary training programs directly, since this specialty has no match.

### PULMONARY DISEASES (INTERNAL MEDICINE)

| | | | |
|---|---|---|---|
| ACGME-Approved Programs | 62 | 1st-Yr Positions (M.D.) | 111 |
| AOA-Approved Programs | 6 | 1st-Yr Positions (D.O.) | 7 |
| PGY-1 Positions | 0 | Part-Time Programs | 2 |
| % Women Residents | 17 | % IMG Residents | 69 |
| Avg. Res. Work Hours/Week | 48.5 | Avg. Days Off Per Month | 6.4 |
| Positions through NRMP Specialties Matching Services | 301 | Programs Offering Multiple Start Dates | 1 |

### PULMONARY DISEASES (PEDIATRICS)

| | | | |
|---|---|---|---|
| ACGME-Approved Programs | 45 | 1st-Yr Positions (M.D.) | 43 |
| AOA-Approved Programs | 0 | 1st-Yr Positions (D.O.) | 0 |
| PGY-1 Positions | 0 | Part-Time Programs | 9 |
| % Women Residents | 43 | % IMG Residents | 46 |
| Avg. Res. Work Hours/Week | 47.1 | Avg. Days Off Per Month | 8.0 |
| Positions through NRMP Specialties Matching Services | 0 | Programs Offering Multiple Start Dates | 5 |

| PULMONARY DISEASES/CRITICAL CARE (INTERNAL MEDICINE) | | | |
|---|---|---|---|
| ACGME-Approved Programs | 100 | 1st-Yr Positions (M.D.) | 269 |
| AOA-Approved Programs | 0 | 1st-Yr Positions (D.O.) | 0 |
| PGY-1 Positions | 0 | Part-Time Programs | 13 |
| % Women Residents | 25 | % IMG Residents | 45 |
| Avg. Res. Work Hours/Week | 52.3 | Avg. Days Off Per Month | 5.9 |
| Positions through NRMP Specialties Matching Services | 268 | Programs Offering Multiple Start Dates | 7 |

## *For more information, contact:*

- American College of Chest Physicians, 3300 Dundee Road, Northbrook, IL 60062-2348; www.chestnet.org.
- American Thoracic Society, 1740 Broadway, New York, NY 10019-4374; www.thoracic.org.

# Radiation Oncology ***

**Specialty Overview:** Radiation Oncologists use radiation therapy in the treatment of malignancies and other diseases. Until about 25 years ago, training in Radiation Oncology was combined with Diagnostic Radiology. A flood of new information about radiation and cancer biology has made Radiation Oncology a rapidly changing field. As new knowledge about cancer emerges, changes in the use of therapeutic radiation will also occur.

While there has previously been a scarcity of Radiation Oncologists, the specialty is now close to equilibrium. Radiation Oncology has relatively little night call.

**Specialists' View:** According to recent AMA surveys, 69% of Radiation Oncologists in academic and clinical positions felt that their practice activities met their expectations. On a scale of 1=very unsatisfied with their current practice position to 5=very satisfied, those surveyed averaged 3.5. They average 50 hours per week doing patient care. Among new residency graduates, 45% had difficulty finding a job they preferred; 8% were unemployed at graduation.

**Training:** Training lasts four years after internship.

**Match:** Currently, medical students obtain PGY-2 positions through the NRMP Match (this was not true in the past). The internship year is generally acquired separately in the Match. In recent years, of the PGY-2 positions available through the NRMP Match, about 79% filled in the Match and about 91% subsequently filled.

**RADIATION ONCOLOGY**

| | | | |
|---|---|---|---|
| ACGME-Approved Programs | 82 | 1st-Yr Positions (M.D.) | 128 |
| AOA-Approved Programs | 0 | 1st-Yr Positions (D.O.) | 0 |
| PGY-1 Positions | 100 | Part-Time Programs | 2 |
| % Women Residents | 28 | % IMG Residents | 10 |
| Avg. Res. Work Hours/Week | 49.0 | Avg. Days Off Per Month | 7.5 |
| % Pursuing Additional Specialty Training | 5 | Programs Offering Multiple Start Dates | 6 |

*For more information, contact:*

- American Osteopathic College of Radiology, 119 E. Second Street, Milan, MO 63556.
- American Society for Therapeutic Radiology & Oncology, 12500 Fair Lakes Circle, Fairfax, VA 22033-3882; www.astro.org.

# Radiology, Diagnostic ***

**Specialty Overview:** Diagnostic Radiologists use x-rays, ultrasound, magnetic fields, and other forms of energy to make diagnoses. While they still train to read basic radiographs, Diagnostic Radiologists must now also learn how to interpret nuclear scans, PET scans, ultrasonography images, CT scans, and MRI images. Additionally, they are trained to perform diagnostic and interventional procedures, such as angiography, guided biopsy and drainage procedures, and non-coronary angioplasty. This is an enormous body of knowledge to learn during a residency.

**Specialists' View:** According to recent AMA surveys, 74% of Diagnostic Radiologists in academic and clinical positions felt that their practice activities met their expectations. On a scale of 1=very unsatisfied with their current practice position to 5=very satisfied, those surveyed averaged 3.6. They average 48 hours per week doing patient care. Among new residency graduates, 33% had difficulty finding a job they preferred; 8% were unemployed at graduation.

Among Neuroradiologists in academic and clinical positions, 72% felt that their practice activities met their expectations. On a scale of 1=very unsatisfied with their current practice position to 5=very satisfied, those surveyed averaged 3.7. They average 50 hours per week doing patient care. Among new residency graduates, 57% had difficulty finding a job they preferred; 3% were unemployed at graduation.

Among Pediatric Radiologists in academic and clinical positions, 81% felt that their practice activities met their expectations. On a scale of 1=very unsatisfied with their current practice position to 5=very satisfied, those surveyed averaged 3.9. They average 52 hours per week doing patient care. Among new residency graduates, 50% had difficulty finding a job they preferred; all were employed at graduation.

Among Vascular and Interventional Radiologists in academic and clinical positions, 76% felt that their practice activities met their expectations. On a scale of 1=very unsatisfied with their current practice position to 5=very satisfied, those surveyed averaged 3.8. They average 57 hours per week doing patient care. Among new residency graduates, 27% had difficulty finding a job they preferred; all were employed at graduation.

The numbers for Nuclear Radiologists were too small to interpret.

**Training:** Diagnostic Radiology programs are generally four years of training following internship. Most Diagnostic Radiology programs require completion of a clinical first year before starting the residency. Only about 15% of individuals entering Radiology residencies do so without doing an initial clinical year, either as part of the program or separately. Most practitioners are hospital-based, although there is a growing movement for Radiologists to practice out of freestanding diagnostic facilities. Because of the increased demand for emergency CT and ultrasound studies, as well as for interventional procedures, Diagnostic Radiology night call has become very active in many hospitals, although increasingly many studies are being read at home via teleradiology. Radiology has also joined Obstetrics and Gynecology as one of the most frequently sued specialties.

Osteopathic training is four years after internship. Some ACGME-approved residencies in Diagnostic Radiology provide special competence in Nuclear Radiology after an additional formal year of training. This should not be confused with a residency in Nuclear Medicine—a distinct specialty with training only in that area.

The field of Diagnostic Radiology is rapidly filling up, with the number of available positions for residency graduates decreasing each year. Many residents are gaining an employment edge by taking yearlong fellowships in Musculoskeletal Radiology (2 programs), Neuroradiology, Nuclear Radiology, Pediatric Radiology, or Vascular and Interventional Radiology.

**Match:** Where a clinical year is required before beginning a Radiology residency, it is obtained through the NRMP PGY-1 Match. Unlike previous years, the vast majority of Diagnostic Radiology positions are now offered through the NRMP PGY-1 Match. In recent years, about 69% of the available PGY-1 positions filled through the NRMP Match and 89% were subsequently filled. Of the PGY-2 positions available through the NRMP Match, about 58% filled in the Match and about 74% subsequently filled.

## RADIOLOGY, DIAGNOSTIC

| | | | |
|---|---|---|---|
| ACGME-Approved Programs | 201 | 1st-Yr Positions (M.D.) | 884 |
| AOA-Approved Programs | 16 | 1st-Yr Positions (D.O.) | 30 |
| PGY-1 Positions | 161 | Part-Time Programs | 13 |
| % Women Residents | 26 | % IMG Residents | 11 |
| Avg. Res. Work Hours/Week | 50.8 | Avg. Days Off Per Month | 7.1 |
| % Pursuing Additional Specialty Training | 63 | Programs Offering Multiple Start Dates | 7 |

## NEURORADIOLOGY (F)

| | | | |
|---|---|---|---|
| ACGME-Approved Programs | 90 | 1st-Yr Positions (M.D.) | 160 |
| AOA-Approved Programs | 0 | 1st-Yr Positions (D.O.) | 0 |
| PGY-1 Positions | 0 | Part-Time Programs | 5 |
| % Women Residents | 23 | % IMG Residents | 12 |
| Avg. Res. Work Hours/Week | 45.1 | Avg. Days Off Per Month | 8.0 |
| Programs Offering Multiple Start Dates | 3 | | |

## NUCLEAR RADIOLOGY (F)

| | | | |
|---|---|---|---|
| ACGME-Approved Programs | 34 | 1st-Yr Positions (M.D.) | 54 |
| AOA-Approved Programs | 0 | 1st-Yr Positions (D.O.) | 0 |
| PGY-1 Positions | 0 | Part-Time Programs | 1 |
| % Women Residents | 15 | % IMG Residents | 20 |
| Avg. Res. Work Hours/Week | 47.4 | Avg. Days Off Per Month | 6.5 |
| Programs Offering Multiple Start Dates | 1 | | |

## PEDIATRIC RADIOLOGY (F)

| | | | |
|---|---|---|---|
| ACGME-Approved Programs | 49 | 1st-Yr Positions (M.D.) | 64 |
| AOA-Approved Programs | 0 | 1st-Yr Positions (D.O.) | 0 |
| PGY-1 Positions | 0 | Part-Time Programs | 7 |
| % Women Residents | 50 | % IMG Residents | 13 |
| Avg. Res. Work Hours/Week | 46.3 | Avg. Days Off Per Month | 6.9 |
| Programs Offering Multiple Start Dates | 6 | | |

## VASCULAR AND INTERVENTIONAL RADIOLOGY (F)

| | | | |
|---|---|---|---|
| ACGME-Approved Programs | 83 | 1st-Yr Positions (M.D.) | 183 |
| AOA-Approved Programs | 0 | 1st-Yr Positions (D.O.) | 0 |
| PGY-1 Positions | 0 | Part-Time Programs | 6 |
| % Women Residents | 11 | % IMG Residents | 4 |
| Avg. Res. Work Hours/Week | 50.0 | Avg. Days Off Per Month | 6.4 |

## *For more information, contact:*

- American College of Radiology, 1891 Preston White Drive, Reston, VA 22091-4397; www.acr.org.

- American Osteopathic College of Radiology, 119 E. Second Street, Milan, MO 63556.
- American Roentgen Ray Society, 44211 Slatestone Court, Leesburg, VA 20176; 222.arrs.org.

# Rheumatology (F) *

**Specialty Overview:** Rheumatologists diagnose and treat patients with a wide variety of diseases of the joints, soft tissues, and blood vessels. These include the various types of arthritides, both acute and chronic, which can affect individuals. The field has grown in recent years with the increased interest in the autoimmune diseases underlying many rheumatologic conditions. Rheumatology is one of the quieter subspecialties of Internal Medicine and Pediatrics. Yet Rheumatologists often care for very ill patients with various autoimmune and acute joint diseases. There is usually little night call and small primary or consultative inpatient services for those not mixing their Rheumatology practice with General Internal Medicine or Pediatrics.

**Specialists' View:** According to recent AMA surveys, 50% of Rheumatologists in academic and clinical positions felt that their practice activities met their expectations. On a scale of 1=very unsatisfied with their current practice position to 5=very satisfied, those surveyed averaged 3.2. They average 48 hours per week doing patient care. Among new residency graduates, 27% had difficulty finding a job they preferred; 14% were unemployed at graduation.

The numbers for Pediatric Rheumatologists were too small to interpret.

**Training:** Training consists of a two-year fellowship following completion of an Internal Medicine residency or three years following a Pediatric residency. For Osteopathic physicians, training follows internship and two years of an Internal Medicine residency.

**Match:** Applicants should contact programs directly.

### RHEUMATOLOGY (INTERNAL MEDICINE)

| | | | |
|---|---|---|---|
| ACGME-Approved Programs | 107 | 1st-Yr Positions (M.D.) | 167 |
| AOA-Approved Programs | 0 | 1st-Yr Positions (D.O.) | 0 |
| PGY-1 Positions | 0 | Part-Time Programs | 11 |
| % Women Residents | 43 | % IMG Residents | 59 |
| Avg. Res. Work Hours/Week | 45.4 | Avg. Days Off Per Month | 6.7 |
| Programs Offering Multiple Start Dates | 16 | | |

| RHEUMATOLOGY (PEDIATRICS) | | | |
|---|---|---|---|
| ACGME-Approved Programs | 16 | 1st-Yr Positions (M.D.) | 17 |
| AOA-Approved Programs | 0 | 1st-Yr Positions (D.O.) | 0 |
| PGY-1 Positions | 0 | Part-Time Programs | 1 |
| % Women Residents | 42 | % IMG Residents | 33 |
| Avg. Res. Work Hours/Week | 46.5 | Avg. Days Off Per Month | 6.1 |
| Programs Offering Multiple Start Dates | 1 | | |

*For more information, contact:*

- American College of Osteopathic Internists, 3 Bethesda Metro Center, Suite 508, Bethesda, MD 20814; www.acoi.org.
- American College of Rheumatology, 1800 Century Place, Suite 250, Atlanta, GA 30345; www.rheumatology.org.

# Sports Medicine (F) ***

**Specialty Overview:** Sports Medicine is a new fellowship available under the auspices of Emergency Medicine, Family Practice, Internal Medicine, and Pediatrics. This specialty is sometimes called (by the NRMP as well as others) "Primary Care Sports Medicine" to distinguish it from Orthopedic Surgery's Sports Medicine subspecialty. Specialists in this area prevent, diagnose, and treat non-operative sports-related injuries. Sports Medicine specialists emphasize prevention and rehabilitation in addition to acute treatment. Some perform epidemiological studies to determine the best preventive methods. Many practitioners incorporate Sports Medicine into their existing practices. They offer fitness evaluations, act as team physicians, and work with recreational athletes.

Orthopedic Sports Medicine is a subspecialty of Orthopedic Surgery. These practitioners perform many of the same preventive and therapeutic measures as other Sports Medicine physicians; in addition, they treat injuries surgically when necessary.

**Specialists' View:** According to recent AMA surveys, 8% of new residency graduates had difficulty finding a job they preferred; 11% were unemployed at graduation. Other numbers for this specialty were too small to interpret.

Among Orthopedic Sports Medicine physicians in academic and clinical positions, 60% felt that their practice activities met their expectations. On a scale of 1=very unsatisfied with their current practice position to 5=very satisfied, those surveyed averaged 3.3. They average 55 hours per week doing patient care. Among new residency graduates, 19% had difficulty finding a job they preferred; 8% were unemployed at graduation.

**Training:** Training in Orthopedic Sports Medicine is a one-year fellowship following the completion of an Orthopedic Surgery residency. Primary Care Sports Medicine (primarily in Family Practice) is one year after the initial residency.

**Match:** Primary Care Sports Medicine applicants should contact individual training programs directly, since this specialty has no match.

Most positions in Orthopedic Sports Medicine are obtained through the NRMP Combined Musculoskeletal Match. About 72% of enrolled applicants found a position through the Match and 88% of available positions filled through the Match.

### PRIMARY CARE SPORTS MEDICINE

| | | | |
|---|---|---|---|
| ACGME-Approved Programs | 33 | 1st-Yr Positions (M.D.) | 44 |
| AOA-Approved Programs | 3 | 1st-Yr Positions (D.O.) | 4 |
| PGY-1 Positions | 0 | Part-Time Programs | 4 |
| % Women Residents | 16 | % IMG Residents | 0 |
| Avg. Res. Work Hours/Week | 47.1 | Avg. Days Off Per Month | 5.7 |
| Positions through NRMP Specialties Matching Services | 0 | % Pursuing Additional Specialty Training | 2 |

### ORTHOPEDIC SPORTS MEDICINE

| | | | |
|---|---|---|---|
| ACGME-Approved Programs | 58 | 1st-Yr Positions (M.D.) | 121 |
| AOA-Approved Programs | 0 | 1st-Yr Positions (D.O.) | 0 |
| PGY-1 Positions | 0 | Part-Time Programs | 8 |
| % Women Residents | 8 | % IMG Residents | 3 |
| Avg. Res. Work Hours/Week | 52.4 | Avg. Days Off Per Month | 7.4 |
| Positions through NRMP Combined Musculoskeletal Match | 115 | | |

## For more information, contact:

- American College of Sports Medicine, P.O. Box 1440, Indianapolis, IN 46206; www.acsm.org.

- American Orthopaedic Society for Sports Medicine, 6300 N. River Road, Suite 200, Rosemont, IL 60018; www.sportsmed.org.

- American Osteopathic Academy of Sports Medicine, 7611 Elmwood Avenue, Suite 201, Middletown, WI 53562.

# Surgery, General ***

**Specialty Overview:** General Surgeons primarily diagnose and treat diseases and injuries to the abdominal organs and to the soft tissues and vasculature of the neck and trunk. They are also usually called in to manage, often in concert with other surgical specialists, patients suffering injuries to more than one body area. In rural settings, the General Surgeon may still be "General," doing Orthopedic, Urologic, and, occasionally, Thoracic or Neurosurgical procedures. But for the most part, today's General Surgeon primarily works in the abdomen, on the breast, on the peripheral vasculature, on the skin, and, in some cases, on the neck. Increasingly, endoscopic and other minimally invasive surgical techniques are being used. Not all General Surgery residencies are prepared to thoroughly teach these techniques as they are perfected.

In the average 60-hour work week of all Surgeons in private practice, 47% of the time is spent on office visits, 29% in surgery, 16% on hospital rounds, and 8% on other patient visits. The field of General Surgery is overcrowded; job opportunities for residency graduates are relatively scarce.

Nearly all surgical specialties are oversupplied with practitioners for the perceived need in the population. Yet there are still many areas of the country that are underserved by surgeons.

**Specialists' View:** According to recent AMA surveys, 69% of General Surgeons in academic and clinical positions felt that their practice activities met their expectations. On a scale of 1=very unsatisfied with their current practice position to 5=very satisfied, those surveyed averaged 3.7. They average 58 hours per week doing patient care. Among new residency graduates, 21% had difficulty finding a job they preferred; 8% were unemployed at graduation.

**Training:** Training in General Surgery is usually five years after medical school. It is four years after internship for Osteopathic physicians. "Categorical" General Surgery residency positions, designed for those interested in completing an entire General Surgery residency, have become relatively difficult to obtain. About one-third of the available Surgery PGY-1 positions are "Preliminary," which only guarantee training for one or two years; they are designed for those wishing to enter other fields, particularly other surgical specialties. Subspecialty fellowships and certification are available in Surgery of the Hand, Pediatric Surgery, Surgical Critical Care, and General Vascular Surgery. Some educators now feel that the lack of continuity of care has harmed surgical training programs in markets dominated by managed care. Residents infrequently see the same patients in the clinic, in the hospital, and during follow-up visits.

**Match:** In recent years, about 96% of the available PGY-1 positions filled through the NRMP Match and 99% of these positions were subsequently filled. Of the Preliminary General Surgery positions, about 40% filled through the NRMP Match and 53% subsequently filled.

| SURGERY, GENERAL | | | |
|---|---|---|---|
| ACGME-Approved Programs | 266 | 1st-Yr Positions (M.D.) | 2,040 |
| AOA-Approved Programs | 36 | 1st-Yr Positions (D.O.) | 72 |
| PGY-1 Positions | 2,033 | Part-Time Programs | 1 |
| % Women Residents | 21 | % IMG Residents | 12 |
| Avg. Res. Work Hours/Week | 80.1 | Avg. Days Off Per Month | 4.5 |
| % Pursuing Additional Specialty Training | 52 | Programs Offering Multiple Start Dates | 3 |

### For more information, contact:

- American College of Surgeons, 633 N. Street Clair Street, Chicago, IL 60611-3211; www.facs.org.
- American College of Osteopathic Surgeons, 123 N. Henry Street, Alexandria, VA 22314-2903.

# Thoracic Surgery (F) ***

**Specialty Overview:** Thoracic or Cardiothoracic Surgeons operatively treat diseases and injuries of the heart, lungs, mediastinum, esophagus, chest wall, diaphragm, and great vessels. The most common surgery that specialists in this field perform is coronary artery bypass grafting. The other common procedures include cardiac surgery for acquired valvular disease or congenital cardiac defects, pulmonary surgery for malignancies, and surgery for trauma to intrathoracic organs. Post-operative care for all these patients is usually the responsibility of the Thoracic Surgeon. As might be expected from the nature of the patients treated by Thoracic Surgeons, very long and erratic hours are often necessary. This results in Thoracic Surgery being one of the most time-consuming and stressful of all the specialties. Those in the field, though, generally feel that the rewards are worth the price.

**Specialists' View:** According to recent AMA surveys, 70% of Thoracic Surgeons in academic and clinical positions felt that their practice activities met their expectations. On a scale of 1=very unsatisfied with their current practice position to 5=very satisfied, those surveyed averaged 3.4. They average 67 hours per week doing patient care. Among new residency graduates, 23% had difficulty finding a job they preferred; 4% were unemployed at graduation.

**Training:** Thoracic Surgery is a subspecialty of General Surgery, and certification in General Surgery is required to take the Thoracic Surgery Boards. Training lasts two to three years after completion of a General Surgery residency. Since the process of going through a General Surgery residency is itself grueling, this acts as a major deterrent to many individuals who might otherwise enter this field. Osteopathic programs are two years in length after three years of General Surgery and one year of internship.

**Match:** Thoracic Surgery Applicants should contact individual training programs directly, since this specialty has no match.

| THORACIC SURGERY (F) | | | |
|---|---|---|---|
| ACGME-Approved Programs | 91 | 1st-Yr Positions (M.D.) | 149 |
| AOA-Approved Programs | 2 | 1st-Yr Positions (D.O.) | 4 |
| PGY-1 Positions | 0 | Part-Time Programs | 7 |
| % Women Residents | 6 | % IMG Residents | 15 |
| Avg. Res. Work Hours/Week | 74.3 | Avg. Days Off Per Month | 5.4 |
| % Pursuing Additional Specialty Training | 13 | Programs Offering Multiple Start Dates | 4 |
| Positions through NRMP Specialties Matching Services | 0 | | |

*For more information, contact:*

- American College of Osteopathic Surgeons, 123 N. Henry Street, Alexandria, VA 22314-2903.
- Society of Thoracic Surgeons, 401 N. Michigan Avenue, Suite 2200, Chicago, IL 60611-4267; www.sts.org.

# Trauma Surgery (F) **

**Specialty Overview:** While not yet an official subspecialty, Trauma Surgery is one of the fastest growing areas in Surgery. With the wide institution of trauma centers, there is an increasing need for Surgeons with training in the treatment of the multiple-injury patient. Trauma Surgeons not only are generally the operating Surgeon for patients with major injuries, but also help coordinate the large team responsible for both the initial and the postoperative care. In-hospital call is usually required on a frequent basis. As with firefighters, there is often the need to immediately go to full speed from a dead stop. Long hours are required, and family life can be difficult. Most Trauma Surgeons now are in medium- to large-sized cities.

**Training:** Training normally consists of a one- or two-year fellowship at a major trauma center following a General Surgery residency. Many Trauma Surgery fellowships are combined with training in Critical Care or with research opportunities. At the present time, most Trauma Surgeons have not completed such a fellowship. The necessity for such a fellowship in the future is currently unknown. A current list of fellowships can be found at www.aast.org/fellow.html. This site contains both those fellowships that comply with AAST guidelines and other available fellowships.

**Match:** Fellowships are arranged on an individual basis during the third or fourth year of General Surgery training.

| TRAUMA SURGERY (F) | | | |
|---|---|---|---|
| Programs (Comply with AAST Guides) | 25 | 1st-Yr Positions (M.D.) | 44 |
| AOA-Approved Programs | 0 | 1st-Yr Positions (D.O.) | 0 |
| PGY-1 Positions | 0 | | |

### For more information, contact:

- American Association for the Surgery of Trauma, Harborview Medical Center, Dept. of Surgery, 325 9th Avenue, P.O. Box 359796, Seattle, WA 98104-2499; www.aast.org.

# Urology *****

**Specialty Overview:** Urologists diagnose and treat diseases of and injuries to the kidney, ureters, bladder, and urethra. In males, they also treat disorders of the prostate and genitals. Often they work in concert with Nephrologists (Internists) and have both a surgical and non-surgical practice. Investigations into fertility and male sexuality, and the use of non-invasive techniques, such as lithotripsy, are expanding areas within the field. Urologists have a moderate amount of night call and often have small inpatient services, since much of Urologic Surgery is now done in an ambulatory setting.

**Specialists' View:** According to recent AMA surveys, 68% of Urologists in academic and clinical positions felt that their practice activities met their expectations. On a scale of 1=very unsatisfied with their current practice position to 5=very satisfied, those surveyed averaged 3.7. They average 58 hours per week doing patient care. Among new residency graduates, 15% had difficulty finding a job they preferred; 2% were unemployed at graduation.

**Training:** Urology training generally consists of two years of General Surgery followed by at least three years of Urology. The preliminary (first two) surgical years are at the same institution as the Urology training in about half of the programs. Eight programs offer a total of 10 Pediatric Urology fellowships. Osteopathic residents who take a "specialty-track" internship in Urology can shorten their training by one year.

**Match:** Urology has a separate match run through The American Urological Association Residency Matching Program (P.O. Box 201820, Houston, TX 77216-1820; www.auanet.org). It requires submission of Rank-Order Lists by mid-January, releases the results in late January, and charges a $50 application fee. Participants in the Urology Match get their results before they must submit their NRMP Rank-Order Lists. They also run a vacancy hotline after the Match: (713) 622-2700 or (800) 282-7077, ext. 88.

Applicants generally must participate in the NRMP PGY-1 Match to obtain the preliminary surgical positions. Most of the Urology positions listed as being available to medical students through the NRMP PGY-1 Match are for individuals who have matched at that institution in Urology through the specialty's Match, since most programs require the "pre-Urology" training to be at their institution. These are usually Preliminary Surgery positions.

### UROLOGY

| | | | |
|---|---|---|---|
| ACGME-Approved Programs | 121 | 1st-Yr Positions (M.D.) | 249 |
| AOA-Approved Programs | 13 | 1st-Yr Positions (D.O.) | 7 |
| PGY-1 Positions | 62 | Part-Time Programs | 2 |
| % Women Residents | 10 | % IMG Residents | 5 |
| Avg. Res. Work Hours/Week | 68.3 | Avg. Days Off Per Month | 5.5 |
| % Pursuing Additional Specialty Training | 12 | | |

*For more information, contact:*

- American College of Osteopathic Surgeons, 123 N. Henry Street, Alexandria, VA 22314-2903.
- American Urological Association, 1120 N. Charles Street, Baltimore, MD 21201-5559; www.auanet.org.

## Vascular Surgery (F) ****

**Specialty Overview:** As subspecialists of General Surgery, Vascular Surgeons diagnose and treat diseases of the arterial, venous, and lymphatic systems. Unless they are associated with very large medical centers, specialists in this field often have to perform General Surgery in order to make a living. This is, in part, because so many General Surgeons also continue to perform Vascular Surgery as a routine part of their practice.

**Specialists' View:** According to recent AMA surveys, 64% of Vascular Surgeons in academic and clinical positions felt that their practice activities met their expectations. On a scale of 1=very unsatisfied with their current practice position to 5=very satisfied, those surveyed averaged 3.4. They average 59 hours per week doing patient care. Among new residency graduates, none had difficulty finding a job they preferred; all were employed at graduation.

**Training:** Training for both M.D.s and D.O.s is generally one year following completion of a General Surgery residency.

**Match:** The NRMP conducts the General Vascular Surgery Specialty Match for residents already in a General Surgery residency. Fourth-year General Surgery residents generally apply for these positions. About half of the available positions are in this Match. Non-participating programs should be contacted directly. In recent years, about half of all applicants successfully matched. Results of the Match are announced in May, one year prior to the start date. Applications for the Match are available between November and April from the NRMP. In recent years, 63% of enrolled applicants found a position through the Match and 97% of the available positions filled in the Match.

### VASCULAR SURGERY (F)

| | | | |
|---|---|---|---|
| ACGME-Approved Programs | 80 | 1st-Yr Positions (M.D.) | 89 |
| AOA-Approved Programs | 8 | 1st-Yr Positions (D.O.) | 19 |
| PGY-1 Positions | 0 | Part-Time Programs | 4 |
| % Women Residents | 11 | % IMG Residents | 9 |
| Avg. Res. Work Hours/Week | 62.5 | Avg. Days Off Per Month | 6.0 |
| Positions through NRMP Specialties Matching Services | 0 | Programs Offering Multiple Start Dates | 1 |

## For more information, contact:

- American College of Osteopathic Surgeons, 123 N. Henry Street, Alexandria, VA 22314-2903.
- Society for Vascular Surgery, 13 Elm Street, Manchester, MA 01944-0314; www.vascsurg.org.

FIGURE 3.1

## Length of Postgraduate Training for M.D. Physicians*

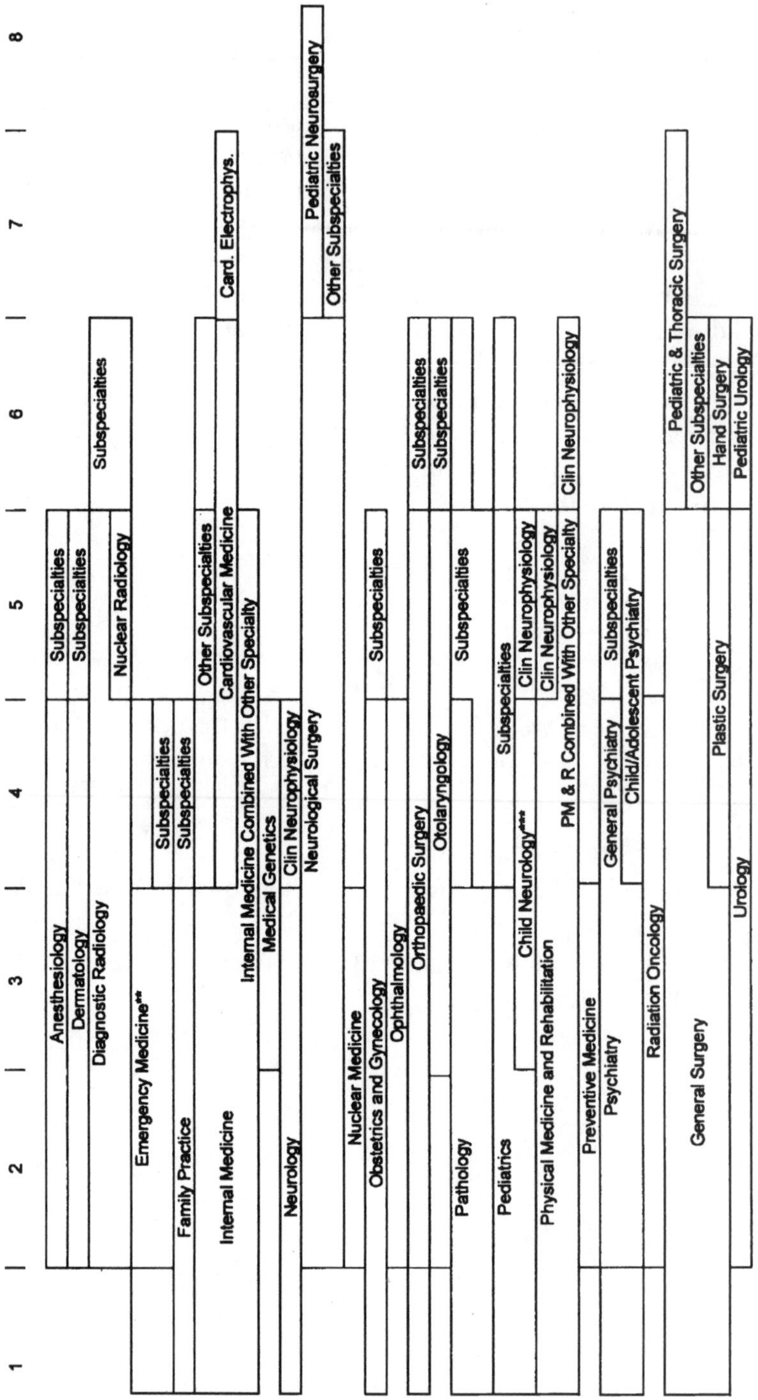

*Many programs offer a broad-based GY-1 and GY-2 years as part of their residencies.
**Emergency Medicine programs may include GY-1 through GY-3, GY-1 through GY-4, or GY-2 through GY-4.
***One broader, adult medicine year may be substituted for one year in Pediatrics.

FIGURE 3.2

## Length of Postgraduate Training for Osteopathic (D.O.) Physicians

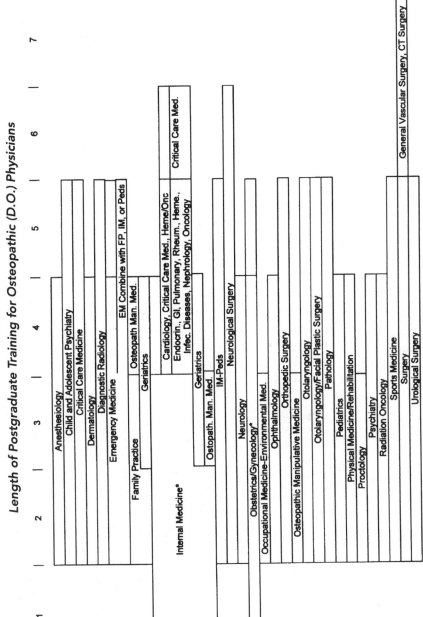

*Nearly all Internal Medicine and OB/Gyn residents take AOA-approved "specialty track" internships to shorten their training by one year.

FIGURE 3.3

### Is This Specialty For You?

| | Percent practitioners saying that the specialty meets their expectations | How satisfied with *current* practice position (1=unsatisfied to 5=very satisfied) | Hours per week doing patient care |
|---|---|---|---|
| Geriatric Psychiatrists | 87.5% | 4.4 | 40.7 |
| Emergency Medicine | 87.4 | 3.8 | 38.5 |
| Hematologist (Path) | 85.7 | 3.6 | 45.0 |
| Pediatric Radiologists | 81.3 | 3.9 | 51.9 |
| Pediatric Surgery | 80.0 | 3.9 | 62.3 |
| Family Practice | 77.4 | 3.6 | 46.3 |
| Pediatric Cardiologists | 77.3 | 3.2 | 49.8 |
| Orthopedic Surgery | 76.9 | 3.8 | 61.1 |
| Internal Medicine-Pediatrics | 76.5 | 3.5 | 48.7 |
| Vascular/Interventional Rad | 76.2 | 3.8 | 56.9 |
| Hand Surgery (Orth) | 75.8 | 3.5 | 57.9 |
| Obstetrics & Gynecology | 75.8 | 3.6 | 50.3 |
| Pathology | 75.7 | 3.5 | 45.4 |
| Child Neurology | 75.0 | 3.4 | 63.8 |
| Hematologist (IM) | 75.0 | 3.5 | 46.5 |
| Cardiology | 74.5 | 3.7 | 60.0 |
| Radiology, Diagnostic | 74.3 | 3.6 | 48.1 |
| Pediatrics | 74.0 | 3.5 | 42.8 |
| Cytopathologists | 73.7 | 3.7 | 49.7 |
| Neuroradiologists | 72.1 | 3.7 | 50.1 |
| Dermatology | 71.2 | 3.8 | 40.0 |
| Otolaryngology | 71.2 | 3.7 | 52.9 |
| Neonatal-Perinatal Medicine | 70.6 | 3.5 | 45.0 |
| Geriatric Medicine (IM) | 70.3 | 3.4 | 40.3 |
| Thoracic Surgery | 70.2 | 3.4 | 66.6 |
| Dermatopathologists | 70.0 | 3.9 | 36.5 |
| General Surgery | 69.4 | 3.7 | 58.2 |
| Oncologist (IM) | 68.9 | 3.1 | 49.2 |
| Infectious Diseases (IM) | 68.8 | 3.5 | 45.6 |
| Radiation Oncology | 68.7 | 3.5 | 50.0 |
| Gastroenterology | 68.6 | 3.7 | 54.3 |
| Urology | 68.1 | 3.7 | 57.5 |
| Pulmonologists-Critical Care | 67.4 | 3.6 | 55.8 |
| Pediatric Gastroenterologists | 66.7 | 3.5 | 45.0 |
| Forensic Pathologists | 66.7 | 4.0 | 32.0 |
| Ophthalmology | 66.1 | 3.5 | 46.1 |

FIGURE 3.3 (continued)

| | Percent practitioners saying that the specialty meets their expectations | How satisfied with *current* practice position (1=unsatisfied to 5=very satisfied) | Hours per week doing patient care |
|---|---|---|---|
| Psychiatry | 65.9% | 3.5 | 43.5 |
| Physical Medicine & Rehabilitation | 65.5 | 3.5 | 47.3 |
| Neurology | 64.8 | 3.6 | 49.1 |
| Plastic Surgery | 64.5 | 3.7 | 59.1 |
| Pulmonary Diseases | 64.4 | 3.3 | 52.4 |
| Vascular Surgery | 64.1 | 3.4 | 58.8 |
| Internal Medicine | 62.9 | 3.3 | 48.7 |
| Neurological Surgery | 62.8 | 3.5 | 62.7 |
| Anesthesiology | 61.6 | 3.3 | 53.9 |
| Nephrology | 61.4 | 3.4 | 55.4 |
| Colon & Rectal Surgery | 60.7 | 3.5 | 60.0 |
| Hematology-Oncology | 60.5 | 3.5 | 54.9 |
| Allergy & Immunology | 60.0 | 3.4 | 42.0 |
| Geriatric Medicine (FP) | 60.0 | 4.0 | 36.4 |
| Adult Reconstructive Orthoped Surg | 60.0 | 3.4 | 49.4 |
| Pediatric Orthopedic Surgery | 60.0 | 3.6 | 52.6 |
| Preventive Medicine | 60.0 | 3.3 | 32.6 |
| Orthopedic Sports Medicine | 59.5 | 3.3 | 55.1 |
| Child & Adolescent Psychiatry | 58.3 | 3.4 | 45.0 |
| Endocrinology, Diabetes, Metabolism | 57.4 | 3.2 | 44.1 |
| Hand Surgery (Plastic Surg) | 57.1 | 3.1 | 56.4 |
| Pediatric Nephrologists | 57.1 | 3.6 | 44.3 |
| Critical Care (Anesth) | 55.6 | 3.1 | 48.8 |
| Critical Care (IM) | 55.2 | 3.2 | 55.4 |
| Nuclear Medicine | 55.0 | 3.2 | 46.9 |
| Critical Care (Ped) | 50.0 | 3.2 | 57.5 |
| Pain Management | 50.0 | 3.1 | 54.3 |
| Pediatric Pulmonologists | 50.0 | 3.0 | 48.3 |
| Rheumatology | 50.0 | 3.2 | 48.3 |
| Critical Care (Surg) | 44.4 | 3.1 | 58.1 |
| Pediatric Hematologist-Oncologists | 44.4 | 3.6 | 36.3 |
| Orthopedic Spinal Surgeons | 44.4 | 2.6 | 51.3 |
| Pediatric Endocrinologists | 42.9 | 3.1 | 36.0 |
| Blood Banking/Transfusion Pathology | 37.5 | 2.6 | 41.3 |
| Hand Surgery (Surg) | 33.3 | 3.3 | 74.0 |

Adapted from AMA statistics, 1999. (To order specialties, numbers were not rounded, as they were in the specialty descriptions.)

# 4

# Choosing A Specialty

*"Cheshire puss," she [Alice] began . . .,*
*"would you please tell me which way I ought to go from here?"*
*"That depends on where you want to get to," said the cat.*
– Lewis Carroll, *Alice's Adventures in Wonderland*

## Your Personal Aptitudes— Assess Them Honestly

There are several methods you can use to assess your interests when deciding which specialty is best for you. The first one is the "try it and like it" method. Using this option, a student does a clinical rotation, likes the limited experience, and decides to make that specialty his or her life's work. This can be very misleading.

A single exposure to a specialty can be particularly stimulating because of the attending, resident team, and selection of patients—or unrealistically dismal for the same reasons. In either case, the experience may have very little to do with how well you are suited to the specialty or what the practice of the specialty is really like outside of the halls of academia. Yet this is the traditional procedure medical students have used to make their career choices.

The method has, until recently, worked to the entire medical system's advantage. Most students entered the specialties to which they were exposed. Since these specialties (the third-year required rotations at most schools are Internal Medicine, Surgery, Pediatrics, Psychiatry, Neurology, Obstetrics and Gynecology, and, most recently, Family Practice) were the specialties that needed the most practitioners, this worked well. However, some of these specialties are currently, or will shortly be, oversubscribed. The available first-year positions in the various specialties (Figure 4.1), though, do not necessarily reflect this.

Approximately 10% to 18% of the first-year slots go unfilled each year. Specialties with more "entry-level positions" open than "PGY-1" positions generally require other training, such as an internship, before entering the residency. In 2000, approximately 22,000 positions were offered at the PGY-1 level, not counting newly accredited programs. Of these, about 3,000 were not filled. Many of the specialties listed in Figure 4.1 have positions beginning in the PGY-2 or subsequent years that are available to medical students through the NRMP or other matching programs. Also, about 1,150 one-year Transitional PGY-1 positions were available.

FIGURE 4.1

### Number of PGY-1 and First-Year
### Specialty Positions Offered 2000-2001

| Specialties in Shortage | Positions Available to PGY-1s | All Entry-Level Positions |
|---|---|---|
| Internal Medicine (C & P)* | 7,517 | 8,263 |
| Family Practice | 3,365 | 3,365 |
| Pediatrics | 2,314 | 2,515 |
| Psychiatry | 1,080 | 1,158 |
| Emergency Medicine | 967 | 1,157 |
| Internal Medicine-Pediatrics | 454 | 463 |
| Physical Medicine & Rehabilitation | 76 | 330 |
| Preventive Medicine/Public Health | 15 | 299 |
| **Specialties Near Equilibrium** | | |
| Pathology | 452 | 549 |
| Neurology** | 56 | 432 |
| Dermatology | 41 | 291 |
| Radiation Oncology | 100 | 128 |
| **Surplus Specialties** | | |
| General Surgery (C & P)* | 2,033 | 2,040 |
| Obstetrics and Gynecology | 1,135 | 1,246 |
| Orthopedic Surgery | 560 | 601 |
| Diagnostic Radiology | 161 | 884 |
| Anesthesiology | 381 | 1,075 |
| Urology** | 62 | 249 |
| Otolaryngology** | 44 | 277 |
| Neurosurgery** | 34 | 136 |
| Ophthalmology** | 9 | 467 |

*"C" are Categorical positions; "P" are Preliminary positions.
**Most positions go through the specialty's own matching program.
Adapted from: Appendix II, Table 10, JAMA. 1999;282(9):904-6.

After looking at Figure 4.1, you may also want to look at Figure 22.2 to see the total number of positions available to medical students (PGY-1 and Advanced Matches), and the total number of entry-level positions that are available to both medical students and those with additional training.

## Specialty Interest Tests

The second, and more scientific, method (remember, physicians are supposed to be applied scientists) is to test yourself for your interest profile. This can be done either by taking a formal, standardized test or by self-testing.

The standardized test, the Strong Vocational Interest Inventory: Gough Medical Subspecialty Scales (a Meyers-Briggs-type preference test), is available through many Dean of Students' offices. This test compares your interests with those of current practitioners in approximately seven major specialties. It has been tested and validated on large numbers of individuals practicing in the various specialties and administered to many medical students, most of whom have found it very useful. Some schools have other Meyers-Briggs-type tests that they use. One warning: If you take any Meyers-Briggs-type test in your first or second year of medical school, it has only a fair predictive value. The farther along you are in your training, the more valid the results will be.

A quicker but less-accurate way of assessing your interests is to test yourself by using either of two handbooks. The first is *How to Choose a Medical Specialty* by Anita Taylor (most medical libraries have a copy). This book contains short descriptions of all the approved specialties and sub-specialties with a self-assessment quiz for each one. If you do the assessment quiz for all the specialties in the book, you will be able to rank your interests. You can then compare your interests with those of practitioners in the specialty.

## Glaxo Welcome Medical Pathway Evaluation Program

The second book, actually part of a course available free to medical students, is the *Glaxo Welcome Medical Specialty Profiles*. Now on CD-ROM, participants in the Glaxo Welcome Medical Pathway Evaluation Program receive it at no cost.

The profiles, which can be printed out, provide a comprehensive look at the specialties and major subspecialties from the average practitioner's viewpoint. Significant research went into preparing this material. Not only is there a complete description of the specialty, including both the likes and dislikes of the specialists, but also personal anecdotes on why practitioners initially entered the field. Seventeen characteristics are described for each specialty and rated, on a linear scale, by the degree of their importance to practitioners. These factors include personal autonomy, patient care, use of manual skills, professional respect, income, and work schedule. An exercise at the end of each section allows you to compare your results with those of physicians practicing in that field.

The Glaxo Welcome Pathway Evaluation Program, given at over 123 medical schools, is a 3½ hour interactive workshop supervised by a faculty or staff member at your school. It helps medical students to choose the specialty career path most suitable to them by teaching a decision-making process and analyzing students' decision-making styles. Participants also examine "critical factors" that are important in making a specialty choice, such as the type of medical practice, the components necessary for personal satisfaction, and lifestyle. The program consists of lectures, videotapes, and decision-making exercises designed to teach five steps in the career decision-making process:

1. Appraising the decision-making challenge.
2. Assessing self, goals, and priorities.
3. Surveying alternatives and options.
4. Evaluating alternatives and options.
5. Achieving commitment to an optimal course of action.

Preparation takes about an hour for the 3½-hour session, and the program is designed to be followed by subsequent counseling from advisers. Ideally, only 20 students participate in each session, since it is designed to be interactive.

I highly recommend that students take the course. Most students who have taken it say they have benefited. The course is free both to the school and to participants. (This represents one of the best, and most ethical, uses of drug company funds directed at medical schools and medical students.) If your school has not yet offered this course, find out from your Dean's office when it is planned, or call (800) 444-PATH for information about where it will be given. Generally, students take the program during the first half of their third year. It could, though, also be useful to first- and second-year students. In all likelihood, if taken early, it would have to be repeated during the third year.

These resources and the Glaxo Welcome Pathway Evaluation Program will broaden your field of vision beyond that which you have already experienced. Your whole professional life is at stake. Take the time to think your choice through carefully.

You can also quickly assess the medical specialty areas, which interest you by completing the Personal Trait Analysis, Figure 4.2.

## Personal Trait Analysis (Figure 4.2)
As you can see in the example (Figure 4.3) completed by a sample medical student, you should put a "+" next to each "Characteristic" that you "Like" or feel is one of your "Strengths." If you neither "Like" the "Characteristic" nor consider it one of your "Strengths," put a "0" in the appropriate place. Note that you may "Like" some of the Characteristics, but not feel that they are "Strengths." Others you may feel are personal "Strengths," but you do not particularly "Like" them. In these cases, just mark the form accordingly. The statements are purposely broad, so do not be alarmed by their general nature.

Once you have completed your Personal Trait Analysis in Figure 4.2, use the Personal Trait Synthesis form (Figure 4.5) to rearrange the "Characteristics" (as our sample student has done in Figure 4.4) under the following four categories:

**High Priority**—Characteristics you marked (+)"Like," (+)"Strength"

**Priority**—Characteristics you marked (+)"Like," (0)"Strength"

**Acceptable**—Characteristics you marked (0)"Like," (+)"Strength"

**Reject**—Characteristics you marked (0)"Like," (0)"Strength"

Next, look at Figure 4.6, which summarizes the characteristics that practitioners in some major specialties feel relate to their area. Then go to Figures 4.7 and 4.8, "Selecting a Specialty for You."

These forms are also available on the *Companion Disk for Getting Into A Residency*. This is a program that has many of the blank forms found in this book, including the forms needed for the "Personal Trait Analysis." The program will even perform all the calculations for you! DOS- and Windows-based programs are available from Galen Press. See the *Annotated Bibliography* for more information.

FIGURE 4.2
## *Personal Trait Analysis*

| Characteristic | Like | Strength |
|---|---|---|
| 1. Deal with Many Major Diseases | | |
| 2. Treat Infectious Diseases | | |
| 3. Treat Incurable & Disabling Diseases | | |
| 4. Evaluate Neurological Functions | | |
| 5. Evaluate Reproductive Functions | | |
| 6. Deal with Complex Problems | | |
| 7. Life-Threatening Problems | | |
| 8. Treat Psychosomatic Problems | | |
| 9. Deal with Intimate Personal Problems | | |
| 10. Deal with Emotional Reactions to Illness | | |
| 11. Older Age Patients | | |
| 12. Child & Adolescent Patients | | |
| 13. Dying Patients | | |
| 14. Many Patients Daily | | |
| 15. Give Comprehensive Care | | |
| 16. Home Health Care | | |
| 17. Do Preventive Care | | |
| 18. Do Genetic Counseling | | |
| 19. Marital & Sexual Counseling | | |
| 20. Family Planning Counseling | | |
| 21. Discuss Personal Relations | | |
| 22. Patient Participation in Care | | |
| 23. See Beneficial Treatment Results | | |
| 24. Use Knowledge of Musculoskeletal System | | |
| 25. Use Knowledge of Circulat., Resp., Digest., & Excretory Systems | | |
| 26. Use Knowledge of Anatomy & Physiology | | |
| 27. Do Extensive, Precise Workups | | |
| 28. Use Lab Tests | | |
| 29. Use Proctoscopies & Arteriograms | | |
| 30. Use Complex Equipment | | |
| 31. Use Your Hands | | |
| 32. Do Repetitive Standard Procedures | | |
| 33. Do High-Risk Procedures | | |
| 34. Do Outpatient Operative Procedures | | |
| 35. Get & Use Family Information | | |
| 36. Use Socioeconomic Information | | |
| 37. Use Rehabilitation Services | | |
| 38. Use Social Services | | |
| 39. Give Psychological Services | | |
| 40. Get Referrals & Give Consultations | | |

FIGURE 4.3
### *Personal Trait Analysis–An Example*

| Characteristic | Like | Strength |
|---|---|---|
| 1. Deal with Many Major Diseases | + | + |
| 2. Treat Infectious Diseases | 0 | + |
| 3. Treat Incurable & Disabling Diseases | 0 | 0 |
| 4. Evaluate Neurological Functions | 0 | 0 |
| 5. Evaluate Reproductive Functions | 0 | 0 |
| 6. Deal with Complex Problems | + | + |
| 7. Life-Threatening Problems | + | + |
| 8. Treat Psychosomatic Problems | + | 0 |
| 9. Deal with Intimate Personal Problems | 0 | 0 |
| 10. Deal with Emotional Reactions to Illness | 0 | 0 |
| 11. Older Age Patients | + | + |
| 12. Child & Adolescent Patients | 0 | + |
| 13. Dying Patients | 0 | + |
| 14. Many Patients Daily | + | 0 |
| 15. Give Comprehensive Care | + | + |
| 16. Home Health Care | 0 | 0 |
| 17. Do Preventive Care | 0 | 0 |
| 18. Do Genetic Counseling | 0 | 0 |
| 19. Marital & Sexual Counseling | 0 | 0 |
| 20. Family Planning Counseling | 0 | 0 |
| 21. Discuss Personal Relations | + | 0 |
| 22. Patient Participation in Care | + | + |
| 23. See Beneficial Treatment Results | + | + |
| 24. Use Knowledge of Musculoskeletal System | + | + |
| 25. Use Knowledge of Circulat., Resp., Digest., & Excretory Systems | + | 0 |
| 26. Use Knowledge of Anatomy & Physiology | + | + |
| 27. Do Extensive, Precise Workups | 0 | + |
| 28. Use Lab Tests | + | + |
| 29. Use Proctoscopies & Arteriograms | 0 | 0 |
| 30. Use Complex Equipment | + | 0 |
| 31. Use Your Hands | + | + |
| 32. Do Repetitive Standard Procedures | 0 | 0 |
| 33. Do High-Risk Procedures | 0 | 0 |
| 34. Do Outpatient Operative Procedures | + | + |
| 35. Get & Use Family Information | 0 | + |
| 36. Use Socioeconomic Information | + | 0 |
| 37. Use Rehabilitation Services | 0 | 0 |
| 38. Use Social Services | 0 | + |
| 39. Give Psychological Services | + | + |
| 40. Get Referrals & Give Consultations | + | 0 |

FIGURE 4.4

### *Personal Trait Synthesis–An Example*

Our sample student has taken his results from Figure 4.3 and grouped them according to their priority for him.

| Characteristic | Like | Strength |
|---|:---:|:---:|
| **HIGH PRIORITY (4)** | | |
| 1. Deal with Many Major Diseases | + | + |
| 6. Deal with Complex Problems | + | + |
| 7. Life-Threatening Problems | + | + |
| 11. Older Age Patients | + | + |
| 15. Give Comprehensive Care | + | + |
| 22. Patient Participation in Care | + | + |
| 23. See Beneficial Treatment Results | + | + |
| 24. Use Knowledge of Musculoskeletal System | + | + |
| 26. Use Knowledge of Anatomy & Physiology | + | + |
| 28. Use Lab Tests | + | + |
| 31. Use Your Hands | + | + |
| 34. Do Outpatient Operative Procedures | + | + |
| 39. Give Psychological Services | + | + |
| **PRIORITY (3)** | | |
| 8. Treat Psychosomatic Problems | + | 0 |
| 14. Many Patients Daily | + | 0 |
| 21. Discuss Personal Relations | + | 0 |
| 25. Use Knowledge of Circul., Resp., Digest., & Excretory Systems | + | 0 |
| 30. Use Complex Equipment | + | 0 |
| 36. Use Socioeconomic Information | + | 0 |
| 40. Get Referrals & Give Consults | + | 0 |
| **ACCEPTABLE (2)** | | |
| 2. Treat Infectious Diseases | 0 | + |
| 12. Child & Adolescent Patients | 0 | + |
| 13. Dying Patients | 0 | + |
| 27. Do Extensive, Precise Workups | 0 | + |
| 35. Get & Use Family Information | 0 | + |
| 38. Use Social Services | 0 | + |
| **REJECT (1)** | | |
| 3. Treat Incurable & Disabling Diseases | 0 | 0 |
| 4. Evaluate Neurological Functions | 0 | 0 |
| 5. Evaluate Reproductive Functions | 0 | 0 |
| 9. Deal with Intimate Personal Problems | 0 | 0 |
| 10. Deal with Emotional Reactions to Illness | 0 | 0 |
| 16. Home Health Care | 0 | 0 |
| 17. Do Preventive Care | 0 | 0 |
| 18. Do Genetic Counseling | 0 | 0 |
| 19. Marital & Sexual Counseling | 0 | 0 |
| 20. Family Planning Counseling | 0 | 0 |
| 29. Use Proctoscopies & Arteriograms | 0 | 0 |
| 32. Do Repetitive Standard Procedures | 0 | 0 |
| 33. Do High-Risk Procedures | 0 | 0 |
| 37. Use Rehabilitation Services | 0 | 0 |

## FIGURE 4.5
### *Personal Trait Synthesis*

Now list your likes/strengths from Figure 4.2 in priority.

### HIGH PRIORITY (4)

_____     _____

_____     _____

_____     _____

_____     _____

### PRIORITY (3)

_____     _____

_____     _____

_____     _____

_____     _____

### ACCEPTABLE (2)

_____     _____

_____     _____

_____     _____

_____     _____

### REJECT (1)

_____     _____

_____     _____

_____     _____

_____     _____

FIGURE 4.6

## Characteristics Strongly Associated with the Practice of Some Major Specialties

The following seven charts summarize the "Characteristics" practitioners feel relate to their specialties in Emergency Medicine, Family Practice, Internal Medicine, Obstetrics and Gynecology, Pediatrics, Psychiatry, and Surgery. While there are *many more specialty fields than are listed here*, these charts should give you a starting point from which to look into similar, related specialty areas.

When you finish looking these over, turn to Figures 4.7 and 4.8 "Selecting a Specialty For You," to determine how your own rating of the Characteristics compares to those of specialists practicing in these fields.

### Emergency Medicine

*Very Common*
- Life-Threatening Problems
- Many Patients Daily
- Use Your Hands

*Common*
- Use Lab Tests
- Child and Adolescent Patients
- Use Knowledge of Musculoskeletal System
- Use Knowledge of Circulatory, Respiratory, Digestive, & Excretory Systems
- Use Knowledge of Anatomy & Physiology
- Many Major Diseases
- Beneficial Treatment Results
- Outpatient Operative Procedures

*Rare*
- Deal with Emotional Reactions to Illness
- Preventive Care
- Use Proctoscopies & Arteriograms
- Incurable & Disabling Diseases
- Discuss Personal Relations
- Use Rehabilitation Services
- Family Planning Counseling
- Use Psychological Services
- Evaluate Reproductive Functions
- Home Health Care

*Very Rare*
- Marital & Sexual Counseling
- Genetic Counseling

### Family Practice

*Very Common*
- Comprehensive Care
- Use Lab Tests
- Outpatient Operative Procedures
- Child & Adolescent Patients
- Older Age Patients
- Many Patients Daily
- Intimate Personal Problems
- Use Family Information
- Treat Infectious Diseases

*Common*
- Many Major Diseases
- Deal with Life-Threatening Problems
- Psychosomatic Problems
- Dying Patients
- Home Health Care
- Preventive Care
- Marital & Sexual Counseling
- Family Planning Counseling
- Discuss Personal Relations
- Patient Participation in Care
- Beneficial Treatment Results
- Repetitive Standard Procedures
- Use Socioeconomic Information
- Use Rehabilitation Services
- Use Social Services

*Rare*
- Genetic Counseling
- Use Complex Equipment
- Do High-Risk Procedures
- Get Referrals & Give Consults

FIGURE 4.6 (continued)

| *Internal Medicine* | *Obstetrics & Gynecology* |
|---|---|
| *Very Common* | *Very Common* |
| • Complex Problems | • Marital & Sexual Counseling |
| • Use Lab Tests | • Use Your Hands |
| • Get Referrals & Give Consults | • Family Planning Counseling |
| | • Intimate Personal Problems |
| *Common* | • Evaluate Reproductive Functions |
| • Many Major Diseases | |
| • Treat Infectious Diseases | *Common* |
| • Incurable and Disabling Diseases | • Many Patients Daily |
| • Life-Threatening Problems | • Preventive Care |
| • Psychosomatic Problems | • Beneficial Treatment Results |
| • Intimate Personal Problems | • Use Lab Tests |
| • Older Age Population | • Repetitive Standard Procedures |
| • Dying Patients | • Get Referrals & Give Consults |
| • Comprehensive Care | |
| • Patient Participation in Care | *Rare* |
| • Knowledge of Circulatory, | • Incurable & Disabling Diseases |
|    Respiratory, Digestive, | • Older Age Patients |
|    & Excretory Systems | • Dying Patients |
| • Extensive, Precise Workups | • Home Health Care |
| • Proctoscopies & Arteriograms | • Use Knowledge of Musculoskeletal |
| • Use Family Information |    System |
| | • Use Complex Equipment |
| *Rare* | • Do High-Risk Procedures |
| • Child & Adolescent Patients | • Use Socioeconomic Information |
| • Genetic Counseling | • Give Psychological Services |
| • Family Planning Counseling | |
| • Psychological Services | *Very Rare* |
| • Use Knowledge of Musculoskeletal | • Use Rehabilitation Services |
|    System | • Use Proctoscopies & Arteriograms |
| • Evaluate Reproductive Functions | • Evaluate Neurological Functions |
| | |
| *Very Rare* | |
| • Outpatient Operative Procedures | |

FIGURE 4.6 (continued)

## Pediatrics

*Very Common*
- Preventive Care
- Comprehensive Care
- Many Patients Daily
- Child & Adolescent Patients
- Treat Infectious Diseases

*Common*
- Beneficial Treatment Results
- Use Lab Tests
- Repetitive Standard Procedures
- Use Family Information

*Rare*
- Incurable & Disabling Diseases
- Family Planning Counseling
- Deal with Emotional Reactions to Illness
- Use Knowledge of Musculoskeletal System

*Very Rare*
- Older Age Patients
- Marital & Sexual Counseling
- Use Complex Equipment
- Do High-Risk Procedures
- Dying Patients
- Evaluate Reproductive Functions
- Use Proctoscopies & Arteriograms

## Psychiatry

*Very Common*
- Psychosomatic Problems
- Intimate Personal Problems
- Emotional Reactions to Illness
- Discuss Personal Relationships
- Patient Participation in Care

*Common*
- Get Referrals & Give Consults
- Give Psychological Services
- Use Social Services
- Use Socioeconomic Information
- Use Family Information
- Marital & Sexual Counseling
- Complex Problems

*Rare*
- Use Lab Tests
- Extensive, Precise Workups
- Genetic Counseling
- Home Health Care
- Life-Threatening Problems
- Evaluate Reproductive Functions
- Use Knowledge of Anatomy & Physiology
- Use Rehabilitation Services

*Very Rare*
- Use Your Hands
- Do High-Risk Procedures
- Outpatient Operative Procedures
- Many Patients Daily
- Use Complex Equipment
- Use Proctoscopies & Arteriograms
- Treat Infectious Diseases
- Use Knowledge of Musculoskeletal System
- Use Knowledge of Circulatory, Respiratory, Digestive, & Excretory Systems

FIGURE 4.6 (continued)

### Surgery

*Very Common*
- Life-Threatening Problems
- Beneficial Treatment Results
- Get Referrals & Give Consults
- Use Your Hands
- Outpatient Operative Procedures
- Use of Knowledge of Anatomy
  & Physiology
- Use Proctoscopies & Arteriograms

*Common*
- Many Major Diseases
- Complex Problems
- Dying Patients
- Extensive Precise Workups
- Use Lab Tests
- Use Knowledge of Musculoskeletal
  System
- Use Knowledge of Circulatory,
  Respiratory, Digestive,
  & Excretory Systems

*Rare*
- Comprehensive Care
- Preventive Care
- Deal with Emotional Reactions
  to Illness
- Intimate Personal Problems
- Evaluate Neurological Functions
- Psychosomatic Problems
- Evaluate Reproductive Functions
- Use Socioeconomic Information

*Very Rare*
- Genetic Counseling
- Marital-Sexual Counseling
- Family Planning Counseling
- Psychological Services

Adapted from: Zimny GH. *Manual for the Medical Specialty Preference Inventory.* (revised draft) St. Louis, MO, 1977; and Zimny GH, Iserson KV, Shepherd C. A characterization of emergency medicine. *JACEP.* 1979;8(4):147-49.

FIGURE 4.7

### *Selecting a Specialty for You–An Example*

This form summarizes the prior pages (Figure 4.6) and briefly describes those characteristics favored by current practitioners in seven common specialties. Our sample student, whose Personal Trait Synthesis can be found in Figure 4.4, would fill out the blank Figure 4.8 as seen below.

Every characteristic that the student rated as a "*High Priority*" [Like (+), Strength (+)] gets *4 points*; each one rated as "*Priority*" [Like (+), Strength (0)] gets *3 points*; each one rated as "*Acceptable*" [Like (0), Strength (+)] gets *2 points*; and each one rated "*Reject*" [Like (0), Strength (0)] gets *1 point*. That student would then fill in the numerical values for each of the characteristics [rated as Very Common (VC), Common (C), Rare (R), or Very Rare (VR)] in each of these specialties.

Once the individual numbers are filled in, a score can be calculated based upon the correlation of personal traits with the specialty characteristics.

| Characteristic | IM | SUR | FP | PED | OB | PSY | EM |
|---|---|---|---|---|---|---|---|
| 1. Deal with Many Major Diseases | C 4 | C 4 | C 4 | – | – | – | C 4 |
| 2. Treat Infectious Diseases | C 2 | – | VC 2 | VC 2 | – | VR 2 | – |
| 3. Treat Incurable & Disabling Diseases | C 1 | – | – | R 1 | R 1 | – | R 1 |
| 4. Evaluate Neurological Functions | – | R 1 | – | – | VR 1 | – | – |
| 5. Evaluate Reproductive Functions | R 1 | R 1 | – | VR 1 | VC 1 | R 1 | R 1 |
| 6. Deal with Complex Problems | VC 4 | C 4 | – | – | – | C 4 | – |
| 7. Life-Threatening Problems | C 4 | VC 4 | C 4 | – | – | R 4 | VC 4 |
| 8. Treat Psychosomatic Problems | C 3 | R 3 | C 3 | – | – | VC 3 | – |
| 9. Deal with Intimate Personal Problems | C 1 | R 1 | VC 1 | – | VC 1 | VC 1 | – |
| 10. Deal with Emotional Reactions to Illness | – | R 1 | – | R 1 | – | VC 1 | R 1 |
| 11. Older Age Patients | C 4 | – | VC 4 | VR 4 | R 4 | – | – |
| 12. Child & Adolescent Patients | R 2 | – | VC 2 | VC 2 | – | – | C 2 |
| 13. Dying Patients | C 2 | C 2 | C 2 | VR 2 | R 2 | – | – |
| 14. Many Patients Daily | – | – | VC 3 | VC 3 | C 3 | VR 3 | VC 3 |

FIGURE 4.7 (continued)

| Characteristic | IM | SUR | FP | PED | OB | PSY | EM |
|---|---|---|---|---|---|---|---|
| 15. Give Comprehensive Care | C<br>4 | R<br>4 | VC<br>4 | VC<br>4 | – | – | C<br>4 |
| 16. Home Health Care | – | – | C<br>1 | – | R<br>1 | R<br>1 | R<br>1 |
| 17. Do Preventive Care | – | R<br>1 | C<br>1 | VC<br>1 | C<br>1 | – | R<br>1 |
| 18. Do Genetic Counseling | R<br>1 | VR<br>1 | R<br>1 | – | – | R<br>1 | VR<br>1 |
| 19. Marital & Sex Counseling | – | VR<br>1 | C<br>1 | VR<br>1 | VC<br>1 | C<br>1 | VR<br>1 |
| 20. Family Planning Counseling | R<br>1 | VR<br>1 | C<br>1 | R<br>1 | VC<br>1 | – | R<br>1 |
| 21. Discuss Personal Relationships | – | – | C<br>3 | – | – | VC<br>3 | R<br>3 |
| 22. Patient Participation in Care | C<br>4 | – | C<br>4 | – | – | VC<br>4 | – |
| 23. See Beneficial Treatment Results | – | VC<br>4 | C<br>4 | C<br>4 | C<br>4 | – | C<br>4 |
| 24. Use Knowledge of Musculoskeletal System | R<br>4 | C<br>4 | – | R<br>4 | R<br>4 | VR<br>4 | C<br>4 |
| 25. Use Knowledge of Circul., Resp., Digest., & Excretory Systems | C<br>3 | C<br>3 | – | – | – | VR<br>3 | C<br>3 |
| 26. Use Knowledge of Anatomy & Physiology | – | VC<br>4 | – | – | – | R<br>4 | C<br>4 |
| 27. Do Extensive, Precise Workups | C<br>2 | C<br>2 | – | – | – | R<br>2 | – |
| 28. Use Lab Tests | VC<br>4 | C<br>4 | VC<br>4 | C<br>4 | C<br>4 | R<br>4 | C<br>4 |
| 29. Use Proctoscopies & Arteriograms | C<br>1 | VC<br>1 | – | VR<br>1 | VR<br>1 | VR<br>1 | R<br>1 |
| 30. Use Complex Equipment | – | – | R<br>3 | VR<br>3 | R<br>3 | VR<br>3 | – |
| 31. Use Your Hands | – | VC<br>4 | – | – | VC<br>4 | VR<br>4 | VC<br>4 |
| 32. Do Repetitive Standard Procedures | – | – | C<br>1 | C<br>1 | C<br>1 | – | – |
| 33. Do High-Risk Procedures | – | – | R<br>1 | VR<br>1 | R<br>1 | VR<br>1 | – |
| 34. Do Outpatient Operative Procedures | VR<br>4 | VC<br>4 | VC<br>4 | – | – | VR<br>4 | C<br>4 |

FIGURE 4.7 (continued)

| Characteristic | IM | SUR | FP | PED | OB | PSY | EM |
|---|---|---|---|---|---|---|---|
| 35. Get & Use Family Information | C 2 | – | VC 2 | C 2 | – | C 2 | – |
| 36. Use Socioeconomic Information | – | R 3 | C 3 | – | R 3 | C 3 | – |
| 37. Use Rehabilitation Services | – | – | C 1 | – | VR 1 | R 1 | R 1 |
| 38. Use Social Services | – | – | C 2 | – | – | C 2 | – |
| 39. Give Psych Services | R 4 | VR 4 | – | – | R 4 | C 4 | R 4 |
| 40. Get Referrals; Give Consultations | VC 3 | VC 3 | R 3 | – | C 3 | C 3 | – |

FIGURE 4.8

## Selecting a Specialty for You

Your rating number, *taken from Figure 4.5,* for each "Characteristic" is inserted below the associated strength of the characteristic ("VC"= Very Common; "C"= Common; "R"= Rare; "VR"= Very Rare) for each specialty. Note that your rating number for each characteristic will be the same under each specialty. (See Figure 4.7 for the numbers to use.) Once the individual numbers are filled in, a score can be calculated based upon the correlation of personal traits with the specialty characteristics.

| Characteristic | IM | SUR | FP | PED | OB | PSY | EM |
|---|---|---|---|---|---|---|---|
| 1. Deal with Many Major Diseases | C | C | C | – | – | – | C |
| 2. Treat Infectious Diseases | C | – | VC | VC | – | VR | – |
| 3. Treat Incurable & Disabling Diseases | C | – | – | R | R | – | R |
| 4. Evaluate Neurological Functions | – | R | – | – | VR | – | – |
| 5. Evaluate Reproductive Functions | R | R | – | VR | VC | R | R |
| 6. Deal with Complex Problems | VC | C | – | – | – | C | – |
| 7. Life-Threatening Problems | C | VC | C | – | – | R | VC |

FIGURE 4.8 (continued)

| Characteristic | IM | SUR | FP | PED | OB | PSY | EM |
|---|---|---|---|---|---|---|---|
| 8. Treat Psychosomatic Problems | C | R | C | – | – | VC | – |
| 9. Deal with Intimate Personal Problems | C | R | VC | – | VC | VC | – |
| 10. Deal with Emotional Reactions to Illness | – | R | – | R | – | VC | R |
| 11. Older Age Patients | C | – | VC | VR | R | – | – |
| 12. Child & Adolescent Patients | R | – | VC | VC | – | – | C |
| 13. Dying Patients | C | C | C | VR | R | – | – |
| 14. Many Patients Daily | – | – | VC | VC | C | VR | VC |
| 15. Give Comprehensive Care | C | R | VC | VC | – | – | C |
| 16 . Home Health Care | – | – | C | – | R | R | R |
| 17. Do Preventive Care | – | R | C | VC | C | – | R |
| 18. Do Genetic Counseling | R | VR | R | – | – | R | VR |
| 19. Marital & Sex Counseling | – | VR | C | VR | VC | C | VR |
| 20. Family Planning Counseling | R | VR | C | R | VC | – | R |
| 21. Discuss Personal Relationships | – | – | C | – | – | VC | R |
| 22. Patient Participation in Care | C | – | C | – | – | VC | – |
| 23. See Beneficial Treatment Results | – | VC | C | C | C | – | C |

FIGURE 4.8 (continued)

| Characteristic | IM | SUR | FP | PED | OB | PSY | EM |
|---|---|---|---|---|---|---|---|
| 24. Use Knowledge of Musculoskeletal System | R | C | | R | R | VR | C |
| 25. Use Knowledge of Circul., Resp., Digest., & Excretory Systems | C | C | | | | VR | C |
| 26. Use Knowledge of Anatomy & Physiology | | VC | | | | R | C |
| 27. Do Extensive, Precise Workups | C | C | – | – | – | R | – |
| 28. Use Lab Tests | VC | C | VC | C | C | R | C |
| 29. Use Proctoscopies & Arteriograms | C | VC | – | VR | VR | VR | R |
| 30. Use Complex Equipment | – | – | R | VR | R | VR | – |
| 31. Use Your Hands | – | VC | – | – | VC | VR | VC |
| 32. Do Repetitive Standard Procedures | – | – | C | C | C | – | – |
| 33. Do High-Risk Procedures | – | – | R | VR | R | VR | – |
| 34. Do Outpatient Operative Procedures | VR | VC | VC | – | – | VR | C |
| 35. Get & Use Family Information | C | – | VC | C | – | C | – |
| 36. Use Socioeconomic Information | – | R | C | – | R | C | – |
| 37. Use Rehabilitation Services | – | – | C | – | VR | R | R |
| 38. Use Social Services | – | – | C | – | – | C | – |
| 39. Give Psych Services | R | VR | – | – | R | C | R |
| 40. Get Referrals; Give Consultations | VC | VC | R | – | C | C | – |

FIGURE 4.9

## Correlation of Personal Traits and Specialty Characteristics

It is now time to see how your own traits, likes, and strengths match with the seven specialties analyzed. Using Figure 4.8, add the numbers associated with a particular rating for each specialty and put the result in the appropriate box in the chart below. For example, our sample student (Figure 4.7), in the Internal Medicine column, put two "4" and one "3" rating for traits listed as Very Common (VC). This equals "11." So our sample student would put the number "11" in the top left box in the chart, labeled "Very Common, IM." (See Figure 4.10 for an example.) The *Companion Disk* will do these calculations for you.

Complete the remainder of your chart in a similar manner. Then, to get the scores you will need, divide by the number specified in the box. This will give you an average score for the traits in that category.

As you can see, the higher the scores in the "Very Common" and "Common" boxes, and the lower the scores in the "Rare" and "Very Rare" boxes, the better your personal traits, strengths, and likes correlate with the practice in a particular specialty.

For an example of this form filled out by our sample student, turn to Figure 4.10.

| | IM | SUR | FP | PED | OB | PSY | EM |
|---|---|---|---|---|---|---|---|
| **Very Common Total:** | | | | | | | |
| Divided by: | 3 | 7 | 9 | 5 | 5 | 5 | 3 |
| Score = | | | | | | | |
| **Common Total:** | | | | | | | |
| Divided by: | 14 | 7 | 15 | 4 | 6 | 7 | 9 |
| Score = | | | | | | | |
| **Rare Total:** | | | | | | | |
| Divided by: | 6 | 8 | 4 | 4 | 9 | 8 | 10 |
| Score = | | | | | | | |
| **Very Rare Total:** | | | | | | | |
| Divided by: | 1 | 4 | – | 7 | 3 | 9 | 2 |
| Score = | | | | | | | |

FIGURE 4.10

## Correlation of Personal Traits and Specialty Characteristics–An Example

|  | IM | SUR | FP | PED | OB | PSY | EM |
|---|---|---|---|---|---|---|---|
| **Very Common Total:** | 11 | 24 | 26 | 12 | 8 | 12 | 11 |
| Divided by: | 3 | 7 | 9 | 5 | 5 | 5 | 3 |
| Score = | **3.67** | **3.43** | **2.89** | **2.40** | **1.60** | **2.40** | **3.67** |
| **Common Total:** | 37 | 23 | 35 | 11 | 16 | 19 | 33 |
| Divided by: | 14 | 7 | 15 | 4 | 6 | 7 | 9 |
| Score = | **2.64** | **3.29** | **2.33** | **2.75** | **2.67** | **2.71** | **3.67** |
| **Rare Total:** | 13 | 15 | 8 | 7 | 23 | 18 | 15 |
| Divided by: | 6 | 8 | 4 | 4 | 9 | 8 | 10 |
| Score = | **2.17** | **1.88** | **2.00** | **1.75** | **2.56** | **2.25** | **1.50** |
| **Very Rare Total:** | 4 | 7 | – | 13 | 3 | 25 | 2 |
| Divided by: | 1 | 4 | – | 7 | 3 | 9 | 2 |
| Score = | **4.00** | **1.75** | – | **1.86** | **1.00** | **2.78** | **1.00** |

This example demonstrates a pattern, which should point our sample student toward a specialty choice. Surgery and Emergency Medicine have characteristics closest to the student's likes and strengths. These two specialties also seem to rarely deal with many of the aspects of medicine the student feels are neither personal "Likes" nor "Strengths."

In general, you should look for the highest scores in the "Very Common" and "Common" characteristic areas, and the lowest scores in the "Rare" and "Very Rare" areas. A specialty that shows a reversal of this trend will be a poor match for you. The presence of very similar numbers in all four categories indicates that you may be able to generate little enthusiasm for the specialty.

However, there is one major caveat to using this scoring sheet: the subspecialty areas are not really considered in this schema. For example, while Internists very rarely do outpatient operative procedures, the subspecialty of Cardiology, especially those Cardiologists who do heart catheterizations, considers this a "Very Common" aspect of their practice. So, use these charts to get an estimate of areas that you would like to explore further. *Do not use them rigidly or without thinking beyond the results.*

# 5

# Important Factors When Choosing A Specialty

*The more alternatives, the more difficult the choice.*
– Abbé D'Allainval, *L'embarras des richesses*, 1726

Many factors come into play when you are trying to choose a specialty. The elements you find important may not be the same ones that your classmates value. Yet it might be instructive to look at what recent graduates felt were important factors in their choice of specialty.

The most important factors that students believe influenced their specialty choice relate to how they will interact with patients. *Interest in helping people, the opportunity to make a difference in people's lives, and the type of patient problems encountered* in the specialty were the major influences for most students. This suggests that most students' altruistic reasons for entering medicine still influence them after the four-year grind of medical school. Very reasonably, most students say other persuasive factors are whether their own *personality fits with the specialty* and whether they *possess the required skills or abilities.*

Medical students seem to make bad specialty choices—either being attracted to or rejecting specialties—based on the nature of the people with whom they work, especially in their third-year rotations. There are, however, personalities inherent in different specialties—especially at each institution. Associating with specialists both at the academic center and in the community, for example at the regional society meeting, may help you decide whether your personality fits that specialty.

Other very common factors considered when making a specialty choice are the *intellectual content* of the specialty and whether the specialty has *challenging diagnostic problems.* Basically, students prefer not to be bored by the career path they take. Interestingly, these are the same factors cited by physicians in practice who still enjoy their specialty 20 and 30 years after completing residency.

Unlike previous generations of medical students, recent graduates have wisely relied much less on a particular physician or a specific medical school course when determining their choice of specialty. However, they do still rely a bit too heavily on their experience during subspecialty clerkships. Brief and isolated experiences such as these can be misleading—both positively and negatively. Beware. Other factors also influence career choices, but few people readily acknowledge being swayed by them. These include income, the length of training, the work hours, whether there will be jobs in the specialty in the future, and the difficulty of getting a residency position.

## Monetary Rewards

One aspect of selecting a specialty, which is rarely, if ever, spoken about except in a humorous fashion, is the financial remuneration you can expect. While it may be both noble and consistent with the values that brought you into the field of medicine to try to ignore financial considerations completely, it is unrealistic. No physician is likely to be poor, but many medical students accrue enormous debts in order to finance their education.

### Specialty Income

Many medical students seem to believe that their educational investment will pay off handsomely. More than one-third of graduating medical students expect to be earning more than $200,000 annually within ten years of completing their postgraduate training.

In general, the Surgical specialties are the most lucrative. And the difference between the income of a Surgeon and his or her non-surgical colleagues can be truly amazing. This is because, at present, the insurance payment schemes reward *doing* (procedures) at a much higher level than *thinking* (cognition). While Pediatricians have a median annual income of $144,000, Radiologists earn about twice as much (Figure 5.1).

According to recent estimates, new Internists will earn only one-fourth to one-half of the starting salary received by physicians who are trained in more procedurally or technically oriented areas. This may change somewhat in the future as mechanisms for physician payment are rearranged at the federal, state, and private levels through "health-care reform." Across the United States, the highest physician incomes are in the West-South-Central states (AR, LA, OK, TX), while the lowest are in New England (CT, ME, MA, NH, RI, VT) and the Pacific states (AK, CA, HI, OR, WA). Real physician income (adjusted for inflation) has remained relatively unchanged for the past decade.

If the past is any indicator, though, the disparity in salary between doers and thinkers will persist. For example, a major income realignment was to occur in the early 1990s with the implementation of the Resource Based Relative Value Scale (RBRVS). It never materialized. Despite predic-

FIGURE 5.1

**Mean Physician Annual Income After Expenses and Before Taxes**

| Specialty | Income |
|---|---|
| Orthopedic Surgeons | $ 331,000 |
| Cardiologists | 284,000 |
| Diagnostic Radiologists | 276,000 |
| Surgeons (All) | 261,000 |
| Urologists | 238,000 |
| Anesthesiologists | 236,000 |
| Otolaryngologists | 230,000 |
| Obstetrician/Gynecologists | 229,000 |
| General Surgeons | 226,000 |
| Dermatologists | 224,000 |
| Ophthalmologists | 222,000 |
| Gastroenterologists | 222,000 |
| Pathologists | 201,000 |
| **All Physicians** | **$ 200,000** |
| Emergency Physicians | $ 197,000 |
| Neurologists | 188,000 |
| General Internists | 176,000 |
| Pediatricians | 144,000 |
| Family Physicians | 141,000 |
| Psychiatrists | 136,000 |

Adapted from: American Medical Association. *Physician Socioeconomic Statistics 1999-2000*. Chicago, IL: AMA, 1999.

tions from the government, the American Medical Association, and other reputable sources that primary care practitioners would benefit, they didn't. In fact, it has been shown that primary care physicians have a substantially lower return on their investment in professional education than do medical or surgical subspecialists, attorneys, dentists, and individuals in business. Yet no matter which specialty a physician chooses to enter, he or she is in no danger of going on the dole.

The changing health care environment, however, should eventually decrease the need for, and the income of, many specialists. This is because managed care organizations generally make money by keeping their patients away from medical specialists. So far, they have been only partially successful at doing this.

Other changes may also affect physicians' income in certain specialties. Recent rules concerning physician reimbursement have severely reduced the income of Clinical Pathologists. The government unilaterally disallowed payment for a large portion of their practice. This, as is usually the case, was followed by a similar move by all other insurers. The government is now seriously looking at making similar changes in reimbursement for other hospital-based specialists, such as Anesthesiologists, Radiologists, and Emergency Physicians. How this will affect their income is uncertain.

Then there is the malpractice insurance dilemma, cycling from a crisis level to merely being uncomfortable, which will continue to affect some specialties until broad tort reform is enacted. Obstetricians still find it difficult in some locales to deliver babies at a cost that new families can afford, while paying the ever-increasing premiums for their malpractice insurance.

In many cases, Family Practitioners have completely given up the portion of their practices that previously included Obstetrics, outpatient Orthopedics, and Surgery. Radiologists have recently joined the luckless group of most-frequently sued specialties, mainly from inaccurately reading mammograms. Neurosurgeons, Plastic Surgeons, and many other specialists now face similar stiff increases in the already astronomical cost of malpractice insurance. While the highest-income specialties are still lucrative, even after subtracting the cost of their malpractice premiums, the net remuneration is not quite as attractive as it would first appear.

Overall, physicians earning the highest net income live in metropolitan areas with fewer than one million people, are not in solo practice, are not linked to a managed care group, and are between 46 and 55 years old.

## Debt & Specialty Choice

No one has consistently shown that most medical students make career choices based on the level of their debt. Some studies, such as that shown in Figure 5.2, suggest a trend in that direction. Most of the highest-paying specialties, though, have also been the most difficult to enter. Perhaps many medical students simply are attracted to those specialties, or to the promise of a nice income, whether or not they have large debts.

In 1998, medical students received nearly $1.5 billion in educational loans. The 83% of 1999 medical school graduates who borrowed money to pay for their education owed an average of more than $90,000. This debt level has increased nearly 300% since 1985! (For perspective, the average graduating student's debt in 1971 was only $8,435.) Students in private medical schools have debts nearly 50% higher than those in public schools.

This debt level will rise, given that the 1999 annual tuition/fee costs at more than sixty-three medical schools were $25,000, and eighteen of these now exceed $30,000. In addition, nearly 16% of medical-school-graduates' spouses have debts exceeding $50,000. Also, nearly 15% of medical students take more than four years to graduate, thus increasing their debt load.

Because of the interest accruing on their loans, many medical students eventually pay back up to three dollars for every dollar they borrow. Therefore, selecting a poorly remunerated specialty without understanding

FIGURE 5.2

**Influence of Indebtedness as it Relates to Medical Students'
Career Choices**

| | Percentage of Medical Students | | |
| --- | --- | --- | --- |
| | No Influence | Minor/Moderate | Major |
| **Debt <$50,000** | | | |
| Gen specialty | 73 % | 24 % | 2 % |
| Med specialty | 77 | 19 | 5 |
| Surg specialty | 79 | 19 | 3 |
| Support specialty | 70 | 24 | 5 |
| **Debt $50-$75,000** | | | |
| Gen specialty | 77 | 18 | 5 |
| Med specialty | 66 | 29 | 5 |
| Surg specialty | 65 | 28 | 7 |
| Support specialty | 53 | 36 | 12 |
| **Debt >$75,000** | | | |
| Gen specialty | 59 | 33 | 8 |
| Med specialty | 61 | 31 | 8 |
| Surg specialty | 52 | 34 | 14 |
| Support specialty | 41 | 39 | 20 |

May not total 100% due to rounding.

Adapted from: Kassebaum DG, Szenas PL. Relationship between indebtedness and the specialty choices of graduating medical students. *Acad Med.* 1992;67:700-7.

the ramifications may lead to a rude awakening at the end of residency training.

During part or all of residency, physicians may either avoid paying and accruing interest on some student loans (deferment) or avoid paying them off while still accruing interest (forbearance or "deferment" of unsubsidized loans), depending on their overall financial situation. The requirements for implementing these options have become stricter in recent years. The rules will certainly continue to change over time, so check with your loan officer to find out the current regulations. Note that, unlike other government loans and most felonies, there is no "statute of limitations" on government loans to students. You owe them the money until it is repaid; even bankruptcy doesn't automatically banish these debts.

Many residents find it wise either to apply for forbearance from their lenders or to consolidate their loans and extend their payment schedule through the Federal Loan Consolidation Program. You should be aware that the federal government now publishes the names of individuals who default on student loans. There has been a move to have all residency training programs provide financial advice and administrative assistance in managing resident education indebtedness. The wise programs are beginning to do this.

## Importance of Income

A final note is in order about the importance of income at various career stages. For the entry-level physician, income is extremely important. This makes sense, since most new physicians have enormous debts, no money, and increasing financial responsibilities. At mid-career, however, income is of only medium importance—with job security being the most important factor keeping the physician in practice. At this stage of physicians' careers, job satisfaction is equally as important as income. Job satisfaction becomes of overwhelming importance for physicians in the last third of their career. Those who have high job satisfaction presumably keep working longer than those who do not, and have more fun while they are working.

# Length of Training

The majority of medical students do not make specialty choices based on the length of required training. The pleasure they get out of practicing a specialty, which interests them generally, pays them back for the added training.

The length of training does seem to influence some medical students, particularly those selecting generalist or support specialties. The amount of this influence increases as the student's debt rises, becoming particularly strong at debt levels above $75,000. While this may be understandable, it is sad to think that after expending so much effort, an individual might make a life-long career decision on such a flimsy basis.

One point worth noting, however, is that longer training does not always equate to additional income. In the medical subspecialties, for example, Gastroenterologists have large incomes because they spend some time specializing, but Rheumatologists make scarcely more than a General Internist. This doesn't mean that those who have a calling in Rheumatology should not pursue this specialty, only that extra education does not always equate to an increased income.

# Work Hours

Income must not be the only factor you consider. Work hours and lifestyle also become important once you complete residency. Even during residency, the hours worked by PGY-2 and higher-level residents in a specialty often mimic the work hours expected in that specialty. Figure 3.3 shows the hours different specialists work doing patient care, and Figure 5.3 shows patient-care hours in relation to the total time some specialists devote to professional activities. A comparison with Figure 5.1 shows that the hours worked do not correlate with income.

The hours a physician puts into his or her work will markedly influence his or her type of family life and extracurricular activities. If you expect to have any life outside of medicine, consider this carefully. Also, note that

FIGURE 5.3
### *Average Weekly Work Hours of Different Specialists*

| Specialty | Patient Care | All Professional Activities |
|---|---|---|
| Obstetrics/Gynecology | 59.9 | 64.3 |
| Radiology | 56.5 | 60.7 |
| Cardiovascular Diseases | 55.9 | 61.7 |
| Gastroenterology | 55.9 | 60.0 |
| Anesthesiology | 55.5 | 60.0 |
| Orthopedic Surgery | 55.0 | 55.0 |
| Gen Internal Medicine | 53.8 | 59.0 |
| General Surgery | 53.1 | 58.2 |
| Family Practice | 51.3 | 55.0 |
| Pediatrics | 48.6 | 54.2 |
| Psychiatry | 44.5 | 50.2 |
| Pathology | 42.9 | 49.0 |
| Emergency Medicine | 41.0 | 47.4 |
| Dermatology | 40.7 | 45.6 |

Adapted from: American Medical Association. *Socioeconomic Characteristics of Medical Practice, 1999-2000.* Chicago, IL: AMA, 1999, pp. 4-0-1.

much of the time a Surgeon or Obstetrician spends at work may be "down time" spent waiting for an available operating room or for a woman in labor. Much of this time may also be in the middle of the night, on weekends, and on holidays.

Many specialists now join group practices to decrease their work hours and on-call time. Depending on the nature of the group, some physicians have found this quite helpful. This has resulted in a large variation in work hours not only among specialties, but also within each individual specialty. Therefore, a specialty's work hours should not be your only consideration when choosing a specialty—but they are a factor that should be taken seriously.

## The Potential Future

It is difficult to predict either the need for or the supply of U.S. physicians in the future—either in total or by specialty. Physician oversupply and maldistribution has been an issue in the United States at least since an 1895 *Journal of the American Medical Association* discussion of the topic, which concluded, "our 'excess of doctors' would disappear at once" if the physician population was equitably distributed.

In the early 1990s, experts predicted an oversupply of as many as 165,000 physicians by the year 2000. Yet these dire predictions have not come to pass. *Anticipating future physician and specialty supply and demand is a very inexact science.*

There have also been suggestions that there will be an increasing physician shortage, becoming serious around the year 2011. Factors cited in support of this hypothesis are:

- The aging of the population.
- A decreasing workload for residents.
- An increasing supply of women in medicine (with a documented decrease in the average total lifetime years working in the profession).
- An increasing number of AIDS and other, similar disease cases.
- Shorter working hours for all physicians due to the increase in alternative health plans, legislative requirements, and changing lifestyles.

Physicians may also continue to retire earlier. In recent years, physician retirement rates have increased significantly. The probability of a physician retiring between the ages of 55 and 74 increased by 60% in the past decade. Above the age of 60, employed physicians consistently retired earlier than those in solo or group practices. According to AMA estimates, increasing retirement rates may absorb as much as one-third of the projected growth in physician supply by the year 2020.

Figure 5.4 shows estimates of the increase of physicians in the major specialties over the next ten and twenty years. Of particular note is that most of the non-primary care specialists will "max out" around 2010 and then the supply will begin to decrease. But again, these are only estimates.

Even though they are based somewhat on projected future needs, the numbers in Figure. 5.4 are highly speculative. While a decreasing birth rate may suggest a need for fewer Pediatricians, a new health care system allowing children greater access may increase the need. No one knows whether advances in the treatment of coronary artery disease will favor a need for more Invasive Cardiologists (those who pass catheters under x-ray guidance) rather than for more Thoracic Surgeons. Changes in both the treatment of chronic renal disease and the government's and public's attitude toward chronic renal dialysis programs will profoundly affect the need for Nephrologists. Finding an organic basis for more major psychoses may reduce the need for Psychiatrists, while increasing the need for (and effectiveness of) Neurologists.

And, if history is any guide, AIDS will be only one of many epidemics requiring more Family Physicians, Internists, and Infectious Diseases specialists. Primary care physicians will clearly increase in numbers. Whether that will result in too many primary care physicians is uncertain.

FIGURE 5.4

*Change in Number and Percentage of M.D. Physician Specialists, 2000, 2010, and 2020*

| Specialty | Number of (Percent of All) Physicians | | | | | |
|---|---|---|---|---|---|---|
| | 2000 | | 2010 | | 2020 | |
| **PRIMARY CARE** | **249,406** | **(34.6)** | **300,590** | **(37.3)** | **339,038** | **(40.1)** |
| Gen/Family Practice | 87,803 | (12.2) | 107,052 | (13.3) | 123,339 | (14.6) |
| Gen Internal Medicine | 109,264 | (15.2) | 128,938 | (16.0) | 142,047 | (16.8) |
| Gen Pediatrics | 52,339 | (7.3) | 64,601 | (8.0) | 73,652 | (8.7) |
| **NON-PRIMARY CARE** | **470,435** | **(65.4)** | **504,702** | **(62.7)** | **505,454** | **(59.9)** |
| Medical Subspecialties | 76,751 | (10.7) | 91,823 | (11.4) | 98,734 | (11.7) |
| Pediatric Subspecialties | 10,115 | (1.4) | 13,519 | (1.7) | 15,854 | (1.9) |
| Obstetrics/Gynecology | 41,759 | (5.8) | 46,088 | (5.7) | 48,009 | (5.7) |
| General Surgery | 34,229 | (4.8) | 34,452 | (4.3) | 33,739 | (4.0) |
| Surgical Subspecialties | 83,185 | (11.6) | 84,214 | (10.5) | 80,515 | (9.5) |
| Emergency Medicine | 21,755 | (3.0) | 23,497 | (2.9) | 22,644 | (2.7) |
| Psychiatry | 47,452 | (6.6) | 49,275 | (6.1) | 48,183 | (5.7) |
| Radiology | 34,866 | (4.8) | 35,057 | (4.4) | 32,972 | (3.9) |
| Anesthesiology | 37,073 | (5.2) | 41,949 | (5.2) | 43,120 | (5.1) |
| Pathology | 20,013 | (2.8) | 20,483 | (2.5) | 19,686 | (2.3) |
| Other Specialties | 63,238 | (8.8) | 64,344 | (8.0) | 61,997 | (7.3) |

Data supplied by the Center for Health Policy Research, American Medical Association, Chicago, IL: December 1999.

Basically, medicine does not remain static. Rather, it is an ocean of care with many storms and currents. The storms are the major new medical discoveries, new diseases, and changes in the demographics of the population. The currents are the changes in attitudes, within both the medical community and the public concerning the popularity of various medical practices. (Yes, unfortunately, medicine is guided by more than pure science.) Your ship will sail this ocean. Care, foresight, and a willingness to occasionally alter course slightly will keep you afloat.

## Difficulty of Getting A Residency Position

The difficulty you have in getting an individual residency position will vary with the amount of preparation you do, including correctly matching your aptitudes and accomplishments with a program's needs. However, you can "guesstimate" how difficult it will be to match with each specialty using the tables in the *NRMP Data Book*, or the NRMP "Results Book," each of which is published annually by the National Resident Matching Program, 2501 M Street N.W., Suite 1, Washington, DC 20037-1307.

For example, in 1999, the average specialty offering PGY-1 positions through the NRMP PGY-1 Match filled 89% of the available spots (although additional spots were filled outside of or after the Match). Those filling higher percentages, and thus being more difficult to match in, were Orthopedic Surgery (527 spots; 99%); Pediatrics-Categorical (2,104 spots; 99%); Emergency Medicine (912 spots; 97%); General Surgery-Categorical (1,009 spots; 96%); Internal Medicine-Categorical (4,753 spots; 95%); Psychiatry (908 spots; 94%); and Obstetrics and Gynecology (1,127 spots; 93%).

These numbers, and those in the charts available in the *NRMP Directory,* do not include all the positions available to you. A more accurate picture can be seen by comparing some of these numbers with those in Figure 22.2. Several specialties, including Ophthalmology, Neurology, Neurosurgery, Otolaryngology, Plastic Surgery, Urology, and some of the Internal Medicine subspecialties, hold separate Matches for some or most of their positions at the PGY-2 or higher level (see Figure 22.8). These Matches occur both through the NRMP and outside of it. Many programs in Child Neurology, Preventive Medicine (Aerospace, Occupational, and Public Health/General Preventive Medicine), Nuclear Medicine, and Osteopathic residencies require direct application to the programs.

Usually, programs accepting students for an advanced-level position require applicants to match separately in a Preliminary or Transitional internship program for their first year. The students themselves must usually arrange for this training, which means going through the NRMP Match to get a first-year slot. On occasion, the specialty program will arrange the first-year position. Find out how it usually works in the specialty of your choice by writing the specialty's board or society. However, you also need to check with the individual programs, as first-year arrangements may vary from program to program, even within the same specialty. Note that the rules for some specialties change yearly.

# 6

# Starting The Process

*There are three types of people: those who make things happen,*
*those who watch things happen, and those who wonder what happened.*
– Anonymous

## Choosing An Adviser/Mentor

Selecting a mentor *is one of the most important career decisions you will ever make*. Most students, however, don't have mentors—they only have "advisers." These faculty members, usually chosen by the Dean, often have multiple advisees and little time for any of them. They may not even have any interest in actually helping students advance their careers in the right direction. *You need a mentor!*

Selecting a mentor is serious business. When you were born, you could not choose your parents. You now, however, have a choice of mentor. And make no mistake about it, you are choosing a surrogate parent. At best, your mentor can simplify the whole process of selecting your specialty, choosing a desirable residency program, and getting into that program. At worst, a mentor can obstruct your decision-making process by putting the roadblocks of guilt and favors in the way of a correct personal choice.

Your mentor is the individual who will help you make the most of your medical school education. He or she will get you over the rough spots, show you opportunities that you otherwise might miss, guide your career, and generally think of your interests above those of other medical students. Your mentor is your guide, your teacher, your role model. But finding one is up to you. It will take effort, initiative, and assertiveness on your part to locate the right individual. The choice is yours—you can either find a mentor or resign yourself to struggling through on your own.

## Choose Early

You should select your mentor early to have the widest possible selection and to fully use his or her expertise. "I'm only in my second semester," you say. "I'll wait until I have had some clinical experience." Baloney! The longer you wait, the less likely it is that your mentor will be:

- your first choice
- a mentor, rather than a standard "adviser"
- able to actually help you very much

A young man showed up in my office one day. Asking if he could have a few moments to talk to me, he explained that he had just been accepted into medical school. He would be starting classes in about six months and wanted to know if I would be his adviser. (His approach was correct. Using the word "mentor" often frightens faculty members.) He explained that he was not sure what field of medicine he wanted to enter, but thought that he had an interest in Emergency Medicine. I agreed to "advise" this student. As his mentor, I was able to introduce him to early clinical experiences, guide him to research opportunities, and help him over some rough spots in his life.

During his clinical years, I showed him alternative paths to enable him to get the most out of his clinical experiences, prepared him for the entire residency matching process, and used personal contacts to get him interviews that he desired. He got into his first choice of residency programs. That, in part, was because he was savvy enough about both medical school and the residency selection process to have a mentor help him get the most out of those experiences. But, in fact, getting a supportive mentor is no different in medicine than it is in any field of endeavor. The trick is, start early!

## What Type of Person?

When Odysseus went on his travels, Mentor was the person he entrusted with caring for his house and son. He looked for a wise and faithful counselor. That is also what you seek.

The individual you want as your mentor has five characteristics: clinical experience, approachability, the understanding and willingness to work through your insecurities, the character to act as your personal and professional role model, and a vested interest in helping you become successful, regardless of the specialty you ultimately choose.

How do you find a mentor? This will take some effort on your part. Start by making contacts with upper-level (third- and fourth-year) students. They should be doing clinical rotations, and so can be found at the hospital in the evening and at night. Two good places to make contact are in the hospital cafeteria and in the library. Introduce yourself as a fellow medical student and tell them that you need some advice. Unless they are in a rush to get somewhere (the life of a medical student is a harried one) they will be honored by your interest. The question you need to ask is, "Who are the best clinical teachers at the school?" Ask several students for their opinions. This will get you started.

### Usually Clinical

Some students select their advisers by picking faculty members with the highest professorial rank in their College of Medicine catalog. Some students may be lucky enough, using this method, to get counselors who are both interested in them and still knowledgeable about what they will need to do as medical students to get into a residency. But the primary requirement for becoming a full professor is research. Teaching really plays very little, if any, part in their promotion. So, choose a mentor from the faculty members who are still involved in teaching, rather than from those who have "retired" to their offices and laboratories. *Your mentor must be reasonably accessible.*

Why choose a clinician rather than a basic scientist? There are three reasons. First, the career that most students plan to enter is clinical medicine. You need someone who knows the clinical ropes—not just those in the lecture hall and the lab. Second, the most difficult decisions you will face as a student will revolve around your clinical rotations. In what order should you take the required rotations? What should you do in your senior year? Clinicians are the most qualified people to answer such questions. Finally, your role model should live in the same world that you plan to enter—clinical medicine.

### Pick a Known Teacher

Now you have a list of clinical teachers that other students consider excellent. Why did they choose these people? Being an excellent teacher takes effort. This effort stems from an interest in helping students to learn. It is also based on a deep and abiding interest in student welfare. Doesn't this sound like the type of person you want for a mentor?

Of course, given the recognition of their excellence by other students, some of these individuals may already have many students whom they are counseling. If they cannot add another student, ask if they can recommend an individual whom they feel would be an excellent adviser. These people can usually spot the gems among their faculty, so take their suggestions seriously. If one of them feels that they can add you to his or her group, go for it. You already stand out by showing initiative so early. You can now do several other things to enhance that positive image.

*Be visible.* This means showing up with some regularity at your adviser's doorstep. The best and most productive way to accomplish this is to spend clinical time with him or her. This could mean doing afternoon or Saturday morning ward rounds, scrubbing in on a Saturday morning operation, or tagging along during an evening clinic or an emergency department shift. Since you have chosen a great teacher, it probably will be no time at all until you are actively participating (at your level of expertise) in patient care. If you do this, be sure to wear appropriate attire. This is the time to start looking professional. And bring along a stethoscope. Here is where you will begin to learn to use it.

*Develop an image in your mentor's mind of a likable, courteous, and considerate individual.* It is always pleasant to have a cheerful person around. But fawning and flattery generally have a negative effect. Mentors can see through these false habits in a minute.

*Be respectful of your mentor's time.* Once a clinician has agreed to be your adviser/mentor, make an appointment to see that individual whenever necessary. This is the professional thing to do and your mentor will appreciate your consideration of his or her valuable time.

*Be clear about what you desire from your mentor* (advice) and what your mentor can expect from you (hard work and dedication). Don't push for anything else. If you demonstrate the hard work and dedication, all else will follow.

Notice that nothing has been said yet about your mentor's area of specialty. Having examined your options, you probably have a general idea of what you are aiming for in the future. But, at best, it will be a very rough guess at this point. Try to select a mentor who is in a field close to your interest. For example, if you are contemplating Thoracic Surgery, a Dermatologist should probably not be your first choice as a mentor. If you do get a mentor who is in the specialty you finally choose, so much the better. However, *your choice of the appropriate person as your mentor actually depends more upon the individual than on his or her specialty.*

## Steer Clear of Those with Blinders

Selecting someone who cannot see beyond his own chosen field of specialization is a real danger. You may discover this attitude early from such comments as, "The only real doctors are Surgeons," or "The only satisfaction in medicine comes from delivering babies." The key here is the word "only." At this point in your career, there is no "only," merely a lot of "maybes."

Too many medical school advisers and other faculty say "That's a bad career move" as they denigrate other specialties that students are considering. This statement is often accompanied by incorrect information about the other specialty. Instead, they should be supporting their students as they search for the best fit of a specialty with their personality, needs, and abilities.

If you find that your selection for mentor wears specialty blinders, bail out—fast. This is the right time to get another adviser—one with a broader outlook about medical practice.

## Supplement Later, If Necessary

Congratulations! You have gone through the process of getting a mentor early. This should help you through many of the rough spots in the road ahead. But now, after your exposure to Pediatrics, you are certain that you are destined to be a Pediatrician. Your mentor is an Anesthesiologist. What should you do?

First, make an appointment with your mentor. Explain that you have given the question of specialty choice a great deal of thought, and have decided on Pediatrics. If you have chosen your mentor correctly, he or she will understand and support your decision.

Next, ask if your adviser knows any Pediatricians, either from within the faculty or in the community, who could assist you in gathering more specific information about the specialty. Could he or she arrange an introduction or telephone ahead to say that you will be calling for an appointment? Then, visit these referrals. Get all the information and special help from them that you can.

But don't forget your mentor! He or she is still the physician who has your interests most at heart. Keep in close contact, and continue to run your major decisions by him or her for an honest appraisal. Your mentor can be a close contact and source of advice for the rest of your career—don't abandon that individual now.

## No Available Specialty Adviser?

While most students will have at least one local physician in their specialty of interest to act as a mentor, no medical center has specialists in every field. Therefore, some students will be faced with the problem of no one practicing that specialty (or trained in the field) at their medical school. What do they do? First, get an adviser who is sympathetic to your plight rather than someone who wants to steer you toward his or her specialty. Talk with the Dean of Students about this to get an appropriate person.

Next, contact the geographically closest physician practicing that specialty. If you have difficulty locating such a person, contact the national specialty organization for assistance. You can also check the "Physician Finder" section of the American Medical Association's website (www.ama.org). Contact that individual and see if they are willing to both give you long distance advice (E-mail, phone, mail) and have you visit their practice when you have time (weekends, holidays).

## Testing Your Specialty Choice

Once you think you know which specialty you might like, why don't you give it a try? Would you buy a car without taking it for a test drive? Of course not! Then why consider investing time, effort, and money to train in a specialty when you really don't know if you have found the correct one?

At graduation, only 20% of medical students are still interested in entering the same specialty that they wanted when they entered medical school. That is certainly understandable. But nearly 25% of all physicians change their specialties after graduation, either during their training or shortly thereafter. In many cases, this is due to poor planning. Be smart. Test your specialty choice before you invest too much of yourself in it.

### Volunteer Time

One of the best ways to learn about a specialty is to spend some of your free time on that clinical service. This is especially true if that specialty rotation is not available early in your third year of medical school. If your mentor is in this field, you should have no problem arranging this. Otherwise, he or she might help you contact a physician in that specialty with whom you can work.

No matter where you are in your training now, you are probably saying, "What free time?" The answer is that you have time to do anything that is important to you. *This is important.* Certainly you can arrange to have a half-hour or 45 minutes to participate in a portion of morning rounds before class. How about Saturday mornings?

What information are you seeking? Look at the specialists around you. Do they seem happy in what they do? Would you enjoy what they do? Do you want to have the same type of clinical practice? What don't you like about it? Could you put up with it for your entire career? These are just a few of the questions that you should ask yourself during your volunteer stint. Some of the questions you will ask yourself, and the clinical experiences that you will have, will differ depending upon your level of training and prior clinical experience. The farther along you are in your training, and the more in-depth your clinical experiences have been, the more subtle the questions you will be able to ask yourself about the specialty.

But this doesn't mean you should delay volunteering for clinical experiences to explore your choices. Rather, it means you should start early. The more of this type of volunteer time that you spend, the faster you will gain experience and be able to probe your specialty choice in depth. *Spend some of your time in a community hospital or office setting.* This will give you a broader view of how the specialty is practiced away from the academic medical center.

### Pre-med

This is an excellent time to volunteer in a specialty. You have time to spare. And you can find out something even more important than what specialty you want to enter: *You can determine if you really want to become a physician.* This must be your choice, not your parents', teachers', or friends' choice for you. And in volunteering, you will be able to see the amount of dedication, hard work, and commitment to continued learning that the profession requires. If a medical career is really what you want, this experience will renew your motivation. If not, it may save you a lot of frustration and help you to redirect your energies.

How do you volunteer at this stage of your training? Undoubtedly, it will be more difficult to get a volunteer position in a specific specialty now than it will be after you enter medical school. You may have fewer contacts in the medical field and less knowledge upon which to base a specialty decision.

Your best bet is to first approach your own family's doctor. Tell him or her of your interest in the medical profession and of your desire to experience medicine firsthand by "tagging along and helping out." Usually the clinician will be flattered that you asked, and will let you participate in at least a limited fashion. After a few months of this (stick it out, you are learning vital information on which to base life-long decisions), it may become obvious that you have progressed beyond the level of knowledge that this practitioner can offer. If the practitioner does not spontaneously suggest it, you should inquire as to whether there is a more in-depth (read "active") medical experience available to you. If you know this physician really well, you might even address the possibility in your first meeting. In many cases, of course, working with a practitioner of this sort will be interesting and intriguing. If that is true for you, stick with it.

Okay, you don't have a family physician and neither of your parents are physicians. (Physician-parents should generally be able to help you to arrange these experiences.) What do you do now? If you are not quite gutsy enough to walk in on a physician unannounced, try to get some leads from the staff at your college's student health center. If this does not prove useful, go to a major hospital in your area and volunteer to work in a clinical area.

The hospital you choose depends upon your interests. To start, you may want to pick the hospital that gets most of the accident victims (Level I Trauma Center). Ask to work in the emergency department. There you will see both a wide variety of illnesses and injuries and some of the activities of practitioners in many different specialties. You may even make some contacts that you can use in the future. If you have the opportunity and the time, it might even be useful for you to work as an emergency department aide. These positions are often available to individuals with little or no experience. Then you will really be part of the team and be able to interact with patients in an even closer manner. You will also get paid.

## Preclinical Years

If you are reading this between studying for Physiology or Pharmacology, you may question where you will find time to volunteer clinically. Nights, weekends, and holidays can all be used for this clinical activity, after the demands of studying (and the absolute imperative to find some time for yourself) have been satisfied.

Volunteering to work clinically during the preclinical years is an essential part of your career preparation—not only to help you choose a specialty, but also to remind you of why you struggled so hard to get into medical school. You have more clinical opportunities available than does an undergraduate student. Remember, you are a medical student. You will soon be a physician, and the entire profession stands ready to help you.

Basically, you will find yourself in one of two situations, depending upon the nature of your medical school. The first is a result of the traditional medical school structure, in which the major teaching hospital is adjacent to the school. There you will bump into "white coats" every day. And you will have little difficulty finding the time between classes to approach clinicians about working with them. The hospital and the physicians working there are oriented toward education and will, in general, be ready to accommodate you.

The second type of medical school is less consolidated than the first type. This makes it somewhat more difficult to get a meaningful early clinical experience. Either the basic science and clinical campuses are geographically separated or there is no specific or adjacent teaching-oriented hospital. (These latter are the "community-based" medical schools.) A mentor, if you have one, can be invaluable in assisting you here. If you don't have a mentor, you will have to approach local hospitals and practitioners on your own. In the case of widely separated campuses, success will often depend upon your persistence—keep trying if you are initially turned down.

With community-based medical schools, there are several options for locating volunteer opportunities. As when choosing a mentor, you can get leads from upper-level medical students. If your school offers Physical Diagnosis courses in the first and second years, use your instructor as a resource. He or she might actually be an individual with whom you can work in a real clinical setting. You can also approach physicians at the largest of the affiliated community teaching hospitals. They are more attuned to education than other practitioners. And even if the first physician you contact can't help you, that clinician can probably give you some excellent leads. If nothing else proves fruitful, try the county or state medical societies. Some branches have programs designed to pair students with practitioners.

The most important reason to obtain clinical experience in your preclinical years is to learn the relationship of the basic sciences to the practice of medicine. "But why will this be important to me as a physician?" asked a first-year medical student after a rather mystifying biochemistry lecture. The lecturer, a Ph.D. who proudly proclaimed whenever he had the chance that he had never been in a hospital as an adult, could not answer the student's question. He did not even understand it.

You are in medical school to become a physician. In almost every case, physicians interact with the ill and injured on a daily basis. If you wonder why the basic sciences are important, you may find the answers in the real and immediate classroom of clinical experience. Spend some time in clinical activities. It's worth it.

### Clinical Years

If you are already in your clinical years, mere additional clinical exposure is not what you need. You must spend time testing your tentative specialty choices.

"But when do I have the time?" you ask. The answer is, during "slow" rotations, on weekends, and in the evenings. If you find this to be too much work, rather than a joy, perhaps you have discovered the answer to whether you are really interested in that specialty. If you don't enjoy the work now, how will you feel about it in 20 years? Or 20 years after that?

By your fourth year, you should have made a reasonably definite and educated decision regarding a specialty choice. Some students wait until their elective time to test their specialty choices. That is too late. Unless there is an elective opportunity in the third year, you cannot afford to wait that long to make a decision. You should use the prime elective time early in your fourth year both to take rotations, such as an Internal Medicine or a General Surgery subinternship, which will help you to be a "star" when you take an elective in your chosen specialty, and to "show your stuff" to the specialists who will be writing your letters of recommendation.

At many schools, students are now allowed to postpone some required clerkships, such as Psychiatry, Neurology, and Family Practice, until their fourth year. This allows them time to experience other fields, such as Anesthesiology and Radiology, which have traditionally been reserved for fourth-year elective time. If it is not overdone, this may be a good chance to get a more in-depth look at an area you have strongly considered as a career.

### Reading (see the *Annotated Bibliography*)

There are several sources for material dealing with particular specialties. The first, and often easiest-to-access, source is your medical school's library. If you are interested in any of the more popular specialties, there should not only be factual material on the specialty but also biographies of individuals in the field. Also, look for articles highlighting the specialty in *The New Physician*, which regularly prints reviews of major specialties. Specialty journals, especially the "throwaways," may also give you an idea of the breadth of the discipline. This is particularly true for some of the smaller specialties, which do not get significant coverage in journal articles that usually discuss only the larger specialties.

Each fall, *JAMA* has a "Contempo" issue devoted to many of the major, and often some of the minor or developing, specialties. Narratives written by prominent individuals in each field discuss new and upcoming developments. They are generally well written and quite interesting.

Two other excellent sources of information are the Specialty Profiles from the American Medical Association and the *Glaxo Welcome Medical Specialties Survey*. They review the history, economics, and practice of most of the medical specialties.

For information about the smaller or newer specialties, you may have to turn to other sources. One, discussed in greater detail in Chapter 9, is the *Directory of Graduate Education Programs* which, in its sections on "Requirements for Accreditation of Programs" and "Certification Requirements," provides a wealth of information about each officially recognized specialty. The specialty societies themselves are usually eager to send interested medical students information about their field. Most also have websites with a great deal of information. Their addresses and websites are listed at the ends of the specialty descriptions in Chapter 3.

Ask your mentor or adviser for material about the specialty that you are considering. This individual may have information from a variety of sources, or may have produced some herself. Finally, you may want to borrow a standard text for the field (assuming that you are considering a lesser-known specialty that is not well-represented in the library). This should also give you a broad idea of the discipline's scope.

## Talk To Many Specialists In The Field

Specialty choices are often based on a student's interaction with one physician in a given field. Often this specialist is a parent or the family's doctor. Other times it is an assigned adviser or a respected member of the faculty. But no matter who the role model is, basing your entire career on only one individual's experiences can lead to disaster.

It is essential that you get input from a wide variety of practitioners as you try to decide on your medical specialty. If your interest is Dermatology, this does not mean talking only with the Dermatologists on the faculty at your school. You should also visit Dermatologists in private practice, group practice settings, and health maintenance organizations in your community. If there is a county or state society meeting for the specialty, try to attend it as a student observer. Normally, these specialty societies will warmly welcome you. You will then have a chance to talk with a variety of specialists practicing in that field, and will also hear about the problems they face in their practices and about their general attitude toward their own specialty choice.

Many physicians practicing today would not choose the same specialty if they had it to do over again. While some of this may be due to "the grass is always greener" syndrome, in large part it is because they made career decisions without adequate information and with inappropriate expectations. Get as much information as you can directly "from the horses' mouths." The grief you save will be your own.

## Match Your Choice To Your Needs

It is vital, when choosing the direction your career will take, to consider your personal desires.

Abraham Maslow, in his famous book, *Motivation and Personality* (Harper & Row, New York, 1954), sought to explain why people are driven by particular needs at particular times. He felt that all human needs are arranged in a hierarchy, from the most pressing to the least pressing (Figure

6.1). As each level of need is satisfied, it is no longer a driving force for that individual. For nearly all medical students, the basic physiological needs, such as hunger and thirst, have been satisfied. The safety needs of security and protection will be satisfied if you believe you will complete medical school, get into a residency program, and earn a living. The factors on this level, plus those on the next most important level, the esteem needs of recognition, self-esteem, and status, are very often the driving forces behind a medical student's specialty choice. (Most medical students can see that the social needs of love and belonging will be fulfilled in the future, if not now.)

What you must do, however, is look beyond these levels and try to visualize what you will need to reach the highest level—*Self-Actualization.* Basically, you must try to determine *what will be fulfilling to you for the rest of your life.* Will you be happy in your specialty choice at age 40? Will you be able to meet your life goals? (You are about to be a doctor so you have essentially achieved that goal.) This is something that, though easily stated, is very hard to do. Yet, if you give it some serious thought—reflecting on it and talking it over with those close to you—you may very well make a much better decision than you otherwise might have made.

FIGURE 6.1

**Maslow's Hierarchy of Needs**

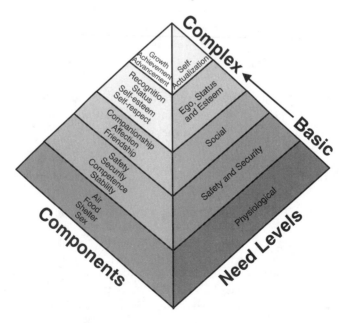

# 7

# Grades, Tests, & Clinical Clerkships

*Whether you think you can or think you can't, you're right.*
– Henry Ford

## Putting Your Effort Where It Counts

Succeeding in medical school takes a lot of work. But since there are many areas in which to work hard and only a finite amount of time and energy available to put into them, it is important to determine where you should put your greatest effort—and how to make it pay off.

Residency programs will use your grades, test scores, and, occasionally, "audition electives" to evaluate your medical school performance. Different institutions, and specific residency programs within those institutions, vary widely in how they assess the individual components of any candidate's application. How a particular program will evaluate different criteria is almost impossible to ascertain. The best you can do is to put as much effort as possible into each of the following areas. Your own personal strengths will help determine the areas in which you excel. The point to remember is that to do really well, you will have to put much effort into each of these elements.

### Honor Grades Are Important

Grades reflect your abilities over a wide range of activities. Therefore, they are one of the major factors used to differentiate you from other applicants. In the basic sciences, grades reflect your ability to gather, memorize, regurgitate, and occasionally (especially in schools with problem-based learning) synthesize information. Grades from clinical services reflect your ability to perform basic patient care and to memorize information. This is measured by how well you regurgitate the information for exams and synthesize it on the wards. Most important, grades from clinical rotations also reflect your social and interactive skills.

Getting "Honors" (equivalent to an "A" or a "4.0" on a four-point scale; also equivalent to "High Honors," "Outstanding," or "Superior" in some schools) sets you apart from your classmates—and, more important, other applicants. But it will be the rare individual, indeed, who will be able to get all, or even a majority of, "Honors" grades. So, it may benefit you to set your sights on particular courses and clerkships in which to make an all-out effort for "Honors," and to settle for "Pass" or average grades in the remaining classes.

If your school happens to be on a strict pass-fail system, you will have a slightly lower chance of getting into the most competitive residencies. You cannot change the grading system your school uses—at least not by yourself. So, you will have to concentrate on other demonstrable honors, awards, and letters of recommendation.

## Order of Importance
Okay, so you have decided to put extra effort into certain courses to get "Honors" grades in them. How do you decide which ones? Actually, it is not that difficult.

### Third-Year Required Clerkships
Your grades (not to mention your letters of recommendation) in required third-year clerkships are the most important. While the level of difficulty and type of experience you get in your preclinical years can vary widely among medical schools, junior-year clinical experiences are, for the most part, very similar—even though their grading varies greatly from school to school. Therefore, residency programs find them the easiest way to compare applicants. Also, unless you are going into Pathology, clinical work is the job for which you will be applying. Therefore, residency programs must know whether you are competent in this area. Since you will apply to the programs very early in your fourth year, most of the clinical grades that the evaluators see when selecting candidates for interviews will be those from the third year.

If you are entering one of the specialties that is required in the third-year curriculum, such as Internal Medicine, General Surgery, Pediatrics, Psychiatry, Obstetrics and Gynecology, and often Neurology or Family Practice, it will obviously be to your advantage to do well in that area. Otherwise, the two clerkships that normally carry the most weight in residency selection are Internal Medicine and Surgery. Make an extra effort to do well on these rotations.

Here is a note about your third year in general. You will probably find your junior year of medical school to be both the most exciting and the most confusing time during your professional career. You will be barraged by the different attitudes, rules of behavior, and personalities of the various specialties through which you rotate. Even if you have a good idea about which discipline you want for a career, don't close your mind to the experiences that you encounter. You might find a field that interests you more than your original choice. But don't rely on a single experience at a single institution with a single group of physicians to make your career decision. It may be very misleading.

In what order should you take your junior clerkships? Basically, it boils down to deciding whether to take Medicine and Surgery early in your year or later, after you have been "seasoned" by completing the "lesser" clerkships. The answer for you depends upon two things:

1. **How much clinical experience have you obtained during your preclinical years?** If you have had significant clinical experience, it matters little when you take any particular clerkship.

2. **Do you want to go into a specialty that is offered in the third year?** If you think you do but you are not sure, take that clerkship early to find out if you like it. On the other hand, if you are sure, take it at a time when you can be certain of doing well on the rotation. Again, if you already have a great deal of clinical experience, take it when it is convenient. If you are a clinical novice, then wait until later in your third year to "show your stuff." Going through other clinical areas first will improve your performance—and your grade.

### Specialty Clerkships

Next in importance to your third-year clerkships, and often of equal or greater importance in some specialties (such as Ophthalmology and Orthopedic Surgery), is your performance in your chosen specialty's senior clerkship. Where and with whom you take this clerkship is critical. If you plan on going into Radiology, taking a Radiology clerkship at the local suburban hospital won't work, no matter what the quality of teaching or your experiences. Use that site for extra volunteer time.

For a senior specialty elective "Honors" grade that residency programs view favorably, and to obtain a beneficial recommendation letter, take this rotation *at a major teaching hospital with an attending physician who is well-known to residency directors in the field.* Since you have ample leeway in setting up your senior schedule, there is no reason why you cannot find a suitable clerkship.

Remember that smaller specialties (e.g., Neurosurgery, Otolaryngology) and smaller programs prefer to take applicants they know. Use this to your advantage.

### Preclinical

Third on the list of priorities for getting "Honors" grades are the preclinical courses. This, of course, does not include those of you who are interested in going either into Pathology or into a research-oriented career. In both of these cases, "Honors" grades in the preclinical years are very important. For a Pathology residency, preclinical "Honors" grades will often be the most important selection factor.

If you are interested in a clinically oriented career, you should pick and choose carefully where to focus your main effort during the first two years. For those entering the Surgical specialties, "Honors" in Anatomy and Pathology are very helpful. Those contemplating any of the Neurosciences (including Psychiatry) should strive for excellence in their Neuroscience course. And for almost everyone else, the key courses are Pharmacology and Physiology. This is not meant to imply that you shouldn't try to make a clean sweep by getting more "Honors" grades. But in reality, this is just not possible for most mortals. So, direct your effort where it will count the most.

A strategy that some students find successful is to pick one major course each semester (or quarter) in which to try to achieve an "Honors" grade. Then, when you have a little extra time to study, concentrate on that course. While this strategy does not always work, many individuals have found that it gives them motivation to study just a bit harder.

### Senior Electives

The grades from senior electives are the least significant to most programs when choosing residents. *This does not include electives in your chosen specialty*. Other senior grades are considered very minimally—except in extraordinary cases, such as getting all "Honors" or, at the other extreme, failing or getting "Incomplete" in a course. All experienced residency directors know that "grade inflation," that is, a higher percentage of excellent scores than is warranted, is rampant on senior electives. This is especially true for electives taken outside the main teaching hospitals. So, don't expect to correct a dismal record with a lot of "Honors" grades from fourth-year electives known to be easily graded. Everyone will see through that ploy.

One problem for some individuals is that the grades for senior specialty electives will not be recorded in time to affect your selection for an interview. If you have done very well on a rotation in your chosen specialty, have your Dean's office send an updated transcript to the programs to which you are applying. Of course, if you didn't do well in some senior electives (too much time at the beach?), not having the grades on the mailed transcript will work to your advantage.

## Clinical Honors = Effort + Effort + Effort

Since so much emphasis is placed on doing well during clinical rotations, understand that you do not have to be either a genius or a saint to get "Honors" grades. All it takes is a realization that you will have to expend *effort, effort, and more effort*. This includes *in-depth reading* about the patients that you have seen, are taking care of, or will see (such as those in the operating room). If you have time, also read about the other patients on the ward. If you are scheduled to do a procedure, read about it ahead of time. And don't just scan the *Cliff's Notes*; get a book that will give you detailed information. If you can, also learn a few pieces of arcane trivia about the disease or procedure. These are always fun to introduce into discussions when making rounds.

*Know the ropes.* New rotations initially confuse all students and residents. Each service has its own culture, its own rules, its own body of basic knowledge, and its own stumbling blocks for the unwary. One way to ease your transition into a new rotation is to discover exactly what the service expects of you. (See Figure 7.1 for a list of questions to ask.) If you don't receive this information at least a week before the rotation, call or visit the rotation director's office to ask your questions. Often, the secretary will have a pre-printed list of the answers that are normally handed out the first day; get them in advance.

*Round early and stay late.* If you show up before the rest of your team to find out what happened on the ward overnight, you will be able to help the housestaff immeasurably. This often translates into glowing recommendations about you to the attendings. Stay late to complete any work that was left undone. If you are still there (doing something useful, not just hanging around) when the other students are gone, you will stand out as the hard worker you are.

*Volunteer for extra or onerous work.* Of course no one wants to put an IV into Mrs. Smith for the twentieth time or to push Mr. Jones down to radiology, but volunteer to do it with a *smile*. Not only will you make points, but you also may get priority in doing things that you want to do, such as the next thoracentesis or hernia repair.

In everything that you do on the clinical services, *show enthusiasm*. Be pleasant. Smile, even if it is after your bedtime (or maybe you haven't been to sleep and it's 6 A.M.). Everyone gets tired, but if you use the energy you still have to bolster everyone's spirits, you will earn big points—and will have a better time doing it than if you are sullen.

FIGURE 7.1

### Questions About Clerkship Expectations

- What are the goals and objectives of the rotation?
- What clinical responsibilities do students have?
- Where and when should I report the first day?
- At which facilities will I work?
- What is the call schedule? Is this in-house call?
- Is there a conference and lecture schedule?
- Do students carry pagers?
- Are there non-clinical responsibilities (such as a presentation)?
- Who is the attending? How often will I meet with him or her?
- Who will be the senior resident on the service?
- Which other students will be on the rotation?
- Is there a list of required or suggested readings?
- Are there printed descriptions of special clinical procedures?
- Are there study questions?
- Will there be written or oral exams? How many and when?
- Who evaluates students? On what basis?
- Can I see a copy of the student-performance evaluation form?
- Is housing available for out-of-town students?
- Can I interview for a residency position during the rotation?

Clinical services are increasingly using problem- and case-based small-group instruction during clerkships. How can you best perform in these groups? The hints below have helped other students perform well in these groups.

### Small Group Participation
- Show up for all sessions.
- Read required material in advance.
- Listen actively.
- Participate an appropriate amount of the time.
- Ask questions that improve discussion and understanding.
- Show respect for other group members' opinions.
- Relate positively and constructively to other group members.
- Encourage other group members to participate.
- Help to keep the discussion on track.

### Problem-Based Learning Hints
(Also useful for presenting cases on the wards.)

- Show up for all sessions.
- Read and research the Problem Case(s) and Learning Issues in advance.
- Prepare using MEDLINE, textbooks, journal articles, and expert faculty.
- Critically interpret information and information sources.
- Identify case issues that may lead to Learning Issues.
- Share information appropriately.
- Identify pertinent facts in the case.
- Present information in an organized manner.
- Formulate hypotheses.
- Identify the information needed to progress further with the case.
- Apply previously learned and new information to the case problems.

Finally, if there are written or oral exams at the end of the rotation— *study*. Find out early if there will be such a test (there usually is) and try to ascertain what will be on it. Then use your extra time (believe it or not there will usually be a lot of "down time" on the wards) to study. If you know what you have to study at the beginning of the rotation, the reading that you do about your patients will complement, enhance, and, often, shorten your study time.

The key to success on clinical rotations, as one student wrote in her personal statement, is to "Work like a duck: appear smooth on the surface, but paddle like crazy underneath."

## Licensing Examinations

The United States Medical Licensing Examination (USMLE) is now the standard licensing examination for M.D.s who wish to practice in the United States or Canada, no matter where they were educated. Osteopathic physicians may take either their own licensing examination or the USMLE.

Licensing examinations, however, are not used solely to obtain medical licenses; residency programs use them as screening devices to select applicants, many medical schools require students to pass them to advance or graduate, and some states require that physicians pass specific USMLE Steps before beginning or continuing residency training.

Many schools use Steps 1 and 2 as a part of their student evaluation system: 104 (of 128 total) U.S. schools require students to pass Step 1 to be promoted or to graduate; sixty-seven schools require passing Step 2. Pennsylvania requires residents to have passed Steps 1 and 2 (or equivalent) before beginning their PGY-2 year. Some residency directors are becoming hesitant to "rank" applicants who have not completed their school's graduation requirements.

The Federation of State Medical Boards now recommends that all medical students pass USMLE Steps 1 and 2 prior to entering residency programs. This means that applicants may have to prove that they passed both Steps before the date that residency directors submit their Rank-Order Lists to the NRMP (or earlier for the "early" matches). If they fail to do this, even if the students complete the Steps before graduation, they will have to either scramble to fill positions left vacant by their peers or lose a year while waiting for an acceptable position.

More than 60% of residency programs require applicants to submit Step 1 USMLE scores; approximately 40% require scores from both Step 1 and Step 2. Applicants who have taken both Steps 1 and 2 before applying to residencies may have a better chance of matching with the programs they rank highly—if they have done well on the exams. As a result of the rapid scoring possible after a computer-based exam and the automatic transmission (if requested by the applicant) of scores to residency programs, increasing numbers of applicants are reporting their Step 2 scores.

Steps 1 and 2 are also administered by the Educational Commission for Foreign Medical Graduates (ECFMG). They fulfill the medical science examination requirement for ECFMG certification. All international medical graduates should apply directly to the ECFMG to take the USMLE.

## United States Medical Licensing Examination (USMLE)

The USMLE (which some students paradoxically call "You Smile") has been given twice annually since 1992–94, when it replaced the old "National Board" exams. The computerized versions were introduced sequentially, with Step 1 beginning in May 1999, Step 2 in August 1999, and Step 3 in November 1999. The advantages of computerizing the exams are:

- Enhanced security (questions are drawn from a large pool of content-parallel questions in a very large question bank).
- Increased flexibility for examinees in scheduling their exam time (since all Steps are now offered throughout the year).
- Shorter testing times for Steps 1 and 2.
- Wider access to the exam.
- Faster score reporting.
- The ability to add new assessment methods to the exams.

The downside to computerization is the fear engendered in those who do not feel that they are computer literate. This was not a problem when the exam was tested. This "problem" should disappear as more computer-based learning and testing is used in schools at all levels. Some IMGs with less computer experience, however, may still feel threatened by the computer-based format.

### USMLE: An Overview

The computerized Step 1 is a one-day (eight-hour) examination consisting of seven 60-minute blocks of approximately 50 multiple-choice questions ("one-best answer" or "extended matching") each. Step 2 is a one-day (nine-hour) examination consisting of eight 60-minute blocks of approximately 50 multiple-choice questions each. Step 3 is a two-day exam, with a day and a half of multiple-choice questions and half a day of computer-based case simulations (CCS). All three Steps have many tables and graphs to interpret.

While the exact questions each examinee gets will vary, everyone is tested on equivalent content. The difficulty of the questions may vary, but the results are statistically adjusted so that all examinees are treated fairly. How well an examinee does on the initial blocks of questions may determine which subsequent blocks he or she gets. Within the time period allowed for a block, examinees may answer questions in any order, go back to review responses, and change their answers. However, once the block is over, the questions and responses in that block cannot be accessed.

One of the keys to doing well on the USMLE is time management. By doing the tutorial in advance, you save 15 minutes for lunch and breaks. By limiting the number of breaks you take, you save time signing in and out (and have longer breaks). Completing sections early also gives you additional time for breaks or lunch. Those who have taken the computerized USMLE recommend that you pre-plan when and for how long you will take your breaks, so that, under stress, you do not shortchange yourself on the allotted time for the test sections.

When taking the test, two-thirds to three-fourths of examinees who go back and change their answer for a prior question go from a wrong to a right answer. This is true if they change the answer because they (1) reread and better understand the test item, (2) use clues or cues in subsequent items, or (3) are correcting a clerical error. Examinees are less likely to select a correct answer if they are replacing one wild guess with another or if they just have a "gut feeling" that the new answer is better.

In Step 3, clinical case simulations (CCS) are scored against answers given by practicing clinicians and experts in the field. The closer you come to matching the ideal management, the higher your score. Potentially dangerous and unnecessary actions significantly lower the score.

The pass/fail standards for all Steps are set before the exam begins. There is no set percentage of examinees that must pass or fail. This standard is statistically maintained at the same level across administrations. Generally, examinees must correctly answer 55% to 65% of the questions on each Step to pass. Although the USMLE program recommends a minimum passing score for each Step, each medical licensing authority may establish the passing scores for their own jurisdiction. With computerized testing underway for about a year in early 2000, the recommended passing scores were 179 for Step 1, 170 for Step 2, and 177 for Step 3. These corresponded to 75 on the 2-digit scale.

**Scores** are mailed about two weeks after the exam. How do you interpret the scores? It has become rather difficult to do, other than knowing that you passed or failed. The formerly reported percentile score that rated examinees against a standard group is no longer being reported, resulting in a more-or-less "Pass-Fail" system. This makes it more difficult for residency directors and licensing boards to determine how well examinees who passed the exam did on the USMLE (although many residency directors will try to interpret the relative scores individuals get).

Unintended consequences of "Pass-Fail" USMLE scores include bland recommendation letters and an increased number of applicants being interviewed for each residency position (increasing costs for applicants and programs). Figure 7.5 shows past USMLE performance of various groups (although it was on the written version of the test).

### How to Apply?

United States medical students or graduates (M.D.s and D.O.s) apply to the National Board of Medical Examiners (NBME) to take Steps 1 and 2, and to their state medical board for Step 3. Application materials are usually available from their Dean of Students, but they can also be obtained from: NBME, Department of Licensing Examination Services, 3750 Market St., Philadelphia, PA 19104-3190, telephone (215) 590-9700. International medical students and graduates should contact: Educational Commission for Foreign Medical Graduates, 3624 Market St., 4th Floor, Philadelphia, PA 19104-2685, telephone (215) 386-5900.

The fee to take Step 1 or Step 2 is $280 (1999). Note that the fee increases if the test will be taken outside the United States, U.S. territories, or Canada. If you will be doing this, call the NBME Department of Licensing Examinations before submitting your application to determine the correct fee. There is an additional charge if a change of testing center or location is requested less than five working days before the test date or if the applicant does not appear for the exam or comes more than 30 minutes late.

### Steps in applying for and taking USMLE Steps 1 and 2

1. Apply to the proper contact to get an application packet.

2. The application packet includes a current application and return envelope, the *USMLE Bulletin of Information on Computer-based Testing (CBT), the Computer-based Content and Sample Questions* for Steps 1 and 2, and a compact disc (CD-ROM) containing practice materials, including an interactive tutorial and sample test questions. (The information on the CD-ROM is also available for downloading off the USMLE website. You can also obtain a scheduling permit (for an extra cost) to take these same questions during a 3½-hour practice session at a Sylvan Technology Center. These practice session fees are much more expensive outside the United States and Canada.)

3. Complete the application. If you must reapply for the same Step, you must again complete the application and submit a fee.

4. Type or print the answers in *black ink* on your application in *upper case block letters*. The form will be electronically scanned, so it must be in this format to be processed.

5. Follow the instructions next to each item on the application.

6. Select a three-month period during which you prefer to take the exam (Item #3 on the application). Be sure that the three-month time period begins at least six weeks from the date you mail your application to allow time for your application to be processed.

7. Attach a photograph with tape or glue.

8. Have the identification form *certified* by a school official (medical student) or notary public (graduate).

9. *SIGN* the application (Item #14 on the application).

10. Enclose the *fee* as a check or money order in *U.S. currency* with your name and Social Security number, Canadian Social Insurance number, or National Identification number on it.

11. Mail your completed application and fee to the National Board of Medical Examiners, P.O. Box 8500-1330, Philadelphia, PA 19178-1330. If you use an express carrier, mail it to CoreStates Bank, Fourth Floor-F/C 1-2-4-3, NBME LB#1330, 401 Market St., Philadelphia, PA 19106-1330. *Do not use the NBME street address.*

12. *If you do not take the examination during your assigned "eligibility period," or want to change your eligibility period or testing region, you must reapply and pay the full fee again.*

13. If you need special accommodations, such as for physical or learning disabilities, or attention-deficit/hyperactivity disorder (ADHD), get the official request form and instructions from the NBME's website (www.nbme.org) or from their Office of Test Accommodations. Return the form and supporting documents directly to them—not with your application, but mail them at the same time. Special accommodations may include assistance with keyboard tasks, audio renditions of the material, extended testing time, extra breaks, enlarged typefaces, or other adaptations.

14. Once your application is processed, you will receive a "Scheduling Permit" which will include the dates of your three-month eligibility period, your exam code(s), instructions for scheduling your examination with a Sylvan Technology Center, your Scheduling Number (SN), and your Candidate Identification Number (CIN). If you do not receive this material or lose it, call the NBME between 8 A.M. and 5 P.M. Eastern Time.

15. Call the Sylvan Technology Center immediately when your receive your permit. They work on a first-come, first-served basis. Before calling Sylvan, select several alternative dates and testing locations. When scheduling your exam, you will need to have your SN. To unlock your test at the Center, you will need your CIN. (Keep these numbers confidential.)

16. If you want to reschedule your test date within your eligibility period, you must either use Sylvan's automated telephone scheduling system or personally speak to a Sylvan staff member about it at least five working days before your scheduled date—or you will have to pay them an extra fee.

17. On test day, get to the test center at least 30 minutes before the exam. If you are more than 30 minutes late, you will not be admitted and will have to pay a rescheduling fee if you still want to take the test.

18. On arrival, you will sign in, present your Scheduling Permit and a photo/signature ID with the name *exactly matching* that on your Scheduling Permit (such as a driver's license, passport, national identity card, or other form of unexpired government-issued identification). Without these, you will not be allowed to take the test. They will then take a digital photo of you. (There *is* a reason they call this test You-Smile!)

19. You are then required to place all personal items (including digital watches, food, beverages, pagers, cellular phones, brimmed hats, bookbags, handbags, backpacks, books, notes or study materials, calculators, watches with computer communication or memory capability, and radios) in a small locker. If you need to keep a personal item (such as food for a diabetic) with you, you will need to apply in advance for special accommodations (see #13 above).

20. A proctor will offer you a pair of earplugs, will give you an erasable writing board, marker, and tissues to use for erasures, escort you to a testing room, and instruct you how to adjust the mouse and monitor. Entering your CIN will initiate a 15-minute tutorial explaining how the test works. If you wish, you can immediately exit this tutorial and begin the test.

21. *Hint:* During each exam day, there are at least 45 minutes of "break time," including the lunch period, you can take as you wish. Additional break time accrues if examinees skip the 15-minute tutorial (because they are already familiar with the testing method through reviewing the CD-ROM or website or taking a practice session), or if they complete a question block early. Be careful not to use up all the break time early in the testing day. If you leave the testing room during a test block, however, it will be reported as an irregularity.

22. Upon completing the test, give your Permit to the proctor, sign out of the Center, and get a Test Completion Notice.

23. You must complete the entire examination (although you may not have time to answer all questions) to receive a score. If you leave the test early, you will not receive a score. If computer or technical problems develop, notify a proctor and they will make the necessary adjustments.

24. Scores are mailed within two weeks of the exam to examinees and to LCME- and AOA-accredited medical schools for their students and graduates. No scores are ever reported by telephone or fax. (This rapid score reporting and their electronic transmission to residency programs will help those who are worried about taking Step 2 late and not having the scores with their applications.)

### USMLE: Common Questions

*Must I take the Steps in order?* You may take either Step 1 or Step 2 first, but you must pass both before taking Step 3. If you fail a Step, you must resubmit the same application and fee as you did the first time to retake it. You must wait at least 60 days to retake the test and cannot take it more than three times in a 12-month period. While the USMLE program recommends that examinees complete all three Steps within a seven-year period (that begins when you take your first USMLE exam) and not be allowed to take any Step more than six times without evidence of additional education, these requirements vary with each licensing body.

*Can I retake a Step?* If you pass a Step, you may not retake it unless the licensing authority requires you to do so.

*What does the USMLE transcript include?* The USMLE transcript includes your history of all attempts to pass USMLE Steps as well as any previously taken NBME Parts or FLEX examinations (old licensing tests). It also includes notations about any examinations for which no scores were reported (incomplete examinations or indeterminate scores), any test accommodations that were provided (generally to adapt to disabilities), any incidents of irregular behavior (e.g., cheating), and any actions that credentialing or licensing authorities have taken against you.

### USMLE: Irregular Behavior

A USMLE examinee's "irregular behavior" is serious and, if confirmed, becomes a part of his or her USMLE record that is sent to medical licensing authorities and residency programs. The examinee may also be barred from future USMLE exams (if they haven't completed the series) meaning that they cannot be licensed in the United States. if they are an M.D., or they may be required to take the test under special conditions. "Irregular behavior" includes:

- Seeking or obtaining access to examination materials prior to the exam.
- Falsifying information on the application or registration forms.
- Taking the exam without being eligible for it.
- Impersonating an examinee or hiring a proxy to take the exam.
- Copying answers from another examinee or looking at another examinee's computer screen.
- Allowing your answers to be copied.
- Making notes of any kind during the exam except on the non-removable, erasable writing surface provided examinees.
- Failure to adhere to test center staff's instructions.
- Disruptive behavior at the test center.
- Possessing photographic, communication, or recording devices, including electronic pagers and cellular telephones.
- Altering or misrepresenting examination scores.

- Theft of or other unauthorized possession of examination materials.
- Any unauthorized reproduction (including memorizing and distributing) of examination materials.

## USMLE: The Steps

### Step 1

Step 1 is a one-day, eight-hour multiple-choice examination that assesses examinees' understanding of and ability to apply key basic biomedical science concepts. It emphasizes the principles and mechanisms of health, disease, and therapeutic modalities. Integrating material across subject areas, most test items apply basic science principles to clinical situations and include interpreting illustrations or other problem-solving skills. "Multiple-choice" on all parts of the USMLE includes both single-answer questions and "extended-matching" questions. (Extended-matching questions have one long list of answers available for each series of questions.) Step 1 covers anatomy, behavioral sciences, biochemistry, microbiology, pathology, pharmacology, physiology, and interdisciplinary topics such as nutrition, genetics, and aging (Figure 7.2).

---

**FIGURE 7.2**

**USMLE Step 1 Content Outline\***

**1. Systems**
General Principles
Normal and abnormal processes not limited
to specific organ systems        40%-50%
Organ Systems
Normal and abnormal processes that are
system specific        50%-60%

- Cardiovascular
- Gastrointestinal
- Musculoskeletal
- Renal / Urinary
- Reproductive
- Endocrine
- Hematopoietic / Lymphoreticular
- Nervous / Special Senses
- Pulmonary / Respiratory
- Skin / Connective Tissue

**2. Process**
Normal structures and functions        30%-50%
Abnormal processes        30%-50%
Principles of therapeutics        15%-25%
Psychosocial, cultural, occupational and
environmental considerations        10%-20%

---

\*All percentages are subject to change.
Adapted from the NBME materials, August 1999.

The test is given in seven 60-minute blocks; each block of from 25 to 50 questions that cover all the subjects. The test items include pictures and tables, requiring the identification of normal and pathologic gross and microscopic specimens, and integrating basic science with clinical problems. Over recent years, the number of factual-recall questions has been declining while more questions that require examinees to answer based on integrating information from various subject areas have been added.

Most U.S. medical students take this Step after completing their second preclinical year. The NBME's Comprehensive Basic Science Subject Examination (CBSE)—given at most U.S. medical schools—seems to predict whether students will pass the USMLE Step 1. Like the USMLE, these tests have become computerized.

### Step 2

Step 2 is a one-day, nine-hour multiple-choice examination. It assesses whether examinees have sufficient knowledge and understanding of the clinical sciences to provide safe and competent patient care under supervision. It emphasizes health promotion, disease prevention, and clinical situations commonly seen during a primary care internship (Figure 7.3).

---

**FIGURE 7.3**

**USMLE Step 2 Content Outline**

**1. Normal Conditions and Disease Categories**
Normal Growth and Development and General Principles of Care
Individual Organ Systems or Disorders

- Blood & Blood-forming Organs
- Cardiovascular Disorders
- Endocrine & Metabolic Disorders
- Gynecologic Disorders
- Immunologic Disorders
- Mental Disorders
- Musculoskeletal System & Connective Tissue
- Nervous System & Special Senses

- Nutritional & Digestive Disorders
- Pregnancy, Childbirth, & Puerperium Disorders
- Renal, Urinary, & Male Reproductive Systems
- Respiratory System
- Skin & Subcutaneous Tissue

**2. Physician Task\***

| | |
|---|---|
| Applying Principles of Management | 15%-25% |
| Establishing a Diagnosis | 25%-40% |
| Promoting Preventive Medicine & Health Maintenance | 15%-20% |
| Understanding Mechanisms of Disease | 20%-35% |

\* These percentages may change.
Adapted from the NBME materials, August 1999.

---

Many questions require the interpretation of tables, laboratory data, imaging and other diagnostic studies, and gross and microscopic pathology specimens. Specific content areas include material from Internal Medicine, Obstetrics and Gynecology, Pediatrics, Preventive Medicine and Public Health, Psychiatry, and Surgery.

Nearly all questions are clinical scenarios where the examinee must provide a diagnosis, a prognosis, an indication of the underlying disease mechanism, or the next step in medical care, including preventive measures. Examinees must interpret tables, laboratory data, imaging studies, photographs of gross and microscopic pathology specimens, and the results from other diagnostic studies.

This Step is designed to be taken near the end of the final year of medical school, although many U.S. medical students take it at the end of their first clinical year (year 3 in most schools).

## Step 3

Step 3 is a two-day examination administered after graduation and usually during the PGY-1 year. It assesses whether examinees have sufficient knowledge and understanding of biomedical and clinical science to practice medicine without supervision. The knowledge base is what would be expected of a generalist physician, including non-emergency and emergency encounters with regular and new patients in various settings, such as clinics, offices, nursing homes, hospitals, emergency departments, and via telephone. It is heavily weighted toward clinically oriented knowledge and situations (Figure 7.4).

Candidates can take this exam after they have passed both Steps 1 and 2, received an M.D. or D.O. degree from a school accredited by the Liaison Committee on Medical Education (LCME) or the American Osteopathic Association (AOA), and completed their state medical board's required amount of graduate medical education (Figure 7.8). Graduates of foreign medical schools must have an ECFMG Certificate or have completed a "Fifth-Pathway" program. (See Chapter 14, "International Medical Graduates.")

Registered applicants should write to their state's board for the additional information contained in *USMLE Step 3 General Instructions, Content Outline, and Sample Items.* The address and telephone numbers of individual state licensing boards are listed in the USMLE *Bulletin of Information* or can be obtained from the Federation of State Medical Boards of the United States, Inc., 400 Fuller Wiser Road, Suite 300, Euless, TX 76039; telephone (817) 735-0722. Depending on state requirements, this Step can be taken during or after the PGY-1 year.

---

FIGURE 7.4

### USMLE Step 3 Content Outline*

**1. Physician Tasks**
Applying Scientific Concepts and Mechanisms
of Disease                                                    8%-12%
Formulating Most Likely Diagnosis                            8%-12%
Evaluating Severity of Patient's Problems                    8%-12%
Managing the Patient                                         45%-55%
  • Health Maintenance      • Clinical Intervention
  • Clinical Therapeutics   • Legal and Ethical Issues

Obtaining History and Performing Physical Examination   8%-12%
Using Laboratory and Diagnostic Studies                  8%-12%

**2. Clinical Encounters**
Continued Care                                               55%-65%
Emergency Care                                               10%-20%
Initial Workups                                              20%-30%

---

*These percentages may change.
Adapted from the NBME materials, August 1999.

Note that the application material for Step 3 is sent to your residency program director. If you change training programs after the Match or, if for some other reason, you do not receive an application, contact your state licensing board or the Test Administration Office, Step 3, National Board of Medical Examiners, 3750 Market St., Philadelphia, PA 19104-3190. Include your full name as it appeared on Steps 1 and 2, your NBME Identification Number which is on your Step 1 and 2 results (if known), your medical school and year of graduation, and your current address.

Since individual state licensing boards administer Step 3, the cost and rules vary. In 1999, the minimum cost was $150 (Virginia) and the maximum was $800 in Texas, with North Carolina close behind at $755. The average fee was $481. The number of times candidates can take Step 3 varies from once (Alaska) to no limit (in 18 states). Candidates generally have seven years to complete all USMLE Steps, although Rhode Island only allows six years, California gives candidates ten years, and four states (MI, NV, NY, NC) have no limit.

Scores are mailed approximately two weeks after the examination. Most state licensing boards have the results sent simultaneously to them and to the examinee. Some state boards have the scores reported to them first, and they then send results to the examinee.

Three types of questions (described below) make up the multiple-choice part of the exam: single item, multiple-item sets, and case clusters. The questions concentrate on therapy and management. They are based upon pictorial and graphic presentations of data (radiographs, EKGs, pictures of patients, photomicrographs, patient charts, etc.) and patient management problems designed to simulate actual patient encounters.

## Single-Item Questions

Single-item questions are typical multiple-choice questions in which you must select the one best answer. The question can be phrased in the positive, such as "What is the next appropriate laboratory test?," or in the negative, such as "What organism is NOT likely to cause the patient's problem?" For both types of questions, first read the case and the question carefully and eliminate the answers you know are wrong. Then, from those remaining, select the answer you think is the most correct. (This strategy does not work for extended-matching questions where there are up to 20 choices.) A typical single-item question is:

1. A 32-year-old man comes to your office with severe flank pain radiating into his right groin. The pain began suddenly about one hour before his arrival. On physical examination, you find normal bowel sounds, no abdominal wall guarding, rigidity or mass, no costovertebral angle tenderness, and no evidence of a hernia. His chest and rectal examinations are normal. The most appropriate next step is to:

    (A) do an intravenous pyelogram.
    (B) get a surgical consultation.
    (C) obtain abdominal radiographs.
    (D) obtain blood for a complete blood count and electrolytes.
    (E) test his urine for blood.

    *(Answer: E)*

## Multiple-Item Sets

Multiple-item sets resemble the single-item questions. The difference is that several questions stem from the same case description. These questions will usually flow in an orderly pattern, so you should answer them in order. An example of this format is:

1. A 15-year-old honor student's parents bring her into your office because one side of her face is drooping. They noticed this only this morning. She has no complaints. On physical examination, the right side of her face sags and she is unable to smile fully or close her right eyelids. Another likely physical finding is that she:

(A) cannot control her bowel or bladder.
(B) cannot wrinkle the right side of her forehead.
(C) has an unsteady gait.
(D) has difficulty completing a mental status examination.
(E) has dysphagia.

*(Answer: B)*

2. The most appropriate next step is to:
   (A) admit her to the hospital for further evaluation.
   (B) check for corneal abrasions.
   (C) do a CT scan.
   (D) get Doppler imaging of her carotids.
   (E) order a complete blood count and serum porphyrin levels.

*(Answer: B)*

3. In describing the prognosis for her condition, you would say that she:
   (A) may be all right after surgical intervention.
   (B) should be fine in several hours.
   (C) will need admission to intensive care unit for respiratory monitoring.
   (D) will need care for her eyes.
   (E) will need several days of intravenous medications.

*(Answer: D)*

END OF CASE

**Case Clusters**

Case clusters are vignettes followed by from four to nine questions. Additional information is supplied as the case develops, so it is extremely important to answer these questions in the order presented. Occasionally a question will be enclosed in a box. These are hypothetical questions related to the case's topic but based upon the information in the box. An example of this format is:

1. A 5-year-old girl's parents bring her to the emergency department because of difficulty breathing. She has previously been in good health and began complaining of pain in her throat about three hours ago. She now is wheezing, sitting forward, and drooling. When auscultating her lungs, you most likely hear:
   (A) diminished breath sounds.
   (B) expiratory wheezes.
   (C) inspiratory wheezes.
   (D) rales in both bases.
   (E) unilateral inspiratory wheezes.

*(Answer: B)*

2. The patient's oxygen saturation on room air is 87%. She does not want an oxygen facemask and pushes it away. Your next step should be:

(A) admit her to the intensive care unit.
(B) do an arterial blood gas analysis.
(C) examine her throat for a foreign body.
(D) have her parent hold the oxygen near her mouth.
(E) perform a thoracostomy.

*(Answer: D)*

3. If you obtained a chest radiograph on a similar patient that showed "steepling" of the tracheal shadow, immediate treatment might include:

(A) endotracheal intubation.
(B) immediate tracheostomy.
(C) inhaled albuterol.
(D) inhaled racemic epinephrine.
(E) topical cocaine.

*(Answer: D)*

4. Soft-tissue radiographs demonstrate [a swollen epiglottis. On the test, you would interpret the radiograph.] The most likely etiologic agent is:

(A) Bacteroides melaninogenicus.
(B) Haemophilus influenzae, type B.
(C) Mycoplasma pneumoniae.
(D) Parainfluenza virus, type 1.
(E) Staphylococcus aureus.

*(Answer: B)*

END OF CASE

## Step 3: Computer-Based Case Simulation (CCS)

In the CCS, the examinee provides care to simulated patients. Given the information in the clinical problem, examinees decide what treatment to give and when to initiate it. They must also monitor patients' responses to their interventions (or non-interventions).

During the CCS, examinees type on the "order sheet" their requests for information from the history and physical, order laboratory studies and procedures, request consults, and begin medications and other therapies. These are drawn from thousands of possible entries. As the case progresses, you can advance the time clock and re-evaluate the patient, check on test results, and learn the results of any interventions. By looking at the patient's chart, you can review vital signs, progress notes, nurses' notes, and test results—all under different tabs. Time is suspended (neat idea) as you consider what steps to take next. You cannot go back in "time," but you may change orders as the situation changes and as you move the patient between the office, home, emergency department, intensive care unit, and ward.

The computer monitors each action the examinee takes, with the highest score being given for thoroughness, efficiency, avoiding risks, timeliness, and avoiding unnecessary or potentially dangerous actions.

*To do well, you must become familiar with the Computer-based Case Simulation (CCS) software and understand how the simulated cases work before taking the exam.* Review all the orientation materials and do all the practice cases sent in your application packet or available at the USMLE website (www.usmle.org) or at LCME- and AOA-accredited medical schools.

Currently, the passing scores as set by the USMLE program are 179 for Step 1, 170 for Step 2, and 177 for Step 3 on the 3-digit scale, or 75 on the 2-digit scale. Each of these corresponds to answering 55-65% of the items correctly. Figure 7.5 shows past performances for various groups, although it was on written, not computer-based, tests.

### Sending USMLE Results

Unless an examinee writes to request that test scores not be sent, they will be automatically sent to M.D. and Osteopathic schools. Requests that scores be sent to others depend on which Step(s) you have taken and where you want to send them. Most residency applicants now have their results sent electronically via ERAS. Other requests must be made in writing to the appropriate body (Figure 7.6).

Upon receiving your written request plus a small fee, the NBME (ECFMG for international medical graduates) will send copies of your USMLE scores to residency programs. The form to use and the current cost can be obtained from the NBME or your Dean of Students. This "NBME transcript" includes not only your passing USMLE scores, but also any failing scores or "incompletes"; your results from any previous NBME licensing examinations (National Boards, FLEX) even if these scores were not originally reported; and notations about any special testing accommodations, "indeterminate" scores, test irregularities, and any actions taken against the individual by medical licensing authorities or other credentialing entities. After physicians take the USMLE Step 3, the Federation of State Licensing Boards, rather than the ECFMG or USMLE, sends out their transcripts.

FIGURE 7.5

## *Recent USMLE Pass Rates*

| Examinee | Pass Rate |
|---|---|
| **STEP 1 (A score of 179 is passing)** | |
| **U.S./Canadian M.D. Students** | |
| First-time taker | 95% |
| Repeater (overall) | 51% |
| Repeater (prior score 176-178) | 85% |
| Repeater (prior score 173-175) | 76% |
| Repeater (prior score 170-172) | 66% |
| Repeater (prior score 165-169) | 52% |
| **D.O. Students** | |
| First-time taker | 82% |
| Repeater | 28% |
| **ECFMG-registered** | |
| First-time taker | 62% |
| Repeater | 32% |
| **STEP 2 (A score of 170 is passing)** | |
| **U.S./Canadian M.D. Students** | |
| First-time taker | 95% |
| Repeater (overall) | 55% |
| Repeater (prior score 167-169) | 91% |
| Repeater (prior score 164-166) | 83% |
| Repeater (prior score 159-163) | 80% |
| Repeater (prior score 150-158) | 57% |
| **D.O. Students** | |
| First-time taker | 82% |
| Repeater | 50% |
| **ECFMG-registered** | |
| First-time taker | 56% |
| Repeater | 32% |
| **STEP 3 (A score of 177 is passing)** | |
| **U.S. M.D. Graduate** | |
| First-time taker | 95% |
| Repeater (overall) | 65% |
| Repeater (prior score 174-176) | 87% |
| Repeater (prior score 170-173) | 82% |
| Repeater (prior score 165-169) | 75% |
| Repeater (prior score 160-164) | 43% |
| **D.O. Graduate** | |
| First-time take | 94% |
| Repeater | 97% |
| **ECFMG-registered** | |
| First-time taker | 56% |
| Repeater | 41% |

Adapted from information on the USMLE materials, August 1999.

FIGURE 7.6

## USMLE Eligibility Requirements and Contacts

| USMLE Step | Type of Applicant | Contact to Take Examination | Contact to Send USMLE Transcript |
|---|---|---|---|
| **Step 1 or Step 2 only** | Students officially enrolled in and graduates of medical schools in the U.S. and Canada accredited by the Liaison Committee on Medical Education (LCME) or the American Osteopathic Association. | Dean of Students at your medical school  – or – NBME Department of Licensing Examination Services 3750 Market St. Philadelphia, PA 19104-3190 (215) 590-9700 www.nbme.org | NBME If registered through the NBME (as are most U.S. and Canadian medical students) and going to recipients (e.g., residency programs) other than licensing bodies (e.g., state medical boards). Results can also be sent through ERAS. |
| **Step 1 or Step 2 only** | Students officially enrolled in and graduates of Foreign Medical Schools. A "foreign" medical school is one that is located outside the United States, Canada, and Puerto Rico that, at the time of application to take the USMLE (student) or of graduation is listed in WHO's *World Directory of Medical Schools*. | ECFMG 3624 Market St. Philadelphia, PA 19104-2685 (215) 386-5900 www.ecfmg.org | ECFMG If registered through the ECFMG (as are most international medical graduates) and going to recipients (e.g., residency programs) other than licensing bodies (e.g., state medical boards). Results can also be sent through ERAS. |
| **Step 3** | All medical graduates who have: (1) Passed Steps 1 and 2, (2) Met their licensing authority's requirements (varies in different locales), and (3) If an international medical graduate, obtained an ECFMG Certificate or successfully completed a Fifth-Pathway program. | Medical licensing Authority (State Medical Board)  – or – FSMB Department of Examination Services 400 Fuller Wiser Rd., Ste. 300 Euless, TX 76039-3855 (817) 571-2949 www.fsmb.org | FSMB For any transcript going to a medical licensing body (e.g., state medical board). |

*Special accommodations*, such as separate rooms or increased examination time limits for students with disabilities can be arranged. If you have special needs due to a documented disability, contact the group that administers the Step (NBME, ECFMG, state medical board) as early as possible. They will then supply you with additional information. Of note, at least one medical school, Brown University School of Medicine, dropped USMLE Step 2 as a graduation requirement because of the National Board of Licensing Examiners' refusal to grant special accommodations for their students with disabilities ranging from slow reading speeds to vision problems.

*Future exams* will be different in both format and content. The NBME is exploring the use of "standardized patients" to simulate real patient encounters. These changes will probably first occur in Step 3; the patient simulators will be similar to those in the Objective Structured Clinical Examination (OSCE) already being given at many medical schools. (See the discussion of this test below.)

## COMLEX (Comprehensive Osteopathic Medical Licensing Examination)

COMLEX is the medical licensing examination path open only to Osteopathic medical school graduates. It replaced the old NBOME exam. Similar to the old USMLE written examination, it is taken in three parts (Levels). It is designed to assess whether the Osteopathic physician has the knowledge to practice medicine without supervision. Each COMLEX contains a variety of "Clinical Presentations" and "Physician Tasks" that get progressively more clinically oriented. Detailed topics covered in each test are available in the annual *Examination Guidelines and Sample Exam* booklets available from the National Board of Osteopathic Medical Examiners (NBOME), 8765 W. Higgins Rd., Suite 200, Chicago, IL 60631-4101, Phone: (773) 714-0622, Fax: (773) 714-0631; www.nbome.org.

All three COMLEX Levels are written multiple-choice examinations given in four 4-hour blocks over two days. The Level 1 and Level 2 examinations are given at Osteopathic medical schools or testing sites arranged by the NBOME. The Level 3 examination is administered at regional test sites near the largest concentrations of Osteopathic interns. Testing centers are listed on each application.

*Level 1,* usually taken in June of the sophomore year, covers the basic medical sciences of anatomy, behavioral science, biochemistry, microbiology, osteopathic principles, pathology, pharmacology, and physiology. Examinees must demonstrate that they understand the mechanisms of medical problems and disease processes.

*Level 2,* usually taken in August of the senior year, covers the clinical disciplines of Community Medicine/medical humanities, Emergency Medicine, Internal Medicine, Obstetrics and Gynecology, Osteopathic Principles, Pediatrics, Psychiatry, and Surgery. Examinees must demonstrate clinical concepts and principles necessary to make appropriate medical diagnoses through patient history and physical examination findings.

*Level 3,* usually taken in February of the first internship/residency year, covers the clinical disciplines of Community Medicine/medical humanities, Emergency Medicine, Internal Medicine, Obstetrics and Gynecology, Osteopathic Principles, Pediatrics, Psychiatry, and Surgery. Examinees must demonstrate that they can make the appropriate patient management decisions and solve medical problems at the level of an independently practicing Osteopathic generalist physician.

Examinees must complete each COMLEX Level in the proper sequence. Candidates who fail any part must retake and pass it to proceed with the next Level. Once passed, no exam can be retaken.

Each exam is scored on the number of items answered correctly, which is then converted to a standard score and a percentile score. The percentage of examinees who pass or fail the examination is not predetermined. The passing score for all Levels is based solely on a candidate's performance on the total examination, not on the performance of individual content areas. Examinees' standard scores are based on information about the performance of examinees who have taken the same examination in the current year.

The mean standard score for each Level is 500. A minimum standard score of 400 on Level 1 or Level 2 is required to pass the exam. A standard score of at least 350 on Level 3 is required to pass the exam. All COMLEX score reports are mailed to both the candidates and their medical schools' Dean within eight weeks of the examination. Level 3 score reports may also be released by the NBOME to the examinees' Directors of Medical Education. No scores are reported by telephone.

### Licensure

Passing all three parts of the USMLE or COMLEX (for D.O.s only) and completing the required amount of ACGME-approved or AOA-approved graduate medical training can be used to gain an initial medical license (Figures 7.7 and 7.8).

In most states, since the licensing bodies are the same for both M.D.s and D.O.s, physicians can use either examination for licensure. However,

---

### FIGURE 7.7
### *Examination Pathways for U.S. Licensure*

**U.S. Graduate Pathway**

| M.D. Student | D.O. Student |
|---|---|
| USMLE Step 1* | USMLE Step 1* |
| USMLE Step 2* | USMLE Step 2* |
| USMLE Step 3 | USMLE Step 3 |
| | – or – |
| | COMLEX Levels I-III |

**IMG Pathway**

ECFMG Certification:
USMLE Step 1*[+]
USMLE Step 2*
English Language Exam[+]
Clinical Skills Assessment
USMLE Step 3

---

\* May be taken in any order.
[+]Must be taken prior to the Clinical Skills Assessment.

Arizona, California, Connecticut, Florida, Hawaii, Maine, Michigan, Nevada, New Mexico, Oklahoma, Pennsylvania, Tennessee, Utah, Vermont, Washington, and West Virginia have separate Osteopathic licensing boards. Each has distinct requirements for licensure (Figure 7.9).

USMLE certification is also acceptable for initial licensing in the Canadian provinces of Alberta and Ontario. For further information about licensure, see U.S. Medical Licensure Statistics and Current Licensure Requirements, published by the American Medical Association.

One important note. NBME policy states that individuals who demonstrate "irregular behavior" and/or those who "subvert the NBME assessment or certification process" (i.e., cheat), will be permanently barred from certification by the Board. In addition, reports will be sent both to the individual's medical school and to the Federation of State Medical Boards. Don't say that you weren't warned.

FIGURE 7.8

### Graduate Education Requirements for M.D. Licensure

Number of years of accredited U.S. or Canadian graduate medical education (residency) required for a medical license.

#### One Year

| | | | |
|---|---|---|---|
| Alabama[1] | Idaho[1] | Nebraska[1] | Texas[1] |
| Alaska | Indiana[1,4] | New Jersey[1] | Utah |
| Arizona[1] | Iowa | New York[1] | Vermont[1] |
| Arkansas | Kansas[1] | North Carolina[1] | Virgin Islands |
| California[1] | Kentucky[1] | North Dakota[1] | Virginia[1] |
| Colorado[1] | Louisiana[1] | Ohio[1] | West Virginia[1] |
| Delaware[1] | Maryland[1,4] | Oklahoma[1] | Wisconsin |
| District of Columbia | Massachusetts[1] | Oregon[1] | Wyoming[1] |
| Florida[1] | Minnesota[1] | Puerto Rico | |
| Georgia[1] | Mississippi[1] | Rhode Island[7,8] | |
| Guam[1] | Missouri[1] | South Carolina[1] | |
| Hawaii[1] | Montana[1] | Tennessee[1] | |

#### Two Years

| | | | |
|---|---|---|---|
| California[2] | Indiana[2] | Minnesota[2] | Pennsylvania[1] |
| Connecticut[8] | Kansas[2] | New Hampshire | South Dakota[5] |
| Guam[3] | Maine[1] | New Mexico | Utah |
| Hawaii[2] | Massachusetts[2] | Ohio[2] | Washington |
| Illinois | Michigan | Oklahoma[2] | Wyoming[2] |

#### Three Years

| | | | |
|---|---|---|---|
| Alabama[2] | Kentucky[2] | Nebraska[2] | Pennsylvania[2,8] |
| Arizona[2] | Louisiana[2] | Nevada | South Carolina[2] |
| Colorado[2] | Maine[2,7,8] | New Jersey[2] | Tennessee[2,8] |
| Delaware[2,8] | Maryland[2] | New York[2,8] | Texas[2] |
| Florida[2] | Mississippi[2] | North Carolina[2] | Vermont[2,6,8] |
| Georgia[2] | Missouri[2] | North Dakota[2] | Virginia[2] |
| Idaho[2] | Montana[2] | Oregon[2] | West Virginia[2] |

[1]Graduates of U.S. medical schools only.

[2]International medical graduates.

[3]Canadian training not accepted.

[4]An additional year of residency is required if the applicant failed any Step of their licensing exam three or more times.

[5]Must complete a residency program.

[6]Canadian training accepted only from Canadian medical school graduates.

[7]May accept graduate medical education completed in England, Scotland, and Ireland for credit toward a license.

[8]May accept specialty certificates granted by non-U.S. boards for credit toward a license.

Adapted from: *State Medical Licensure Requirements & Statistics: 1999-2000.* Chicago, IL: AMA, 1999, Tables 5 and 7.

FIGURE 7.9
**Requirements for Osteopathic Physician Licensure**

Requirements for Licensure

| Do Not Accept USMLE | Accept AOA-approved training only | Two years GME required for license |
|---|---|---|
| CA, FL, MI, PA, | FL, MI, NV, | CT, DC, IL, |
| TN, VT, WV | OK, PA, WV | NH, SD*, UT |

*Must complete an entire residency program.
Adapted from *1999 Yearbook and Directory of Osteopathic Physicians, 90th ed.* Chicago, IL: American Osteopathic Association, 1999.

## Suggested New Medical Licensing Requirements

Medical licensing, the resident experience, and the prospect of resident moonlighting all were shaken by the Federation of State Medical Boards' (FSMB) May 1998 "Recommendations on Licensure." This body, comprised of representatives of all state medical licensing bodies, recommended that these boards adopt the following policies:

1. All M.D. and D.O. students be required to pass Steps 1 and 2 of the USMLE (M.D. or D.O.) or Parts 1 and 2 of the COMLEX (D.O.s only) prior to entering residency training.

2. Residents must complete three years in an ACGME- or AOA-approved postgraduate training program before becoming eligible to apply for full licensure.

3. Residents must apply to their state board for a state permit to practice as a resident, with the program director reporting to the board annually on any disciplinary problems or other problems that could impair the resident's ability to function.

4. All residents seeking training permits will undergo a criminal background check.

Some medical boards have either accepted these recommendations or are considering adopting them. This will mean that all physicians will need at least three years of residency training to practice medicine in the United States. It will also mean that, in states that adopt these recommendations, residents will only be able to moonlight (and begin paying back their enormous debts) at their own institutions. This may conflict with the ACGME's requirements, thus leaving residents no moonlighting opportunities.

## Special Purpose Examination (SPEX)

State licensing authorities use this one-day examination, containing 450 multiple-choice questions, to test the knowledge-base of physicians who seek licensure in a new state or relicensure in the same state *at least five years after graduation from medical school.* Increasingly, state medical boards require that physicians who were previously licensed in another state pass the SPEX before getting a license in their state. Medical boards also use the test before reinstating the license of physicians who have been inactive for a period of time. The pass rate is about 68%. This was the first examination for licensing physicians to be computerized. This test is *not* available as a licensing mechanism for graduating medical students.

## Importance of Passing The Tests

Residency directors are just learning that if applicants they match with do not pass the tests their schools require for graduation, they may not have enough residents in July. That is why even moderately competitive residencies may require you to submit evidence that you have passed any examinations (Steps 1 or 2 or the OSCE) required for you to graduate from medical school. Students at schools that require passing Step 2 to graduate may need to take this Step in August/September of their senior year. That way, they will be able to assure residency directors that they have passed the test and presumably will graduate on time. In addition, if you do not eventually pass the USMLE (or the equivalent examinations for Osteopaths), you will never practice medicine in the United States.

### How Important are the Scores in the Resident-Selection Process?

Although the tests are not designed for this purpose, many, if not most, residencies use applicants' USMLE or COMLEX examination scores as a *primary screening device.* Because of the unavailability of other information about candidates, the scores on licensing examinations, especially Steps 1 and 2 of the USMLE, become outrageously important. This is not the fault of program directors. They would like nothing better than a useful transcript (not all "Pass" grades), a specific Dean's letter (not saying that everyone "will be a fine clinician"), and school honors (such as AOA election) that are given out before they make Match decisions. However, even in this, the best of all possible worlds, the licensing examination scores are often the only objective way to evaluate a large pool of candidates from multiple schools with varying amounts of background and support material.

Residency directors know that when their program is reviewed, they will be judged, in part, on how many of their residency graduates pass the specialty's Board examination. (This information is also in *AMA-FREIDA®*, the AMA's *Fellowship and Residency Electronic Interactive Database Access.*) As one residency director said, "Our residency program is judged, in part, on how well our graduates do on their Board examinations. Doing well on the USMLE says that they are at least good test takers—and that's important." Good USMLE scores do correlate with passing specialty board examinations. In general, they also correlate with students' clinical performance in at least their PGY-1 year.

Although this practice has been officially condemned, the NBME has sent residency directors information on how to interpret the USMLE scores to screen applicants. At the most competitive programs and in the most competitive specialties, you must obtain minimum scores on these exams for them to consider you, despite any other credentials. The specific minimum scores vary directly with the specialty's and the program's competitiveness. Scores may not be considered at all in non-competitive programs, while some very competitive specialties and programs reportedly use USMLE scores greater than 210 to determine whether they grant applicants an interview (200 is the mean score; 20 points is the standard deviation). This alone suggests that the scores may be very important to you and that you should take the test very seriously.

For most applicants to programs in the NRMP PGY-1 Match, and for nearly all those applying to specialties with an advanced Match, only Step 1 scores will be available, since most students do not take the August/September Step 2 administration. This magnifies the problem of placing so much emphasis on these scores; for all but the future Pathologists among you, clinical experience is the most important factor in your success as a resident. Step 1 emphasizes the basic sciences. Much of the tested material is not clinically applicable. Nevertheless, Step 1 is an important part of most residency programs' selection process.

### How Much Effort Should You Expend?

Since the Boards are so important to your career, it is worthwhile to expend the extra effort to do well on them. Educators refer to these tests as "high-stakes evaluations," because they may determine whether you graduate from medical school, the type and quality of the residency program you enter, and whether you are ever licensed to practice medicine. Take heed.

To prepare for Step 1, begin by reviewing your notes and books from your two basic-science years. The key is to *review* material, rather than trying to learn it for the first time. This builds on your strengths and minimizes your weaknesses. It may be more difficult to prepare for Steps 2 and 3, however, since these require you to integrate material from several sources.

Most medical schools use USMLE-type questions for many of their examinations, so you will already be familiar with the format. (Some courses, however, have not changed their examinations in years, so they still use the old question format that the USMLE has abandoned, i.e., single questions with multiple true-false options.) You have probably also learned some of the tricks about how to take these kinds of tests. A few basic tips are listed in the next section.

Each of you knows how you learn best. For some, it is by reviewing notes and textbooks. For others, it may be by going over any one of the available specialized review texts. Many students recommend using the books from the National Medical Series for Independent Study (NMS; John Wiley & Sons, Publishers). These may, however, be too extensive and detailed for most students. Some students find that they do better studying from their own notes. The well-publicized national review courses are primarily for those students whose academic performance has been marginal, those who have failed the test once, or for IMGs who are not native American-English speakers. The five-week Medical H.E.L.P. Program at Marshall University in West Virginia is for those with learning disabilities and dyslexia. They can be contacted at (304) 696-6315; www.marshall.edu/medicalhelp.

These courses can be expensive. *Whatever the method or methods you use, it is important for you to take this test seriously and to do the best that you possibly can.*

If you did not do as well as you thought you should or could have the first time, *you do not have the option of repeating the test.* You can retake the exam only if you fail (Step 1, less than 179; Step 2, less than 170). If you retake and pass a Step, the passing score becomes the official National Board record, although transcripts that are sent out, will list all your attempts to pass the USMLE. Even if you successfully complete several subsections of a Step on the initial attempt, the entire Step must be retaken. Steps 1 and 2 may be taken as many times as are needed to pass.

Many of the students who fail Step 1 may do so because of reading problems or learning disabilities. Most medical schools are not prepared to deal with these difficulties. If you fail Step 1 and feel that a learning disability is the reason, you might want to contact either your school's education department or ArcVentures Education Services, 820 W. Jackson Blvd., Suite 800, Chicago, IL 60607. ArcVentures has a program, initially developed at Rush Medical College in Chicago, that has been very successful in helping medical students from around the country pass a retake of Step 1.

If an applicant fails Step 3, the licensing board may require evidence of additional training before allowing him or her to retake the exam. For licensure, most states require that all Steps be completed within a seven-year period, although some have longer limits (California, 10 years; Rhode Island, 12 years).

## Tips For Taking USMLE-Type Examinations

There are several things you can do to maximize your scores on licensing examinations They are listed below. The first, of course, is to know the material as well as you can. If you don't know the material, there are few tips that can help, especially on tests that have been written and field-tested by experts.

1. Know the material.

2. Get enough sleep the night before.

3. Follow a normal routine the day of the exam.

4. Wear comfortable clothing.

5. Arrive early enough to sign in and get your entire allotted time for the exam.

6. Check the test information to be certain that you bring all needed materials, e.g., admission card or identification with picture.

7. Be familiar with the test format so that you don't waste time taking the tutorial or floundering with the computerized test. (Do this by taking a computerized practice test and the tutorial on the CD supplied with the registration materials.)

8. Be familiar with the types of questions (single answer) that will be used.

9. Know how the test will be scored.

10. Use your time efficiently.

Mental preparation is the next key. Most people are familiar with pretest anxiety. Butterflies in the stomach, sweaty palms, rapid heartbeat and respiratory rate, and fear of failure do not necessarily mean you have lost the war of nerves. You merely have to steady yourself. It is said that Johnny Carson (during whose show you were probably conceived) had a heart rate approaching 160 just before he went out to do his monologue. And he did this for 25 years! The trick for you is to do everything as normally as possible. Get enough sleep the night before the exam and follow your normal routine the day of the test. Dress in comfortable clothes. Large testing sites are often either too warm, too cold, or alternate between these extremes. Wear clothing that can be removed or loosened to cool off and bring something extra to wear in case it gets too cold. Arrive at the testing site early to avoid hassles.

Read over testing materials well in advance of the exam date. Do not be caught short by failing to bring your picture ID or the admission card.

The testing materials you receive in advance will also tell you how the test will be scored and explain the types of questions used on the exam. The USMLE is scored by crediting the correct answers; there is no numeric penalty for getting a question wrong, although it will affect the subsequent questions you get for that block. If you don't know the answer, it pays to guess. Therefore, you need to know how to guess effectively.

Guessing effectively means knowing how to best answer the types of questions on the test. As medical students, most of you will be very familiar with the standard A-Type (single-answer, multiple-choice) questions used on the exams. These are essentially variations of simple true-false questions. To answer them correctly, use the following hints:

1. Even if "A" seems to be the correct answer, look over the other answers to be certain that a more correct answer does not exist. This is especially important on USMLE Steps 2 and 3.

2. If you cannot spot which answer is "true," read each alternative and mark the ones you believe are "false." If you can mark three answers (out of five) as "false," you have increased your chance of correctly answering the item from 20% to 50%.

3. Use the information you get from other parts of the test to help answer questions you otherwise would not know. A great deal of information is given in the stems (first part) of the exam's questions. Use this to your advantage.

4. Try not to change your answers. Change an answer only if you are *certain* that your initial answer was incorrect.

5. Look for long introductory clauses (foils) or the qualifying word "may" in true answers. Look for the limiting words "never" or "always" to spot false answers.

When faced with questions concerning a clinical case, first review the questions. These will often suggest the parts of the case that are most important and the key points to look for when reading the clinical description.

Finally, use your time effectively. This is possibly the most important strategy for successful test-taking. Do not spend too much time on any one question. If you don't pace yourself and then have to randomly guess the answers to too many questions, you will fail the exam. On the USMLE, you have only about one minute per question. Since each question counts the same, if a question is too difficult to be answered in a reasonable amount of time, make an educated guess at the answer immediately and make a note to go back to it for further work after you have finished the rest of the test. Initially skipping difficult questions is like a military force bypassing the enemy's stronghold—it is good strategy. Since you have taken examinations of this sort in medical school, you should know which path works best for you.

If you run out of time in a module, but are still working on a question, you are allowed to finish that question. The time, however, is deducted from your total time allotment, although it is generally worthwhile to try to answer that last question.

## If You Don't Have To Take The USMLE

A number of schools do not require their students to take Steps 1 and 2 of the USMLE. Some only require that the student pass Step 2. But unless you are an Osteopathic student, there is only one route to getting a medical license in the United States—the USMLE. You must pass all three USMLE Steps. In general, you will never be as prepared to take the basic-science-oriented Step 1 as you are during medical school. Take the test; not all residency programs require that you send a copy of your scores—and you must remember your priorities. While a low score on Step 1 might put you out of the running for a residency position, you will have passed the first hurdle to practicing medicine. Take Steps 1 and 2 while you are in medical school. Taking the USMLE during your preclinical years may well result in a high USMLE score to promote your candidacy for a residency position.

"But I took Subject Exams (also called "Shelf Exams") in my pre-clinical courses," you say. Residency directors place little stock in these test results, with good reasons. Performance on these tests, taken from prior Board examinations, is not directly comparable to performance on the USMLE Step 1. That is because rather than having to study for, and know, all the basic sciences at once, you take the Subject Exams immediately after you have intensively studied each subject, usually as a final examination for the course. These exams also do not contain the newer type of test questions or the inter-subject questions now found on the USMLE. This is similarly true for Subject Exams given in the clinical years. For example, students with marginal passing scores on the Subject Exams for Biochemistry, Physiology, Pathology, Pharmacology, and Microbiology still had a 25% or greater chance of failing the same section when they took their licensing examination.

## Are The Examinations Fair?

Some subgroups have consistently different results when taking both the USMLE and the COMLEX. This has raised some doubts about these exams' fairness.

Both gender and race seem to influence students' USMLE scores, at least on Steps 1 and 2. (These findings were actually drawn from the very similar NBME Parts I and II exams.) White men have the highest pass rate, followed in order by Asian/Pacific Islander men, White women, Asian/Pacific Islander women, and Hispanic men. Trailing badly are, in order, Hispanic women, Black men, and Black women. Many of the differences in test results could be predicted from the MCAT scores for reading or science problems.

On the COMLEX precursor, the NBEOPS examination, men consistently scored higher on Part I, and women scored higher on Part III. Men and women perform equally well on Part II. These findings remained consistent across all Osteopathic schools. Some researchers suggest that these findings result from a difference in men's and women's academic growth rates. The debate continues as to whether or not the variance in scores on the USMLE or COMLEX reflects real differences in individuals' clinical competence.

## Objective Structured Clinical Examination (OSCE)

Relatively new in medical schools, the Objective Structured Clinical Examination (OSCE) tests a student's clinical abilities. The OSCE uses "standardized patients"—either patients with stable physical findings (e.g., arthritis, heart murmurs) simulating disease symptoms or staff members trained to simulate such symptoms. These standardized tests evaluate how well students deal with real patients' problems, not just how well they score on tests, in class, or on the licensing examinations. Ideally, the OSCE tests whether a student can

- perform a focused history and physical examination.
- recognize pathological processes.
- interpret laboratory data.
- establish a relevant differential diagnosis.
- develop a management plan.
- clearly document clinical findings and plans.

OSCE examinations normally take about 6 hours (including breaks), with each station requiring from 5 to 40 minutes to complete. Some stations may be coupled, so that the second station relies on clinical information from the first station. Time and the number of stations are the two variations that do not seem to affect the test's validity. Students are scored at each station using a standardized checklist of tasks.

More than 89 (of 128 total) U.S. and all 16 Canadian medical schools now use the OSCE for clinical evaluations. Several require their students to pass it before graduation. In the future, more schools will undoubtedly use this test. The results will also appear in Deans' letters, most probably showing the student's results in comparison to his or her classmates. Since all specialties value clinical abilities in their residents, these test results may carry enormous weight with residency directors.

OSCE-type "simulated patient" encounters (probably computerized) may eventually be part of the USMLE. They already are part of the Medical Council of Canada's licensing exam and international medical graduates now must pass a similar test, the Clinical Skills Assessment Examination, to get an ECFMG Certificate.

## Summer Work

The Beach Boys sang that "you'll have fun, fun, fun 'til your daddy takes your T-Bird away." Even if you do not have any idea what a T-Bird is (a car) or who the Beach Boys are (a California singing group), you certainly know about summer fun. Unfortunately, now that you are in medical school, the sun and fun will have to be put in proper perspective. Summer, especially the summer between your first and second years of school, is your only free time to explore the tentative selections you have made concerning a specialty choice. But it also will probably be the last "free" summer that you will have for many years. The question for you is, "What is most important?"

There is no question that the pull to escape from the bookwork and laboratories of your first year is great. That is only natural. But escape into the world of clinical medicine. This should be an exciting and interesting experience on several counts.

First, it will be completely different from the classroom you have labored in for the past nine-plus months. Second, it will allow you to do what you got into medical school to do—practice medicine. This might rejuvenate you for your second year of studies. Third, it will enable you to see in more detail just what aspects of medicine you enjoy and what parts you dislike. Finally, you might even make some money.

The two places to start when exploring options for summer work are your mentor and the Student Affairs office. The latter will probably have lists of those clinical (and research) fellowships that are offered to medical students. While some fellowships are available through national programs (though not necessarily to first-year students), others are generally specific to a particular institution.

What you are looking for is *clinical experience.* In some cases, this will be obvious, e.g., it is labeled as a student clinical fellowship. Other times the clinical experience may come disguised as research, as in a Pediatric project where you will have to do specific parts of a physical examination on children to collect the necessary data. The point in summer work is to try, if at all possible, to be around clinicians, learning and doing some of what they do.

The second source to use for finding a summer clinical experience is your mentor. This individual may not only be aware of opportunities at your institution of which the Dean's office is uninformed, but also may know of opportunities in the community or at other institutions. Your mentor may also invite you to work with him or her during the summer. This could be an outstanding experience. But you may not receive any money for it.

If you are in serious need of money to continue living through the next year, you may have to balance the time you spend in an unpaid clinical experience with time spent in a paying job. However, do not neglect this unique opportunity to get your feet wet and your hands dirty in the clinical sphere. It will help crystallize your idea of what you want to do when you finish medical school, as well as improve your attitude and ability to learn in your second year.

## Research

Common wisdom nowadays, meaning the scuttlebutt among the rest of your class, is that it is vital to do research if you are going to get into a good residency program—especially if it is in one of the competitive specialties like Emergency Medicine, Orthopedics, Neurosurgery, or Otolaryngology. As with all rumors, there is a kernel of truth imbedded in the lie. It isn't mandatory to do research. If you have no desire to do research at this time, and if you have no knack for it and no convenient route to performing it, forgo it for now. Put your energy into some of the other areas in which you do have an interest and that, therefore, will pay off more handsomely for the amount of energy that you expend.

If you do have an interest in research, it is important to make any such endeavor a meaningful experience. First of all, *try to do a project that is clinically related to the field to which you will be applying.* Too many applications list research projects dealing with such obscurities as the genetic makeup of the hummingbird. This is not the kind of research that will endear you to most clinicians. Though that type of research can be important and the students who do it probably learn many fine laboratory techniques, they are misdirecting a lot of energy if their goal is to get into a clinical residency program. So, how do you go about getting the most out of your research effort?

First, you must choose the correct preceptor. Hopefully, your mentor either will be willing to act as your research preceptor or can direct you to someone else who is suitable. Make certain the individual you choose has previously worked on student and resident research projects. Many students suffer under the tutelage of either experienced researchers who see medical students only as "gofers," or individuals without adequate research experience (the blind leading the blind).

## Doable Project

Next, select the project. It can be your idea or, more likely, it will be your preceptor's idea. The key to choosing the correct project is to *select one that interests you.* You should also be able to do the project with relatively little assistance. This usually rules out the use of a linear accelerator or other complicated instruments unless you have prior experience, or the time and interest to learn how to use such equipment. It must be a project that you can do in the time that you will have available to you. If you will only be working on it at night and during weekends, it is foolish to take on a project that requires your intervention six times a day for a month. If you have a period of time, say a month or six weeks, that you want to block out to do the research, make sure that you plan to do the work in less time than that. Research *always* takes much more time and energy than is initially allotted.

Finally, make sure that your research is at least somewhat related to your specialty choice. If you are not 100% certain yet of what that is, aim for something with broad clinical applicability—something that affects all aspects of medicine. Projects dealing with a specific (very, very specific) aspect of hypertension, diabetes, wound healing, or sepsis are some examples.

## Make It Count

Other than the factors listed above, there are several key parts of the project that will provide extra impact for you. There are *two things that must be decided before any work is performed.* The first is to make sure that a *publication* will come out of the research, and that the work won't just be either relegated to the circular file or used as a footnote in a larger piece of work. While nearly half of all medical students are involved in research projects, only one-third of this group get listed as authors on publications. The issue of *authorship* is very important. Even if you do 90% of the work, you may only get fifth billing on any publications, meaning that you will be listed after four other individuals. You would like to be listed first, or at least second, on the paper that comes out of the research. Of course, make sure that you do enough work on the project to warrant this.

You should also be aware that clinical research seems to be much easier to publish than basic science research. It also often seems to require less time to actually perform the research—particularly if you retrospectively study already available data, such as in a chart review. And, if you do not wish to or do not have the time to do actual research, a case report with a literature review is a reasonable alternative. All these are excellent learning experiences. Okay, so you won't get a Nobel Prize for it, but that publication will help you get the prized residency you want. If you broach this subject at the start of discussions about your research project, you may find that you will have a much easier time getting both a publication and appropriate authorship.

The other item to arrange ahead of time is the question of *presentation at a scientific meeting*. A scientific article may take a long time to get published, often a year or more after submission. And the words "submitted for publication" next to an article on a résumé or application are not as impressive as "published" or "presented." The quickest way to upgrade the firepower of your paper and the research behind it is to present the findings at a national scientific meeting. If the research is of decent quality, you should have no problem doing this. If it is to be presented, an abstract of your paper is normally published ahead of time in a scientific journal; you will still be able to submit the entire paper later for publication. But if you are considering this, be sure to think, early in the planning stages, about both the project's content and the deadlines for the meeting. That way you will be able to finish the project in time to meet the meeting's deadline. Plan ahead.

## Sources of Funding For Student Research

Several sources provide funding for students with identifiable research projects. These include the:

- Alpha Omega Alpha (AOA) Student Research Fellowships
- American Heart Association Student Scholarships in Cerebrovascular Disease
- American Medical Association Foundation
- American Federation for Aging Research (AFAR)

Some sources provide funding for students who will devote a year or more to specific research projects:

- Howard Hughes Medical Institute Medical Student Research Training Fellowships
- Stanley J. Sarnoff Fellowships
- National Institutes of Health Predoctoral (IRTA) Fellowships

For those with no clue about a project, but who would like some research experience over a one- to two-month period, the following may be of interest:

- American Medical Student Association (AMSA) Washington Health Policy Fellowship Program
- American Medical Student Association (AMSA) Health Promotion Disease Prevention Project
- Bristol-Myers Squibb Pharmaceutical Research Institute
- Centers for Disease Control and Prevention, Epidemiology Elective Program
- Memorial Sloan-Kettering Cancer Center
- National Institutes of Health Summer Research Fellowship Program
- Society for Pediatric Research and American Pediatric Society Research Program
- U.S. Public Health Service Commissioned Officer Student Training and Extern Program (COSTEP)

## Arranging Your Senior Schedule

One of the major questions that medical students ask their advisers is "How do I arrange my senior schedule?" Although there is a movement away from the previous *laissez faire* attitude toward the senior year at many medical schools, most, if not all, of the senior year is still wide open for anything that the student wants to take. But, by now you understand that you will need to arrange your schedule so as to maximize the results of your hard work and have the best chance of getting into a residency. So, your choices, or at least your timing, become somewhat more limited. How do you arrange your schedule?

Let's start with the second half of your senior year. Mid-February until June of your fourth year is when you should take the balance of your allotted vacation, any exotic international electives for which you have a yearning, and electives in areas in which you feel that you need more training. The average senior medical student takes more than seven weeks of electives outside his or her medical school, with the average school allowing students to take 24 weeks of electives. A good source for electives somewhat out of the ordinary is Iserson KV: *Non-Standard Medical Electives in the U.S. and Canada*, Second Edition (Galen Press, Tucson, AZ).

Many senior students bolster their training in Radiology, Anesthesiology, Emergency Medicine, Pediatrics, Orthopedics, Cardiology, and Critical Care with senior electives. This is definitely not the time to take more electives in your chosen specialty. It is, instead, an opportunity to fill in some of the gaps in your training. However, when planning these exciting electives, remember that there is a cost to traveling, housing, and maybe even tuition for some electives away from your school. (Some electives now charge medical students from other schools.) Look into it before you sign onto an away experience.

Working backward, you need to block out the next period for interviews. Remembering that you want to interview as late as possible, this means January and early February for those matching through the NRMP, and December for those in one of the early Matches. You will either have to use up some of your vacation or be on a *very* flexible rotation during this period.

Now for those *critical months* at the beginning of your fourth year. *First, do not take any vacation between your third and fourth years.* Immediately following the end of your third-year clerkships, start your subinternship (described below). You will need both the intense experience of this rotation and an excellent reference letter from it for your application. Next, take a rotation in the specialty that you have chosen. If you think it will be useful to you, opt for more than one. But remember, your time is limited to those months between the end of your subinternship (often up to eight weeks long) and the beginning of your interviews.

Now that these rules for arranging your senior year have been laid out, it doesn't seem so difficult, does it? If you remember that your twin goals are to use the first half of your senior year preparing to get into a residency and the second half obtaining training in your areas of clinical deficiency, you won't go wrong. And as you can see, the rotations that you should be taking in the first half of the year, no matter what the reason, will give you the type of solid clinical experience that no adviser can fault.

## Subinternship

As a subintern, medical students have more responsibility and authority than they have had before. This is the rotation, if done correctly, in which the student assumes all or part of the intern's role on a clinical service. This is where learning how to practice medicine actually takes place. Advisers often scorn the subinternship (a.k.a., junior internship, advanced clerk-ship). They say, "Why do your internship early?" Your answer is that you need to learn how to practice medicine, and that *you learn when you take responsibility.*

The most effective subinternships for senior students to take, there-fore, are the ones that offer the most responsibility for patient care. These are often located at the municipal or Veteran's Administration hospitals. While these rotations are never as "cushy" as others that are available, they do provide the experiences that teach you the independence of thought and action which a good clinician, and a "standout" senior student, must learn.

Most frequently the rotation, no matter what career specialty you have selected, will be on an Internal Medicine service. Because of these services' large patient loads, and the difficulty of doing any major damage before being stopped, students often can be given enough responsibility to become effective clinicians. In some cases, this will also be true of other services, but it is less likely. For the most part, because so much of the decision making on Surgery services is irreversible, the staff will be less likely to offer this kind of responsibility to students. But this varies from institution to institution.

Try to get information from the class ahead of you and from your Dean of Students about the nature of the various subinternships available. If possible, get a prestigious individual as an attending so he or she can write a letter about your performance. You can do this primarily by investigating who will attend at the institutions that are available to you during the appropriate time period. *But don't pick a stellar attending over a stellar experience.* The latter is much more important.

A second option available to some of you may also give you the same responsibility. This is working at a medical mission in a remote, usually foreign, area. While this is often an exciting and broadening learning experience, it is not available universally, it may not be affordable, it may teach you some thought processes and methods that are frowned upon in the United States (at a time in your training when it may be hard to distinguish these adequately), and most important of all, many faculty may look upon it as mere senior-student flightiness.

## Senior-Year Specialty Rotations

Questions constantly arise about whether, when, and how many rotations you should take in your chosen specialty field. You have by now, of course, heard at least some snatches from the debate on this subject. From the halls of academia, the pronouncement often goes something like, "Don't use your senior electives to train in the specialty for which you are applying. You will get enough of this training in your residency. Use your senior year to broaden your medical education." This, of course, is advice from academicians who are firmly ensconced in tenured posts. But is this the advice that they followed as medical students? Is it advice that they would give to their children? Probably not. Nearly 95% of medical students take electives in their first-choice specialty, and more than a third take three or more such electives.

What should you do? This depends first upon your perceived competitiveness for the specialty. As a candidate for a particular specialty, you fall into one of three categories: a star, middle-of-the-pack, or a struggler. How should students in each of these categories approach the idea of a senior-year specialty rotation? Assuming that you have done adequate preparation and now are reasonably certain that you do want to enter a particular area of medicine, your use of the senior specialty rotation should be directed toward maximizing your chance of getting the residency you want.

### Advantages & Disadvantages

For the few of you who qualify as *stars*, you can use the rotation to demonstrate to residency programs that you are as good as your file says. Physicians, being generally conservative in nature, tend to prefer working with people whom they know, in lieu of those whom they have not met or have met only briefly in interviews. Some residency directors require that candidates do student rotations at their program if they wish to be considered. More than 35% of programs suggest to applicants that they are more likely to be seriously considered for selection if they take an elective at that program. If you truly are a "star" academically, personally, and clinically, show them your stuff!

If you fall into the *struggler* category, where it is obvious that your paperwork will not even get you an interview, much less the residency slot of your choice, you will need to do more than one specialty rotation. Putting your greatest effort forward, you need to demonstrate to the faculty at the residency programs not only that you are capable of doing a solid job as a resident, but also that you will fit in well with their department. Demonstrate to them that you are a pleasure to have around and that you will acquit yourself well now that you have found the area of medicine for which you have been searching. Many students, after doing poorly in medical school, have used this strategy to land excellent residency positions. The key to succeeding with this strategy, however, is to work very hard—both clinically and at fitting in with the team.

Most of you are in the *middle-of-the-pack* group. While you should do at least one senior specialty elective, both to confirm your interest in the specialty and to get an additional reference letter, you run a great risk if you do more than that. There are only two types of performance for senior students doing electives in their chosen specialties. They are either "standouts" or "shutouts." There are relatively few individuals who shine both clinically and personally. If you can achieve that status, you are as good as in the residency. But even the "stars," and these are the best of the best, cannot always achieve that ranking in the minds of the specialty faculty during a rotation.

If you do not become a "standout," you are a "shutout." As Dr. Alan Langlieb wrote just after he went through the interviewing process, "One experience shared by me and other students I have met on interviews was the 'so-this-is-what-we're-getting' or the 'we-can-do-better' phenomenon. Faculty are honored that someone took the trouble and had the interest to spend from four to six weeks at their institution, but often do not know the best place to put you. They don't want to work you too hard. Anyway, you spend half your time getting accustomed to a new hospital . . . The program may see too much of the student and feel as though they could do better . . . My advice is to spend a night or weekend on call. This lets the program know of your interest and makes you stand out from other applicants, but you are not around long enough to become a part of the wallpaper."

The student who looks really good on paper, but who has not rotated though the department, will be seen as a potentially much stronger candidate than one who has rotated through and done anything less than a stellar job. Simply getting "Honors," while essential, does not necessarily mean that you were perceived as a "standout." It may only be a reflection of easy grading or it may have been based upon your clinical performance alone. The faculty may have thought that you would be impossible to work with for the duration of a training program. And there is no way to really know this. So, you take a big risk by doing a rotation at a residency where you would like to go.

But if programs require that all applicants do a rotation at their facility, you are stuck. More than one-third of students report that programs to which they applied at least suggested that they were more likely to be considered if they did a rotation with them. If you really want to go into such a program, you will need to do the rotation. These are normally rather small programs in selected specialties. In most cases, Orthopedics, Ophthalmology, and Neurosurgery only rank students who have done an "audition clerkship" at their program. However, this requirement severely limits their applicant pool and, therefore, you may stand a better chance than you would otherwise expect. There are, of course, ways to improve your clinical performance on the specialty rotation. This takes a little preparation.

## Preparation

How do you prepare for an elective rotation in the specialty that you have chosen? First, of course, you should have been preparing over the past several years by reading about the specialty, talking with many practitioners in the field, and spending volunteer time with physicians in the specialty.

But now you are getting ready to "show your stuff" to a residency faculty and you want to be a "standout." Clinically, a residency faculty is looking for an individual who

1. Knows enough of the specialty's factual material to have a solid basis for future training.

2. Is able to utilize these facts in an intelligent manner to deliver good patient care.

3. Delivers patient care in a manner consistent with the specialty's personality.

This almost sounds as idealistic as "motherhood and apple pie." But it is what you have to achieve.

The first requirement, **knowing the basic facts**, can be satisfied through exposure to specialists in the field, reviewing your notes from the relevant basic science courses, and reading specialty textbooks. (Make sure to read at least one cover-to-cover prior to taking the rotation. If you are pressed for time, it can be the shorter "Essentials of . . ." version.)

The second requirement, **using those facts in an intelligent manner to deliver good patient care**, is more difficult to achieve. This means having the skill to integrate the facts that you have learned and then apply them in clinical situations. It also means, in almost all cases, demonstrating a certain degree of independence by devising and carrying out diagnostic and treatment plans without guidance, though not without supervision. How, as a fourth-year student, will you possibly be able to do this? The answer is because of the training and experience you gained while doing a sub-internship.

The third attribute specialty faculties look for is whether you **deliver care in a manner consistent with that field's personality**. What does this mean? One of best examples of this is expressed in a story about a new General Surgery intern at a prestigious institution.

As he was walking across the hospital's cafeteria one day, he was pointed out to the surgical chief residents by the chairman of the department with the comment, "He's just not aggressive enough to be a *real* surgeon. He'll have to go." Perhaps this quiet, studious physician was too stubborn to be kicked out (also maybe too good), but he didn't go. And, as is true in all such stories, he went on to succeed—in fact he became a world-famous Cardiovascular Surgeon. But the fact remains that each specialty is peopled by a particular type of person, and the medical care in that field is generally given with a certain overlay of that personality.

While there are many exceptions (you probably know of some), a certain aggressiveness is expected in applicants for Surgery, most Surgical subspecialties, and Emergency Medicine. Warmth and understanding is looked for in applicants to programs in Psychiatry, Pediatrics, Family Practice, and Physiatry. Calmness and a low-key nature are often sought in applicants for Internal Medicine, Radiology, Anesthesiology, Pathology, and Neurology residencies. It is not clear whether current practitioners' personalities guide the specialty's personality, or whether the nature of each specialty attracts and molds particular individuals. But the important point to remember is: if you stand out as a significantly different personality type than individuals already in the specialty, it will be more difficult for you to get a training position in that specialty.

### Home or Away?

Many factors involved in taking a specialty rotation at home or away have already been discussed. However, there are still three points worth noting.

**First: There can be significant expenses** involved in the travel, meals, and lodging associated with taking an away rotation. While you may assume that there is housing available for rotating medical students, and some of you might even expect free meals, much of the time you would be mistaken. Find out about these costs before arranging the rotation.

**Second: The expense might be worth it.** If you rotate at the site of your first-choice residency only to find out that it really does not meet your needs, you have spent the money wisely. In such a case, the one-month rotation may possibly save you several years of unhappiness. Remember, specialty rotations work both ways—they look you over and you look them over.

**Third: Apply for externships early!** Very popular clerkships, either at your own school or away, are often filled a year or more in advance. Even if you make your specialty choice at a late date, you may still have a good chance of obtaining a rotation in the specialty at your own school. This is not true of away rotations. If you are strongly considering doing an away elective in your chosen specialty, get information and sign up for the externship as early as possible. If you change your mind later, you can always cancel. The Association of American Medical Colleges, 2450 N Street

N.W., Washington, DC 20037-1126, keeps a list, categorized by state and medical school (updated annually), of available electives. Many specialty societies have lists of available electives in their specialty.

### Timing

When should you do your specialty rotation? If you are applying to one of the specialties that does not match early, you have some leeway. But if you will be in an early Match, you may be pressed for time. In either case, you should do a strong subinternship immediately following your junior year, usually on an Internal Medicine service. That's right—no vacation for now; you will have to wait until much later in the year.

A subinternship is usually a six- or eight-week block, so you should finish near the end of August. Then you should take a specialty rotation. If you take it at a program to which you are applying, you will probably be able to interview near the end of the rotation—especially if you notify them of your desire to do this in advance and reconfirm your intent upon arrival. If you have the time, and you feel that you will be exceptionally weak clinically for a fourth-year student in your selected specialty, you may want to first do a specialty rotation at a program that you do not rank highly. Then, if you think that doing another rotation will help your individual chances, you can do it at one of your top choices. Consider, though, that many students have found that the programs that they thought would be lowest on their Rank-Order List ended up at or near the top.

As you did with your third-year clinical rotations, try to arrange your schedule so you can work with an attending who is well-known by residency directors in the specialty. Ask that individual at the start of the rotation if, contingent upon your performance, he or she would be willing to write you a letter of recommendation. Attendings are normally very amenable to this. Then make sure that you supply the necessary names and addresses so that the letters can be sent. There won't be much time. These letters will have to go out *fast*.

You will have now used up all the time that you have available for rotations that will be of any help (or hindrance) in getting into a residency. You can finally spend some time broadening your medical horizons and, certainly, taking a well-deserved vacation.

## Awards

Not everyone receives awards during medical school. But getting them may help you obtain a residency position, and make you feel good in the process. Who doesn't like getting an award? The acknowledgments you received as an undergraduate are passé. Not that you shouldn't list Phi Beta Kappa or other undergraduate achievement awards on your résumé, but remember that everyone else has similar achievements. That is why you were accepted into medical school. And anyway, you received those awards a long time ago. Residencies want to know what you have done recently. Awards, in part, answer that question. They are also an important factor in making you and your application stand out as being unique among the crop of applicants to the programs.

## AOA

Alpha Omega Alpha is the national M.D. medical school honorary society. (Note that this is not the American Osteopathic Association [AOA]. Residency directors know the difference.) Students are elected to AOA based primarily on their grades. In most schools, students can be elected to AOA either at the end of their third year or during their fourth year. Because it is found in most schools, AOA is the best-recognized medical school award. Students elected to the honorary are generally assured of serious consideration by residency programs. This means that many will get most of the interviews they desire. After that it will, of course, be up to them to do well in these interviews.

Some schools do not have AOA chapters. Generally, this is due to the philosophy that the school should attempt to reduce competition among students. Other schools do not elect anyone to AOA until late in the senior year. Their assumption is that this gives those students at the bottom of the class a better chance of competing against their classmates for residency slots. It is, however, not just your classmates but, rather, all medical students who are the competition.

If your school has an AOA chapter, find out from the Dean of Students what the requirements generally are to be elected. If you think that you can satisfy these requirements, then go for it. Getting into AOA can somewhat ease the burden and anxiety of getting a residency position.

If you are elected to AOA after your applications have been sent, or even after you have been interviewed, send the programs an official notification from the registrar. Most schools will ask you for the necessary addresses since they know this is very important.

But AOA is not the only award that you can get.

### Just For Women

The American Medical Women's Association gives several awards to its members. These include a merit-based scholarship, an essay award, a certificate to top medical school graduates, and a research award. They also occasionally have month-long, special-project "internships." For further information, contact: AMWA, 801 N. Fairfax St., Suite 400, Alexandria, VA 22314-1767, or call (703) 838-0500.

## Special Opportunities

Many other awards are given out both nationally and locally. However, they may have to be sought out. Your Dean of Students should have a list of the awards given at your school, and probably knows a good bit about other national prizes.

The most obvious awards are those that you in all probability investigated as soon as you were accepted into medical school. These are *scholarships*. Since these are awards, they should be noted as such on program applications. If you were given renewals of these scholarships because of your good performance in medical school, so much the better. Note, however, that bartering service for money, such as signing up for the Health Professions Scholarship Program, doesn't count.

Another type of award given in most schools is for *excellence in particular courses or clerkships*. For example, the outstanding student in Anatomy or in Family Practice may get an award (often with money as well as a plaque). If you have been selected for such recognition, it is a big deal! Note it prominently on your applications. If the specialty for which you are applying has an award, by all means find out the requirements for it and see if you can be the one to receive it. Your interest in the specialty alone should go a long way toward getting you this honor. Unfortunately many schools do not announce award recipients until graduation. This is long past the time when it will help you to get a residency position. While speaking to your Dean of Students about awards in general, find out if this is your school's policy. If it is, can it be changed? If it can't, and you know that you have been designated for such an award, try to at least have it mentioned in your Dean's letter or in a separate letter that you can include with your applications.

One way you can get recognition and also buff up another area of your application is to receive a *research grant*. Very often either medical schools or individual departments, or both, have monies specifically set aside for medical student research. If you plan to do research anyway, it wouldn't be a bad idea to apply for some of this research money. Not only is it a significant accolade, but it will also make your foray into research much easier.

There are also awards, usually given by major drug companies, for *medical writing, biomedical illustration*, and other specialized endeavors. If you have talent in any area where such a prize is given, go after it. You will often be able to find out about these awards from your Dean of Students, notices on your class's bulletin board, or advertisements in *The New Physician*.

# 8

# Putting Off A Decision

*If you carry a lantern, you will not fear the darkness.*

– Folk Saying

Not making a decision about a specialty choice is, as the saying goes, equivalent to deciding not to go into a specialty—at least for the present. In the past (forty or more years ago), medical students routinely put off choosing a specialty until they were well into their internship year. This is the tradition of Ben Casey and Marcus Welby (maybe you saw them in reruns) and of *Arrowsmith* (perhaps you read it in high school). This tradition stemmed from a time, now happily past, when many, if not most, physicians went into practice with little more than an internship as their postgraduate training.

Today, it is dangerous—if not insane—to go into practice so unprepared. Advanced training is now necessary to understand the increasing complexity of medical practice. Without advanced training, today's medical school graduates will usually neither qualify for malpractice insurance nor be granted hospital privileges.

Sadly, we still routinely allow physicians with only an internship to practice in both our Public Health Service (treating Native Americans and poor people) and the military. If you plan to follow these career paths, you can do so with only a PGY-1 year of training. Without advanced training, however, you will probably not progress very far within these services.

Admittedly, making a specialty choice is difficult. It is yet another step in the maturation process, and will remove you from the comfort you have felt for a number of years—ever since you made the decision to enter medical school.

Now, instead of seeing yourself as "a doctor," you must generate another image of yourself. Looking in the mirror, you now must see a Pediatrician, a Pathologist, a Family Practitioner, a Surgeon, or another specialist.

This much narrower focus may be an uncomfortable fit if you have envisioned yourself as the omniscient healer. But it is a fit to which you are going to have to adjust. The only question is, when should you make the decision?

More medical students make their initial specialty decision during their third year of medical school (46%) than at any other time. Another 24% select a specialty during their fourth year, while 23% make a decision before beginning their clinical years of medical school.

## The Fine Art of Procrastination

Despite the common wisdom, making a life-changing decision is not easy and may not completely succumb to rational analysis. A decision about which specialty to enter is just such a decision. Writing a list of pros and cons will often just not hack it. Such decisions also must include many intangible factors, such as your past experiences, willingness to take risks, and unspoken dreams.

Everyone has, at one time or another, procrastinated about making a major decision. The question to ask is, why are you procrastinating? Usually it is fear of making a "wrong" decision, especially if that decision seems irrevocable. Any major decision involves risk—personal, financial, or both. Some decisions don't work out the way you planned. That's okay. Obviously, choosing a specialty to enter is a gigantic step. It is not, however, unchangeable, since up to 20% of physicians change their career direction at least once.

Several techniques may help you make a decision, especially if you have already spent the necessary time to gather the basic information about the specialties you are considering, including time with both academic and community physicians practicing those specialties.

*Discuss your options* with close friends and family. Allow yourself to express your emotions, not just "the facts." Your career choice is emotional, so "let it all hang out."

*Weigh what is most important* in your own life: personal satisfaction, family, money, prestige, time off. Actually give them a weight (like in the "Must-Want" Analysis) and see how each specialty you are considering will fulfill them.

When you are quietly alone, *imagine yourself* in each of the specialties you are considering. Are you enjoying yourself or stressed out? Do you feel satisfied or frustrated? Maybe most important, do you want to go to work tomorrow?

## Taking Time Off

There are several reasons to take time off during or immediately after medical school. Residency directors are used to seeing this type of hiatus in medical training, and most should not hurt an applicant's chances of getting into a program.

If you have a choice, when should you take time off? One student suggested that if she took time off between her first and second years, she could go straight into third year without losing any clinical skills or knowledge. Some students take time off between their second and third years, others between the third and fourth years. Few take time off immediately after graduation.

Leave for medical, personal, and family reasons, especially to have a baby, is now fairly common. Simply put that into your personal statement so the reason is clear. With the increasing debt load many medical students carry, some schools now allow students to take a year off to work. In the long run, this is probably not a wise financial decision, but it should not penalize residency applicants. If you put something in your personal statement, however, it is fair game to ask about during the interview. If you describe a chronic illness, they may ask if it is under control or how often you have exacerbations requiring time off.

If the time off is to acquire another degree, do extended research, or have an unusual medical experience (such as doing a volunteer year in a disaster area), that should probably be the focus of your personal statement, describing what you learned and why you did it. This may also be the focus of most of your interviews. In many cases, this type of extra experience and knowledge may make you an even *more desirable* candidate.

Others taking time off may have less-clear motivations. Often, it is because the individuals are not sure whether they really want to pursue a medical career or because they have had so much academic difficulty that they were asked to temporarily drop out. These types of breaks in training may seriously hurt applicants' chances of getting a desirable residency position, especially if they cannot demonstrate that they have used the time off to make certain that medicine is the career they want or that they have corrected their academic deficiencies.

## Win-Win Decisions

Fear of making decisions often keeps people from moving ahead with their lives and their careers. The motto for most medical students—those who have traveled the normal route to medical school—is often "Be careful! You might make the wrong decision." They believe that, at any juncture, an incorrect career choice could deprive them of those things that the "correct" decision is supposed to bring—money, love, respect, security. They may also, by making the "wrong" decision, find that they are neither perfect nor in complete control of their lives. But, like the donkey that couldn't choose between two bales of hay, it is possible for them to waiver in their decision just long enough to starve to death.

To feel better about making a career decision, you must adjust your view of the possible outcomes. First, realize that your decision will not determine your life or death. The decision need not be permanent. It can be reassessed at a later time when you have more information. Second, instead of thinking of your career decision in terms of the "right" path— you win versus the "wrong" path—you lose, consider that any of the paths you have reasonably investigated can offer you exciting, although not necessarily equivalent, opportunities.

By thinking of your career decision as a Win-Lose situation (Figure 8.1), you will doom yourself to forever thinking, "What if I had taken the other route?" every time something in your career, or your life, is not perfect. This results in a life of misery and depression. By following a Win-Win model (Figure 8.2), you allow yourself to feel good and gain the rewards you desire from whichever path you take.

FIGURE 8.1

**Win-Lose Decision-Making Model**

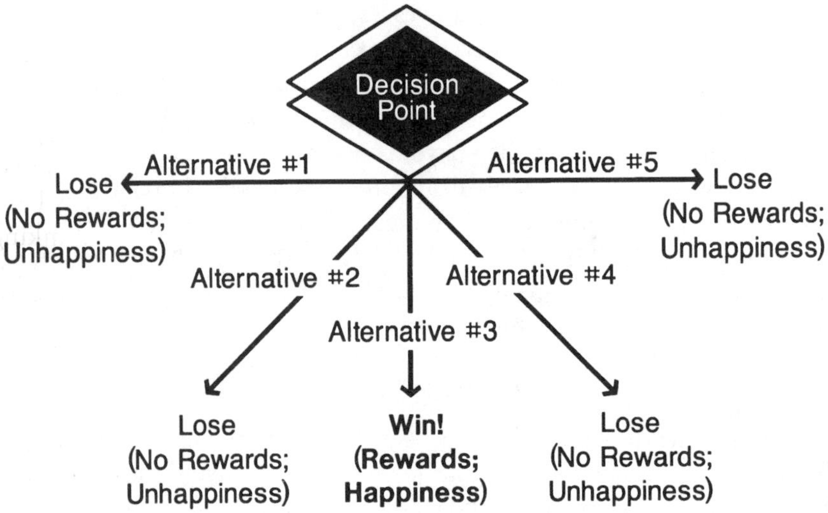

FIGURE 8.2

*Win-Win Decision-Making Model*

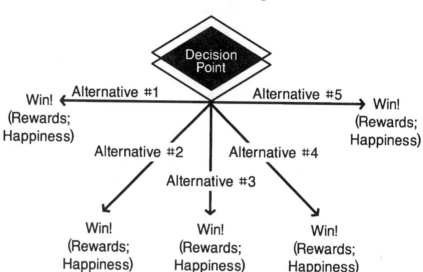

## Advantages & Disadvantages of A Transitional Year

Taking a transitional internship without having obtained a commitment for PGY-2-level training has both advantages and disadvantages.

The Transitional internship is similar to internships of old. It exposes physicians to Medicine, Surgery, Emergency Medicine, Obstetrics and Gynecology, Pediatrics, and perhaps Psychiatry. Very similar in many ways to a repeat of your third year of medical school, albeit with upgraded responsibility, it provides another general overview of the practice of medicine. The additional knowledge and abilities you acquire may be very useful throughout your career. This is especially true if you are thinking of using this as your first year of training prior to beginning a program that starts in the second year, such as Anesthesiology, Radiology, or Ophthalmology. But if you are merely postponing a decision about which specialty to enter, and assume you will use the Transitional year to decide, you may be in for a rude awakening.

First, look at the time schedule for the NRMP application process (Figure 22.5). You will see that, at best, going into a Transitional year allows you to put off making a decision only until the end of your senior year of medical school. Matching in the advanced Matches (PGY-2 and above) and with programs not participating in the Match usually occurs even earlier. If you plan to start specialty training the year after your internship, you will have to have made a decision before the end of your senior year. So, what price do you pay by procrastinating?

Internship is tough on both body and soul. It doesn't matter whether you are in a Transitional program or in a Categorical internship. (For an explanation of the types of internships, see Chapter 22.) You will work long hours and get little sleep. That is the nature of the beast. So, now you have moved the very grueling process of applying for a training position to what will probably be the most difficult time in your entire life—the first half of your internship. Not a pretty prospect. It is so difficult to deal with the added stress that many interns basically give up and take the easiest route to a decision. That is, they agree to take virtually any open position, even if it is not in the specialty they want. They promise themselves that they will look for a better position later. They rarely do.

Another problem relates directly to the Transitional year. Many specialties, including most Surgical areas, Internal Medicine, Pediatrics, and Family Practice, will not accept a Transitional year as counting toward completion of a residency (Figure 22.1). Therefore, you may have to either avoid going into these specialties or repeat your internship—a dismal thought and nearly always an unhappy experience. No matter how much you think you won't mind repeating the intern year—you will hate it. I have seen many individuals, all of whom truly believed they would not mind going through internship again, be absolutely miserable when having to repeat the experience. Most people emerge from their internship with a wealth of new clinical knowledge, and an ability to make clinical decisions and work in a clinical setting. Repeating this experience will not substantially increase these abilities. Instead, it will often cause frustration, since your supervising residents may not have the same level of skills that you do.

An alternative, if you can at least decide between Surgery and Medicine, is to take a "Preliminary" Surgery or Medicine internship. These are not broadly based, as are Transitional years. They are essentially the same programs as those the Categorical Medicine or Surgery interns go through. The benefit is that more possibilities exist for you following such training. Surgery and its associated areas will accept a Preliminary Surgery internship; Medicine will accept a Preliminary Medicine internship. Preliminary spots also may be relatively easy to obtain, with only 85% of those in Medicine and only 57% of those in Surgery filling in the 1999 Match. Specialties that accept Transitional programs will also accept either of these. So, perhaps part of a decision is better than none.

You may still decide to do a Transitional year, as did about 5% of 1999 graduates, either because you cannot make up your mind about a specialty or because your specialty requires a preliminary clinical year before beginning specialty training, such as in Anesthesiology (21% of Transitional interns), Radiology (14%), and Ophthalmology (11%). About 80% of residents in a Transitional year plan to follow that year with a residency. Another 12% intend to follow the year with obligated federal service, and a small number plan to go into research. With more confidence than common sense, 1% plan to go into practice after just this one year of training!

If you intend to do a Transitional year, a good information source, aside from the *FREIDA* system, is the *Transitional Year Program Directory* (formerly called *The Purple Book*), published by the Association for Hospital Medical Education. See Chapter 9 for descriptions of both of these sources.

## Quick Decisions & Forty Years of Sadness

More than half of all medical school graduates believe that deciding on a specialty before beginning their third year gives them an advantage in obtaining their choice of residency program. While this may have some validity, there are dangers in making a specialty decision too quickly. Many physicians with whom I have come in contact or have counseled over the years are disappointed, if not frankly frustrated and bored, by their specialty (see Figure 3.3). This is not as surprising as it may seem. When asked how they had made a specialty decision in the first place, many said that they were influenced by an exciting third-year rotation, a dynamic teacher in medical school, a childhood physician, or a physician-parent.

During training, some got a hint that the specialty was not for them. They may have lacked a feeling of excitement when they were about to go to the operating room. Or they became depressed taking care of patients with chronic illnesses on the wards. But they did not listen to their feelings and continued their training. By the time they finished their residencies, they felt that they had too much time committed to the specialty to change.

Others liked their training immensely. The diagnostic challenges and therapeutic dilemmas seen in the tertiary-care teaching facility stimulated them. But once they got into practice, they found that they rarely used most of their skills. Rather, they dealt with a parade of patients with the same mundane problems. And this was not what they had anticipated.

Physicians also change specialties because of the process of self-discovery that accompanies most educational endeavors. It is not uncommon for medical students (maybe not you, but certainly most of your friends) to be service-oriented, obsessive-compulsive individuals. They receive much of their stimulus to achieve from a self-sacrificing posture designed to win approval from superiors, relatives, and friends. Yet while training in clinical medicine, some individuals find that their route to personal satisfaction is not through their chosen specialty; some find that the route does not include medical practice at all.

In the past, I have gotten calls not only from physicians in practice, but also from their spouses. Our discussions were always variations on the same theme. The physicians had been in practice from eight to ten years and were very unhappy, even though they were often in what most people consider to be very desirable specialties. The physicians repeatedly stated that life would be much better if only they could change their specialty. The caller now wanted advice about how to make that change. What could not be ascertained, however, was whether the initial specialty choice, or something much more profound, was the problem.

I am saddened when I see a 45-year-old physician who is unhappy that he or she ever entered the field of medicine. It is less sad, but still somewhat unnerving, to see the same physician reenter a training program to change specialties at such an advanced stage in his or her career. So, there definitely can be reasons to wait to make a specialty decision. Investigating your options early will help to prevent you from making a foolish or uninformed choice. But just procrastinating in making that decision will not make the final selection either easier or better.

Residency programs may now hesitate to take physicians who have completed too much prior residency training. The federal government, through the Medicare program, reimburses hospitals for much of the cost of resident education. This support is at its maximum for the time required to meet the requirements for initial Board certification—with a maximum of five years. They calculate this time period beginning with the first year of Categorical residency (not counting a Transitional or Osteopathic internship year). Although the amount of money is relatively small, the impact makes some programs wary of accepting residents who have already done training in another specialty or in a transitional year. An exception, of course, is where that year is required as part of the training, such as is required before beginning Otolaryngology, Urology, Neurology, etc. This also applies to those who have entered another field, even decades ago, and now want to retrain in another specialty.

In reality, however, the Medicare payments hospitals receive for these residents are not decreased as much as one might believe. They continue to get the substantial "indirect" reimbursement; it is only the "direct" payment that is partially decreased. While programs and hospitals may consider this as one factor, generally it will not prevent residents from changing their residency program. *This relatively minor reduction in hospital reimbursement should never cause residents to work for free, as some have suggested.*

## Switching Careers

Medicine, more than any other profession, tenaciously hangs onto its practitioners. Physicians are expected to remain committed to the field until death or voluntary retirement, either through a sense of altruism, because of the benefits they gain, or simply because they believe that their focused education eliminates other forms of employment.

Yet numerous physicians have successfully either combined other careers with medicine or switched completely. Most of these names are well known to you, although you may not know that they were physicians. These include:

- **Philosophers:** John Locke and Oliver Wendell Holmes, Sr.
- **Astronomer:** Nicholas Copernicus (physician to the Heilsberg Bishopric)
- **Scientists:** Luigi Galvani (Italian physiologist), Carol Linnaeus (Swedish taxonomist), and Thomas Huxley (English biologist)
- **Politicians:** Jean Marat (French Revolution), Georges Clemenceau (World War I French Premier), Sun Yat Sen (first president of the Chinese Republic), and Che Guevara (modern communist revolutionary)
- **Writers:** Arthur Conan Doyle, Tobias Smollett, A.J. Cronin, Thomas Campion, Anton Chekhov, Johann Schiller, John Keats, William Somerset Maugham, and Michael Crichton
- **Others:** Galileo, Charles Darwin, and Gertrude Stein went on to fame after dropping out during medical school. (In Ms. Stein's case, it was during her 4th-year OB/Gyn clerkship at Johns Hopkins.)

So there is life outside medicine. However, one of the most common alternative careers physicians now consider is the law. There are about 2,000 physician-lawyers in the United States. Each year, many physicians enter law school for uncertain reasons, but drop out because they find it tedious or boring. If you consider changing from a medical career, go towards a positive goal, don't just run away.

## Dangers of Waffling

Some students think that because they have been unable to make a specialty decision, they will let the luck of the Match—not at all like the luck of the Irish—decide for them. They interview in two or more specialties. And, although they may give preference in their Rank-Order List to one field or another, it is clear that they are not committed to a particular specialty. (This is not to say that you should not list some appropriate internships at the bottom of your Rank-Order List—that is just being careful. See Chapter 22.)

In such cases of indecision, the question must be raised, "Is the indecision based upon a lack of knowledge about the specialties, or about one's self?" Unfortunately, it is fairly common for students to apply to multiple types of specialties. If you are contemplating such a move, it is time to get some serious counseling. And one of the items that needs to be discussed is *whether you really want a career in medicine.* But if you still think you really do want to work as a physician (of course you have already spent a lot of time in school, but residency will be another three to seven years), and you intend for some reason to apply to multiple specialties, consider the two biggest problems involved.

The first, and most obvious, problem with applying to multiple specialties is the time and cost involved. If you plan to research the specialties, and perhaps take senior electives in them, you will use up your available time very quickly. Expenses also mount up rapidly if you are applying to multiple specialties.

The second problem is that you will have broken a basic tenet of the residency application process. You will have shown that you are not committed to a specialty. And if the reason you are applying to multiple specialties in this fashion is to stay within a defined geographic area, be assured that most of the programs will know or soon discover this. If the programs are anything more than "bottom-rung" and you are anything less than a "star," they probably will not consider you seriously. Consequently, you may very well end up in a poor, nondescript program, which probably will, either then or later, make you very unhappy. It is better to make an informed choice about a single specialty and then go after the position with maximum effort.

# 9

# Gathering Information

*Just to look costs nothing.*

– Folk Saying

Now that your specialty decision is made, it is time to collect information, not on the specialty in general, but on that specialty's individual training programs. You need to discover the differences among training programs, where they are located, how difficult it is to get a position at each, and what variables and options exist for completing your training.

With the limited time and money you have to invest in searching for the best programs for you, it is essential that you do some priority shopping—spending your resources in a manner to give you the highest probability of finding what you want. To do this, you must get enough information about each program that you seriously consider to allow you to complete your own "Must/Want" Analysis (Figure 10.1). If you know where to look, much of this information is readily available.

You will be sifting through a lot of information, so get organized first! One method that many students find useful is to set up a file for each program they consider. If you do this, then you can put the material in the file as you collect it. Paste a copy of your "Must/Want" Analysis on the *inside* cover of each file folder.

When you take this file with you to your interview (or "audition" elective), you can fill in your "Must/Want" Analysis as you go along, and no one else will see it. It would be a good idea to also paste in a copy of "Interview Notes" (Figure 17.2). (The *Companion Disk* contains these two vital forms for you to customize and print out.) Since most students do not have their own filing cabinet, you may find it useful to purchase a sturdy cardboard file box (sometimes called a "bankers box"). A 12″ X 15″ X 10″ box can hold about 35 files.

Now that you have a method for organizing program information, let's consider some of these sources in detail. (For more sources and how to get them, see the *Annotated Bibliography*.)

## Graduate Medical Education Directory

This substantial book, usually referred to as the "Green Book," is issued annually by the American Medical Association (AMA), 515 N. State St., Chicago, IL 60610. It lists all "approved" training programs, i.e., those accredited by the Accreditation Council for Graduate Medical Education (ACGME). Most of the information in this book has been supplanted by the *AMA-FREIDA* system (see below). However, there are a few areas that are still important to residency applicants, mainly at the beginning (Section II) and the end (Appendix: Board Requirements) of the book.

## Section I: Information Items

This section contains an abbreviated list of requirements for international medical graduates (IMGs) who are attempting to obtain residency positions in the United States. It includes basic details about visas, the differences between immigrant and exchange-visitor IMGs, and Fifth-Pathway students. This section also includes a general description of residency training in the Armed Services, and information about the National Resident Matching Program.

## Section II: Requirements for Accreditation of Programs

This section has the "Institutional Requirements" (also called "General Requirements") to which residencies must adhere for accreditation, including the responsibilities of institutions, program organization and responsibilities, the eligibility and selection of residents, and the relationships between programs and residents. This section also includes information about the eligibility of international medical graduates and U.S.-citizen graduates of medical schools not approved by the LCME or AOA to enter into U.S. training programs. There is also a list of the minimum elements for contracts between the residency programs and the applicants.

More important, this section includes the "Program Requirements" (also called "Special Requirements") for each specialty. These requirements detail each specialty's training philosophy, programs' expected general characteristics, the required scope of training (including special exceptions, acceptable prerequisite training, and alternative routes to accomplish training, if they exist), programs' expected content, the nature of the teaching staff and facilities, and any other requirements unique to the specialty.

**One caveat**, however: When reading the Program Requirements, remember that you will be reading what the specialty's leaders would like their ideal residency program to encompass. Few, if any, training programs ever meet all these requirements. To be accredited, they are expected to have met most of them and, where possible, to work on meeting the others. The pertinent questions for you to ask will be: (1) Does the program meet enough requirements so that it will most likely remain accredited throughout my period of training?, and (2) Are the factors that I consider important present at that program?

### Section III:
### Accredited Graduate Medical Education Training Programs
This section constitutes the bulk of the book and was once the most familiar to medical students. It contains a listing of residency programs and some basic contact information. It has been supplanted by *FREIDA*. The "Supplement" that comes out each year may prove useful, however, since it includes programs that are too new to be in *FREIDA*.

### Section IV:
### Graduate Medical Education Teaching Institutions
This is a listing, city by city, of the institutions participating in graduate medical education. The first part of this section lists the primary sponsoring institutions. The second part lists other participating institutions where often only a few or elective rotations are taken.

### Appendices
Several of these appendices are useful. Most important for all applicants are the requirements for certification by the recognized American Specialty (M.D.) Boards. Now would be a good time to look at these requirements, especially if you are not going directly from medical school into the residency for which you are applying, or if you are anticipating something out of the ordinary for your training experience. Better to learn the rules now than to suffer later.

This section of the book contains a listing of combined specialty training programs, such as Pediatrics-Emergency Medicine. *FREIDA* contains the specifics. For those who want to apply to shared-schedule (part-time) residency positions, another appendix contains a specialty-specific list of these programs.

This section also includes the licensure requirements of the various U.S. licensing jurisdictions and the addresses for all state medical boards. If you plan to moonlight during your residency, look over these requirements and make certain that you qualify in the locales in which you are interested. Also, if you still need the information, there is a list of all U.S. medical schools with their addresses.

## AMA-Fellowship and Residency Electronic Interactive Database Access (FREIDA)

*The AMA-Fellowship and Residency Electronic Interactive Database Access* (officially called *AMA-FREIDA®* but from here on we'll use her more familiar name, *FREIDA*) is an applicant's major source of information about training programs. Instituted at the request of the AMA's Resident Physician Section, the system provides students with a wealth of information. Indeed, so much information is available that the unprepared can be overwhelmed. It now lists about 7,500 ACGME-approved residency and fellowship programs and about 200 programs for combined specialty residencies. It also offers specialty-specific and compensation workforce information and the results of residents' and graduates' job satisfaction surveys.

Before using this database, the prudent move would be to review the section on the "Must/Want" Analysis to determine which characteristics of residency programs are of importance to you.

*FREIDA* can be accessed either through a computerized version on a medical school computer (often at the library) or through the American Medical Association's website. The system supports both Netscape and Internet Explorer. The recommended hardware is a Pentium machine with 32MB RAM and a modem of at least 28.8 kbps. There is NO CHARGE to applicants to use this system!

To access *FREIDA* on the Web, go to either www.ama-assn.org/FREIDA or the American Medical Association's main page at www.ama-assn.org. On their first page, highlight the section labeled "Ethics, Education, Science, Accreditation." This will bring up a short menu that includes a listing for "FREIDA online."

At the main *FREIDA* screen, you have three primary choices and a number of lesser ones, such as "frequently asked questions." To begin searching in the specialties, click "GME Programs and Main Institutional Search." Use the other main categories, "Physician Workforce Information" and "Specialty Statistics," to add to your knowledge about the specialties you are considering.

Once you get there, click on "GME programs" to start the program. You can limit your search by specialty(ies), location, program size, or a particular program if you have their identification number.

When you select a program in which you are interested, rather than wasting time looking at each individual category of information, simply click on "View All Program Info" to see everything about the program on the system. The same goes for information about the program's "Sponsoring" and "Participating" institutions.

Each program with a complete *FREIDA* listing has about ninety information items available in the database. *FREIDA* divides the data into:

1. **Basic information:** the name, E-mail, Web, and snail-mail addresses, and telephone number of the program director and contact person (if different); program length; whether they are accepting applications for the current and following years; program start date, whether they participate in ERAS; and which institutions are sponsors and participants. You can access extensive information about each listed institution from this location.

2. **General information:** the number of positions in each PGY year; whether prior residency training is required; availability of "preliminary" positions; if a non-accredited fellowship year is offered; participation in and code for the NRMP; the number of applications and interviews in the past year; the ratio of applicants to enrollees (the higher the ratio; the more difficult the program is to enter); the number of required reference letters; the deadline for applications; and the interview period.

3. **Program faculty:** the number of physician/non-physician full-time, part-time, and volunteer faculty; percentage of full-time female physician faculty; and the ratio of full-time-equivalent paid faculty to residents.

4. **Work schedule:** average hours on duty per week excluding beeper call; maximum consecutive hours on duty during first year excluding beeper call; number of 24-hour off-duty periods per month during first year; and work, beeper, and call schedules for each year of the program.

5. **Educational environment and features:** educational conference frequency; hospital/non-hospital ambulatory experience; time in HMO settings; and special education features of the program including whether there are written evaluations, research experiences, an ethics curriculum, a primary care track option, or teaching/communication skills programs.

6. **Policies and board information:** whether written policies exist on substance abuse, mental health impairment, physical disability, and cross-coverage for illness; medical student supervision; in-service examinations; and the percentage of residents completing the program, taking specialty board examinations, and passing the boards on their first try.

7. **Program benefits:** salary and vacation/leave/sick days policy for each year in the program; paid liability insurance; availability of part-time/shared positions; on-site childcare; educational leave and reimbursement; paid professional memberships; computerized records of resident clinical experiences; and the length of and pay during maternity/paternity/family/medical leave.

8. **Institutional information** (available for each clinical site in the program): hospital size; size of the medical staff; annual admissions, percentage of HMO admitted patients; patient demographics; emergency department and non-emergency department outpatient visits; specialized inpatient units and services; and whether there is an organized medical group.

9. **Major medical benefits** (available for each clinical site in the program): major medical, dental, disability, and life insurance.

10. **Specialties in institution** (available for each clinical site in the program): all accredited graduate medical education programs at the clinical site.

There is an enormous amount of information, but the necessity of molding the database to all specialties has resulted in a poor fit for some. For example, for some specialties (especially Surgery, Radiology, Anesthesiology, and Pathology), applicants want to know the number of procedures performed. This information is not available. Yet the *FREIDA* system represents a vast improvement over the "Green Book."

**Two caveats:** Residency directors supply their own program information and no one verifies that it is true. When using *FREIDA*, applicants should be careful about how they interpret the information, and should double-check it if it seems questionable. Verify all important information before and during your interview. Programs can update their information using a password, but may not have done so recently. Note the date listed under "Basic Information," which tells you the last time the information was updated. Also, *FREIDA* may not list very new programs and programs (e.g., Maternal-Fetal Medicine, Trauma Surgery) which are not ACGME-approved or for which there are not yet approved program requirements. You need to contact these programs directly for their information.

The AMA asks every graduate medical education program to provide data for its listing. However, while all ACGME-approved graduate education programs are listed, some fellowships, small residencies, and residencies with few positions have incomplete listings, showing only their name, information on how to contact them, and the number of positions offered. This suggests that you should double-check the "Green Book" to be certain that you locate all the programs in which you may be interested.

**Mailing Labels.** *FREIDA* also allows you to print mailing labels for the programs in which you are interested. AMA student and resident members can print two sets of mailing labels for free (up to 30 programs), and can get them for 70 more programs for $50. Non-members can E-mail *FREIDA@ama-assn.org* to find out how much it costs for these labels. (It is usually a much better deal to join the AMA for this service plus *JAMA* and other benefits.) Another option is to print the program information for each program in which you are interested and cut out the address information.

*FREIDA* is remarkably easy to use, even for the computer illiterate. Just turn on the machine or connect to the website and follow the instructions. Have fun with it.

### National Residency Matching Program (NRMP) Directory

The *NRMP Directory* is posted annually (and updated weekly during the Match "season") on the National Resident Matching Program (NRMP) website (www.nrmp.aamc.org). This is another important source of information about residencies, especially about programs in the NRMP's PGY-1 and Specialties Matches. It is a crucial book to have if you plan to go through the NRMP Match.

Information available to everyone at the website includes the NRMP rules, how to apply as a medical student or Independent Applicant, and several useful work forms and applications. By the 2002 Match, the NRMP plans to have phased out paper applications, and work solely on-line. The site also has the Schedule of Dates important to those participating in the Match. This will be your guide to timing the Match-related events in your senior year—including which day to set aside to party when the Match results are posted.

Once you enroll in the NRMP Match, you have access to the specific program information, including their program numbers (which you list on your Rank-Order List—see Chapter 22), and the current number of positions at each program. Note that this may change up until late January. The original number of listed positions often varies by as many as 2,000 by the time the NRMP runs the matching algorithm.

Both medical student and Independent Applicants (IMGs, Osteopathic students, and non-medical-school-sponsored physicians) use the same general website.

### NRMP Program Results—Listing of Filled and Unfilled Programs

This information, released on the NRMP website two days before Match Day each year, shows geographically and by specialty which programs matched and which did not—*through the NRMP Match*. This is vital information for you to read, especially if you think that you might have difficulty getting a position. It shows you which programs might be a bit easier to enter in the coming year.

### Council of Teaching Hospitals Directory

Published by the Council of Teaching Hospitals (COTH), a section of the Association of American Medical Colleges, 2501 M Street N.W., Suite 1, Washington, DC 20037-1307, this volume contains detailed information on the more than 400 individual hospitals that are COTH members. It often includes different information than is on *FREIDA*. This is where you may be able to validate some of the information provided by the programs themselves. The *Directory* (along with the AHA's reference, below) also can give you information about the workings of the entire hospital. This may be very important to the type and quality of training that you can get.

The *Directory* is issued each year, and includes information on admissions, affiliations, bed capacity, physical facilities, clinical services provided, composition of housestaff, and the residency positions offered at the institution. The most important information for you will be the type of residencies, the total number of residents, and the total number of international medical graduates in residency positions at each hospital. It is available through your medical school's library or Dean's office.

### American Hospital Association Guide to the Health Care Field

This annual publication of the American Hospital Association (AHA), 325 7th Street N.W., Suite 700, Washington, DC 20004-2802, gives a detailed listing and description of over 7,000 member hospitals. Virtually all hospitals involved in teaching are members of the AHA, even if they are not all members of the Council of Teaching Hospitals (COTH). This is especially true of hospitals that are not considered primary or base teaching hospitals, but where you still may spend a great deal of time and receive a substantial part of your training. These are the institutions that you will be particularly interested in getting information about from this book. You can find it at virtually any medical or major public library.

## Council of Teaching Hospitals Survey of Housestaff Stipends, Benefits, and Funding

This annual survey, also published by the COTH section of the Association of American Medical Colleges, is perhaps the only independent source of compiled national and regional information concerning the salaries and benefits offered by programs. While these are not your first considerations when making a decision about residencies, they are certainly important.

The manual breaks down salaries and benefits for housestaff in a variety of ways. While it does not list individual programs, it does list the salaries paid and the benefits provided by region of the country, type of hospital, and postgraduate year of training. You can compare these figures to the figures supplied by the various programs to see how far they are from the mean.

You really should not ask questions about salary and benefits during your interview. It's better that you get information such as this from the *COTH Survey*, which should be available in the medical library, your Dean's office, or on the AAMC website (www.aamc.org). As an added bonus, the book also lists the ratio of housestaff to patients in the various areas of the country and by type of hospital. This is a very important statistic for determining the number of hours you will work and the responsibility you will have.

### Transitional Year Program Directory

If you are searching for information sources on a Transitional PGY-1 year, this annual publication (formerly called *The Purple Book*) of the Association for Hospital Medical Education, 1200 19th Street N.W., #300, Washington, DC 20036-2412, will be very useful to you.

This book lists most of the available Transitional programs, their contact information, the number of months of required and elective rotations, the presence of other training programs, the demographics of the individuals who match with the programs, the difficulty of getting a position, the night-call frequency, and the opportunities for a PGY-2 year at the institution. This book remains an excellent source of hard-to-come-by information to supplement that found in *FREIDA*.

## Individual Programs

Once you have used the information from the sources described above to narrow your program choices at least a little, acquire additional information directly from the programs themselves. To get this information, send them a letter, postcard, or fax. While the rumors about programs keeping this first request letter on file are not true—they start a file when they actually receive application materials—it doesn't hurt to make the requests legible. Also, include a legible return address. Each year our program receives about ten requests without legible, or even any, return addresses. It also helps to print or type your name. Many information requests have only signatures. And true to form, fewer than half of these can be deciphered.

By far the easiest way to send a request for information to a residency program is by filling out a preprinted postcard (Figure 9.1). These are often available from your Dean's office. Another easy solution to the problem is to photocopy a typed request and paste these copies on multiple postcards. Then all you have to do is address the cards. This has also become easier now that *FREIDA* will automatically print out mailing labels for programs. If you are interested in programs in your geographic area, or if you have access to inexpensive telephone service, call the programs and request the information.

If you write or call early, that is, before the interviewing process is over for the prior year, be prepared to get material applicable to trainees a year ahead of you. Usually this will not be much different from the material that is finally ready for your year, but be sure to compare the information you received with more current information for those programs with which you interview. In some cases, however, there may be substantial changes from year to year. Also, if you request your information during the early part of the year (February to April), be prepared for some delay while new

FIGURE 9.1

**Format for a Pre-Printed Postcard to Request Information from Programs**

```
                                        _____
                                            (Date)

To:  [Program Director's Name and Address]

     I am a medical student at the _____

     College of Medicine with an expected graduation date of _____.

     I am interested in receiving information and an application about your

     _____ [Externship,

     Internship, Residency, Fellowship] in _____

     [Specialty]. Please send the information and application to:

     _____

     _____ [Your Name and Address] _____
```

material is being prepared. It is best to get preliminary information that describes the year before you wish to enter the program, and then update the materials for the "short list" of programs to which you intend to apply.

Information from residency programs varies widely. It ranges from glossy brochures with lots of pictures and very little solid information to very detailed descriptions of the program, institutions, faculty, and resident responsibilities and benefits. You will probably not be able to tell the good programs from the marginal ones based only on the material you receive. Essentially, that is because the information is not of uniform quality. Also, some residency programs are good at marketing, others are not. Nevertheless, the information sent directly from the programs may assist you in working out your own "Must/Want" Analysis (Figure 10.1) and in winnowing the programs down to a reasonable number for further consideration.

The *FREIDA* system, described earlier in this chapter, supplies information in a uniform style that is more readily available to you than that from the individual programs and institutions. Yet the programs' materials may supply you with more recent, as well as additional, information, so requesting it is worthwhile.

### The Internet

The Internet has exploded with information in recent years. Nearly every specialty now has a website with extensive information, and increasing numbers of individual residencies also have websites. Check the "Important Contacts" at the end of this book for some of these Web addresses.

One good website that may be around longer than some others is www.aamc.org/medcareers/tools/resources.html. It contains, among other things, links to specialty organizations and some career planning tools.

Many specialties have not only websites but also listservers that you may be able to join. These may provide you with much valuable information. The listservers can be found most easily through the specialties' national organizations. They may require you to join their medical student/ resident organization (usually very inexpensive).

### Specialty Society Publications

At least six specialties publish directories of residency programs. These are Family Practice, Internal Medicine, Psychiatry, Preventive Medicine, Physical Medicine and Rehabilitation, and Urology. Each source contains significantly more information than can be obtained by writing to the residency programs. And, though they are not all published annually, they are excellent places to get a good picture of both the scope of residencies in the specialty and the individual programs in which you might be interested. Each is described in the *Annotated Bibliography*.

## Specialty Faculty

Your mentor or specialty adviser will obviously be another source of information about programs. This individual may have enough knowledge about some, or in the case of small specialties, most or all programs in the specialty to reasonably assist you in your search. Usually, he or she will be familiar with programs in one or more specific geographic areas. If your mentor has been in the field for some time, he or she may have also visited other training programs in the course of professional activities. This will provide a wider knowledge base from which to counsel you. But an adviser's input must still be considered in light of both your personal needs and the other information you collect.

Remember, no matter what your specialty adviser thinks is the best program, you are the one who will be going through the training. However, do not discount his or her inside information and contacts at specific programs. You will not find this in any book. And this is what may get you an interview at your most desired program.

## Journals

If you are looking for programs with a strong academic or research bent, you may want to scan the major specialty journals to see which programs are most heavily represented. In addition, either from these journals or from mailings your specialty adviser receives, you can discern which programs are most heavily represented at national scientific meetings. Obviously, this will only be supplemental knowledge. But it may come in handy not only when selecting programs, but also by giving you an inside track (with your special information) during interviews.

If you seek a program that will be relatively easy to match with, look at the advertisements in *The New Physician*. Programs normally advertise here if they have difficulty filling their slots. Many such programs are at well-known institutions, and some are even in hard-to-match-with specialties, such as Orthopedic Surgery or Otolaryngology. Similar advertisements also appear, although not in as great a quantity or with as much information, in *JAMA* and the *New England Journal of Medicine*.

A program's or institution's national reputation is not usually of major importance unless you are shooting for an eventual high-profile research or academic position. In that case, your training institution's reputation may play a role in landing you that position. Information about some institutions and their reputations for treating certain disease processes can be found in the annual "Best of" issue of *U.S. News & World Report.* This issue normally comes out in late July. Note that this listing says nothing about the quality of their training programs.

## Dean of Students

Another source of information about specific residencies is your Dean of Students. You should already have had numerous opportunities to contact him or her while you were searching out a mentor, trying to decide upon your interests and how they matched with different specialty fields, and arranging your schedule to best meet your needs. While this person may not know very much about specific programs in the specialties, he or she is usually very conversant about the difficulty or ease of getting into the various fields. Often, he or she can be invaluable if you perceive that you will have difficulty in getting a position in your chosen specialty. The Dean of Students often knows, or can find out, where extra positions will open up, and about Transitional programs and other first-year slots that you might be able to fill.

Some Student Affairs offices have a "contact book" which lists the contacts various faculty members have with programs around the country. So, especially if you think you are in really big trouble, go see your Dean of Students. The sooner the better.

## Residency Fairs

Many medical schools and some hospitals have residency fairs where students have an opportunity to hear residency directors talk about their specialties. Students can also often talk with and question physicians involved in several specialties' training programs. Some schools combine these fairs with the distribution of NRMP Match materials. Often, residency programs from within the institution (and elsewhere) have booths set up with glossy materials and people to answer questions. These fairs may give you some leads, as well as some additional program and specialty information.

# 10

# Finding Programs That Meet Your Needs

*If the doors of perception were closed, everything would appear as it is–infinite.*
– William Blake, *A Vision of the Last Judgement*

## The First Cut

Now that you have some initial information about residency programs, it is time to start weeding. But like any good gardener, be cautious. Don't be so anxious to get rid of the "bad choices" that you inadvertently discard the daffodils with the dandelions. Be prudent when eliminating potential programs from your list. Only reject them after you have carefully reviewed their information. Don't eliminate programs you want to enter simply because you suspect you are not a strong enough candidate—at least wait until after they tell you they do not want to interview you.

You will probably want to consider about thirty programs seriously enough to get all their information. Out of this group, apply to about fifteen programs (more if you are really stretching to get into some very competitive programs) and interview at ten. These numbers will vary somewhat depending upon your personal needs and the difficulty of getting a residency slot in the specialty of your choice. Nearly 40% of medical students interview at ten or fewer programs, and nearly two-thirds interview at fifteen or fewer.

There are good reasons to be liberal in your selection criteria and leery of discarding programs from consideration too soon. The main reason is that often residencies that appear superficially unacceptable may actually be the ones that really will fit your personal needs. Written material from programs varies greatly with the marketing sophistication of the residency and hospital. You want to neither miss a great opportunity just because a program does not know how to present itself on paper, nor only pursue programs at institutions with excellent marketing personnel.

## What Do You Want In A Program?

What do *you* want in a residency program? You can't get to the right place until you figure out what the "right place" looks like. Your situation is similar to that of a pilot who says to his passengers over the intercom, "I have good news, and I have bad news . . . We are making good time, but I have no clue where we are going." Take the time to know where you want to go.

Both your residency and your subsequent career will differ markedly from medical school. In deciding about the best residencies for you, you will consider a large number of factors that you may never have had to think about previously. Most of these factors apply to everyone. But how much weight you put on each factor will be a function of your personal needs. Although it may be somewhat onerous to find some of the information you need to make a decision, the information sources listed in the previous chapter, especially *FREIDA*, make it much easier than it was in the past.

### Weighing The Factors—The "Must/Want" Analysis

How do you weigh the many factors involved in deciding to which residencies you apply (and then how do you rank them in the Match)? The simplest method is to use a "Must/Want" analysis.

As shown in Figure 10.1, you make a list of all the possible factors that could influence your decision about the type of program that you would like. (Do not complete your own "Must/Want" Analysis or fill in Figure 10.1 now; wait until after you have read all the following descriptions of the factors to consider.) Some of the items may be absolute necessities for you, such as full family health care. *If an item is an absolute, a "Must," you have decided that the factor is so important that it must be present or else you will eliminate the program from consideration regardless of the program's other qualities.*

Other items will be relatively more or less important to you. For example, you may have important personal reasons for living in a certain part of the country or a certain city. In that case, you would rate "geography" relatively higher than other factors. However, if where you live is less important than other factors, you would give "geography" a low rating, or you might even eliminate it from your list. Assigning "Weights" to each factor rates their relative importance to you. Refer to Figure 10.2 and see how a sample student assigned "Weights" to the factors important to her. After you have read the descriptions, you will use Figure 10.1 as a master form from which to build your own list.

## Deciding What You Want—The Most Difficult Task

Completing the "Must/Want" Analysis has consistently been each student's most arduous task in the residency selection process. It is not because the concept is difficult, but because it requires you to assess what you really are searching for in a training program. It helps you answer three questions:

1. What "Must" I have to go to a program?

2. What do I "Want" in a program?

3. How important are the various elements to me?

I require my advisees to complete their own list of important factors and assign "Weights" to each before discussing which programs they might want to consider. (Our medical students get this book free from the Arizona Medical Association.) This process often precipitates important discussions between students and their families, significant others, and mentors, especially about where they feel they would like to (or must) live during residency training.

Once students have puzzled through what is important to them, they find that they are much better prepared to discuss why they might want to apply to certain programs. The focus of the discussion changes from what the adviser thinks are the "best" programs to which programs best meet the needs described by a student's "Must/Want" Analysis.

I have talked with numerous students who followed much of the advice contained in this book, got the residency they wanted, and then found that it did not meet their needs or expectations. As the old saying goes, "Be careful what you wish for—you might get it." In nearly every case, they neglected to complete their "Must/Want" Analysis, and found out that their "wish" was not what they really wanted. In many cases, the programs' reputations or their locations overwhelmed every other consideration, to the individual's subsequent regret. Take the time to complete your own "Must/Want" Analysis. And once you complete it, be sure to use it! Avoid years of dissatisfaction.

Now, skim Figure 10.1 and read through the descriptions of the various factors you may want to consider. Then I will explain in detail how to complete your own "Must/Want" Analysis using Figure 10.1 as a base.

---

FIGURE 10.1

### *"Must/Want" Analysis–The Instructions*

Read the following instructions *before* filling this form out. Once you have adapted this form to reflect your needs and wants, you should make several copies. One copy of this form will be used for each residency program you consider.

1.  Add any personal factors to the list that are not already listed.

2.  Select any factors that absolutely MUST be present for you to consider the program. Put the word "MUST" in the "Weight" column instead of assigning it a number value. This means the factor is so important to you that if it is not present, you will not go to that program.

3.  Next, select those factors that are not at all important to you and, therefore, that you will not consider in making your decision. Put a "0" next to these in the "Weight" column. Delete these factors from your final list.

4.  Finally, determine how important each of the remaining factors is to you in selecting a residency position. Put a number next to each remaining factor in the "Weight" column, so the *total of all the "Weights" equals 100.* To do this easily, first rate factors of minimal importance with a "1," and rate those of slightly more importance "2." Continue in this fashion until the total for all assigned "Weights" equals "100." You will probably need to make multiple changes until you are happy with the result.

Congratulations! You have now completed the most difficult part of the process. Make multiple copies of your "Must/Want" Analysis Form with the "Weight" column completed. You will use one of these for each residency program you consider. (The *Companion Disk* has this form, see *Annotated Bibliography*.) Figure 10.2 shows how one hypothetical student completed this first step.

Later, as you get information about each program, you will assign a "Score" (on a 1-10 scale; 10 is "perfect") which is your estimate of how well each specific residency program fulfills your initial expectation in that category. Then you multiply the "Weight" by the "Score" to give the factor "Total" for that program. All factor "Totals" are added to get your "Program Evaluation Score." Examples of this are shown in Figures 10.9, 10.10, and 10.11. These "Program Evaluation Scores" will be what you use to make your Rank-Order List (ROL) for the Match. (Don't worry, I'll explain this in more detail as we get to it.)

FIGURE 10.1

### *"Must/Want" Analysis–The Form*

PROGRAM _____

| Clinical Experience | WEIGHT | X SCORE | = TOTAL |
|---|---|---|---|
| On-Call Schedule | | | |
| Patient Population | | | |
| Responsibility | | | |
| Setting | | | |
| Volume | | | |
| **Geographic Location** | | | |
| Inner City, Suburb, Rural | | | |
| Part of Country | | | |
| Specific City | | | |
| Spouse/Mate/Dependent Needs | | | |
| **Reputation** | | | |
| Institution's Reputation | | | |
| Program's Reputation | | | |
| Program Age and Stability | | | |
| **Faculty** | | | |
| Availability | | | |
| Interest | | | |
| Stability | | | |
| **Curriculum** | | | |
| Curriculum Structure | | | |
| Interaction with Other Specialties | | | |
| Number of Conferences | | | |
| Special Training | | | |
| Types of Conferences | | | |
| **Esprit de Corps** | | | |
| **Research Opportunities/Training** | | | |
| Knowledge | | | |
| Materials | | | |
| Time | | | |
| **Local Job Prospects After Training** | | | |
| **Facilities** | | | |
| Clinical Laboratory Support | | | |
| Computerized Records/Lab Results | | | |
| Hospitals' Ages, Atmosphere | | | |

FIGURE 10.1 (continued)

| | WEIGHT | X SCORE | = TOTAL |
|---|---|---|---|
| Library/Media | | | |
| Parking | | | |
| Resident Call Room Ambiance | | | |
| Safety/Security | | | |
| No Restrictive Covenant | | | |
| **Benefits: Health Benefits** | | | |
| Dental | | | |
| Drug Prescriptions | | | |
| Employee Health Services | | | |
| Health Insurance | | | |
| Health Promotion | | | |
| Hospitalization | | | |
| Optical | | | |
| Psychiatric Counseling | | | |
| Sick Leave | | | |
| **Benefits: Non-Health Benefits** | | | |
| Association Dues | | | |
| Childcare | | | |
| Disability Insurance | | | |
| Educational Leave: Funding Available | | | |
| Time Off | | | |
| Family Educational Benefits | | | |
| Housing (Allowance) | | | |
| Laundry/Uniforms | | | |
| Liability Insurance | | | |
| Life Insurance | | | |
| Parental Leave | | | |
| Meals | | | |
| Photocopying | | | |
| Vacation | | | |
| Organized Housestaff/Union | | | |
| **Moonlighting** | | | |
| **Shared/Part-time Positions** | | | |

TOTAL OF ALL WEIGHTS   =   100

**PROGRAM EVALUATION SCORE  =  _____**

FIGURE 10.2

*"Must/Want" Analysis–An Example*

| Clinical Experience | WEIGHT | X SCORE | = TOTAL |
|---|---|---|---|
| On-Call Schedule | 5 | | |
| Patient Population | 2 | | |
| Responsibility | 14 | | |
| Setting | 7 | | |
| Volume | 10 | | |
| **Geographic Location** | | | |
| Part of Country | 1 | | |
| Specific City | 1 | | |
| **Reputation** | | | |
| Program Age and Stability | 2 | | |
| **Faculty** | | | |
| Availability | 5 | | |
| Interest | 7 | | |
| Stability | 3 | | |
| **Curriculum** | | | |
| Number of Conferences | 1 | | |
| Special Training | 6 | | |
| Types of Conferences | 2 | | |
| **Esprit de Corps** | 8 | | |
| **Research Opportunities/Training** | | | |
| Knowledge | 5 | | |
| Materials | 2 | | |
| Time | 7 | | |
| **Facilities** | | | |
| Clinical Laboratory Support | 1 | | |
| Library/Media | 2 | | |
| Safety/Security | 3 | | |
| No Restrictive Covenant | MUST | | |
| **Benefits: Health Benefits** | | | |
| Health Insurance | MUST | | |
| Hospitalization | MUST | | |
| **Benefits: Non-Health Benefits** | | | |
| Childcare | MUST | | |
| Disability Insurance | MUST | | |

FIGURE 10.2 (continued)

| | WEIGHT | X | SCORE | = | TOTAL |
|---|---|---|---|---|---|
| Educational Leave: Funding Available | 1 | | | | |
| Time Off | 2 | | | | |
| Liability Insurance | MUST | | | | |
| Vacation | 1 | | | | |
| **Moonlighting** | 2 | | | | |

TOTAL OF ALL WEIGHTS  =  100

Note that this individual, who is a single mother, feels that disability, liability, and health insurance, as well as childcare are absolute necessities for any position she might take. She also gives rather a high priority to research and subspecialty training since she plans an academic career. However other educational benefits, local job prospects after training, and the availability of a shared-schedule position are of no interest at all, and her interest in the geographic location of the program is minimal. This allowed her to shorten her "Must/Want" Analysis form to include only the items she considered important. How this individual will score specific programs will be discussed in Figures 10.9, 10.10, and 10.11

# Factors To Consider

The following is a discussion of the most common factors encountered when choosing a residency program. The importance of some factors, which may not seem obvious at first, is explained. Read the discussion carefully. Next, complete your own "Must/Want" Analysis form (Figure 10.1) by adding any factors that are applicable to your situation and deleting those factors that are not. Then assign either a "Must" rating or a "Weight" to each factor on your list.

Medical students are often given the advice about big name programs that "If you can get into that program, go for it!" Fellow students, residents, and faculty give the advice. This advice is worth just what you have paid for it: Nothing! No residency program, no matter what its reputation, is right for everyone. You are an individual. Start treating yourself like one. Look at your own needs, both for now and those you can foresee for the future. Examine your personal desires and your dreams. The program you choose, the contacts you make during training, and the type of training you receive will determine the course of your future professional and, possibly, your personal life.

A resident I knew at a very prestigious, high-powered, research-oriented institution spent most days moping through the halls. She was halfway through her second year of training and completely miserable. She confided that she had come to this program because of its great reputation, but was now completely disheartened because she was not receiving the "nuts and bolts" primary care experience she knew she would need when she went into rural practice. Rather than deciding for herself what needs she wanted filled by a residency program, she had let others make her choice for her. Luckily, after some soul-searching and counseling, she switched to a program that emphasized rural primary care—where she was much happier. Choose carefully. Choose for yourself. It's your life, not your peers', friends', mentor's, or family's.

## Clinical Experience

Clinical experience is the basis of any residency program. This is true whether you go into a field that acts as a primary provider, such as Family Practice or Internal Medicine, or one that acts as a consultant, such as Radiology or Pathology. It is important to your training that the entire clinical experience, from the volume and types of patients treated to the setting of the program and the amount of responsibility that you are asked to assume, is as close to optimal as possible for your needs. *If the clinical experience isn't right for you, it is unlikely that any other factor or combination of factors can make up for it.*

### On-Call Schedule

The frequency of night and weekend call varies enormously, depending upon the specialty, type of institution, specific service, and year of training. Every-other-night call is still common, and being on-call every night is still the norm for Chief Residents in some locales. ACGME guidelines for all specialties now suggest that residents have one day off each week, and that they are on-call no more often than once every third night. Yet General Accounting Office investigators indicate that these work limits "will be loosely applied, and residents in some specialties or geographic areas will continue to work 96 or more hours per week."

Even in New York, the only state to mandate an 80-hour maximum workweek for residents, there has been substantial noncompliance, especially in New York City's private hospitals. As of 1998, more than one-third of all New York hospital residents worked more than 85 hours per week and 20% exceeded 95 hours per week. Surgery was the worst offender, with about two-thirds of residents in New York City and one-third elsewhere in the state working more than 95 hours per week. It is likely that inner-city hospitals throughout the country will have difficulty complying with any new work-hours standard, since they rely heavily on housestaff for service needs.

All Internal Medicine programs must limit residents to 80-hour workweeks (averaged over four weeks), with at least one full day out of seven away from the hospital. (Even this is not particularly enlightened. The British implemented a 72-hour maximum work week for their residents in 1991, and hired enough new residents to take up the slack.) How this is accomplished varies at different institutions.

Some programs also designate a person as a "night float" to handle excess new admissions for the on-call resident. This may relieve much of the stress of being on call at busy institutions—until you get tapped to be the night floater.

Carefully investigate the call schedules at the programs to which you apply. Be certain that you will be able to survive with the amount of rest that these schedules imply. In general, Surgery programs, particularly in the PGY-1 and Chief Resident years, have more brutal call schedules than other specialties. But this is certainly not always the case. And remember to also ask about the amount of call "from home." No matter how benign this sounds, it will also deprive you of sleep. The key is to investigate the call schedule thoroughly—by asking the residents.

### Patient Population

The types of patients and their prevalent problems vary greatly among institutions and in different parts of the country. Consider whether the institution offers the diversity of patients and diseases necessary for your training. Knowing only the number of patients seen tells you nothing about this important element.

Will you see a general cross section of patients that are normally encountered by practitioners in your specialty? Or will you see a population restricted to the narrow subspecialty or tertiary care interests of a particular program or institution? Will you see only middle-class neurotics at a Psychiatry program in a well-to-do suburb? Or will you see the full range of psychiatric diseases?

Will you see only tertiary referrals for complicated procedures at the world-famous mecca of surgery? Or will you get to see patients with "hot" appendices and gallbladders as well? Are virtually all the admissions scheduled and the major procedures done electively? Or is there a large population with unexpected, urgent, or traumatic disease? In large part, these answers can be ascertained from the type of institution in which a program resides.

## Responsibility

As the traditional expression says, a physician "sees one, does one and then teaches one." This is how you will learn in the medical field. Yet it is not only learning to do procedures, but also deciding *whether* to do procedures (or admit patients, or pursue "work-ups") that constitute the essence of clinical maturity. Performing the procedures is relatively easy, making the hard decisions is difficult. To learn this, trainees must (with adequate backup, of course) assume responsibility for all aspects of patient care for many patients. What does this mean?

First, this means having primary clinical responsibility. Will you be the one to make the moment-by-moment decisions necessary for acute patient care? Or will every decision have to be approved in advance? Will you really be responsible for the management of a group of patients? Or will you only be the "scut puppy" for attendings and the more senior residents? Will you be doing the critical care procedures, or are these relegated to the sub-specialty fellows? Will you be responsible for your patients when they enter the intensive care unit? Or will they be turned over to another specialty team? You learn by taking responsibility. In any program that you investigate, find out if you will have actual responsibility for patient care.

Second, if you choose a specialty in which procedures are a large part of the practice, make certain that you will do those procedures. Procedures are essential in all Surgical specialties, including Obstetrics and Gynecology. But procedures are also a vital part of Anesthesiology, Emergency Medicine, Radiology, Cardiology, Internal Medicine, Family Practice, Gastroenterology, and Pathology.

Not only do you need to perform an adequate number, but you also need to do the types of procedures that you expect to be doing when you go into practice. It does you little good as an Ophthalmology resident to become an expert at drilling burr holes, or as a Family Practice resident to refine your laminectomy skills. You certainly will not be performing these operations when you go into practice. You need to gain proficiency in at least those skills that all Board-Certified specialists in your field are expected to know. A list of these procedures can, in most cases, be obtained from the specialty Board. Concentrate on finding out whether the procedures you will need are offered in sufficient quantities so you can hone these skills during your training.

If you are going into a Surgical specialty, you may want to know not only how many and what type of procedures you will perform as a resident, but also how soon you will get to operate. In many programs, the first-year residents, though working harder than they may have thought possible, get little or no actual operating experience. They certainly go to the operating room often, but only to watch and hold retractors. At some programs, this can last well into the second or third year. Remember, unless you are a very unusual individual, you will not only become very frustrated by this, but you will also not learn very much. For Surgeons, the question "When do I actually operate?" is vital. However, be smooth about when and where you ask this question, since it can raise the hackles of many faculty members. If you cannot ascertain this from the program's literature, find out from the residents when you make your visit. It will save you a lot of frustration in the future.

**One caveat:** Personnel other than resident physicians should be available to do minor procedures, such as blood draws and the placement of peripheral intravenous lines or routine catheters, once these have been mastered. While it is necessary for most clinicians to learn to do these procedures, constant repetition serves little purpose and may become an impediment to a resident's education. It is worthwhile to find out how this is handled at each institution.

### Setting

The institution(s) at which a residency program is located often determine the volume of patients that you will personally see, the responsibility that you will have for these patients, and the procedures that you will perform. Hospitals in large urban settings tend to offer more patients and more responsibility to the resident physician. They are often understaffed with attendings and have an overabundance of patients. At the other end of the spectrum, are those community hospital programs with an abundance of attendings and a dearth of patients.

Neither situation is ideal. What you should look for is something in-between—enough patients to satisfy your personal training needs, and enough attendings to give you adequate guidance without taking away your responsibility for most of the decisions and procedures.

Sometimes major deficiencies, such as the lack of major trauma in a Surgery program, are corrected by using "away" rotations. These are designed to supply the necessary training that the home institution lacks. These short stints are often at institutions particularly known for their expertise in the deficient areas. How well these "away" rotations work varies widely. It depends upon the residents, the "away" institution, the deficient areas, and the amount of time spent away. To evaluate this type of rotation with any accuracy, you will need to speak to the residents in the program who have already "been there and done that."

Adequate training in ambulatory, rather than inpatient, settings is becoming more desirable due to changes in the practice of medicine. It is vital in all specialties that you have significant exposure to the specific methodologies used, the problems encountered, and the patients that can be treated in an outpatient setting. The type of outpatient setting is also important. If you are planning a primary care practice, it may be helpful, for example, to have some experience working at a managed care facility. (Less than 20% of all teaching hospitals have residents spend time in health maintenance organizations.) Find out how high the acuity is in the program's outpatient clinics. This can be measured by the ratio of admissions to those seen. Emergency departments usually admit from 15% to 18% of the total patients they see. Judge from that number.

## Volume

The actual volume of patients to which you will be exposed, either as the primary provider or as a consultant, is of paramount importance to the quality of your training. However, information about numbers of patients can be very misleading—and often is deliberately skewed in order to attract medical students to an institution's training programs.

The size of a particular institution, the number of patients seen at the facility or by a particular service, and the number of procedures done only indirectly give you, a prospective trainee, the information you need. You also need to know the ratio of house officers to patients. If you are going into General Surgery, and the hospitals used by a training program do a total of 4,000 resident-performed operations per year, it sounds like an adequate number. But if there are fifty General Surgery residents, each resident only does eighty cases—with probably only about forty of these being major cases. This means that at the PGY-1 and PGY-2 levels you will rarely, if ever, hold a scalpel.

At other programs, where ward and outpatient activities comprise most of the training, there is another danger. That is, *while it is important to guarantee that there will be enough patients, it is also necessary to find out if there are enough residents.* Both extremes can be harmful to your training. If the ratio of residents to patients is too high (too few patients), you may not be exposed to enough medical activity to get the training you desire. But if the ratio of residents to patients is too low (too few residents), you will be robbed of valuable reading, thinking, and discussion time. You will use this time attempting to care for an ever-multiplying patient load.

The ratio of postgraduate trainees to inpatient beds is highest at training programs in the Western United States (0.34 residents per bed), programs at university-operated institutions (0.65), and those at state-owned institutions (0.62). Programs in the Southern United States (0.24), with limited university affiliation (0.15), and that are church-owned (0.14) have the lowest ratios.

Numbers can also deceive in another way. While a residency program may note that there are over 1,500 babies delivered per year at the hospital, it may not tell you that over private practitioners deliver half of these with no resident involvement. This is, in part, related to the amount of responsibility that you can assume as a resident. But it also impacts greatly on the volume of patients that you will personally encounter. Your individual patient load should be at the forefront of your mind while assessing any residency training program.

## Geography

Geography often plays a more important role in the selection of a residency program than it rightfully should. But, probably more than any other factor that you will consider in selecting a program, geography will be the most personal for you. Remember, though, that geographical ignorance and prejudices should not be allowed to limit your choice of programs.

If you, like many of your cohorts, have not had time to visit most of our country, then spend some time getting an accurate picture of both the geography and the medicine in different parts of the nation from people who have actually been there. No, it's not true that everything east of the Mississippi River is concrete. Likewise, it's not true that physicians practice "cowboy medicine" between the Mississippi and the Pacific Coast. Wherever you are now, I have no doubt that you have heard horror stories about other areas of the country. Find out about these sections of the country from faculty who have lived and worked there. Don't assume anything. You may be surprised by what you discover.

There may be a special reason to carefully consider the location of residency programs. About half of all physicians remain to practice in the state where they did their residency. Those most likely to stay are those who do their residency in the same state where they went to medical school, generalist physicians, and women.

Note that the number of residency programs varies greatly by region (Figure 10.3). If you concentrate on a region with a small number of residency positions, your chance of matching may decrease.

FIGURE 10.3

*Percent of Residency Programs and Residents by Geographic Region\**

| Region | Programs | Residents |
|---|---|---|
| Mid-Atlantic (NJ, NY, PA) | 23.2% | 24.1% |
| East-North Central (IL, IN, MI, OH, WI) | 17.3 | 17.3 |
| South Atlantic (DE, DC, FL, GA, MD, NC, SC, VA, WV) | 16.2 | 15.1 |
| Pacific (AK, CA, HI, OR, WA) | 10.9 | 11.4 |
| West-South Central (AR, LA, OK, TX) | 9.1 | 9.3 |
| New England (CT, ME, MA, NH, RI, VT) | 7.9 | 7.7 |
| West-North Central (IA, KS, MN, MO, NE, ND, SD) | 6.7 | 6.5 |
| East-South Central (AL, KY, MS, TN) | 4.8 | 4.5 |
| Mountain (AZ, CO, ID, MT, NV, NM, UT, WY) | 3.5 | 3.3 |
| Territories (PR) | 1.0 | 0.8 |

*These are ACGME-accredited residency programs and the residents (M.D.s and D.O.s) in these programs. The location of AOA-accredited programs generally correlates with these numbers.

Adapted from Appendix II, Table 2, JAMA. 1999;282(9):895.

The following factors will determine how important it is for you to obtain a training position in a specific part of the country, a specific city or part of a city, or another area.

### Family Needs

Many students have family obligations which limit where they can go for training. These may include having a spouse or "significant other" in a job that he or she cannot leave or transfer, a spouse or child at a critical point in school, ill parents, or family members who need specialized medical care. In dual professional relationships, the ability of the other partner to meet professional requirements in another locale (often, for the second time) carries great weight. Dentists, lawyers, accountants, architects, and others may find relicensing difficult, if not impossible, in another state. For some people, being near their extended family or coreligionists may also be an important consideration.

One of these factors may make a particular geographic location a "Must" for you. Since this is so personal, little advice can be given. But be sure to talk it over with the individual involved before you assume that you need to limit your search for that person's benefit. You may be amazed at the amount of flexibility you actually have.

## Personal Needs

Other needs may influence how much weight you will give to geography. Besides a need to "see the mountains (or ocean, or trees) everyday," the most common personal geographic need is compatibility with leisure-time activities. Although you probably won't have much spare time, especially during your first year of training, the desire to make the most of the free time that you do have is very reasonable. But even this may not restrict you as much as you think.

Of course, if you are a mountain climber, you need mountains. And if you are a surfer, you will need surf. But if you are involved in running, swimming, hiking, or the more cerebral activities of music, art, and theater, you can find many locations that will meet your needs. By the way, if you are a skier, remember that the snow only lasts a little while—and anyway, you can always fly.

## Range

Although several comments have already been made about expanding your geographic horizons when choosing programs, a word needs to be said specifically about hesitancy to leave the "nest." The "nest" is your medical school, where you know the rules, know the faculty, and generally feel at home. It would be very comfortable to stay. And, unless you are a top student from a highly respected medical school, you may feel that you are not prepared to go out into the world and work with, as I have heard many students say, "students who really know something."

My advice is: *leave if you possibly can.* You are just as capable as the medical students from other or "big name" schools. In fact, you may have much more clinical experience. And, if you stay at your medical school's hospital for residency training, you will probably be working under a handicap that will not afflict your fellow residents. That is the syndrome of "Once a medical student, always a medical student."

The faculty and staff know you as a medical student. Of course, they will know, deep down, that you are now a resident, but you may have some frustrating attitudes directed your way. You certainly will have to work harder for their respect. By the way, this factor has an exponential effect upon residents joining the faculty where they completed their residencies. They spend an inordinate amount of time making the switch, in their colleague's minds, from resident to staff physician. So, if you have aspirations of joining the faculty at a specific institution, especially your medical school, go elsewhere for residency training.

## Salary

In general, resident salaries have remained stable (in constant dollars) since the late 1960s. (This means that although the total amount has increased, when it is adjusted for inflation, its purchasing power has remained unchanged.)

Although it may seem that salary should be discussed under benefits, there is an element of salary that is geography-dependent. The cost of living varies significantly across the country. In general, costs will be lower in the deep South and in the Midwest. The farther Northeast or West you go, the more the average living costs will be. Normally this will not be a significant factor, since residents' salaries usually reflect the local cost of living. If, however, you need to repay a monster-sized school loan, this difference may be important.

For the most current update on resident salaries and other benefits, go to www.aamc.org/hlthcare/coth-hss/start-htm.

## Reputation

The institution's and program's reputations naturally influence applicants. Few reputations derive from excellent education. Rather, other achievements bring recognition to the institution and faculty. Nearly all residency applicants do best if they look beyond a reputation to the factors that are important to their own professional development.

### Institution's Reputation

Some venerable institutions, such as Harvard, Johns Hopkins, Stanford, and the University of Chicago, have built their reputations largely on research over decades or centuries. The prestige envelops all their programs, whether deserved or not. How should this institutional reputation affect an applicant's decision about whether to go there? If the institution has a residency program that is competitive in all aspects with other programs, some applicants may want to consider another factor: prestige. Those physicians aspiring to careers in academia or to clinical practices in posh locales may benefit from "gold-plated" credentials. Problems arise when an applicant sacrifices an excellent education for this prestige, as sometimes happens. In general, it is best to choose programs that provide an optimal educational experience, regardless of their perceived status.

### Program's Reputation

Some programs in every specialty have a reputation for excellence. Many of these provide superior education. But some programs' reputations linger long after the glow has faded. Other programs have not yet acquired a reputation for excellence, either because they are new or because information about program alterations have not permeated the specialty's information network. Changes in the residency director, affiliated institutions, the patient population, and institutional funding may all affect a program. Applicants cannot simply rely on a program's reputation for past excellence, they must analyze each program as it currently exists, on the basis of their personal needs.

Nevertheless, more than one-fourth of all applicants use a program's reputation as their primary factor in deciding among programs. Many later regret this.

## Program's Age & Stability

No one wants to enter a residency program only to learn part way through training that the program will merge with another institution or close, that crucial faculty members are leaving, or that the program has lost accreditation. In these times of financial upheaval within the health care industry, no guarantees exist. Large teaching hospitals and individual residency programs are closing; faculty leave for better personal opportunities.

Increasing numbers of teaching hospitals are now merging for economic reasons. This provides them with economies of scale, may reduce operational expenses by eliminating redundant services, and makes them more attractive for managed care contracts. These mergers, though, may disrupt resident education. Teaching faculty, especially in subspecialty areas, may be diminished, as might indigent or resident clinics and ancillary services that ease the workload. Remaining faculty may be pressured to decrease teaching and increase patient care while shifting many of their duties to physician assistants, nurse practitioners and other allied health personnel. While these changes are going on in many institutions, the rate may be accelerated during and just after large mergers. It would be wise to check to see whether such a merger is in the works at programs to which you are applying.

Although it provides no warranty (e.g., the Mount Sinai Medical Center in Cleveland and the Manhattan Eye, Ear and Throat Hospital in New York suddenly closed their residencies in June 1999, as new residents were arriving), a reasonable method for testing a program's stability is to look at its history. How long has it existed? Has it ever had difficulty with accreditation? Has the program's faculty been stable? The answers to these questions cut two ways. They may indicate a stable program, but they also may point to programs and faculty that are rigid and unable to change with the times. Other than discerning information about an institution's financial soundness (which is difficult to get and often more difficult to believe), information about a program's stability may only be marginally helpful.

## Strong Faculty

A large part of what makes any residency training program unique is the faculty. Their interests, strengths, and involvement in the institution, national specialty activities, and the local community all are important factors in making any residency solid. Without a dynamic faculty, it does not matter what else is present—the residency will be weak.

Current residents can best answer your questions about the faculty. They interact (or don't) with the faculty every day, and will either highly praise them or barely give them a lukewarm endorsement. There is rarely a medium ground.

### Availability

Even if the faculty is intensely interested in teaching, there might either be too few of them or too much extra work, such as administrative duties, added clinical responsibilities, student teaching, research, or writing, for them to be around when you need them. Specifically, you need to know whether teachers are readily available to you in three situations.

*Clinical setting.* Do program faculty just make rounds or take morning report, or are they there for you when you feel that you have gotten in over your head? Can they be relied upon to respond in the middle of the night and on weekends? Will you be left "hanging" in clinics without anyone to guide you through tough or unfamiliar territory? And do they show up promptly when you need to go to the operating room or do a procedure under emergency conditions? Sadly, the answers at many programs are not optimal. Recently, non-physician staff has supervised residents in some programs. While this is not permitted under ACGME rules, find out if it occurs at the programs in which you are interested.

*Personal counseling.* The second time you need faculty to be available is for personal counseling. As with any job, no residency will be without its ups and downs—moments of personal crisis and indecision. More mundane will be the day-to-day administrative problems of scheduling your days off appropriately, getting your research started, or getting a nagging administrator off your back. Eventually, there will also be the question of a job search and the process of going out into the "real world." All of this can, and should, be eased by personal interaction with your faculty. That is one of the reasons they are there. If they are not available for this, you may have nowhere to turn.

*Formal teaching*. Last, and perhaps least important, is the faculty's participation in formal teaching. This includes grand rounds, journal clubs, and other formal conferences. While generally regarded as the most important of a faculty member's duties, it will actually be of less importance to you than the other activities.

The point is, that for faculty to be effective, they not only have to be interested, but they must also be available. Part-time faculty, those with too many other duties, and those who just don't have the concern to be available to residents are not what you are seeking. Reviewing the often-inflated faculty to resident ratios that many programs advertise will not help you to answer this question. Get this information during your program visits.

### Interest

The key ingredient for any individual faculty member, or any faculty group, is that they have a strong interest in training residents.

This may seem to be a foregone conclusion. They are faculty members at a training institution, aren't they? But individuals choose the academic path for a variety of reasons, many of which do not include teaching. They may have a strong research interest, want to avoid night call as much as possible, or just want the easier or more distant clinical experience that teaching institutions often permit. Or, they may have had, at one time, a strong interest in teaching, but are now burned out. This is not to say that there aren't many great and wonderful teachers at residency programs. But the quality varies widely, and it is up to you to check it closely. Without real faculty interest, you will essentially be on your own.

### Stability

Along with faculty interest and a presence, there needs to be some continuity. Look for how long faculty have been with the program. If there is a high turnover, it indicates that there may be significant problems. How much experience have the faculty members had in the specialty? If most of the faculty are fresh out of residency training themselves, you will probably not get the wisdom (yes, indeed—there really is some) that comes with experience, if not age. You may be getting instruction from a group who are themselves still "wet behind the ears" in their practice of medicine. While some individuals at this level may give a program an instillation of vigor and enthusiasm, too many may lead to a less-than-satisfactory training experience. The key, then, is to check into the interest level, availability, and stability of the faculty. They are the residency program's foundations.

## Curriculum

What educational opportunities, in what settings, and with what outcomes does the residency program say it offers? Standard specialty requirements may determine some of this. Some of what they say may be exaggerated. Remember that whatever they say about the curriculum is always subject to modification based on financial changes, institutional reorganization, faculty transitions, and patient care needs.

### Curriculum Structure

What will you do and when? Which services will you be on, for how long, and in which training years? These elements, the most basic part of a program's curriculum, are the easiest to compare among programs. Will you do the intensive care service in the first year? Do you work in the clinic during your second and third years? If particular programs interest you because of either specific rotations or the order or length of rotations, ask about these during your interview to be certain that the program anticipates no changes in them.

Curriculum structure matters in some specialties more than in others. Child/Adolescent Psychiatry programs, for example, may mix the Psychiatry and Child Psychiatry years in different ways. Similarly, all the "hyphenated programs," such as Pediatrics-Physical Medicine and Rehabilitation, Internal Medicine-Emergency Medicine, or Psychiatry-Neurology, may combine time in each specialty in different ways. If this is important to your educational needs, find out how the program has structured its curriculum.

### Interaction with Other Specialties

Few residents get the most from their residency programs unless they have exposure to the knowledge other specialists provide. Usually, much of this exposure comes from interaction with the residents in other specialties. They often provide a non-threatening source for information to expand one's knowledge about the diseases, procedures, and thought processes of other specialties. In addition, other specialty training programs often have organized conferences and teaching rounds that you can attend.

In some cases, the presence of other specialty residencies or fellowships may interfere with your residency training. Family Practice seems to be the most commonly affected, since specialty residents' involvement in cases often precludes Family Practice residents from first-assisting in surgery, delivering babies and doing Cesarean sections, or getting adequate experience in Orthopedics. Many Family Practice programs utilize alternative institutions to work around this problem. Not so obvious may be the decreased experience some residents get due to the presence of subspecialty fellows. Surgery residents may not get a full Thoracic Surgery experience if fellows do or first-assist on most of the cases, and Internal Medicine or Pediatric residents may lack some procedural skills if Critical Care, Hematology-Oncology, or Cardiology fellows constantly upstage them.

The presence of other specialists and subspecialists is a mixed blessing. Consider each institution's blessings in light of your own needs.

## Conferences

How many conferences does the residency program offer? This number is usually a prominent part of the program's literature. Rather than the absolute number, however, look at the amount of time devoted to conferences per month. (Use conferences per month as the comparison figure, since some programs hold their conferences only once or twice a month, while others may have them daily or weekly.)

Also important are the answers to these questions: How many of these conferences will you be able to attend? Is coverage of your clinical duties provided? Which takes precedence, conferences or patient care? (Conferences do you no good unless you can attend.) Also, does the program require attendance at a minimum number of conferences? If so, do penalties exist for non-attendance? Ask residents these questions for a more balanced answer.

Not only is the quantity of conference time important, but so are the *types and quality of these conferences*. Some types of conferences are mandated by the specialty's requirements. Others are at the whim or educational savvy of the residency's faculty.

It is relatively easy to determine what conferences a program holds. More difficult to determine is how good an educational experience they provide. Conference quality varies with the organization, faculty participation, relevance, and ambiance. Relevance refers to the importance of the topics to your education, rather than to the faculty's research interests or a sponsoring drug company's latest wonder drug. Do the conferences regularly enhance your ability to perform patient care or expand your knowledge of the specialty? Are some conferences joint projects between your department and complementary specialties? These are the qualities that make conferences useful.

Ambiance refers to the amount of tension that faculty and senior residents produce, especially during morbidity and mortality conferences. Education need not be an ego-destructive experience, although some residency programs have yet to figure that out.

Lastly, how many of these conferences are resident-run? This is less important than the conference quality, although it points to another area of resident responsibility.

## Special Training

Residency programs differ in their orientation. This is true for all specialties. This orientation depends partly on the values and philosophy of the institution, partly on the residency director, and in large measure on the faculty's interests and abilities.

At present, there are recognized subspecialty areas within nearly all medical specialties (Figures 2.8 and 2.9). Some are well defined, with specialty boards in place. Others, such as Trauma Surgery, have been defined both through need and by the medical community's acceptance. If you think you have a desire for training in a subspecialty, make sure that you will be exposed to it during your residency program. If you are not certain about your long-term goals, you should make sure that you will at least have exposure to several of these areas. You might just develop an interest in one of them.

If you are certain you want to enter a specific subspecialty training program after residency, find out if that area is particularly strong at the institution(s) in which the residency is located. Will you have an easier time getting into the subspecialty training program (if one exists) at that institution if you do your residency there? Find out now. It may save you time, money, and a great deal of effort in the future.

## Esprit de Corps

An important factor for your well being is the amount of esprit de corps, i.e., fellowship and camaraderie, found in the department. This aspect of a training program is hard to measure, and can only be assessed by your perception of the *gestalt* of the program. But it is important to most residents, and affects how much they enjoy their residency experience. About one out of five applicants rate this as their main consideration in deciding among programs.

The attitude that pervades any department helps to determine the ease with which residents, faculty, and staff perform their duties. If there is a feeling of calm serenity, with people genuinely liking and trusting their coworkers, then the resident's job is much easier. But if there is a feeling of strain, anxiety, and perhaps fear, a resident's entire life becomes much more difficult.

The important attitudes are the day-to-day interpersonal interactions at all levels within the department, rather than those during episodic medical crises. Do the secretaries respond to you as if you are a welcome guest, or a miserable underling? Do the residents and faculty seem to get along with each other? Is there an underlying feeling of tension and bitterness?

The problem, of course, is how to assess this nebulous quality. The trick is to open your personal sensors and record your experiences after every interaction, including telephone calls, with each program. When you visit the program, try to discover their feelings. Pump the residents, and if possible the ancillary staff, for their attitudes toward the people in the department. While inexact, this is the best method for assessing the departmental attitudes that may be very important for your happiness during your training.

## Research Opportunities/Training

If you plan to skip this section because you don't have any interest in research, please stop and reconsider. The availability of research opportunities and training at a residency program means that you will

1. Sharpen your ability to critically read the medical literature—as you know, there is a lot of junk out there.

2. Keep abreast of the latest knowledge—at least in the areas being researched.

3. Be exposed to enough research to see if you actually might get "turned on" by it.

Quite a few residents have entered residency programs intending to never do any research after their training, only to discover that they actually liked searching for answers to pithy questions. In fact, some of them found that research actually added a necessary and fulfilling dimension to their professional life.

While they are still in the minority, an increasing number of new medical school graduates seem to be interested in research. More than 40% plan to include a period of research in their postgraduate training.

The presence of research activity suggests that clinical service, such as patient care, is not the only reason that the faculty and residents are at a particular institution. There is more to that department and institution than merely treating patient after patient. To have research, a spirit of learning and education must be present. This is what you are looking for in a training program. Value it highly when you find it.

### Knowledge

No one learns to do research by him- or herself. You may have done some research as a medical student. However, it is unlikely that you either had the primary responsibility for the project or had to acquire the in-depth knowledge of scientific methodology, statistical analysis, writing, or any of the other elements of a successful research project. You are looking for faculty members who are experienced in doing (and publishing) research in your specialty. If you have developed an interest in one particular area, you may look for that. The important thing is to find at least one faculty member experienced in research who will be willing to work with you during your training. This individual will act as a research mentor, much like your mentor in medical school.

Of course, it is best to have a selection of experienced researchers to choose from, but this is not always possible. The things you should learn about research from any particular program are

- How to design a research project.
- How to perform those techniques needed to complete the project.
- How to statistically analyze your research.
- How to coherently write a scientific article.
- Where and how to present and/or publish your results.

How is this information about doing research presented? Is it given as lectures, assigned readings, personal tutelage, or learned by trial and error? Usually, programs use a combination of all these methods. But the most important element is exposure to those who have been there before—a faculty experienced in all phases of research.

## Materials

If you plan to do research, especially if your time will be limited, find out what materials for research are available to you. The more that are readily available, the less time and energy you will have to spend hunting down needed supplies, space, and equipment.

The first, and often the most essential, material is *money*. While it is the root of all evil, money is also the key to getting research done. Does the department or institution have funds set aside for resident research? Are there other sources that can be tapped easily? Are the amounts limited? Does their availability depend on the type of research being done?

The second material you may need is *laboratory facilities*. If you are planning on doing either bench or animal research, you need both laboratory space and equipment at your disposal. You will often be able to "squeeze into" a faculty member's lab and use "borrowed" equipment. But, of course, these first have to be available. Also find out if there are support personnel, such as veterinarians and technicians, available to help you. Are there animals available for research? This will vary markedly due to both state law and the amount of funding you have available. Are there individuals outside the department who are supportive enough of resident research to help with space, equipment, or expertise?

Often forgotten is the question of whether you can get *secretarial support*. Whether or not you are a "hunt-and-peck" typist, those keys can get mighty blurry when you are doing the third revision of a manuscript after making ward rounds at 8 P.M. Although not essential, the availability of secretarial support is a great asset.

Finally, how about *computers*? Are they available? Is training available if you have yet to be indoctrinated? Even if you aren't interested in any other aspect of research, inquire about computers. It is essential for the modern physician, no matter what the specialty, to be acquainted with at least basic computer operation—which means being computer literate. All large hospitals in the country, as well as most physicians' offices, use computers for business management. Most also use them for the management of clinical records and other information, such as lab results. In research, computers are essential. Knowledge of databases, spreadsheets, statistical packages, and word processors is necessary for all but the simplest research being conducted today. Be sure that you come out of your residency training computer literate.

### Time Allotted

If you anticipate doing serious research during your residency training, you will need adequate time. Programs vary widely in how they supply that time. Some assign specific blocks of time in which to do research. Often this is because of, or at least consistent with, specialty board requirements.

Other options are either doing research during an elective time period or working on research while attending to other clinical duties. The former may deprive you of necessary extra clinical experiences, which are often in subspecialty or complementary areas (such as neonatal ICU for an Obstetrics resident). The latter, unless the clinical load is very light, will deprive you of sleep. And during a residency, as you will find out, sleep is a commodity in very short supply. It will be wise to determine, as early as possible, how research time is allotted in the programs that you investigate.

### Local Job Prospects After Training

You may believe that you already know where you want to live and set up practice once you have finished training. If that is true, you might want to reflect on this when selecting a residency training site. But first, consider whether jobs in your chosen specialty are even available in the particular geographic area in which you are interested. More important, with the ongoing changes in health care delivery systems, will jobs still be available by the time you complete training? Will training in that geographic area help you get a local job when you finish? Will you still be interested in living in that area when you finish?

Remember, your attitudes change as you mature. In some instances, residents who train in a particular area have an advantage getting local jobs, since they have been able to make contacts during their residency. In other cases, it may be a better strategy to train at a respected program and then look for jobs in the geographic region that interests you. Determine this by checking with clinicians or the medical society in the communities you are considering. Do not make a residency selection based on erroneous assumptions. Always check the facts first.

Also, career counseling should not end with deciding upon a specialty or entering a residency. With the proliferation of subspecialties and the wide variety of practice options, residents should actively seek advice on career decisions, beginning as soon as they enter their residency program. This may stimulate the faculty to provide some of this information in a stand-ardized fashion, and even if they do not, it suggests to them that you are a top-notch resident who has his or her eyes fixed on having a fulfilling and meaningful career. Is such counseling available at the residency program?

## Facilities
As a resident, many factors will influence your day-to-day stress and comfort levels. The nature and organization of the facilities in which you work, however, are major contributing factors. While many residency applicants discount these elements, you would be wise to consider how important they will be to your education, your lifestyle, and your sanity.

### Clinical Laboratory Support
Waiting for the results of an urgent, pre-operative, or outpatient laboratory test can cost both residents and patients their most valuable resource, time. Delays can frustrate everyone involved. Questions about the speed and comprehensiveness of clinical laboratories may be very important. How extensive are the tests an institution's clinical laboratories run? Is a stat lab available? Can you only get commonly needed tests during certain hours? Will lab technicians (or nursing staff) draw blood at all hours?

The days of running your own laboratory tests came and went, and now have come again—at least to a limited extent. Performing these and similar tests are part of medicine's new age. Can you perform the common tests, such as Strep screens and pregnancy tests, done in your clinic? Some laboratories have stopped clinicians from performing tests in the clinics in the name of quality control (or is it revenues?). Yet you need this experience to be prepared for medical practice after residency.

### Computerized Records/Lab Results

The world is moving toward computerization. While medicine has generally moved more slowly than many other fields, financial pressures have pushed many medical practices to produce first computerized laboratory results and then computerized patient records. Both save physicians an enormous amount of time when waiting or searching for information. While many training institutions have incorporated computerization to at least a limited degree, the more they have done so, the less time you will waste.

### Hospitals' Ages & Atmosphere

The bricks and mortar (and plastic, steel, and wood) that make up the institution(s) in which you work may look chic and modern or staid and ivy-covered on the outside, but you work on the inside. How well is the facility maintained? Is its structure so outmoded that it makes working there difficult? Do its piecemeal additions mean that you will be walking endless miles to do the simplest tasks? Or are the new "modern" conveniences unworkable? Does the place look shabby and unkempt, or does it look neat and clean, despite its age?

You are going to spend many long hours here. The hospital's or clinic's appearance and structure may not be your first consideration, but it will impact your daily existence.

### Library/Media

How good is the *library*? Even if you do not plan to do research, the library is essential for house officers to prepare talks and investigate unusual findings in their patients. Likewise, what facilities are there to do *computer searches*, to learn about and use the *Internet*, and to *photocopy*? These services are now an essential part of medical education and available through most medical libraries.

### Parking

Parking may not only be expensive, but also it can—as you probably already know from your medical school experience—be a hassle. The amount of frustration involved in parking a vehicle can be ascertained by talking to current residents. The cost, though, is a commonly offered benefit. Seventy-four percent of teaching hospitals pay at least part of the parking costs for

PGY-1 housestaff. Additional questions to ask are: How safe is the parking area? How safe is the area between where I will park and the hospital?

### Resident On-Call Room Ambiance

The on-call rooms will be your home-away-from-home. Don't expect them to resemble even the quality or size of a low-rent motel room. They should, however, be clean, quiet, have ready access to a telephone, have reasonable air flow and temperature control, and be private. The rooms should also be cleaned daily and have fresh bed linens, although this is not the case at some institutions. Privacy is necessary so that whatever sleep you get when on call will not be interrupted by telephone calls or pages to other residents sharing your sleeping quarters. The room should also have a lock so that both you and your personal items remain safe. Ideally, these rooms should have access to a bathroom and shower.

These requirements do not describe five-star accommodations, but rather one step above tent camping. Yet, if the on-call rooms meet the above requirements, they should suffice for your nocturnal hospital stays. Ask to see the on-call rooms during your visits.

### Safety/Security

Most medical students feel they are immortal (at least until they take Pathology). Since age brings some form of wisdom, most residents recognize that they must not only learn but also be safe in their clinical environments. Recent news stories about physicians being killed only suggest the level of danger faced by physicians in and around hospitals. Many institutions in traditionally high-crime areas have tight security in place at their facilities. Yet even there, injuries and deaths have occurred. Some institutions have not yet come to grips with their changing environment and lack adequate security. If you recognize that no place is absolutely safe, you can reasonably balance your security concerns with your educational needs.

## Restrictive Covenants

Restrictive covenants, also called "non-compete clauses," are sections of employment contracts that prevent individuals from subsequently working within a specified geographic radius. For residents, this often meant not being allowed to work in the same city where the residency was located or within a specified number of miles of the residency's main clinical site.

The AMA's Council on Ethical and Judicial Affairs has said "it is unethical for a teaching institution to seek a non-competition guarantee in return for fulfilling its educational obligations. Physicians-in-training should not be asked to sign covenants-not-to-compete as a condition of their entry into any residency or fellowship program." According to ACGME rules, residencies must not require individuals to sign these types of covenants in order to become or remain a resident. Even so, program directors are asked to state in their program's description in *FREIDA* whether they have such clauses (because everyone does not follow the rules). Find this under the "Basic Institutional Information."

Unless there are extenuating circumstances, *do not apply* to programs that have restrictive covenants. Therefore, in the Must/Want Analysis, "No Restrictive Covenants" should be completed as a "Must."

## Benefits

The benefits a residency program provides determine your real compensation level, and, in part, how endurable your life will be during residency. They suggest how much of your salary will have to be spent on some of life's necessities, or whether you can afford to do your residency at all.

At present, programs may offer nearly any benefit package that allows them to compete for applicants. They must, however, provide professional liability (malpractice) coverage for the duration of a resident's training and for any lawsuits arising after they leave the program arising from events that occurred as part of their educational program. The AMA, through its representation on the Accreditation Council for Graduate Medical Education (the organization that puts out the "Green Book" and accredits residency programs), is urging that residency programs be required to also provide health, life, and disability insurance for all residents.

When you are told about the benefits that programs offer, be aware of the fine print. Many programs offer certain benefits only if the resident contributes a share of the cost. Often this portion of the cost can be considerable. If you need a particular benefit, such as parking, dental care, or insurance, be sure that you know in advance how much you will need to contribute to get that benefit.

### Salary

It is the bedrock of all other benefits. Unlike nearly all others aspiring to a professional position, residency applicants never negotiate salary—it is fixed in advance. Generally, institutions have the same salary for all residents in the same postgraduate year of training. Yet these salaries can vary considerably from institution to institution, and from one region of the country to another.

In general, PGY-1 residents will receive an average salary of $36,014 in the Northeastern United States, and of $32,250 in the West. Nationwide,

PGY-1 average salaries ranged from $37,167 in church-owned hospitals to $35,882 in Veterans Affairs hospitals.

Regional variations in salaries and variations by type of hospital (federal, university, private) are detailed in the *COTH Survey of Housestaff Stipends, Benefits and Funding.* Salaries rise about 10% per year during training. Housestaff salaries have actually declined slightly over a quarter century, if adjusted for inflation. (A 1999 salary of $34,104, the national average first-year salary, is equal to about $12,413 in 1977 dollars, a bit less than what many of your professors were paid as interns, $13,186.)

If there is a large variation in housestaff salaries among the institutions within a particular region, think about why a particular institution has to pay higher salaries to their housestaff. Often it is because they have a deficient training program or other reasons for housestaff dissatisfaction.

Salary is not an absolute number. Rather, it should be compared to the cost of living in a particular locale. A high salary may not go very far in Washington, DC; San Francisco; Boston; New York City; or parts of Los Angeles. (Los Angeles, by the way, has one of the lowest average first-year housestaff salaries.) However, a much lower salary may allow a rather nice lifestyle in many smaller, southern, or Midwestern cities.

### Health Benefits

Health benefits vary. Since you really are getting older and you probably don't plan to sit in a chair and vegetate during your time off, you need an affordable way to stay healthy and to get necessary medical treatment. This is without even considering the needs of any dependents, e.g., spouse or children, which you have or might acquire along the way.

Health benefits you might find available through your employer at a residency program include coverage for hospitalization, dental services, drug prescriptions, employee health services, psychiatric counseling, vision services (glasses), and additional health insurance. These are often grouped under various types and styles of health insurance. The bottom-line question, though, is: What services are paid for by the employer?

You may never before have had to purchase *health insurance.* In the past, your parents or your school may have picked up your health insurance needs. If so, you will be shocked at the cost. Health insurance is very expensive. And not only does it cost a great deal, but also the permutations in what you get for your insurance dollars vary greatly (Figure 10.4).

The major elements to consider when looking at insurance that a residency program offers are: (1) who is covered, (2) what is covered, and (3) how much you will still have to pay. If you have dependents, it is very important to know whether they will also be covered. If you expect to need

FIGURE 10.4

**Health Benefits Provided to Housestaff and Dependents, Nationwide***

| Benefit | | Res | Fam |
|---|---|---|---|
| **Group Medical Insurance** | Offered/Fully Paid | 61% | 40% |
| | Offered/Cost Shared | 39 | 53 |
| | Not Offered/Not Paid | 1 | 7 |
| **Dental** | Offered/Fully Paid | 40% | 26% |
| | Offered/Cost Shared | 38 | 45 |
| | Not Offered/Not Paid | 22 | 29 |
| **Drug Prescriptions** | Offered/Fully Paid | 56% | 39% |
| | Offered/Cost Shared | 42 | 53 |
| | Not Offered/Not Paid | 2 | 8 |
| **Psychiatric Benefits** | Offered/Fully Paid | 61% | 41% |
| | Offered/Cost Shared | 38 | 53 |
| | Not Offered/Not Paid | 1 | 6 |
| **Vision** | Offered/Fully Paid | 43% | 32% |
| | Offered/Cost Shared | 29 | 39 |
| | Not Offered/Not Paid | 28 | 29 |

*Some totals may not add up to 100% due to rounding.
Adapted from: Association of American Medical Colleges. *Council of Teaching Hospitals Survey of Housestaff Stipends, Benefits and Funding.* Washington, DC: AAMC, 1998.

obstetric care, or if you or a member of your family needs special medical services, be certain that these will be covered by the policy. In addition, are prescriptions, glasses, and dental care covered? If they aren't, these items can take a big bite out of your resident salary.

Finally, if the insurance does cover your specific health needs, what is your copayment? A *copayment is the amount that you must pay*, and may be a flat fee or calculated as a percentage of the charges for specific health services. If the copayment is large or the total amount covered for services is relatively small, you could be put at financial risk if you or your family needs extensive health services. More than half of all institutions charge residents copayments for inpatient medical care, averaging $22 per stay, but ranging from $5 to $1,500. For ambulatory services, about two-thirds have copayments, averaging $16 per visit and ranging from $5 to $45.

*Group medical coverage* is insurance that nearly all teaching institutions offer to residents and their families. Most hospitals have from two to eight plans to choose from; the benefits vary among the plans. More Western hospitals (86%) fully pay for resident coverage than do those elsewhere in the country (<60%). Western programs also most commonly fully pay for a resident's family coverage (76%); this is least frequent in the South (28%). Municipal (city-owned) hospitals were the most likely, and V.A. hospitals the least likely, to fully pay medical insurance for housestaff (68% and 43%, respectively) and their families (53% and 33%). HIV/AIDS coverage is included in most policies.

*Dental* benefits for both housestaff and dependents are provided by about 70%, and *prescription drug* benefits are provided by more than 90% of teaching hospitals. *Psychiatric* benefits are provided to housestaff in 96% of teaching hospitals. The percentage offering this benefit has been gradually increasing in recent years. *Optical services* are provided at low or no cost at many programs. Although this may appear to be a minor benefit, glasses can be very expensive.

*Health promotion* has become a cost-effective benefit for an increasing number of non-hospital employers, and will eventually make its way into the health treatment system. At least one-third of major employers now have on-site exercise facilities and classes. An additional one-third provide employee discounts for health club memberships. The increasing awareness of and interest in fitness should soon make this benefit available at many teaching hospitals. Health promotion comes in two forms: screening and risk-avoidance. Residency applicants dislike pre-employment screening, such as that for drugs or HIV. They respond positively, however, to such things as a smoke-free work environment.

*Sick leave* is one benefit few people look forward to using. Since you will work around ill patients and colleagues, you will probably get sick enough to stay away from work at some point during your residency. What provisions does the program have for this? The other side of the coin is: What requirements are there for you to act as "back-up" for other residents who take sick leave? These requirements are often generally set by the specialty's residency review committee, and more specifically by the institutions and programs.

Note that, just as with most of the other benefits that a program may offer, there is either no tax or very low tax for you on health benefits. And, since these are costs that you otherwise would have to pay, they are, in essence, additional salary. But they are only worthwhile to you if you need the benefit. Obstetric care does you no good if you are a single male. Nearly half of all institutions now offer flexible (cafeteria-style) benefit plans in which the employee selects the specific benefits that he or she wants from a menu of available options. Midwest programs offer flexible plans more often (71%) than other areas; they are least common in the South (46%).

## Non-Health Benefits

Non-health benefits are designed to make your life as an employee easier. They often cover some of the necessities of modern life that you will have pay for if the teaching institution does not pick up the cost. So, in essence, if you need the particular benefit, having it offered by your employer will make your salary go that much farther. Of course, if a particular benefit is of no use to you, it should not be considered as a real part of your benefit package.

Non-health benefits that may be offered to housestaff or their dependents include: life insurance, disability insurance, parking, housing allowance, meals, vacation, educational time off, educational funding, liability insurance, childcare, laundry (uniforms), association dues, family educational benefits, and photocopying allowances. It is important to consider each institution's salary and benefit package to ensure that you will have the means to survive. You may find it useful to compare the benefits with those offered by similar institutions nationwide (Figures 10.5 and 10.6).

*Life insurance* is a necessity if you have dependents (especially if they are children). If anything should happen to you, this is what they will use for survival for the first several months after your death. Premiums are fully paid by 82% of teaching institutions, and partially paid by another 11%. The V.A. hospitals pay the full cost less often (52%) than most teaching hospitals. Most teaching hospitals (77%) have provisions for housestaff to purchase additional life insurance if they so desire. The average amount of life insurance provided is about $48,000, ranging from $1,000 to $600,000.

*Disability insurance* is an absolute necessity for you from now on. You have invested an enormous amount of time, effort, and money getting into and through medical school. Your potential earning power is sizable. However, if anything should happen to you that would prevent you from practicing medicine, or even practicing in your specialty once you have been trained, you will lose it all. Disability insurance will cover some of this loss, although current standard policies for residents pay a maximum of 60% of your salary per year, and may not include increases based on inflation.

It may be worthwhile to consider purchasing additional disability insurance individually, especially since you, like nearly 80% of residents, may have substantial education-associated debts. Depending upon the type of coverage, you will be paid a set amount regularly for a defined period of time if you cannot work as either a physician or a specialist once you have been trained. A special "HIV Indemnity Plan" is available through some insurance companies, including the AMA, to pay a lump sum if a resident

FIGURE 10.5

**Non-Health Benefits for First-Year Housestaff\***

| Benefit | Hospital Contribution | Percentage with Benefit |
|---|---|---|
| Life Insurance | Offered/Fully Paid | 82.0% |
| | Offered/Cost Shared | 11.0 |
| | Not Offered/Not Paid | 8.0 |
| Disability Insurance | Offered/Fully Paid | 77.0% |
| | Offered/Cost Shared | 5.0 |
| | Not Offered/Not Paid | 19.0 |
| Parking | Offered/Fully Paid | 62.0% |
| | Offered/Cost Shared | 17.2 |
| | Not Offered/Not Paid | 20.6 |
| Housing | Offered/Fully Paid | 3.9% |
| | Offered/Cost Shared | 9.7 |
| | Not Offered /Not Paid | 86.5 |
| Meals when on call | Offered/Fully Paid | 85.2% |
| | Offered/Cost Shared | 10.5 |
| | Not Offered/Not Paid | 4.3 |
| Meals when working | Offered/Fully Paid | 24.9% |
| | Offered/Cost Shared | 23.4 |
| | Not Offered/Not Paid | 51.8 |

\*Some totals may not add up to 100% due to rounding.

Adapted from: Association of American Medical Colleges. *AAMC Data Book*. Washington, DC: AAMC, 1999.

becomes HIV-positive. Many disability policies will not pay unless the individual becomes incapacitated.

More than three-quarters (77%) of teaching hospitals pay some or all of the costs for their housestaff's disability insurance. Veteran's Administration and municipal hospitals offer this important benefit least often. Disability policies may also be continued (are "portable") when a resident leaves most programs (77%) if someone (usually the resident) continues to pay the premiums. In 74% of these cases, additional coverage can be purchased.

*Housing* is a necessity, although you may not see much of your personal housing as an intern. Only about 14% of teaching hospitals offer to pay all or part of the costs of housing. This benefit is most common in the Northeast (23%) and least common in the West (4%).

*Meals* are provided at no cost to most (85%) first-year on-call housestaff, and to many (25%) when working but not on call. Many other hospitals subsidize a portion of housestaff meals. Two important considerations are whether the food is edible and whether it will be available when you have time to eat, such as at 3 A.M.

*Vacation and educational leave* (Figure 10.6) are important mind- and body-rejuvenation periods. First-year housestaff typically get 15 days of vacation and PGY-2s typically get 23 days. Educational leave to attend conferences in excess of vacation time is granted by 81% of teaching hospitals. While many institutions have a general vacation policy, two-thirds let individual programs determine the amount of a resident's time off to attend conferences. Most hospitals contribute about $400 toward seminar registration and per diem costs for PGY-1s, and $700 for PGY-2s.

*Lab coats* are less critical than many other benefits, but their purchase and upkeep are often expensive. Will the hospital pay for your lab coats and launder them?

*Liability insurance* (malpractice) is a "Must" for all residents. The cost is astronomical if you pay for it personally, and even higher if you should need it and not have it. This is one expense that *must* be covered by the institution. It is not too difficult to consider as a "Must" since, for their own protection, all teaching institutions cover your insurance. There is no harm in double-checking, however.

House-officer groups have recently questioned whether hospitals are supplying residents with the appropriate type of malpractice insurance. The more inclusive type of coverage is the "occurrence" policy, which covers all alleged negligent acts occurring during the policy period. "Claims-made" policies are less comprehensive, and cover policyholders for all lawsuits filed during the period of coverage. (The alleged negligent act must also have occurred during the period of coverage).

### FIGURE 10.6
### *Vacation and Educational Leave for House Officers\**

| Annual Vacation | 1-10 Days | 11-15 Days | 16-21 Days | 22+ Days |
|---|---|---|---|---|
| PGY-1 | 18% | 42% | 33% | 8% |
| PGY-2 | 7% | 41% | 39% | 13% |
| Educational Leave | None | 1-5 Days | 6-9 Days | 10+ Days |
| PGY-1 | 23% | 60% | 14% | 3% |
| PGY-2 | 4% | 70% | 20% | 6% |

*Some totals may not add up to 100% due to rounding.

Adapted from: Association of American Medical Colleges. *Council of Teaching Hospitals Survey of Housestaff Stipends, Benefits and Funding.* Washington, DC: AAMC, 1998.

In essence, an occurrence policy will cover you for any malpractice allegations that happen during your residency—no matter when the lawsuit is filed. This is the type of professional liability coverage that the General Requirements for residency accreditation strongly suggest all programs have in place. Governing bodies also strongly suggest that occurrence-type professional liability coverage be provided.

The claims-made policy only covers you while you are still at the same institution. If lawsuits are subsequently filed, you are not covered by the insurance unless separate "tail coverage" has been purchased. However, so far no former resident is known to have been forced to pay damages. But it could happen.

Although the General Requirements for all residency training programs mandate that applicants must be provided with the details of the professional liability coverage, programs might forget to do so—especially if the coverage is inadequate. Ask which type of and how much coverage the hospital provides.

*Childcare* is a rather new benefit, offered by a limited number of programs and institutions. Childcare is an outgrowth of the general increase in the number of working mothers. In medicine, approximately 43% of all medical students are now women. Nearly 13% of all graduating medical students have children, and half of these have two or more.

Childcare allows parents to perform their jobs and not spend all their earnings to pay for their offspring's care. Unfortunately, in many cases, childcare services only include normal working hours, meaning Monday through Friday, 8:00 A.M. to 5:00 P.M. As a resident, your hours will be neither that regular nor that short. Only 15% of existing childcare programs are open weekends and holidays, and only 5% are open overnight (6:00 P.M. to 7:00 A.M.).

Some teaching hospitals, in recognition of the growing need for childcare services, especially when parents are working long and irregular hours, are implementing on-site childcare for housestaff. At present, only about 40% of teaching hospitals offer childcare services to their housestaff. These hospitals find that childcare not only helps attract residents, but also decreases absenteeism.

Most teaching institutions will assist residents in finding childcare if they don't offer it. Many institutions subsidize childcare, with the average maximum subsidy being 30% of the cost. Even where institutions offer childcare, 78% have waiting lists for housestaff's children. The average wait to enroll an infant (0 to 1 year) is six months, and to enroll children two years old and above is two months.

Besides its convenience, having childcare as a benefit can be a large savings to you. The hospitals normally charge residents between $45 and $100/week per child for this service. This is usually a marked financial, as well as emotional, savings over having to arrange comparable services outside the institution. The institutional services are reliable (your one sitter does not get sick), often have flexible hours matching yours, do not require transportation for the child to another site, and usually have care for sick children available.

Having childcare available for children even when they are ill is a new movement, in most cases spearheaded by health care facilities. This allows parents to continue working, as they must when a resident, with the assurance that their children are being cared for. If you think you could use this benefit, inquire. But, since children and the responsibility that they entail are sensitive issues, inquire discreetly.

*Parental leave*, once called maternity leave but now also available to fathers, is a rapidly spreading benefit since passage of the federal Family Leave Act. While nearly 94% of teaching hospitals have family leave policies, fewer than 60% of those institutions have had anyone take leave under their policy. (Isn't anyone getting pregnant among their resident staff?)

In 1997, approximately 47% of all residency programs provided "paid" maternity leave, 39% required residents to use vacation time or sick leave, and 3% did not grant maternity leave. In addition, 31% provided "paid" paternity leave, 50% required residents to use vacation time or sick leave, and 19% did not grant paternity leave (see Figure 13.4).

These numbers suggest that all applicants, not only women, need to be aware that regardless of a residency program's stated policy on parental leave, childcare, or other family matters, it is the attitude of the residency director that matters most. If a resident's supervisor is supportive, then the policies work, if not, they fail. Asking current residents during your site visit is the only way to find out just what a particular department's attitude on family-related matters really is. *FREIDA* makes it easy to review any program's childcare services (if they have completed that information). The database includes specific questions on maternity and paternity policy. It also includes the excellent question of whether this time comes out of vacation or sick leave time. If it is important to you, find out by asking the housestaff office or the residents.

*Family educational benefits* are offered by some programs, especially those associated with major universities. In some cases, the benefits include free or markedly reduced tuition for college classes. While this may not be useful to most residents, who may be spending much of their free time sleeping, it may be very helpful to their spouse. Many spouses are at the point in their life when they are interested in pursuing the remainder of either undergraduate or graduate training. If this benefit is useful, the money saved can be substantial.

*Recruitment incentives* (Figure 10.7) are now commonly offered in primary care specialties. While some national groups tried to halt this practice, Justice Department intervention assured that it will continue. Incentives range from supplying an expense account for books and educational courses to subsidizing interview expenses. Many of these incentives are now only offered at marginal programs. In the future, better programs may also begin to adopt these tactics.

*Organized housestaff/unions* have become much more common over the past few years. Often called Independent Housestaff Organizations (IHOs), residents' collective bargaining units have blossomed after the American Medical Association began supporting them and working with residents to get them organized. The AMA began the Physicians for Responsible Negotiations (PRN) to assist this organizing effort.

IHOs have helped the approximately 10,000 resident members in public hospitals address training conditions, salaries and benefits, ancillary support, and patient care with a collective voice. Joining a residency where such an organization exists (if it has been effective) may help lessen the frustrations you experience during residency.

In December 1999, the National Labor Relations Board overturned a 23-year-old precedent by granting medical residents the right to organize in private institutions. They had previously said that interns and residents could not collectively bargain because they were considered students, not employees. The new ruling has been interpreted as meaning that residents should be considered both employees and students.

FIGURE 10.7

### Recruitment Incentives*

| Incentive | Family Pract | Internal Med | Peds |
|---|---|---|---|
| Assist student-loan repayments | 3% | 3% | 1% |
| Forgive medical school loans | 1% | 1% | 1% |
| Financial bonus or added pay | 4% | 3% | 2% |
| Subsidize moving expenses | 5% | 3% | 2% |

*The small number of survey respondents may affect the data.

Adapted from: Association of American Medical Colleges. *Council of Teaching Hospitals Survey of Housestaff Stipends, Benefits and Funding.* Washington, DC: AAMC, 1998.

## Moonlighting

Moonlighting means working for pay during time off during residency or fellowship training. It is not the first thing that most medical students think of when they consider residency programs. Being allowed to work clinically at another site for pay and having opportunities available to do so, however, may make the difference between eating steak or peanut butter sandwiches—or, more important, between buying gasoline for your car so you can drive to work or having to walk.

Moonlighting also offers residents an opportunity to broaden their clinical experiences, learn about communities in which they might want to practice, let the communities learn about them, and find out what clinical practice is like outside a tertiary-care mecca. Most important, it lets you experience, maybe for the first time, what it feels like to be treated like a professional—and to take on a professional's responsibilities.

Most residency programs have rules about moonlighting. Some allow all moonlighting. Others don't allow any. Most restrict moonlighting to either specific amounts of time or situations where it will not interfere with resident activities. Most moonlighting occurs in Internal Medicine and Family Practice programs, with about 30% of Internal Medicine residents and 18% of Family Practice residents moonlighting. If you think that you might want to moonlight, find out under what conditions it is allowed.

States also may regulate moonlighting through licensure. A number of states now require two or more years of postgraduate training prior to licensure—a requirement that is more common and more stringent for IMGs (Figure 7.8). This either discourages most moonlighting in these states or limits it to those in their last years of residency. The Federation of State Medical Boards has recommended that all state licensing boards require at least three years of postgraduate training for licensure.

The next question is whether moonlighting jobs are available. In some institutions, moonlighting opportunities exist within the institution itself or at the institution's satellite facilities. In other hospitals, groups of residents have acquired moonlighting opportunities that are available to the entire group. In most cases, however, finding moonlighting opportunities is an individual endeavor. Try to find out whether current residents have found such opportunities. If so, have they been within a reasonable distance from the main institution?

Finally, what will moonlighting cost? How expensive is a medical license in the state? How long will it take to get? In some states, it may take six months or more after applying to get a license allowing you to moonlight. How much must you spend for malpractice insurance? If there are moonlighting opportunities within the institution, it may not cost you anything. In other cases, employers furnish insurance (claims-made rather than occurrence—see "Liability Insurance," above). However, if you are forced to get your own insurance, it can be very expensive. Talk to the current residents to find out. The information will be more reliable, and the impression that you leave with the program will be much better than if you asked these questions of faculty members.

In an interesting twist, a substantial number of teaching hospitals now arrange moonlighting opportunities, and even subsidize malpractice insurance for moonlighting, for residents in some specialties. This is thought to entice students to enter these fields, or at least these residencies. Sponsoring or arranging moonlighting opportunities is most common in the primary care fields of Family Practice, Internal Medicine, and Pediatrics. About 20% subsidize malpractice insurance for moonlighting.

## Shared-Residency/Part-Time Positions

It may be important to you, for any number of personal or professional reasons, to do your residency on a part-time basis, even though it takes longer to complete than normal. These part-time programs appear to have worked well for those involved in them. Approximately 11% of programs (1,116) offer "shared-schedule/part-time" positions (Figure 10.8). Of this number, most are in Family Practice, Internal Medicine, Pediatrics, Psychiatry, or Child Psychiatry. The Boards and national specialty societies in other specialties may be unfamiliar with this type of program, even if one or more of their residencies offer it.

A shared-schedule position is one in which two residents, who usually pair up before interviewing and applying to programs, agree to each spend less than full-time in a single residency slot. In essence, they share one position. This can be done either by having each spend less time per day at work, or more easily (and commonly) by alternating weeks or months worked. This requires a great deal of forbearance on the part of a lot of people. First, the partners must be willing to work together and be flexible. Second, the program must be willing to work within the agreed-upon format. No two shared-schedule positions are ever structured exactly the same way. A now-lapsed federal law specified that these types of positions had to be available, with each resident working no more than two-thirds time for no less than half-time pay. You can try to figure that one out for yourself.

*The key is to obtain the arrangement with the program, whatever it is, in writing. Be sure to get it in writing before you rank programs for the Match.* If you require scheduling in a specific manner, then get this agreed to and spelled out in advance. This will not only let you know what the

FIGURE 10.8

## Shared-Schedule/Part-Time Positions Offered by Specialties

| Specialty | Number of Programs with Shared/ Part-Time Positions | Percent of Programs with Shared/ Part-Time Positions |
|---|---|---|
| Aerospace Medicine | 000 | 000% |
| Allergy & Immunology | 14 | 18 |
| Anesthesiology | 19 | 13 |
| Cardiology | 16 | 8 |
| Child/Adolescent Psychiatry | 74 | 64 |
| Child Neurology | 14 | 20 |
| Colon and Rectal Surgery | 3 | 10 |
| Critical Care (all) | 23 | 10 |
| Dermatology | 4 | 4 |
| Emergency Medicine | 12 | 10 |
| Endocrinology | 24 | 18 |
| Family Practice | 109 | 22 |
| Family Practice-Internal Medicine | 2 | 67 |
| Gastroenterology | 15 | 9 |
| Geriatric Psychiatry | 15 | 32 |
| Geriatrics (IM & FP) | 34 | 27 |
| Hand Surgery (all) | 5 | 7 |
| Hematology (all) | 88 | 8 |
| Hematology/Oncology (all) | 21 | 12 |
| Infectious Diseases | 23 | 16 |
| Internal Medicine/Emergency Med | 2 | 18 |
| Internal Medicine/Neurology | 5 | 31 |
| Internal Medicine/Pediatrics | 32 | 30 |
| Internal Med/Physical Med-Rehab | 5 | 33 |
| Internal Med/Preventive Med | 2 | 67 |
| Internal Medicine/Psychiatry | 10 | 38 |
| Internal Medicine | 94 | 23 |
| Internal Medicine, Primary | 29 | 31 |
| Medical Genetics | 0 | 0 |
| Neonatology | 25 | 25 |
| Nephrology | 16 | 12 |
| Neurological Surgery | 3 | 3 |
| Neurology | 16 | 14 |
| Nuclear Medicine | 4 | 5 |
| Obstetrics/Gynecology | 8 | 3 |

FIGURE 10.8 (continued)

| Specialty | Number of Programs with Shared/ Part-Time Positions | Percent of Programs with Shared/ Part-Time Positions |
|---|---|---|
| Occupational Medicine | 17 | 40% |
| Oncology | 3 | 7 |
| Ophthalmology | 8 | 6 |
| Orthopedic Surgery | 5 | 3 |
| Otolaryngology | 5 | 5 |
| Pain Management | 12 | 13 |
| Pathology | 21 | 12 |
| Pediatric Surgery | 4 | 13 |
| Pediatrics | 70 | 32 |
| Pediatrics/Emergency Medicine | 1 | 25 |
| Pediatrics/Physical Medicine-Rehab | 5 | 17 |
| Pediatrics/Psychiatry/Child Psych | 5 | 30 |
| Physical Medicine & Rehabilitation | 5 | 6 |
| Plastic Surgery | 4 | 4 |
| Prevent Medicine, Public Health | 45 | 51 |
| Psychiatry | 90 | 47 |
| Pulmonary Diseases (all) | 11 | 10 |
| Pulmonary Diseases-Critical Care | 13 | 13 |
| Radiation Oncology | 2 | 2 |
| Radiology-Diagnostic | 13 | 6 |
| Rheumatology (all) | 12 | 10 |
| Sports Medicine, Orthopedic | 8 | 14 |
| Sports Medicine, Primary Care | 4 | 12 |
| Surgery, General | 1 | <1 |
| Thoracic Surgery | 7 | 8 |
| Transitional | 6 | 4 |
| Urology | 2 | 2 |
| Vascular Surgery | 4 | 5 |

Data derived from: American Medical Association. *Graduate Medical Education Directory-Supplement 1999-2000.* Chicago, IL: AMA, 1999.

arrangement is, but will also allow your partner and the program to know. Chapters 13 and 22 contain the special rules for interviewing and for entering the NRMP Match for shared/part-time positions.

## Other Factors
While the discussion above has covered the most common factors to consider in choosing a training position, don't forget any other personal

factors that you feel are important enough to guide this decision. One rather exhaustive list of possible factors can be found in "An Applicant's Evaluation of a Medical House Officership," by Martin Raff and Ira Schwartz (1974, *The New England Journal of Medicine*). Even though the article is fairly old, its list is as pertinent today as it was then.

## Narrowing The Choices

If you have read through the description of some of the factors to consider in selecting a residency position, and if you understand the format for "Weighting" the factors in a "Must/Want" Analysis, then you are ready to complete your own "Must/Want" Analysis Form. Use Figure 10.1 as a master form to devise your own list. You will use one "Must/Want" Analysis Form later for each program that you evaluate, so *you should make several copies of the form once you have adapted it for your needs.* They will be completed first using the programs' written information alone, then updated using any additional information you get while interviewing.

The Companion Disk for Getting Into A Residency, available from Galen Press, has a master copy of the "Must/Want" Analysis that you can customize to fit your needs. It will save and print multiple copies of the form. After you enter weights and scores for the programs, it will also calculate the totals for you. (It even keeps track of your "Weights" total so you can easily tell when it reaches "100.") See the *Annotated Bibliography* for more information.

### Personal "Must/Want" Analysis

To decide the programs to which you wish to apply, complete the *Must/Want Analysis Form* (see Figure 10.1). Once you have listed the factors and assigned the "Weights" in your "Must/Want" Analysis, you should be able to go through the mass of information you have collected about the residency programs in an organized and rational manner.

How does the residency that you are assessing stack up against your ideal for that particular item? For each program you evaluate, every factor is given a "Score" ranging from "1" (farthest from your ideal) to a "10" (exactly what you are looking for). You record this result in the "Score" column of the "Must/Want" Analysis. For example, if you ideally would like to have faculty available in the hospital for consultation 24 hours/day, you would score any program in which this was true a "10" for this factor. If faculty were available only every third Thursday, you would probably feel obliged to give this factor a "Score" of "1." (The scores do not have to add up to anything! Feel free to give any applicable score to any factor.) The scoring is subjective, but then, you are the subject and what counts is how you perceive the situation.

Let's see how our hypothetical applicant (from Figure 10.2) filled out her "Must/Want" Analysis Forms for three separate programs. Remember, she has not yet gone for interviews, so some of the information is not yet available. See Figures 10.9, 10.10, and 10.11 for her evaluations of three hypothetical programs.

FIGURE 10.9

*"Must/Want" Analysis–Example #1*

PROGRAM #1–BACKWATER STATE HOSPITAL

| Clinical Experience | WEIGHT | X | SCORE | = | TOTAL |
|---|---|---|---|---|---|
| On-Call Schedule | 5 | | 7 | | |
| Patient Population | 2 | | 7 | | |
| Responsibility | 14 | | 9 | | |
| Setting | 7 | | 8 | | |
| Volume | 10 | | 6 | | |
| **Geographic Location** | | | | | |
| Part of Country | 1 | | 4 | | |
| Specific City | 1 | | 1 | | |
| **Reputation** | | | | | |
| Program Age and Stability | 2 | | 3 | | |
| **Faculty** | | | | | |
| Availability | 5 | | ? | | |
| Interest | 7 | | ? | | |
| Stability | 3 | | 10 | | |
| **Curriculum** | | | | | |
| Number of Conferences | 1 | | 6 | | |
| Special Training | 6 | | 7 | | |
| Types of Conferences | 2 | | 2 | | |
| **Esprit de Corps** | 8 | | 3 | | |
| **Research Opportunities/Training** | | | | | |
| Knowledge | 5 | | 8 | | |
| Materials | 2 | | ? | | |
| Time | 7 | | 9 | | |
| **Facilities** | | | | | |
| Clinical Laboratory Support | 1 | | 2 | | |
| Library/Media | 2 | | 3 | | |
| Safety/Security | 3 | | 9 | | |
| No Restrictive Covenant | MUST | | Yes | | |

FIGURE 10.9 (continued)

| | WEIGHT | X SCORE | = TOTAL |
|---|---|---|---|
| **Benefits: Health Benefits** | | | |
| Health Insurance | MUST | Yes | |
| Hospitalization | MUST | Yes | |
| **Benefits: Non-Health Benefits** | | | |
| Childcare | MUST | **NO!** | |
| Disability Insurance | MUST | Yes | |
| Educational Leave: Funding Available | 1 | Yes | |
| Time Off | 2 | 3 | |
| Liability Insurance | MUST | Yes | |
| Vacation | 1 | 4 | |
| **Moonlighting** | 2 | ? | |

TOTAL OF ALL WEIGHTS  =  100

**PROGRAM EVALUATION SCORE = Not Applicable**

Program #1 is completely eliminated from this applicant's consideration because of the lack of childcare. It doesn't matter what the scores are for any of the other factors—even though it scored well in several major areas. Note that a number of factors are scored as question marks. This is because the information was not available from the written material she received or from her adviser.

FIGURE 10.10

## *"Must/Want" Analysis–Example #2*

PROGRAM #2–MAKO GENERAL HOSPITAL

| Clinical Experience | WEIGHT | X | SCORE | = | TOTAL |
|---|---|---|---|---|---|
| On-Call Schedule | 5 | | 5 | | 25 |
| Patient Population | 2 | | 3 | | 6 |
| Responsibility | 14 | | 9 | | 126 |
| Setting | 7 | | 8 | | 56 |
| Volume | 10 | | 8 | | 80 |
| **Geographic Location** | | | | | |
| Part of Country | 1 | | 2 | | 2 |
| Specific City | 1 | | 1 | | 1 |
| **Reputation** | | | | | |
| Program Age and Stability | 2 | | 5 | | 10 |
| **Faculty** | | | | | |
| Availability | 5 | | ? | | ? |
| Interest | 7 | | ? | | ? |
| Stability | 3 | | 3 | | 9 |
| **Curriculum** | | | | | |
| Number of Conferences | 1 | | 7 | | 7 |
| Special Training | 6 | | 9 | | 54 |
| Types of Conferences | 2 | | 3 | | 6 |
| **Esprit de Corps** | 8 | | ? | | ? |
| **Research Opportunities/Training** | | | | | |
| Knowledge | 5 | | ? | | ? |
| Materials | 2 | | 8 | | 16 |
| Time | 7 | | 8 | | 56 |
| **Facilities** | | | | | |
| Clinical Laboratory Support | 1 | | 4 | | 4 |
| Library/Media | 2 | | 3 | | 6 |
| Safety/Security | 3 | | 5 | | 15 |
| No Restrictive Covenant | MUST | | Yes | | OK |
| **Benefits: Health Benefits** | | | | | |
| Health Insurance | MUST | | Yes | | OK |
| Hospitalization | MUST | | Yes | | OK |

FIGURE 10.10 (continued)

| | WEIGHT | X   SCORE | =   TOTAL |
|---|---|---|---|
| **Benefits: Non-Health Benefits** | | | |
| Childcare | MUST | Yes | OK |
| Disability Insurance | MUST | Yes | OK |
| Educational Leave: Funding Available | 1 | ? | ? |
| Time Off | 2 | 9 | 18 |
| Liability Insurance | MUST | Yes | OK |
| Vacation | 1 | 7 | 7 |
| **Moonlighting** | 2 | ? | ? |

TOTAL OF ALL WEIGHTS  =  __100__

**PROGRAM EVALUATION SCORE  =  505 (+ ?)**

Program #2 has scored very well compared to our applicant's criteria. The "Program Evaluation Score" is at least 505. However, just as in the first program, some factors could not be scored. In most cases, the same or related factors for each program will not be able to be scored without a visit to the program. These include the faculty's availability and interest, the esprit de corps of the program, and the "knowledge" of available research. Other factors may only have partial information available and may need to be further elucidated in person. The scores can then be adjusted as necessary.

If a particular factor is either a "Must" or a very important (high "Weight") element for you, it is worthwhile to call the program and obtain any needed information before you make your decision about where to interview. Failing to do this may either result in wasted interviews or cause you to overlook some programs that might meet your needs.

FIGURE 10.11

## *"Must/Want" Analysis–Example #3*

### PROGRAM #3–SAGUARO COMMUNITY HOSPITAL

| Clinical Experience | WEIGHT X | SCORE = | TOTAL |
|---|---|---|---|
| On-Call Schedule | 5 | 6 | 30 |
| Patient Population | 2 | 5 | 10 |
| Responsibility | 14 | 4 | 56 |
| Setting | 7 | 10 | 70 |
| Volume | 10 | 3 | 30 |
| **Geographic Location** | | | |
| Part of Country | 1 | 10 | 10 |
| Specific City | 1 | 10 | 10 |
| **Reputation** | | | |
| Program Age and Stability | 2 | 7 | 14 |
| **Faculty** | | | |
| Availability | 5 | ? | ? |
| Interest | 7 | ? | ? |
| Stability | 3 | ? | ? |
| **Curriculum** | | | |
| Number of Conferences | 1 | 4 | 4 |
| Special Training | 6 | 6 | 36 |
| Types of Conferences | 2 | 9 | 18 |
| **Esprit de Corps** | 8 | ? | ? |
| **Research Opportunities/Training** | | | |
| Knowledge | 5 | ? | ? |
| Materials | 2 | 8 | 16 |
| Time | 7 | 4 | 28 |
| **Facilities** | | | |
| Clinical Laboratory Support | 1 | ? | ? |
| Library/Media | 2 | 1 | 2 |
| Safety/Security | 3 | 5 | 15 |
| No Restrictive Covenant | MUST | Yes | OK |
| **Benefits: Health Benefits** | | | |
| Health Insurance | MUST | Yes | OK |
| Hospitalization | MUST | Yes | OK |

FIGURE 10.11 (continued)

| | WEIGHT | X SCORE | = TOTAL |
|---|---|---|---|
| **Benefits: Non-Health Benefits** | | | |
| Childcare | MUST | Yes | OK |
| Disability Insurance | MUST | Yes | OK |
| Educational Leave: Funding Available | 1 | 8 | 8 |
| Time Off | 2 | ? | ? |
| Liability Insurance | MUST | Yes | OK |
| Vacation | 1 | 4 | 4 |
| **Moonlighting** | 2 | ? | ? |

TOTAL OF ALL WEIGHTS  =  100

PROGRAM EVALUATION SCORE  =  361 (+ ?)

Since the information that was available for programs #2 and #3 was not the same, they cannot be directly compared (yet). But the information available does give a general ranking for the programs. One piece of information had to be obtained by telephone about program #3, but that residency's secretary was happy to answer a potential applicant's questions. The call provided the facts that our applicant needed in order to make an informed decision. From this group, Program #2 is the one to which our applicant will be sure to apply. Depending upon how the other programs she rates stack up, she also might decide to apply to Program #3. Program #1, of course, has been eliminated for not fulfilling one of her required "Musts." By the time she finishes interviewing at programs, she should have enough information to eliminate the question marks on her forms.

# 11

# Playing The Odds: How Many Program Applications?

*There is no certainty without some doubt.*
— Elias Levita, *Tishbi*

*Forecasting is hard, particularly of the future.*
— Anonymous

Medical students frequently ask, "To how many programs should I apply?" There is no easy answer, since *the real answer depends upon your wants and needs, including your specialty choice.* No magic number exists. No one factor will give you an answer. As with all other aspects of the competition for a residency slot, the number of programs to which you should apply must be individualized. You must consider the competitiveness of the specialty you have chosen, the geographic and academic restrictions you are placing upon a residency choice, and your own competitiveness. Then, after discussions with your mentor or your specialty adviser, apply to a generous number of programs.

## How Competitive Is The Specialty You Want?

First, consider how competitive your chosen specialty is. For example, Otolaryngology, Neurosurgery, and Orthopedics require applications to more programs to be assured of an adequate number of interviews than do Psychiatry or Pathology (see Figures 4.1, 22.2, and 22.9). For many years, students have been told (with only a little exaggeration) that "If your parents did not submit your Ophthalmology application while you were in diapers, it is too late." While the situation for most competitive specialties is not that bad, some remain difficult to enter. Some specialties fluctuate widely in their competitiveness from year to year. Ophthalmology, for example, has become markedly less competitive over the past decade. Also, one of the least competitive specialties in the 1970s, Anesthesiology, became extremely competitive in the 1980s, and now again is relatively easy to enter. Generally, the more competitive the specialty, the more programs to which you should apply. See the specialty descriptions in Chapter 3 for information on each specialty's relative competitiveness.

## How Competitive Are You?

How competitive are you—really? List the qualities that are viewed as plusses in your desired specialty. Do you have strengths or weaknesses in these areas? Be objective. If you cannot be objective on your own, have your adviser or a mentor in the field help you. It is generally inadvisable to have a spouse or close friend help on this—too much honesty from the wrong source can be very ego-destructive.

Do not compare yourself with others in your school who are applying to the same specialty. This will not result in an accurate assessment of your competition. *The competitive pool is made up of all students from all schools who want to enter your chosen specialty.* Your best chance of success lies in assessing your competitiveness as accurately as possible. You do this by comparing the strengths that you have identified in yourself with those that you perceive the residency programs in your desired specialty want. The ideal candidate, the one who fits all the desired qualities, is the one you are competing against (see Chapter 18). But don't worry. That individual probably doesn't exist.

## What Do You Have To Lose?

Professional photographers constantly tell amateurs to go ahead and take lots of pictures. "So what if you blow a few shots? You may end up with some beautiful pictures you wouldn't have gotten if you had been more conservative. Remember," they say, "the film is the least expensive part of system."

Just so with the application process. Applying to a few extra programs, especially those to which you really want to go but are afraid that they won't accept you, makes good sense for at least two reasons. First, you will never have to say to yourself, as so many physicians do in their later years when they meet up with a moron graduate from their most desired training program, that "I could have gotten in if only I had applied." Second, you actually may get an interview (and then a position) at that program. It takes very little extra effort to apply to a few more programs. Since you are applying to some programs anyway, follow your dreams—they may come true. If you can dream it, you can do it!

As a general guideline, the number of applications recent graduates submitted to programs in their first choice of specialty is listed in Figure 11.1. Students submitted an average of 17 applications, although it varied greatly by specialty. Figure 11.2 demonstrates the change in total PGY-1 applicants and positions over the past three decades.

Make up your list once and then apply to those programs. Don't continue to add to it piecemeal. The application process is hard enough and it is very difficult to keep track of the paper shuffle under normal circumstances. Adding programs as you go along will only make the process harder on you, and on the people sending out your reference letters. One request for information to be sent to all your programs usually works well. Dribbling in those requests separately over time can spell disaster.

### FIGURE 11.1
### Number of Applications to Programs

| Number of Applications Submitted | Percentage of Students* |
|---|---|
| None | 0.2% |
| 1-2 | 5.8 |
| 3-5 | 11.1 |
| 6-10 | 22.0 |
| 11-15 | 18.6 |
| 16-25 | 19.2 |
| 26 or more | 18.7 |
| Unknown | 4.2 |

*Numbers do not add up to 100% due to rounding.

Adapted from: Association of American Medical Colleges. *1995 Medical School Graduation Survey Results, All School Summary.* Washington, DC: AAMC, 1995, p. 27.

FIGURE 11.2

**Applicants and 1st-Year Positions
1952-1999**

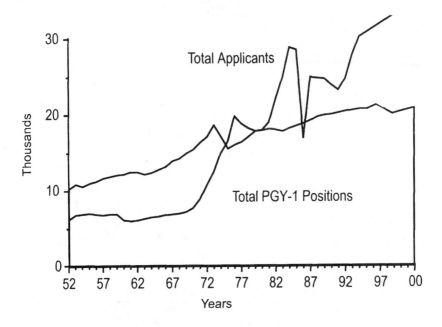

Adapted from: National Resident Matching Program. *NRMP Data, April 1999.* Washington, DC:NRMP, 1999.

# 12

# Buffing Your File: The Paperwork

*A wise man recognizes the convenience of a general statement, but he bows to the authority of a particular fact.*

– Oliver Wendell Holmes, Jr.

The key to success in preparing and gathering the information required by residency programs is the same one that got you into medical school—being compulsive. Four rules that will put you far ahead of the pack are:

1. **Be Thorough**
2. **Look Neat**
3. **Be Early**
4. **Be Organized**

*Thoroughness* means reading the application materials over twice. Dot the i's and cross those t's. If a program requests something out of the ordinary, such as your undergraduate transcript, then make sure that you note the requirement and get them a copy. You can lose lots of points in this game if you don't read each set of rules carefully. No one is prepared to go out of his or her way to accommodate you. Some programs may not even notify you that your application is incomplete, so it's up to you to develop a system to keep track of your applications. Keep photocopies of all correspondence and detailed records of your telephone calls to the programs. Be thorough.

The *lack of neatness* probably destroys more potentially successful candidates than all other factors combined. You are applying for a real job, as well as for your lifelong career. Don't send your potential employers anything unless it looks like it is the work of a professional. This means that your application and résumé should never be completed in a barely legible scrawl, in pencil, or in the middle of ward rounds. Neither should they be hacked out on the old upright manual typewriter in the back office, nor printed on a dot matrix printer. These documents are your representatives, your entries to the goal you seek. Make them look sharp. Make them look professional. Make them look neat.

Although there are many rumors to the contrary, programs rarely keep the correspondence you send to them requesting information and an application. They do not normally start a file on you until something more substantial, such as an application, a reference letter, or a transcript arrives. However, the postcard or short letter that you send to them requesting information must at least be legible and contain your name and address (see Figure 9.1). You would be surprised how many supposedly intelligent medical students send requests that lack one or the other of these necessary items.

Early birds catch the worm and *early applicants get the interviews*. More and more applicants now complete their applications at the beginning of the application "season" (August and September for programs in the NRMP PGY-1 Match). Still, many students have not even gotten application packets and information from the programs at which they wish to interview by the time they should be making decisions about which programs to apply to and completing the necessary paperwork.

No matter how good the program, nor how experienced the residency director, the question that always arises at this time of year is, "Will I get enough good candidates this year?" As a result, programs have rather liberal criteria early on for granting interviews. If you walk on water and fly through the air (without assistance, of course), you can wait and file with the rest of the applicant horde. But if you don't, get your packet completed early. Even if you can do miraculous deeds, however, if you apply late, optimal interview dates may not be available when you're offered one. In fact, some programs may run out of interview slots, since many have only a finite number available. Get your act together early.

*Get organized.* You will, undoubtedly, be flooded with material about residency programs and will be sending out lots of material to these programs (unless you apply to specialties using the Electronic Residency Application Service [ERAS®, described later in this chapter] or the Central Application Service [Ophthalmology, Neurological Surgery, Plastic Surgery, and Otolaryngology]). Therefore, you need to have a filing system that allows you to quickly locate, assess, and track both the material you receive and the material you send. Develop the system before you begin this process. For a system that has worked for many students, see Chapter 9.

## Your Name

Everyone has a name, so what's the problem? The problem is that your name may change or have several variations. In the world of medical credentialing and verification, which you entered when you took USMLE Step 1 or similar exams, variations aren't well tolerated. People using first initials and middle names, changing their names when married or divorced, inverting first and last names, and hyphenating their last names, may all encounter difficulties. The key to avoiding difficulties with the various bureaucrats who must verify that you are who you say you are, is to use the same name on all your paperwork.

For example, you used T. Michael Jones on your medical school entrance materials. (You are not too keen on using Thaddeous.) Your transcript now probably reads that way—but find out from the registrar before you complete the USMLE Step 1 application. When you register for Step 1, use the same form of your name that is on your transcript. Do this for all subsequent official papers. That way, no one will confuse you with Tremont Michael Jones, Thomas Michael Jones, or even Theresa Michael Jones.

The same holds true for those who change their name when they get married or divorced. This has become more common with the increased number of women physicians. Those who get married after medical school usually have two names—their married name that they use in social situations, and their "professional name" that they use for work and for all medically official documents. That way, there is no bureaucratic confusion. Those who marry before or while in medical school often begin using their married name for everything. Unfortunately, many of these marriages don't last, and so confusion may reign when the physician must use both her married and new (or old) names for the inevitable paperwork. As the number of names increases with subsequent marriages, the confusion and resultant difficulties multiply. If possible, the best course is to have a married and professional name. Keep your professional name constant.

In Spanish-speaking countries, and less commonly elsewhere, a person often uses two last names—the first from their father and the second being their mother's maiden name. Therefore, documents may be listed in a variety of ways, for example, Marco T. Velasco, Marco T. Velasco-Lopez, or Marco Velasco-Lopez. Others, such as those with Vietnamese names, may have their last and first names switched in some circumstances.

If you are in this situation, notify all residency programs, ERAS, the ECFMG, and any licensing bodies that the different names on transcripts, Board scores, diplomas, and in reference letters all belong to the same person. You do not want to be refused entrance to the USMLE because the names on your application and your ID don't match exactly. You do not want to lose out on a possible interview because of an "incomplete file" resulting from having your materials filed under more than one name. And once you go through all this hassle, you don't want problems with the matching programs because you are not listed with the residency programs under the same name you used to apply to the Match. The best course is to use only *your full name on all official documents*.

## The Application

Most M.D. residencies now use ERAS or the Centralized Application Service (CAS). They present most information in a standard format. Some M.D. residencies, all fellowships, and all D.O. programs use their own applications or the Universal Application (available from your Dean of Students). If you are in this situation, the first step is to get the program applications from those programs in which you are interested. Some can be downloaded from the program's website.

Generally, the application will be the first piece of paper in your file at residency programs. The front page of the application, above all the other paperwork that you submit, must look as if the person completing is was a professional. Programs ask for data that they feel is necessary to make a choice among candidates. They have put their application together in a specific manner so they can quickly screen it for this information.

Application forms will also, in most cases, specify what other information is needed to complete the application process. Read the fine print. Make a chart of the materials required by each program.

As you can see by the example in Figure 12.1, the requirements for different programs can vary widely. Nearly all will request a Dean's letter, medical school transcript, and application. Make certain that you supply at least the minimum that is required. In most instances, you should send out as many excellent reference letters as you have available. Whether programs ask for one or not, make sure that you send a copy of your résumé. As for a personal statement, if it is not specifically requested, do not send one unless it is really good.

Some applicants will also need to send copies of their ECFMG Certificates, letters of waiver from the military or Public Health Service, letters or evaluations from previous residency training, or other items. Be certain that you list all these items on your own tracking form.

FIGURE 12.1

### Requirements for Applications to Different Programs–Example

| Hospital | Dean's Letter | Transcript | Appli-cation | Under-graduate Transcript | Personal Statement | Résumé | Ref Letters |
|---|---|---|---|---|---|---|---|
| Saw Comm | X | X | X | | | X | A+2 |
| St. Mary's | X | X | U | X | | X | 2 |
| Amhurt Univ | X | X | X | | X | | 3 |
| Smort Med Ctr | X | X | X | | | X | A+3 |
| Arden St. | X | | X | X | X | | 2 |
| Robin Hood | X | X | X | | X | X | 2+P |
| WGMC | X | X | U | | X | X | A+P |
| U of State | X | X | X | X | X | | 3 |

X–Required by program.
U–Requires use of the Universal Application.
A–Indicates a letter from your adviser.
#–Number of additional reference letters required.
P–At least one letter from a physician in the specialty for which you are applying.

On the program's application form itself, fill in all pertinent blanks. And fill them in with the requested information. *Never put in the words "see résumé."* Of course, you will supply a résumé to the program, and there will certainly be some duplication of information. Not filling in the application with the requested information, however, can be the kiss of death. It indicates that you did not think enough of the program to do the specific work required to fill out their application. Instead, you left them to search around your résumé for the information they desire. Is that also how you plan to act as a resident? It is the impression that you have delivered. That is not the impression that you want the residency program to have about you as an applicant.

## Illegal Questions

What about illegal questions? Those are the ones barred from pre-employment screening by federal and state civil rights acts. Questions dealing with race, sex, age, height, weight, national origin, military discharge status, arrest record, marital status or who lives with you, physical disability, and religion are restricted to those situations where they directly impact upon the job requirements or where the applicant raises them. Although they are not legal, many applications still contain those types of questions. How do you handle them?

First, remember that, in general, the programs are not being malicious in their use of these questions. Many times they are merely ignorant of the law. There is a fine line between questions that are illegal and those that are simply inept, curious, or friendly. Don't approach these questions in a hostile manner. Second, look over your Dean's letter, your transcript, and your other reference letters. How much new information are you really supplying by answering these questions? Probably not much. What you are doing is putting the information down in a standard format for easy retrieval and comparison. So, the general advice is to fill in all the blanks.

Before you begin completing a residency program's application, it is a good idea to make copies of the form. Neatly fill out one of these copies, and then have a trusted friend review it for any spelling or grammatical errors. Those errors tend to stand out prominently and will project a poor image of you. The reviewer, who can also evaluate your personal statement, should know you well enough to be able to suggest additions to the information that you were too modest to include. Then, after all your applications are ready, give these copies along with the original blank forms to a professional typist for preparation. This process will give you the best results.

Finally, get your applications in early. It takes quite a bit of time to do the paperwork involved in preparing applications for submission. Since you are going to do it anyway, why not complete it early when you have a much better chance of obtaining the maximum results for your effort.

## The Universal Application

The Universal Application for Residency, now rarely used, was an attempt to limit the amount of medical students' application paperwork. However, as has been noted, relatively few programs use this form. Nevertheless, you will probably encounter it somewhere in your application process. How should you deal with it?

The ERAS and CAS have mostly replaced the Universal Application, as well as individual program applications. If you find that you do need this form, you may get the application from the programs themselves, from your Dean of Students, or with an NRMP application packet. You will usually have to use a photocopy of the original. From this "sow's ear" it may be very hard to make a "silk purse."

Some students who use the Universal Application for multiple programs photocopy one completed copy without the references and type those in individually. This not only looks sloppy, but also shows the program that they may be receiving a different reference list than other programs. Their resulting attitude may be "What is this character up to?" Don't invite this kind of curiosity. Once you have completed the application using a photocopy of your original, give it to a professional typist with clear notes about variations for individual programs. Let the typist do the labor, and make your application look professional.

A note of caution is in order. Some programs specifically give applicants a choice between using the Universal Application or the program's application. If you have that choice, opt for the program's form. It will demonstrate more commitment, satisfy the information needs of the program better and, since it will probably be an original rather than a photocopied application, look neater.

### Electronic Residency Application Service (ERAS)

The Electronic Residency Application Service (ERAS), run by the Association of American Medical Colleges (AAMC), transmits residency applications, recommendation letters, Deans' letters, transcripts, USMLE scores, ECFMG certification, and other supporting credentials to residency programs. Starting with Obstetrics and Gynecology in the 1995-96 Match cycle, the specialties now participating in ERAS 2000 include:

- Diagnostic Radiology
- Emergency Medicine
- Emergency Med/Internal Med
- Emergency Med/Pediatrics
- Family Practice
- Family Practice/Internal Med
- General Surgery
- Internal Med (Preliminary & Categorical)
- Internal Med/Pediatrics
- Internal Med/Physiatry
- Obstetrics & Gynecology
- Orthopedic Surgery
- Pediatrics
- Pediatrics/Physiatry
- Physical Med & Rehab (Physiatry)
- Transitional Year Programs
- All Army & Navy PGY-1 positions

In principle, programs in these specialties will no longer accept paper applications. For the year 2000 application process, more than 2,400 residency programs in 16 specialties used the ERAS system, handling over 25,000 residency applications. However, while about 95% of programs in these specialties participate in ERAS, some programs (listed in grey or italics on the ERAS website's list of programs in each specialty) do not participate in ERAS and only accept paper applications. Others may accept ERAS or paper applications. Carefully review program application materials or websites to determine which they use.

*You cannot apply to non-participating programs using ERAS!* For programs in the participating specialties that do not use ERAS, you need to obtain paper applications. Their contact information is available on *FREIDA* or in the AMA *Green Book.*

One fear that both applicants and program directors had about the system was that the ease of submitting applications would overwhelm the system—especially program directors. While some programs have seen an increase in applications, the overall number of applications has not increased. (Perhaps because of the steep price for applying to more than 30 programs—$30 each.)

## How It Works

**U.S./Canadian Medical Students/Graduates:** Applicants, whether currently third-year students or graduates, receive "Student Workstation Kits" from their school's Dean of Students about the beginning of July. This kit contains a "Student Workstation Data Diskette," a "Student Workstation Backup Data Diskette," the *ERAS Student Workstation Instruction Manual.* (As of the 2001 application cycle, ERAS plans not to use diskettes, but to have applicants enter all information on-line.) International medical students and graduates get the material from and apply through the ECFMG. Osteopathic students and graduates may be able to get this material from their Dean. Canadian students should follow the directions from their Dean of Students, since they will usually be sending their disk to the Canadian Resident Matching Service (CaRMS). Military applicants should contact their military counselor for any special instructions.

Use the *ERAS Student Workstation Instruction Manual* carefully, following each step as outlined. Several helpful hints and program features are described below. Since the system will change from year to year with upgrades, any specific information should be double-checked in the *Manual.*

Your school will establish procedures for distributing packets and processing ERAS applications and materials. They may be slightly different at each school. Their processing will include uploading Student Workstation Diskettes, scanning transcripts (many have backgrounds that make them nearly illegible), recommendation letters and supporting documents, and transmitting the files.

**International Medical Students/Graduates:** To obtain an ERAS Kit from the ECFMG, fax (215) 222-5641 or E-mail erashelp@ecfmg.org. Student Workstation Software can also be downloaded from www.aamc.org/eras/swsdisk. ERAS Kits should arrive after three to five business days (processing plus mailing time). Even if you have a kit from a prior year, you must use a new kit each year, since the program will only recognize the current year's software.

The Kit contains three black System Disks, a white formatted Student Data Diskette, and an empty green Backup Disk. If the white Student Data Diskette is missing or damaged, request a replacement by E-mail from the ECFMG. Put your USMLE number in the E-mail Subject Line. If the green backup disk is missing or damaged, use any blank 1.44MB disk. Label it "Backup Diskette." If the three black discs are missing or damaged, you can request a replacement or download them from www.aamc.org/eras.

### Questions

When installing ERAS, if you have a software problem, go to www.aamc. org/eras and select "Solutions to Problems." If this doesn't help, E-mail swshelp@aamc.org.

The AAMC and ECFMG websites for ERAS also contain sets of frequently asked questions (FAQ) which would be useful to look over before embarking on this process. The AAMC site also lists newly available or newly closed programs in all participating specialties.

### Computer Requirements

You do not need to own a computer, but you do need access to one. This should be a PC-compatible machine running Windows® 3.1 or higher. (Some Mac machines will run this software, but ERAS does not offer support for them.) You also need an E-mail address to receive communications from residency directors. Access to the Web is very helpful so that you can obtain current information from the AAMC or ECFMG sites.

The E-mail address is very important, as is checking your electronic mailbox frequently. Many program directors use this method to ask applicants additional questions and to offer them interview slots.

One glitch that affected medical students at Duke, Indiana, and the University of Osteopathic Medicine in Iowa was that when applicants received E-mail messages from program directors offering them an interview, their university's computer systems rejected the messages as "spam" or junk mail. While that has been corrected at these institutions, if you find that most programs have downloaded your ERAS materials and you haven't heard from any of them, you may want to check to see if they sent you a message that your computer system rejected.

### Costs

ERAS prints a Processing Fee Invoice. Print this invoice only after you have completed your diskette and are ready to turn it in, since fees depend, in part, on the number of residencies to which you apply. The charges will vary each year and are based on the number of programs to which the applicant applies through ERAS.

One confusing point is that once the button is pushed to submit the information, you owe the fees, even if you later withdraw from ERAS.

**U.S./Canadian Medical Students/Graduates:** For the year 2000 cycle, the ERAS fee for medical students and graduates from U.S./Canadian schools is $60, which includes application to up to ten programs. Applying to up to ten more programs costs $6 each, the next ten cost $12 each, and, if you apply to more than thirty programs, each additional application costs $30. Most students elect to have ERAS send all their USMLE transcripts to programs for a single $40 fee. They will not send COMLEX (NBOME) transcripts or scores for D.O. students or physicians. These must be sent directly to programs.

**International Medical Students/Graduates:** IMGs pay an extra fee for the ECFMG's services as their "designated Dean's Office."

### Contents (Help)
This is the most important button. The "?" button opens the "Help" screen from which you can easily navigate to the answer for nearly any question. The screen works like those in any Windows® program. "Help" also contains a glossary of terms used in the program.

### Save
Find this button and use it often to avoid repeating your efforts. Each time you save your work, you will be asked to verify that all the information you save to a disk is true. Be sure you save a copy of all your work on the Backup Diskette!

### Open SWS Application
This button opens the "Common Application Form" (CAF), which will be sent to all programs. Use the numbered buttons at the top of the screen to switch pages. These pages are where you enter the data that is normally found on residency applications. Entering the information is generally self-explanatory. Be careful to type the information accurately.

Some material entered on the application may not be transmitted by some schools if they feel that it is legally problematic (e.g., gender, birth date, citizenship, visa status, photo). This should not cause you any problems, since it is generally illegal for potential employers to request this information.

### New Personal Statement

This button opens a window in which you place one or more personal statements. Each different statement has a label, which is only for identification purposes; it neither prints nor goes to the programs. You can type the statement directly into the window. However, since there is no spelling or grammar checker, it is best to first produce your personal statement using a word processor and import the document into this window using the instructions in the *Manual*. In the future, this program will support limited formatting, but the different fonts and type sizes will be limited so that they are easily readable.

Even though you have the opportunity to write a very long personal statement in this file—don't. Limit your statement to one page. This may be difficult (it is more difficult to write a poem than a novel), but no one wants to read more than this from any applicant.

Since this program does not have a separate place for a résumé, if you wish to include one, attach this file to the end of each personal statement. Many residency directors, however, specifically request that a separate résumé not be included on ERAS, since they feel that the ERAS application contains all relevant information.

### Open Personal Statement

Click this button to see a list of the personal statements you have written. They are listed by the titles you gave them, so it is wise to use descriptive titles. Use this button to review, delete, or edit your personal statements.

### Request Letters of Recommendation

The "envelope" icon allows you to generate requests for recommendation letters. Enter the names of all the people who should get these requests. This could be many names since, while the system will accept only *four* letters for each program, you may want to send different letters to different programs. Also, you must deliver these requests. At this point, when many faculty do not know about ERAS, it may be best to include a cover letter or, even better, deliver the request in person so you can explain about the ERAS system. All letters should be addressed to "Dear Program Director," "Dear Doctor," Dear Colleague, " or "To whom it may concern." The remainder of the format is up to the writer. All applicants should be sure that the letter writers know that they should return *both* their recommendation letter and the bar-coded sheet you sent them to either you or the Dean's Office/ECFMG. The Dean's Letter and transcript do *not* count as one of your four letters.

If your school has special instructions for faculty generating ERAS recommendation letters, however, they should follow these instructions.

U.S./Canadian graduates using ERAS must also be certain that their recommendation letters go to the Dean's office for processing, rather than directly to programs participating in ERAS.

IMGs applying to California programs need to also submit a copy of the "Applicant Evaluation Status Letter" issued by the Medical Board of California. List the "California Letter" as one of your recommendation letters.

### Résumé

ERAS will not easily accommodate your résumé in the system, but will generate one based on the information you provide in the Common Application Form. If you want programs to get a copy of your personalized résumé, you need to send it to them by mail, carry copies with you to the interviews, or send it through ERAS in place of a recommendation letter in excess of the number programs require. However, this is probably not necessary unless you have such a detailed history that ERAS doesn't accurately reflect it.

### Add Programs

This button allows you to select programs to which you want application materials sent. The system contains the names of all programs in each participating specialty that have agreed to use ERAS.

On this screen or the main screen containing your list of selected programs, you can access limited program information (program director's name, address, telephone number, and E-mail address, and the program's ACGME and NRMP numbers). ERAS will not allow you to accidentally select the same program more than once. It also maintains a running total of the number of programs you select.

When applying to more than one track in the same specialty at the same institution, check on the "Add Programs" screen to see how they are listed. Some hospitals may have one listing that includes several tracks, such as Internal Medicine preliminary, categorical, advanced, and primary care, while another hospital lists them all separately.

Although, in principle, it is not a good idea, you can apply to multiple specialties at one time using ERAS.

If a program does not participate in ERAS, their name is grayed out on the screen and cannot be selected. For those programs, applicants must apply directly to the program as do applicants to non-participating specialties.

### Assign Documents

Press this button (it's supposed to look like a paper-clipped memo) to link the various documents (Common Application Form, Letters of Recommendation, Personal Statement, USMLE Transcript) with *each program* to which you are applying. First select the program name from the drop-down list. Then select the documents you want that program to receive. While all your selected programs automatically get your Common Application Form, you select which recommendation letters go to which programs. Also, you select which form of your personal statement and résumé goes to each program. (These are listed by the title you gave them.) Also, you can choose which programs should get your USMLE transcript. If you change your mind, use the "Remove" button to delete an item.

ERAS can transmit USMLE Step 1 and 2 scores. For those who have taken USMLE Step 3, you can enter them into your personal statement and send a copy (or better, have the FSMB send a copy) to the residency program.

### International Medical Graduates: Special Questions

- **What if you cannot supply a Dean's Letter?** If you will not provide these documents, the program allows you to type a short sentence explaining why. If you click "Yes" when asked if a Dean's Letter and medical school transcript will be provided, you can click on "Print Cover Sheet" which will print a bar-coded cover sheet.

- **What if you cannot print a bar-coded cover sheet?** Print your USMLE number (not your ERAS ID) in the upper right-hand corner of your recommendation letters.

- **If your Dean's Letter and transcript are not in English, what do you do?** You should submit only a high-quality, high-resolution copy of the translation. Be prepared, however, to show any residency directors who ask (and all should), the original-language documents and the translator's certificate.

- **Is there anything special for "Fifth-Pathway" graduates?** Those who hold a Fifth-Pathway Certificate may want to enter "Fifth-Pathway Certificate" as one recommendation letter instead of an individual's name. This notifies program directors not to look for an ECFMG Certificate, even though you are an IMG. You can then send the Certificate to the program.

- **What does the ECFMG send the residency programs?** The ECFMG automatically sends a "Status Report" to all residencies to which you apply; you have no choice in this. It lists the most current passing performance on the Clinical Skills Assessment (either N/A or a month/year) and a date through which these results are valid. It also lists your passing score(s) on any tests administered through the ECFMG necessary for their certification. The USMLE transcript, which contains additional information, including all times you took the exam, is only sent to those programs you designate when completing ERAS.

### Print

Save all your work to the Student Data Diskette before attempting to print anything. Test your printer first by printing a document from Windows. If your printer works with Windows, it should work with this program. To test this, turn on the printer and go into Windows' File Manager. Select (by highlighting it) a file to print. On the menu bar, select "File" and then select "Print" from the drop-down menu. If the document prints, the printer should work with ERAS documents.

The Print button allows you to print proof copies of your Common Application Form and Personal Statements. (Your Dean of Students' office prints or electronically transmits the final copy.) You also can print the letters requesting recommendation letters from the people you designated, a list of the programs you selected, and a list of the materials you want sent to each one.

### Transmitting & Receiving Information

Individual programs, rather than ERAS, set residency application deadlines. However, the ERAS "Post Office" opens (usually mid-August) and transmits all applications received to that time. After that, they transmit new applications daily. All Deans' Letters that have been received are transmitted on November 1.

Get your materials to your Dean's office as soon as possible so that they can be transmitted. As the application season progresses, the folks responsible for submitting your information may get a bit bogged down. The ERAS system also reportedly gets a bit slower with masses of applications coming and going. If you submit everything early, you should have rapid and smooth sailing. Even if there are glitches, they can be more easily ironed out when both your school's ERAS staff and the folks at the AAMC have a bit more time to work on them.

Dean's offices receive a confirmation of receipt for the application materials they send. To learn when your application was transmitted to the ERAS PostOffice, and the dates different residency programs downloaded your file, go to the Applicant Document Tracking System (ADTS) located at www.aamc.org/eras/adts. It begins operating each year at the same time, as does the ERAS PostOffice. You need your ERAS ID and password to access the information. If a program seems to have delayed in downloading your ERAS application, you must contact them directly to see why.

If you are ready to submit your completed data disk but have not yet received your NRMP number, leave that field blank and submit your disk and documents. When your get your NRMP number, update your backup disk, and submit it with a new invoice (even if you have not added additional programs or if you owe additional fees).

**U.S./Canadian Medical Students/Graduates:** After completing (and proofing) your application, printing the ERAS Application Invoice, and making a backup disk, take or send your Student Data Diskette and a wallet-sized (2½″ x 3½″) color photo of yourself to your Dean's office. *Do not send your personal password.* Once they transmit your file to the ERAS "PostOffice" via the Internet, all fees as detailed on the Invoice must be paid within two weeks to avoid cancelling your application.

**International Medical Students/Graduates:** After completing (and proofing) your application, printing the ERAS Application Invoice, and making a backup disk, take or send your Student Data Diskette and a wallet-sized (2½″ x 3½″) color photo of yourself to the ECFMG. Send only high-resolution, high-quality copies of your transcripts and Dean's Letters, since these will not be returned. *Do not send your personal password.*

If you send your disks and documents *without* a check or money order, mail it to: ERAS Program, P.O. Box 13467, Philadelphia, PA 19101-3467. Once they transmit your file to the ERAS "PostOffice" via the Internet, all fees as detailed on the Invoice must be paid within two weeks to avoid them cancelling your application. Use this same address if you use a credit card to pay.

If you enclose a check or money order with your disk, mail it to: ERAS Diskettes at PNC, P.O. Box 820010, Philadelphia, PA 19182-0010. For anything sent by courier delivery, use: ERAS Program, 3624 Market St., Philadelphia, PA 19104.

### Future ERAS Changes
In the coming years, ERAS will put the Student Workstation Software on the Web. Most residency programs in the enrolled specialties and more specialties will eventually be enrolled in ERAS, making applicants' lives even easier.

# The Résumé

Your résumé, also known as a *curriculum vitae* or *c.v.*, is a word picture of yourself. It is necessary for most applications (you will want to include it with all your non-ERAS applications whether it is a stated requirement or not), and the process of putting it together will help you organize your thoughts about your past accomplishments and future plans.

Try to tailor the information you provide to the specialty for which you are applying. For example, extracurricular activities and community service may be less important to program directors in Surgery than to those in Family Practice.

While a good résumé will not guarantee that you get into a residency, a poor résumé will certainly eliminate you from consideration. For more detailed information, see also *Résumés and Personal Statements for Health Professionals, 2nd ed.*, by James W. Tysinger, Ph.D. (Galen Press, 1999).

## Misrepresentations

Only include true information in your résumé and personal statement. About 20% of residency applicants, and a much higher number of fellow-ship applicants, who list publications either were not an author of a real paper or listed a non-existent paper. One study, for example, showed that nearly one-third of Gastroenterology fellowship applicants misrepresented their academic accomplishments. Residency directors know this. With the ease of computer medical literature searches, programs commonly check listed publications. Consequently, it is becoming more dangerous for applicants to misrepresent their scholarly writings.

Sometimes, however, applicants misstate their manuscript's status due to not knowing how to cite it. The Council of Residency Directors (Emergency Medicine) suggests the following:

1. **Published manuscript**: give full citation.

2. **Accepted manuscripts (in press)**: list acceptance date.

3. **Submitted manuscripts**: list submission date.

4. **Research experience (or manuscript in progress)**: list research title/hypothesis, time period for the research, and research mentors.

Bring a copy of all published works, acceptance letters, submitted articles with the submission letter, and letters from research mentors listing research dates to all interviews. For presented papers, bring a copy of the published abstract or even better, a copy of the meeting program.

General recruiters estimate that about one-third of résumés include lies. Applicants think that they will be forgiven for embellishing their résumés. At least for residency applicants, forgiveness is rarely granted, and doctors' résumés are part of a paper trail that follows them wherever they go. Aside from any moral question, lying on application materials may result in not getting your desired residency position. It absolutely puts you at risk for immediate dismissal at anytime while you are a resident.

A few people each year try to enter residencies despite never having graduated from medical school; some succeed. Because of the notoriety given such cases, residency programs and state medical boards increasingly check on applicants using databanks run by the Federations of State Medical Boards, the American Medical Association, ECFMG, and the AAMC.

## Résumé Layout

Those using ERAS will have their résumé information entered in a generic style. You can, however, also provide programs with your own, more detailed and personalized, résumé. Those not using ERAS must provide programs with a résumé.

When compiling your résumé, there are several rules to follow, and several pitfalls (Figures 12.2 and 12.5) to avoid:

1. **Emphasize your strengths.** Write the résumé so these aspects of your past are prominent.

2. **Be clear, concise, and accurate.** Unless you are extraordinary, one, or at most two, pages will suffice.

3. **Design your résumé to be pleasant to the eye**, clean, and uncluttered. (See "Résumé Graphics," page 307.)

4. **Use action words** (Figure 12.3) wherever possible. As Mark Twain said, the difference between the right word and the almost-right word is the difference between lightning and a lightning bug.

5. **Follow the standard layout** recommended in the checklist in Figure 12.4. Use the examples (Figures 12.6 to 12.8) when you design your own résumé. These examples are chronological résumés. This is the type preferred by most program directors.

6. **Have it professionally typed**, unless you have a true "letter quality" printer (daisy-wheel, inkjet, or laser) on which to generate your résumé.

---

FIGURE 12.2

*Résumé Disaster Areas*

- Poor Organization
- Poor Grammar
- Handwritten
- Poor Photocopy
- More than Two Pages
- Lack of Name, Address, Telephone Number

- Narrative, Rather than Outline
- Misspellings of Any Kind
- Unexplained Time Periods
- Use of Onionskin Paper
- Exaggerations
- Insufficient Information

---

7. **Do not put "Résumé" or "Curriculum Vitae" at the top of the document** unless you think those reading it are idiots. Résumé formats are immediately obvious, and these words waste valuable space.

Some experts recommend that your first résumé is most easily organized using 3″ x 5″ cards (or their computer equivalent). Simply label one card for each of the topics in Figure 12.4 that applies to you. Then collect the information on each card (including names, dates, addresses, etc.) that you will need to complete the section. Put these cards in the order you want to see them on your résumé, and type the information onto your résumé.

After printing a sample copy, check it carefully for spelling. One medical student wrote, for example, "I am passed USMLE . . ." and "I would like to know weather . . ." As you might expect, he had a difficult time getting a position. Even if you are a native English speaker, have someone literate proofread your materials before you send them.

Only then should you decide on the graphic presentation you want. Once you have written your résumé, ask someone who knows you well to review it to be certain that you have portrayed yourself in the best possible manner. Figures 12.5 to 12.7 demonstrate some positive and negative examples. There is no perfect résumé style.

After further revisions, get some objective feedback, preferably from your adviser, your mentor, or the Dean of Students. If that is not possible, get someone to look at it who has experience with resident applicant résumés.

If you just can't get your act together, another option is to pay a commercial service to produce your résumé. You will, however, still have to provide the information, tell them how you want it organized, and usually proof it for accuracy. (Most of them proofread it for the spelling of common words.) Résumé services can be found in all large cities and around most universities. Their charges vary by location and the amount of work they need to do.

## FIGURE 12.3
### *Action Words for Your Résumé*

| | | | |
|---|---|---|---|
| accelerated | developed | introduced | reorganized |
| accomplished | directed | invented | replaced |
| achieved | discovered | launched | represented |
| active member | distributed | led | researched |
| actively | edited | made | responsible for |
| adapted | effected | maintained | restored |
| adjusted | elected | managed | revised |
| administered | enlarged | modified | scheduled |
| advised | established | monitored | selected |
| analyzed | examined | motivated | served |
| arranged | excelled | negotiated | set up |
| assisted | expanded | obtained | sold |
| awarded | experienced in | operated | solved |
| built | focused | organized | streamlined |
| chairperson | formulated | participated in | strengthened |
| charted | founded | performed | studied |
| compiled | generated | persuaded | successfully |
| completed | guided | planned | supervised |
| conceived | headed | prepared | supplied |
| conducted | identified | presented | taught |
| constructed | implemented | produced | tested |
| controlled | improved | proficient at | trained |
| coordinated | increased | programmed | translated |
| counseled | influenced | promoted to | updated |
| created | initiated | proposed | won |
| delivered | installed | provided | wrote |
| demonstrated | instituted | published | |
| designed | instructed | ran | |
| determined | interpreted | recorded | |

FIGURE 12.4

*A Résumé Checklist*

❑ Name[1]                          ❑ Extracurricular Activities[3]
❑ Address(es)                      ❑ Personal[3]
❑ Telephone Number(s)[2]              ❑ Birth Place & Date
❑ Objective                           ❑ Marital Status
❑ Publications                        ❑ Children
❑ Research                         ❑ Work Experience[4]
❑ Presentations                    ❑ Licenses & Certifications[5]
❑ Language/Computer Skills         ❑ Military[6]
❑ Honors & Awards                  ❑ Education[7]
❑ Reference Statement                 ❑ Medical School
❑ Applicable Jobs                     ❑ Graduate School
❑ Professional Memberships            ❑ Undergraduate

1. If you have changed your name, be certain that there is a clear statement explaining why your name differs on your transcript, licenses, diplomas, etc. If at all possible, it is best to keep one "professional name" throughout your career, even if you plan on changing your name in a social context.

2. Include all addresses and telephone numbers where you can be reached for the *next six months.*

3. Optional information. Include extracurricular activities only if they are extraordinary or applicable to medicine, such as working with the Ski Patrol or a volunteer ambulance service. Personal information can be supplied at your own discretion.

4. Include the dates that you held jobs. Other than military service, include only those jobs that you held for long periods of time, were applicable to medicine, or were full-time positions.

5. List currently held health-related licenses, such as R.N. (give states and dates), and health-related certifications, such as EMT, ACLS, ATLS, and PALS (give expiration dates).

6. The type of discharge that you received is legally privileged information. If it was anything less than honorable, don't include it.

7. Only include undergraduate and graduate school, medical school, and any other medically related course, such as an EMT or ACLS course. You have been out of high school a long time now, and no one is interested in that.

FIGURE 12.5

*Sample Résumé—The Disaster*

*Don't you have a first name?*

*Isn't it obvious that this is your C.V.?*

CURRICULUM VITAE

I. R. Smarte *Phone/Fax/Cell phone numbers? E-mail address?*

405 Campbell Ave. Washinton, DC 20043 *Dates at this address?*

Citizenship: USA *Assumed, unless otherwise stated*
Birthdate: October 27, 1967 *Who cares?*
Spouse's name: Les Smarte, I.R.S. Agent *This will really win points!*
Child: Matthew, age 4
Family:Mother: Helen S. Dingle, age 71, retired
       Sister: Jean Folks, age 45, Prof. Poly Sci

*Irrelevant in all circumstances*

Undergraduate education: Univ. Of Arizona, 1993
       B.S. in Cell Biology
       Honors: Phi Beta Kappa, Cum Laud Graduate. *Spelling!*
       Extracurricular Activities: Pep Squad,
              Marching Band, Biology Honorary, *Which one?*
              Rescue Squad *Which? Where?*
*Spelling!* *When?*
Post graduate ed: Univ. Of Cinti., 1987 (1997) Toxicology *Written corrections are sloppy!*
       Honors: Munroe Scholorship *What is this?*
       Research/Publications: ``The Effect of a Sub-
       freezing Environment on Cellular Metabolism *When & where were these published?*
       in Rats.'' (Thesis); Simons, G., Smarte, I.R.,
       Sullivan, J.P. ``Cellular Inhibition of Rat Tail
       Growth in a Subfreezing Atmosphere.''
*Spell out!* *Capitalize!*
Med School-- U of MD 2001
       Honors: Sherk Scholarship, Ama stud rep
       physiology, social/prventatave med, OB/GYN.
       Electives: forensic sci, experimental sugr lab

*Include only if your transcript is difficult to interpret*

*State that job was medically related*
Employment: 93/95 US Air Force, Staff Sgt.;
       91-93: carpenter (part-time) *Irrelevant*

Interests: Radical Student Alliance; Messianic *Irrelevant Counterproductive*
       Religious Revival

*Spelling!*
References: Ft. John X. Anlen: Our Lady of Sorrow, *Priest*
       31 Ensel Street, Baltimore, MD *Zip Code?*
              Michelle Rout, M.D., Radiology Resident, *Resident*
U. of AZ, 1501 N. Campbell Ave., Tucson, AZ 85724
              Sally Friendly: Director, Messianic *Friend*
       Student Revival, 1 North St., Reuther, MD 20933
*Counterproductive References*

*Why list references?*

*✻ Sloppy & Inconsistent Formatting ✻*

FIGURE 12.6
*A Sample Résumé–Style #1*

──────────────── **IRENE R. SMARTE** ────────────────

| | |
|---|---|
| 405 N. Campbell Ave. | 5573 Chillum Place, Apt. D |
| Washington, DC 20043 | Reading, PA 19380 |
| (202) 555-9087 | (215) 555-1836 |
| [Use: 8/00-10/00 & 4/01-6/01] | [Use: 11/00-3/01] |

**OBJECTIVE**   Superior training in Radiology which will give me the basis from which to practice in either the academic or the private sector for the next forty years.

**EDUCATION**   M.D., University of Maryland School of Medicine
Baltimore, MD
Sept. 1997–June 2001 (anticipated)
M.S., University of Cincinnati
Cincinnati, OH
Major: Toxicology
July 1995–June 1997
B.S., University of Arizona
Tucson, AZ
Major: Cellular Biology
Sept. 1989–June 1993

**HONORS/ AWARDS**   *Medical School*:   Sherk Scholarship (Most promising student in the sophomore class)
Class Vice-President: Junior Year
Student Representative, AMA, 2000-2001

*Graduate School*: Munroe Scholarship (2 years)

*Undergraduate*:   Phi Beta Kappa
Dann-Victor Scholarship (2 years)
Cum Laude Graduate
President, Biology Honorary, 1992-1993

**MILITARY EXPERIENCE**   Staff Sergeant, Medical Service Corps
U.S. Air Force, 1993-1995; Honorable Discharge
Responsible for administering a 40-person Radiology department at a regional hospital.

**PUBLICATIONS**   Simons, G; Smarte, IR; Sullivan, JP: "Cellular Inhibition of Rat Tail Growth in a Subfreezing Atmosphere." *Journal of Arctic Biology*. 2000;3(1):12-16.

**RESEARCH**   "The Effect of a Subfreezing Environment on Cellular Metabolism in Rats." (M.S. Thesis) Adviser: Professor G. Simons, Ph.D.

**EXTRA- CURRICULAR ACTIVITIES**   Member, Wheaton Rescue Squad
(Ambulance and Heavy Rescue)

**PERSONAL REFERENCES**   Married, 1 child; U. S. citizen;  excellent health
Excellent references furnished upon request.

FIGURE 12.7

## *A Sample Résumé–Style #2*

This is a slightly different style than the résumé in Figure 12.6. Some information has been purposely omitted. Other information has been combined. Two new sections have been added for you to use as an example.

## IRENE R. SMARTE

405 N. Campbell Ave.
Washington, DC 20043
(202) 555-9087

### OBJECTIVE
Superior training in Radiology which will give me the basis from which to practice in either the academic or the private sector over the span of my career.

### EDUCATION
M.D., *University of Maryland School of Medicine*, Baltimore, Maryland
September 1997–June 2001 (anticipated)
- Sherk Scholarship (Most promising student in the sophomore class)
- Class Vice-President: Junior Year
- Student Representative, AMA: 2000-2001

M.S., *University of Cincinnati*, Cincinnati, Ohio
Major: Toxicology; July 1995–June 1997
- Munroe Scholarship (2 years)

B.S., *University of Arizona*, Tucson, Arizona
Major: Cellular Biology; September 1989–June 1993
- Phi Beta Kappa
- Dann-Victor Scholarship (2 years)
- Cum Laude Graduate
- President, Biology Honorary, 1992-93

### MILITARY EXPERIENCE
Staff Sergeant, Medical Service Corps
U.S. Air Force, 1993-95; Honorable Discharge
Responsible for administering a 40-person Radiology department at a regional hospital.

### RESEARCH & PUBLICATIONS
Simons G, Smarte IR, Sullivan JP: "Cellular Inhibition of Rat Tail Growth in a Subfreezing Atmosphere." *Journal of Arctic Biology.* 3:1:12-16, 2000.

### PROFESSIONAL ORGANIZATIONS
- American Medical Student Association
- American College of Radiology: Student Member

### LANGUAGES
- Spanish (fluent written and spoken)
- Russian (written only)

### EXTRACURRICULAR ACTIVITIES
- Member, Wheaton Rescue Squad (Ambulance and Heavy Rescue)

### REFERENCES
Excellent references furnished upon request.

FIGURE 12.8

*Two Other Acceptable Résumé Formats*

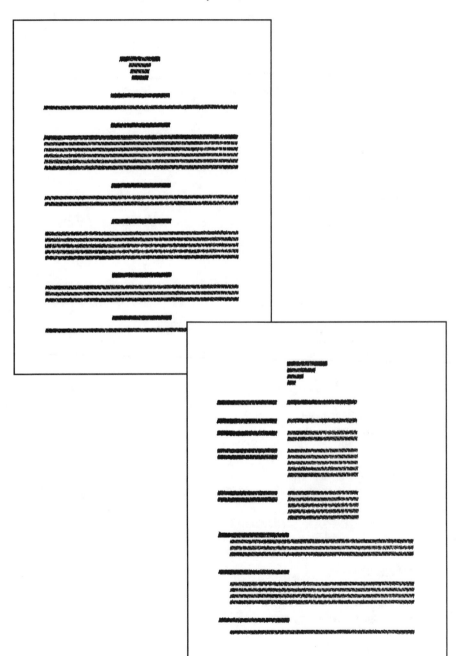

## Résumé Graphics

Avoid having a résumé that looks like every other résumé in circulation! Your résumé must have a clean and distinctive appearance. Like all of your written communications, it must attract attention. Essentially, it must be more attractive than the competition. To accomplish this, you must pay attention to the paper size and appearance, margins and spacing, type size and style, and layout.

### Paper

Most applicants use white bond paper. Your résumé will stand out if you use something different. Gray, ivory, or white paper with a textured or "pebble" finish will stand out among the throng of résumés. The weight of the paper is also important. Use 20- or 24-pound paper. If you plan to print your résumé on both sides of one sheet of paper, which is actually not a good idea, be sure that the paper is opaque enough so that the printing will not show through.

### Paper Size

Again, most of the résumés received by residency directors are on standard 8½" x 11" paper. Several other sizes are available which may serve to help your résumé stand out. The most acceptable is the "Monarch" size of stationery (7¼" x 10½"). Another possibility is using an 11" x 17" sheet, which will fold over into an 8½" x 11" folio. You can then put your name, address, and telephone number on the outside cover.

### Margins & Spacing

No matter how good your résumé is, it will look cheap, rushed, and of poor quality if you do not leave an ample margin. When using a standard 8½" x 11" sheet of paper, leave side margins of 1" to 1½". The space at the top of the page should be at least 1½", and at the bottom at least 1". If you will be using Monarch paper, leave ¾" to 1" margins on either side of the page. A minimum for the top and bottom margins is 1".

### Type Size & Style

Type comes in different sizes, known as "pitch," which designates the number of characters per inch. Either 10- or 12-pitch is standard for most typewriters and printers, and it is also adequate for most résumés. If you use Monarch paper, 12-pitch type is recommended. Type also differs in height. Differing heights, known as "points," can also be used in the résumé.

Various styles of type (fonts), such as Pica, Elite, and Roman, are available. Some variety can be added to your résumé by altering these type styles appropriately. This technique is most effective when used for the captions and subheadings. Make sure that all styles are complimentary to those used for the main body of your résumé. Boldface, underlining, italics, and asterisks or bullets (circles) can also, if used sparingly, successfully highlight important areas of your résumé. The key to an effective résumé is to plan it carefully, and make sure the final product reflects the planning that went into it.

### Laser Printers

Word processors and laser printers can produce amazing variations in type size and style within the résumé. If you have the requisite knowledge and software, you can design a magnificent résumé. If you don't though, you will need to go to a professional—including the secretaries in your adviser's or Dean's office—to get your résumé printed in this manner.

## The Personal Statement

The personal statement requested by many residency programs causes more anguish among applicants than almost anything else in the application process. A great deal of time and effort is often put into these epistles—and, in general, it is mostly wasted. Although some program directors take the time to carefully read applicants' personal statements (especially those in primary care specialties), many use personal statements only to eliminate those individuals who clearly stand out as being: (1) relatively illiterate, (2) pompous or tactless, or (3) outside the mainstream of physicians in the specialty or institution.

The key to writing a good personal statement is to *be honest, but not shy* about trumpeting your virtues. Many students find this hard to do. The elements of a "safe and sane" personal statement include:

1. *Why do you want to go into the specialty?* Briefly explain what has drawn you to the specialty. If there was one particular event that stands out, describe it. Your trait analyses from Chapter 4 may help you out. Do not state that you are interested in the field primarily because of either the monetary rewards you anticipate or the way in which it fits your lifestyle. These reasons are usually considered evidence of a shallow personality and a sloppy decision-making process.

2. *What do you intend to do during your career in the specialty?* Be general. In a community hospital program, it is always safe to say that you are planning on a primarily clinical career with some clinical research and teaching. This question may be difficult to answer in some high-powered academic centers where there is a palpable rift between the researcher-physicians and the physician-occasional researchers. You may want to tailor this part of your personal statement to the institution to which it is being sent, as well as to your particular interests. Do not state, however, that you want to be a small-town practitioner if you are applying to a high-powered research program, or vice versa.

3. *Other interests.* What else do you do with your life? Be brief. Discussing your family, sports, and community activities are safe. This section of your statement should be no longer than either of the previous two sections.

Additional points that may be addressed in the statement include explanations of any major problems, deficiencies, or questions that might arise after a review of your application or transcript. You might want to mention something particularly outstanding from your undergraduate career or your life outside school. *Avoid discussing politics or religion.* Neither has any place in any of your application materials.

The personal statement format is now constrained by the computer limitations of ERAS (unless you apply to a specialty or program that does not participate). You still can make it interesting, and even enjoyable to read. One applicant, for example, had a five-paragraph statement, each paragraph beginning with a key phrase that had been said to her and that related to her specialty of choice (e.g., "Aren't you scared to take care of all those really sick people?"). There are many other interesting ways to write the personal statement. The keys are to make it

- short enough to read easily
- in readable English without spelling or grammatical errors
- based on one or more stories that illustrate your life
- interesting

As with all other materials you send to programs, review your statement for format (Figure 12.9) before you have the final copy typed. Just as with the résumé, there is no one perfect style. (*Résumés and Personal Statements for Health Professionals, 2nd ed.,* by Tysinger has numerous examples of personal statements and details a system for writing these documents.)

---

FIGURE 12.9
**Format for Personal Statement**

One Page

Product of Laser or Inkjet Printer

Proper Grammar, Spelling, and Composition
(Get help with this if you need it.)

---

Occasionally students ask whether they should try to make their personal statement unusual enough to stand out. Literate and witty are the best ways to make a personal statement get noticed. One applicant, for example, vividly wrote, "Activity is my oxygen." The faculty remembered her!

Generally though, you take a big risk by writing a very unusual personal statement. Remember that physicians, in general, are conservative animals. Anything odd or unusual will ordinarily be viewed negatively. "Unusual" in a personal statement is normally interpreted by those reading the statement as something that is cute, flippant, or crass. That is not the impression you want to create. Of course, some applicants have gotten interviews and even positions based, in part, on unusual personal statements. But it is rare. Unless your life story in of itself is unusual, stick with standard and boring.

While most personal statements will be in simple paragraph format, and printed in the ERAS application, which allows little flexibility, those not using ERAS may want to use an alternative format for their statements. An example of another format is shown in Figure 12.10.

## Reference Letters

The reference letters that you have sent to residency programs are reflections of you in other people's eyes. They play an important part in getting you a residency position. Obtaining good reference letters, however, takes advance planning, hard work, and initiative. If you are willing to make the effort, the steps outlined below will help you to get the best possible reference letters. They will also help you make the most of the ones you do get.

FIGURE 12.10

*Alternative Style for a Personal Statement*

---

# MAXWELL I. SMARTE

## — Personal Statement —

| | |
|---|---|
| **hard working** | I grew up in Minnesota, spending summers on my parents' farm. It was here that I learned the value of hard work. |
| **mature** | At age 18, I joined the U.S. Air Force. Rising to the rank of Staff Sergeant, this was a period of personal growth. Four years in the service as a surgical technician and OR supervisor, both stateside and in Japan, gave me a more stable view of life. |
| **academic & clinical skills** | After completing undergraduate school in three years with a Chemistry major, I entered medical school, where I scored 82/200 on Step 1 of the USMLE and achieved Honors in Surgery and in Pediatrics. I spent many evenings working with one of our local Pediatric Surgeons. |
| **career goals** | The latter activity convinced me that Pediatric Surgery will provide me with what I want from a career in medicine—curing sick children, caring for those with both acute and chronic diseases, and involvement in the broadest type of General Surgery. |
| | After residency, I would like to work at a major tertiary care teaching hospital. There I could combine practice, teaching, and research. My choice of residency reflects these long-term goals. |
| **summary** | In summary, I am a hard working, mature individual who has a clear vision of a career in Pediatric Surgery. Both my experiences and training have reinforced my dedication to this dynamic and exciting field of medicine. |

Sincerely,

Maxwell I. Smarte

## Dean's Letter

Each medical school sends about 2,800 Dean's letters each year, averaging 21 letters per student. (This totals more than one million pages per year. What a way to destroy our forests!) These letters follow each school's standard format. Most are relatively long, averaging 3.1 single-spaced pages, and detailed. The material that they contain, however, can vary a great deal (Figures 12.11 and 12.12).

Dean's letters include some personal background information about you, with reference to your undergraduate experience. They then go on to detail your preclinical and, especially, your clinical course work. Most letters include direct quotes from evaluations of your performance.

Based on the Association of American Medical Colleges' guidelines for Dean's letters (Figure 12.14), many create charts which show a student's performance on clinical clerkships compared with that of his or her class-mates or with that of a compilation of several recent classes. Some now also include the student's results on the Objective Structured Clinical Examination (OSCE), a standardized measure of clinical performance being used at more than sixty U.S. medical schools.

### FIGURE 12.11
*Frequency of Appearance of Information in Dean's Letters*

| Type of Information | % Never | % Sometimes | % Always |
|---|---|---|---|
| Research Experience | 0 | 8 | 92 |
| School-Related Extracurricular Activities | 0 | 9 | 91 |
| Academic Background Prior to Med School | 3 | 9 | 88 |
| Interpersonal Skills | 0 | 20 | 80 |
| Personality Descriptions | 3 | 39 | 58 |
| Non-professional Interests (Hobbies) | 5 | 37 | 58 |
| Responsibility to Others* | 0 | 44 | 56 |
| Statements Regarding Professional Growth | 2 | 44 | 54 |
| Personal Background Prior to Med School | 8 | 44 | 49 |
| Work Background Prior to Medical School | 9 | 47 | 44 |
| Statements Regarding Personal Growth** | 5 | 53 | 42 |
| Class Rank | 56 | 16 | 28 |
| Extent of Contact with Student | 37 | 48 | 16 |
| Reasons for Choosing Specialty | 36 | 52 | 13 |
| Reasons for Choosing Medicine | 42 | 49 | 9 |

*Defined as acceptance of responsibility for one's own actions, keeping agreements, and meeting obligations.
**Defined as sense of independence, purpose, and maturity.
Adapted from: Hunt DD, MacLaren CF, Scott CS, Chu J, Leiden LI. Characteristics of dean's letters in 1981 and 1992. *Academic Medicine.* 1993;68(12):905-11.

FIGURE 12.12

**Frequency of Negative Information Known to the Dean's Office
Appearing in Dean's Letters**

| Type of Information | % Never | % Sometimes | % Always |
|---|---|---|---|
| Ethical Problems (e.g., cheating) | 10 | 34 | 57 |
| Substance Abuse | 15 | 46 | 39 |
| Emotional Instability | 4 | 65 | 31 |
| Physical Illness | 2 | 75 | 23 |

Adapted from: Hunt DD, MacLaren CF, Scott CS, Chu J, Leiden LI. Characteristics of dean's letters in 1981 and 1992. *Academic Medicine.* 1993;68(12):905-11.

Most (about 85%) of the letters also include a key sentence at the end that gives an overall or summary recommendation. Because of the overblown syntax used in many recommendation letters, some schools now give an actual numerical breakdown of the recommendations that they use. For example, the top 10% of graduates (from this year or recent years) may be rated "outstanding," while the next 25% of graduates are rated "excellent." There is no question in anyone's mind where you stand (at the very bottom of the class) if you get a "satisfactory" overall evaluation. Little more than one-fourth of Dean's letters actually give a class ranking. The lack of class ranking can hurt top candidates applying for very competitive programs, since it appears that residency faculty will give preference to top-ranked individuals from "average" medical schools over unranked students from "top" schools.

While these letters usually go out over the Dean of Students' signature, they may be written by subsidiary deans or administrative personnel (18%), by faculty committees (3%), or by individual faculty advisers (6%). In a few instances, students themselves get to write the biographical portion of their letter. It is helpful to know the system at your school in case you can supply some additional input. Your Dean's office will be happy to explain the system they use.

As a matter of policy, as well as common courtesy, at most medical schools the Dean's letters are usually shown to students before they are sent out. *Your first responsibility* in regard to your Dean's letter is to *carefully review it.* Check it for mistakes. But more important, check to make sure that all good evaluations and special honors, awards, and activities have been mentioned. If there are problems or discrepancies in the letter, bring them to the Dean's attention at once. This letter will not only be used when you apply for a residency position, but it will also be sent out in the future, at your request, when you are looking for employment after residency.

Virtually all residency programs require a Dean's letter before they invite applicants for an interview. The letters, however, are not always a big help to residency faculty in screening applicants; they do, however, serve as a gross measure of a student's achievements compared with his or her classmates. A group who reviewed Dean's letters from all U. S. medical schools felt that nearly half failed to provide either an adequate format for locating necessary information or the information itself. Nearly one-half of Pediatrics residency directors and about one-third of those in Family Practice say that they do not use the Deans' letters when making decisions about whom to interview.

The medical school deans and faculty who write the Dean's letters want all their graduates to match into the best possible residencies. They are also unreasonably threatened by a fear of tort litigation if they are too candid about a student's performance. The writer's underlying theme is the old adage, "If you can't say something nice, don't say anything at all." A letter to the *New England Journal of Medicine* once remarked that Adolf Hitler's Dean's letter might have read, "A natural leader . . . good communication skills . . . likes to find solutions to problems." The result is a bland, positive, often oblique, and incomplete picture of a graduate.

Even with all the letter's drawbacks, experienced residency directors know that if they read between the lines, the Dean's letters are an effective way of screening candidates. They look for words like "enthusiastic" (manic?), "organized" (obsessive-compulsive?), "colorful" (bizarre?), or "active social life" (flirt?). Letters that dwell on a candidate's dress and punctuality suggest that the author is hunting for something nice to say. They rarely are as explicit as are the comments heard about applicants in conversation (Figure 12.13). Finally, the Dean's letter, in combination with a transcript and a telephone call, is a good method of eliminating any charlatans posing as medical students. (Yes, they really are out there.)

It is particularly disturbing when one or two schools each year cannot seem to get their Dean's letters out on time. In recent years, the schools where this has happened have been among the best in the country. Those who suffered were the medical students who did not get interview spots (most residencies only have a limited number) and therefore did not get to select from many of their top program choices. Therefore, *your second responsibility* in regard to your Dean's letter is to *keep track of when it is supposed to go out.* United States medical school Deans have agreed to a uniform date of November 1—before which no Dean's letters are to be mailed or sent via ERAS—for current medical students. (Nearly half of all

---

**FIGURE 12.13**

**Disparaging Comments About Applicants
(but too witty for most faculty)**

- "Works well when under constant supervision and cornered like a rat in a trap."

- "He would be out of his depth in a puddle."

- "Technically sound, but socially inept."

- "This young lady has delusions of adequacy."

- "He has the wisdom of youth and the energy of old age."

- "The nursing staff would follow him anywhere, but only out of morbid curiosity."

- "This student has reached rock bottom and shows signs of starting to dig."

- "When she opens her mouth, it is only to change whichever foot was previously in there."

- "He sets low personal standards and then consistently fails to achieve them."

---

graduating medical students report that programs are requesting these letters before November 1. Some Deans bypass the spirit, if not the letter, of this requirement by announcing that they are willing to supply verbal information to program directors prior to the November 1 date.) The November date gives the Dean's offices plenty of time to write the letters. Make sure that *your* Dean's letter goes out on or before November 1. (If you have already graduated from medical school, your old Dean's letter can go out whenever you request it.)

*Your third responsibility is, if you are not using ERAS or CAS, to supply the Dean with a correct list of program names and addresses in a timely manner.* If you don't do this, it does not matter how good the letter is, nor how timely the school was in getting it ready. If it cannot be sent for want of an address, you still lose.

FIGURE 12.14

*Suggested Format for Dean's Letters*

| | |
|---|---|
| **HEADING** | _____ |
| | _____ |
| | _____ |
| | _____ |
| | |
| | Dear _____ : |
| | This letter is an evaluation of the achievements of |
| | _____ |
| | Name |

| | |
|---|---|
| **INTRODUCTION** | • This section should provide a concise chronology of the student's progress through medical school.<br>• Indicate and explain irregular progress and any required remediation. |

| | |
|---|---|
| **PRECLINICAL RECORD** | • Avoid course by course descriptions.<br>• Highlight unusually good or poor achievements. |

| | |
|---|---|
| **CLINICAL CLERKSHIP RECORD** | • In chronological order, describe the student's performance in each required clerkship.<br>• Focus on knowledge, data gathering, analytic reasoning, and interpersonal skills.<br>• Cite unusual accomplishments in elective clerkships at the end of this section.<br><br>(First Clerkship:  _____ )<br>(Second Clerkship:  _____ )<br>(Third Clerkship:  _____ )<br>(Fourth Clerkship:  _____ )<br>(Fifth Clerkship: etc.)<br><br>(Elective Clerkships—only list unusual accomplishments) |

| | |
|---|---|
| **SPECIAL ACTIVITIES** | • Report activities reflecting the student's talents (e.g., research experience, volunteer work, leadership roles). |

| | |
|---|---|
| **PERSONAL QUALITIES** | • This section should provide the reader with a sense of the student as a person.<br>• When necessary, include comments about personal limitations. |

| | |
|---|---|
| **SUMMARY** | • The program director most likely will read this section first.<br>• Provide a clear, concise, and balanced synopsis of the above sections. |

_____

Signature

FIGURE 12.14 (continued)

## SAMPLE RATINGS SHEET

CLASS OF

Name_____

### RATINGS OF CLINICAL COMPETENCE IN CORE CLERKSHIPS

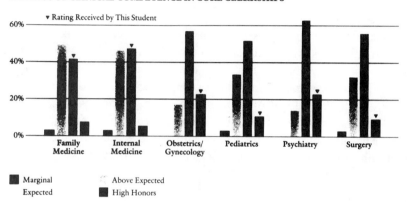

Marginal       Above Expected

Expected       High Honors

### WRITTEN EXAMINATION GRADES IN CORE CLERKSHIPS

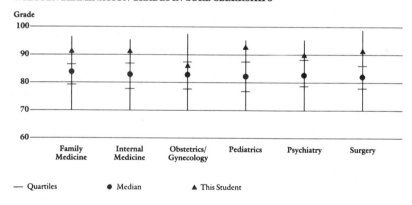

— Quartiles     ● Median     ▲ This Student

# Other Reference Letters

## Whom To Ask

Most of the reference letters you will send to residency programs will come from those individuals you have personally asked to write them. It is essential for you to know whom to ask.

### The Ideal Reference

The ideal reference letter is from an individual who is well-known to program directors in the field—a nationally recognized figure in the specialty of choice, who: (1) has worked with you clinically; (2) thinks you are a "star"; and (3) came from the institution to which you are applying. If the individual works at one of the specialty's residency programs, it is optimal if their letter says that you have been strongly encouraged to apply to his or her program. All this may be difficult to achieve in one letter. But you should think of such a reference as the "gold standard."

### Other Clinical Faculty

Other good reference sources are faculty with whom you have worked clinically and who thought you did a great job. Look for those clinical rotations where you did "Honors" work to get these letters. But don't stray too far afield from your area of interest. Getting letters from a Psychiatry attending will not be too effective if you are applying for a Radiology position. If you have cultivated a mentor early on, whether or not he or she is in your desired specialty, it might be useful to have him or her write you a letter. If your mentor has worked with you clinically (and if they haven't it is *your* fault), his or her opinion will often carry a great deal of weight.

### Preclinical Instructors

How about your preclinical instructors? Weak! Unless you are applying to Pathology, Public Health, or a very heavily research-oriented program these letters should only be used in addition to any required reference letters. Everyone can tell how well you did in Anatomy by your grade. The clinical programs want to know how well you treated live patients.

### Researchers

"But I've done research," you say. "Can't I get a letter from my research preceptor?" Again, unless you are going into an area where this particular research will be central to your training, such a letter should only be considered as additional support. In general, medical students participating in research are used as "scut puppies." They frequently contribute very little except brute labor. Often they actually have little contact with the research director, and consequently, that individual may know very little about their clinical abilities.

### Counterproductive References

Do not get letters from residents, friends, relatives, clergymen, politicians, or patients. You think I'm being funny? Not a bit. I have personally received reference letters for residency applicants from individuals in all these categories. Letters from these sources normally do not help your application. They may, in fact, be detrimental. Residency directors are interested in how well you will do in their program. They want consistent information from reputable, knowledgeable sources. That means your teachers. "If she can't get these letters, there must be something wrong with her," they say. Don't make them think that!

## When To Ask

Don't be a wimp! If you want a letter from a particular individual, ask for it. But ask at the right time and in the right way. When is the right time? If you are on a clinical service with the individual, ask while you are on the service, or soon afterwards. Don't wait until six months or a year later. No matter how great a job you did, the faculty member's memory of you will fade with time. Ask if the letter can be drafted now, saying that you will give him or her the list of programs to send the letter to later.

If it is from a mentor or adviser, ask for a reference letter during a counseling session. If someone has arbitrarily selected your adviser, first think about whether he or she knows you well enough to write a letter.

If the letter you want is from a faculty member in your desired specialty, you will get it either because you have been working with the individual for some time (volunteer, fellowship, etc.), or because of your performance during a clinical rotation. If it is due to the former, just ask. If the latter, do some investigation before you start any clinical work in the department. With whom will you be working? Does this individual meet the qualifications you need for a reference? If not, is there a way of switching the schedule so you can work with someone who will be a good reference? Once you select the individual or individuals, let them know early in the rotation that you are interested in their specialty and you would like them to write you a reference letter if they think you have done an excellent job by the end of the rotation. This motivates both of you. You will know that extra scrutiny is coming your way from the faculty members, and the faculty members will pay extra attention to your performance.

## How To Ask

Several years ago, I received a scrawled letter from a student who had rotated through our department some months before. Addressed to "Residency Director," it asked, "Dear Sir: Please write a letter of reference to:" and proceeded to list a number of programs. There was no return address. Seeing no way to refuse, and personally feeling that the student had done, at best, an adequate job during his rotation, I wrote the following letter: "Mr. Student did a clinical rotation with us in July. He performed adequately." This, if you haven't guessed, is a very negative letter. I don't know if this particular student ever did match in our specialty, but his discourtesy, not to mention lack of insight and poor clinical aptitude, certainly did not help his chances of getting the residency he desired.

Don't send blind letters or coded messages. Ask for a reference letter directly. But phrase it in such a way that neither you nor the faculty member will be saddled with either a negative or a neutral (read: "negative") letter. One way of doing this is to ask if the faculty member "would feel comfortable writing me a strong letter of support?" If the answer is anything other than strongly affirmative, look elsewhere. One of our wisest and most experienced faculty members, Dr. Douglas Lindsey, offers to write letters for every medical student. He writes them honestly. He then shows the student the letter. It is up to the student to decide whether it is sent. This is an excellent policy of a great teacher. Unfortunately, it is probably unique.

One way of circumventing the problem of a poor reference letter is to ask for a copy of the letter for your files. This gambit is somewhat tricky. If you firmly believe that the individual you have asked will write a superlative letter but will not give you a copy, go ahead—at some risk. If the individual agrees to give you a copy of the letter, then you stand a good chance of, at least marginally, upgrading the quality of the letter by discussing the content with the writer. A very few physicians make it a policy to send copies of the reference letters they write to the individuals for whom they write them. In the business world, this is standard practice and common courtesy. Too bad it isn't yet a widespread practice within the medical profession.

If you do happen to get a reference letter that isn't glowing, don't panic. You have one card left to play. If the letter has not yet been sent out, don't give its author any program addresses to which he or she can send it. If you have followed the plan above, you will get a copy of the letter long before you yourself even know where you are going to apply. You will also have plenty of time to collect other, more complimentary letters. By the time you are ready to send out reference letters, you should have a file of copies of letters that have been written on your behalf. Select the best and ask these individuals to mail them to the programs to which you are applying. If you can pull it off, this is virtually a no-lose situation. You might also supply them with mailing labels to save them time. They will appreciate it.

A few students have been asked to sign statements that they have not seen their reference letters. This is ridiculous and unenforceable. Don't sign. However, it is common practice for students to be asked to sign a waiver of their right to request to see reference letters. If you are forced into this type of situation, you may have to sign it and hope for good letters. If possible, you do want to see those letters before they go out.

## The Format

While the Dean's letter will follow the institution's format and will be professionally done on College of Medicine stationery, the same may not be true for your reference letters. It is almost unbelievable that faculty physicians send out reference letters that are not on letterhead, are done on dot matrix printers, or are handwritten. This is a negative reflection not only on these individuals, but also on you. If you believe that any of the individuals from whom you have requested a letter will have difficulty producing a professional-appearing document, either offer to have the letter typed for them or just ask someone else. Physicians working for the federal government and those in solo or rural practice settings seem to have the most difficulty in producing professional reference letters. It should be noted that the best format is the typewritten letter on letterhead stationery with a handwritten note from the writer. That gets attention.

Although most medical school faculty send out many reference letters, they have never been taught what goes in them. They might find it useful if you give them a copy of Figure 12.15, Elements of a Reference Letter, when you ask them to write your reference letter. Better still, especially with older or more experienced faculty members, ask if they would like you to send them a copy. Individuals from outside your medical center whom you are asking for a reference would almost assuredly appreciate a format to guide them in writing the letter.

Some specialties and programs now use a Standard Letter of Recommendation (SLOR). Pioneered by Emergency Medicine, they are designed to improve communication about applicants. These can be more easily scanned into computers and analyzed than can normal reference letters, although many people still send both a standard letter and this form.

---

### FIGURE 12.15

### *Elements of a Reference Letter*

It is very useful to include the following items in reference letters for applicants to residency programs:

**Scholastic Record**

1. Standing in graduating class
2. Honors/commendations in courses
3. Other honors

**Medical Abilities**

1. Interaction with patients
2. Diagnostic ability
3. Physical examination ability
4. Laboratory use and test interpretation
5. Use of pharmacological agents
6. Clarity of oral presentations
7. Clarity/completeness of charts
8. Knowledge of medical literature

**Personal Characteristics**
(List strongest points first.)

1. Relations with peers, faculty, ancillary staff
2. Willingness to assume responsibility
3. Dependability
4. Integrity; moral and ethical qualities
5. Industriousness
6. Initiative
7. Motivation
8. Interest
9. Maturity
10. Flexibility
11. Sense of humor

---

The form includes key information, such as how likely the applicant is to match at the reference's residency program ("guaranteed," "very likely," "likely," etc.), how their grade compares with those of other students from the same year, and how the applicant measures up compared to other applicants for which the reference has written letters. Look for them to be used more frequently in the future.

# A Picture?

Although it remains very questionable whether photographs should be a part of any employment application, including a photograph has become moot for all those using ERAS. To process your application, you must include a photo. However, it just happens to be illegal under civil rights legislation, since it indicates race, gender, and age. The legal point is that since potential employers cannot discriminate against individuals based on race, sex, age, and national background, there is no reason for a picture.

What kind of photograph do you include? As with everything you do in conjunction with your application, your photograph should look professional—especially because the first version they will probably see will be the black and white scanned version from ERAS. Have it professionally done. Don't sit in the drugstore photo machine that gives you five pictures for one dollar. This is your career at stake.

Go to a professional photographer and explain that you need a portrait photo. Unless you are specifically asked for a black and white picture, get it in color. It may be less expensive to order extra copies of the photographs your school takes of students in the second or third year. But if you have noticeably altered your appearance since then, such as with the addition of a beard or a change in hairstyle, get a new set of pictures. The benefit of using a professional photographer is that no matter what you really look like, you will appear much better in the professional's picture. Also, make sure that you look like a neat, clean, professional. As in the interview itself, when getting the photo, don't go in for fancy hairstyles, party or informal clothes, or extravagant jewelry.

You use the color photograph once you have been granted an interview. Have a photograph ready for the program to include with your application material. Actually, it is illegal for a program to request a photograph, even after you have been interviewed in person. But you are not going to wait for them to request it—you will arrive at the interview with the photograph in hand.

Why should you do this? For a very obvious reason. You want to be remembered. Do you really think that an interviewer will remember anything specific about Jerry Glover or Mary Smythe after seeing forty applicants? Probably not. They may even have trouble recalling applicants using the ERAS picture. But with a great color photograph to jog their memory during final selection, the good impressions that you left with the faculty will come flooding back.

Finally, before handing the picture to the residency secretary for your file, make sure that you put a gummed label on the back with not only your name, but also your address, telephone number, and the date that you are interviewing.

Oh yes, remember to say "cheese."

## The Transcript

Your official medical school transcript, which will be required by nearly every program to which you apply, is a coded summary of your progress through medical school. The key word here is "coded." Symbols are used in each transcript. Familiar to most residency directors are such designations as "H" (Honors) or "A" for top grades. These symbols are widely used. Somewhat deceptively however, some schools use "High Honors" for a top grade and "Honors" for the runners-up. Some schools, for their own reasons, use symbols that are distinctly different from those used in most transcripts. A few use "O" (Outstanding), "S" (Superior)—which indicates a less-than-Honors grade in some schools, but the top grade in others—or various numerical systems to designate a top grade. Those using numerical systems also tend to obscure the student grades with multiple columns of irrelevant data.

If you have done well in school, it is important that it be obvious to the faculty members who will review your transcript. No, the school's detailed explanation on the back of or accompanying the transcript does not help. If it needs that much explanation, the school needs to revise its method of recording grades. That, however, is something you cannot do anything about now. What you need to do is to include a separate page which summarizes your transcript with your application materials.

Your transcript summary page, *which is separate from your résumé*, should include all the following:

1. A listing of all courses in which you received "Honors." Clearly specify that the grade, whatever it is called on the transcript, is in fact the top grade given out at your school.

2. A listing of all courses in which you received a "B" grade, if such grades are given out at your school.

3. An explanation of any unusual grades or symbols on your transcript. This means detailing why there was an "Incomplete" listed for Biochemistry. It is very important to do this. If it was because you turned in a required project late, it is far different from what is assumed otherwise—that you failed part of the course and had to make it up.

4. A listing of courses you will take in the balance of the year, but whose grades may not yet have been received or recorded by the registrar. The purpose of this is to alleviate concerns caused by misinterpretation of the transcript. Some schools use a "P" (which generally means "Pass," the average grade) to indicate that a course is "In Progress." If this appears next to the rotations taken early in your senior year (which probably will include your specialty elective), it could mean curtains for any chance to get an interview unless you explain it.

5. An explanation of any leaves of absence taken during medical school. If this needs more than a few words, state that it is further explained in your résumé or personal statement.

6. An explanation of any awards listed on your transcript. This explanation should include who gave the award and the achievement recognized.

7. Identify your class rank if your school notes this on the transcript, or if it will be to your advantage (if you are in the top half of your class) to do so.

Obviously, to intelligently write a personalized explanatory cover letter, it will be necessary for you to review a copy of your transcript. You can get this copy from the registrar's office. Most individuals in these offices will be very happy to help you. Some even suggest that you come in and review your transcript periodically to ensure that they have not erred when recording your grades. Occasionally, however, some registrars may be reluctant to show you your transcript. In those cases, request help from your Dean of Students. After explaining why you want to review your record, you should have no difficulty in obtaining a copy for yourself.

Finally, you may get excellent grades in significant courses after sending in your initial transcript. It would serve you well to send, near the end of the interviewing "season," an updated transcript to the programs where you have interviewed. Make certain that the registrar has received and recorded late grades before the revised transcripts are sent out. Also, see if the Registrar's office can attach a note stating that this is an updated transcript. This will alert the programs to replace the transcript currently in their files with the new one that contains important, updated information.

A word now to those whose grades have not been stellar. An obscure transcript can often work to your advantage. You certainly do not want to call attention to it by enclosing the explanation of the transcript described above. Rather, you would like to have the transcript ignored as much as possible. It is still important, though, to explain in your résumé or personal statement any leaves of absence, failing grades, and courses-in-progress.

Finally, just as with the Dean's letter, make certain, if you are not using ERAS or CAS, that your transcript is sent out on time. Many applicants will be trying to send out transcripts simultaneously. This overburdens the registrar's office. If your transcript is delayed, your work to get the right interviews might go for naught. Try to get your request in a little early. It is acceptable to forward a transcript before you have sent in, or even completed, the program's application. So, get those addresses into the registrar's office as soon as you can. Make sure that one of the addresses is that of your mentor. When he or she receives a copy (discuss this in advance), you will know that the programs should have received their copies as well.

## Timing—It's Your Future At Stake

Now that you have spent a great deal of time getting your material ready, make certain that you send it all in early. One of the primary caveats in sending your material is that the requirements for granting interviews stiffen as the "season" progresses. When the first completed applications arrive, most programs are rather liberal about granting interviews. Later, as the vast influx of applications arrives, applicants are generally compared against those who have already been granted interviews. The requirements, therefore, get more demanding with the passing weeks. Perhaps more important, nearly half of Pediatrics residency directors and about one-fourth of those in Family Medicine and Anesthesiology use a "first-come, first-served" basis for selecting candidates to interview.

It is, therefore, vital to get your materials in as soon as possible. Once you have requested that everything be sent or you have actually sent it to the programs, you can safely sit back and wait for interview requests, right? Wrong! Haven't you ever received a birthday card in the mail two months late, even though it was postmarked before your birthday? Of course you have. Not that the mail is slow or prone to frequent errors. But if your career depends upon the programs receiving all of your materials by a specific deadline, then it behooves you to be sure that they get it. And most programs do have specific deadlines.

If you use ERAS, check on your applications' status by using their tracking system, ADTS, located at www.aamc.org/eras/adts. If you don't use ERAS, keep a log of everything that you assume have been sent to each program. When you think that all of your materials should have arrived at the programs, call and ask. If they say that your file is incomplete, ascertain exactly what is lacking. If the missing document is something that has been sent to multiple programs, check with more than one program. The problem may actually be within one program's filing system. But it may mean that you will have to send duplicates of some material to some programs. Remember that for programs requiring a Dean's letter, the file for graduating students cannot be complete until at least the first week in November, since these letters are not mailed until November 1.

There is another method you can easily use to assure receipt of your materials. You can enclose a self-addressed, stamped postcard with each application for the program to use to notify you when all your materials have arrived. The postcard, with a place to put a date, should say, "All necessary application materials have been received by the (name of residency program) Residency Program for (your name)." *You* should fill out the blanks before you enclose it. Attach a small note asking that the postcard be returned when all of your materials are received. Occasionally, even a small item such as using this postcard will suggest something positive about an applicant. A real example of one such postcard that our program received is shown in Figure 12.16.

In any event, once your file is complete, you should be able to call the programs to find out whether you will be offered an interview. Persistent calling, if you are pleasant about it, rather than making you a pest, may get you an interview you might not otherwise have received.

Some students use registered mail and "return request" slips to ensure that the material they personally send gets to the program. This is probably overkill. Others, at the last minute, send materials by overnight mail/courier services. This is not only very expensive, it is sloppy. The programs may wonder why you couldn't get your act together a few days earlier.

The bottom line, then, is to plan ahead to get all your material to the residency programs on time—and then check to make certain it was received.

FIGURE 12.16
*A Completed-Application Postcard*

---

Date _____

Congratulations! Your application is now **complete**.

❏ Please call to schedule an interview.
❏ We will contact you to schedule an interview.
❏ Sorry buddy. Ever thought about law school?

Thanks for all your help.

Program _____

Telephone _____

Contact _____

---

# 13

# Special Situations

*To be a bullfighter, you must learn to think like the bull.*
— Spanish Folk Saying

*We hold these truths to be self-evident, that all men are created equal;*
*that they are endowed by their creator with certain unalienable rights;*
*that among these are life, liberty and the pursuit of happiness.*
— Thomas Jefferson

The archetypical physician in the United States was, for a long time, a White, Anglo-Saxon male. But this has changed drastically over the last four decades.

There was a large influx of foreign-born, foreign-trained physicians during the perceived doctor shortage in the 1960s and 1970s. Advancements in the rights of women and minorities also were made during this time, and it gradually became easier for all qualified applicants to medical schools to equitably compete for entrance into the profession. This resulted in an increasing number of physicians who did not meet the classic male "WASP" mold. Soon after, these physicians began knocking at the doors of residency programs to get further training. Gradually, the once-barred doors of virtually all specialties have opened. However, many groups still have particular problems gaining entrance into residencies.

Of note is that the federal Equal Employment Opportunity Commission (EEOC) has ruled that once you have obtained a residency position, you are an employee. This means that you are specifically protected under Title VII from discrimination in employment based on race, color, sex, religious beliefs, or national origin. You are also protected under the Equal Pay Act and the Age Discrimination in Employment Act.

Some excellent resources for medical students who don't fit the mold are the American Medical Student Association's (AMSA) groups and computer listservers for those with disabilities; lesbian, gay and bisexual students; minorities; and women. They also publish information about these groups nearly every month in *The New Physician*, often including contact phone numbers, E-mail addresses, and websites.

## Women

The first woman to graduate from a U.S. medical school, Dr. Elizabeth Blackwell, graduated from the Geneva Medical College in upstate New York in 1849. Despite many obstacles, she graduated first in her class. Yet in 1921, more than 70 years later, only 8% of U.S.-hospital internships accepted women. Today, women account for about 22% of practicing physicians, 43% of medical students (44% of first-year students), 36% of residents, and nearly 26% of medical school faculty members. However, on average, there is only one woman department head per medical school and only 7% of medical school Deans are women.

It is no longer unusual for women to constitute the majority of a medical school class; they comprise more than half the 1999 entering class in 40 U.S. medical schools. More than one in five (22%) of all U.S. physicians was female in 1999, compared to about one in 13 physicians (7.7%) in 1970. It is estimated that the number of female physicians will double between 1993 and 2010, when women will constitute almost one-third of all U.S. physicians. Among Osteopathic physicians, the number of women practitioners will more than triple by 2010.

This is a significant advance from the 1890s when the new Johns Hopkins Medical School, because of its need for the funds that women were raising, and then only under duress, agreed to accept qualified women as medical students. Although as recently as 1977 there were no female residents in more than one-third of all specialties, by 1999, women were training in every accredited area except a few minor subspecialties with few total trainees.

Nearly all women physicians say that they are satisfied with their careers. Those most satisfied have more children, less home stress, are strongly religious, and feel in control of their work life. Nevertheless, many would choose a different specialty or another career if given the chance.

Nearly 60% of female physicians under 35 years old are in Primary Care. About 60% of male physicians in this age group are in non-Primary Care specialties. This gender disparity is similar for physicians 35 to 54 years old. Most women physicians tend to specialize in Internal Medicine, Pediatrics, or Family Practice (49% of all women residents, but only 36% of men in 1998). Another 14% of women (7% of men) go into Obstetrics and Gynecology and Psychiatry. However, only 53% of women physicians are Board-certified in their specialty, as opposed to 65% of men.

This does not mean that there is no longer discrimination against women trying to get residency positions—especially in the surgical fields. While the match rate for women is better than for men in the specialties of Family Practice, Internal Medicine, Anesthesiology, Emergency Medicine, and Diagnostic Radiology, the reverse is true in some other specialties. Obstetrics and Gynecology, Pediatrics, Psychiatry, Pathology, General Surgery, and Orthopedic Surgery all have consistently higher match rates for men than for women. It has been suggested that in the first four of the latter specialties, a form of reverse discrimination is occurring. Program directors may be attempting to reverse the preponderance of women in those specialties by giving preference to male applicants (Figure 13.1).

In Surgery, though, while only 5% of all surgical residents are women, 25% of women applicants to General Surgery residency programs have failed to match in recent years, compared with about 15% of men. Women account for less than 2.5% of new physicians entering the field of General Surgery, and less than 3.7% of those entering surgical subspecialties. A recent survey of both male and female physicians cited General Surgery, Orthopedic Surgery, and Urology as the specialties that most restrict opportunities for women.

Respondents in this same survey cited Family Practice, Obstetrics and Gynecology, Pediatrics, and Internal Medicine as having an equal or higher rate of opportunity for female physicians. In Internal Medicine, a much higher percentage of women than men practice General Internal Medicine, despite any subspecialty training.

FIGURE 13.1

### Women's Representation in Selected Specialties

| Specialty | % of physicians in this specialty | % of physicians in the specialty that are women | % of women in specialty less than 35 years old |
|---|---|---|---|
| Internal Medicine | 28% | 25% | 37% |
| Family Practice | 14 | 25 | 35 |
| Pediatrics | 12 | 46 | 33 |
| General Surgery | 9 | 9 | 49 |
| Obstetrics/Gynecology | 8 | 32 | 35 |
| Psychiatry | 7 | 28 | 16 |
| Anesthesiology | 5 | 20 | 20 |
| Diagnostic Radiology | 4 | 19 | 30 |
| Emergency Medicine | 4 | 18 | 32 |
| Orthopedic Surgery | 4 | 3 | ? |

From: Table 9. *Physician Characteristics and Distribution in the U.S., 1999*. Chicago, IL: AMA, 1999, p. 45.

If a woman candidate presents herself as firm and assertive, she is often labeled "strident and aggressive." If she demonstrates a milder, more traditionally feminine image, she runs the risk of a "meek and wimpy" label. In essence, it is often a lose-lose situation.

Greater awareness of federal laws prohibiting discrimination against women in hiring and during employment, as well as a change in social attitudes toward professional women, have made discriminatory practices more complex and subtle. These practices are often based upon the irrational fears of potential employers, which often are not only unfair but also arbitrary. These employers are frequently disturbed by the idea of working with women as equals. One possible result is the under-representation of women on residency faculties. The percentage of women faculty members varies greatly by specialty, and their academic ranks are lower than those of their male colleagues (Figures 13.2 and 13.3).

One example of widespread discrimination is seen in the discrepancy between the average male and female physicians' income. Female physicians in practice (and not working for the federal government) still receive an average of 40%, or about $75,000, less annual net income than their male counterparts. This is only partially explained by differences in specialty, practice setting, age, and productivity. The exact amount varies by specialty, but this trend pervades medical practice.

## Sexual Harassment

Unfortunately, nearly half of women physicians report having been harassed on the basis of gender, and more than one third report having been sexually harassed by patients, peers, or attending physicians. The frequency of both is about the same during medical school and training. (It decreases somewhat when the physicians enter practice.)

FIGURE 13.2
### Gender of Medical School Faculty, by Rank

| Academic Rank | Men | | Women | |
|---|---|---|---|---|
| | number | percentage* | number | percentage* |
| Professor | 19,698 | 23.1% | 2,402 | 2.8% |
| Associate Professor | 15,512 | 18.2 | 4,463 | 5.2 |
| Assistant Professor | 22,964 | 26.9 | 11,595 | 13.6 |
| Instructor | 4,870 | 5.7 | 3,922 | 4.6 |
| Totals | 63,044 | 73.8% | 22,382 | 26.2% |

*Percentages do not total 100% due to rounding.
Adapted from: AAMC Faculty Roster System, 1999.

FIGURE 13.3

**Women Faculty in Various Specialties**

| Specialty | Percentage of all specialty faculty who are women | Percentage of women faculty who are full professors |
|---|---|---|
| Pediatrics | 40% | 18% |
| Public Health | 38 | 64 |
| Physical Medicine | 38 | 15 |
| Obstetrics/Gynecology | 38 | 11 |
| Family Practice | 34 | 15 |
| Psychiatry | 34 | 13 |
| Dermatology | 32 | 12 |
| Pathology (All) | 28 | 14 |
| Anesthesiology | 27 | 11 |
| Other Clinical | 25 | 5 |
| Internal Medicine | 24 | 8 |
| Neurology | 23 | 9 |
| Ophthalmology | 23 | 8 |
| Emergency Medicine | 23 | 7 |
| Radiology | 22 | 9 |
| Otolaryngology | 21 | 9 |
| Surgery | 12 | 3 |
| Orthopedic Surgery | 9 | 2 |

From: Association of American Medical Colleges Faculty Roster System, 1999.

The EEOC defines sexual harassment as:

> Unwelcome sexual advances, requests for sexual favors, and other verbal or physical conduct of a sexual nature constitute sexual harassment when:
>
> 1. submission to such conduct is made either explicitly or implicitly a term or condition of an individual's employment;
> 2. submission to or rejection of such conduct by an individual is used as the basis for employment decisions affecting such individual; or
> 3. such conduct has the purpose or effect of unreasonably interfering with an individual's work performance or creating an intimidating, hostile, or offensive working environment.

The American Medical Women's Association states that women physicians practicing General Surgery report the highest rate of sexual harassment at 50%. About 25% of those in Pediatrics, Obstetrics and Gynecology, Family Practice, and Internal Medicine report being sexually harassed. Only 12% of women in Psychiatry recount having had this problem. Harassment included gender-specific and sexual comments, being touched or pinched, and being pressured for dates. Married women and those with children suffered less harassment than single women. Most women say they don't report harassment because they fear the negative impact and they believe that no action would be taken anyway, even though virtually all teaching hospitals have policies regarding the sexual harassment of residents. While male medical students and residents have also reported being sexually harassed, this occurs at a much lower level than with women. Women more frequently suffer physical harassment, and those who harass them generally have a higher professional status than the harassed woman.

During the residency selection process, women are also often asked sexist, blatantly illegal questions. See "Illegal Questions" in Chapter 20 for more information.

Even without discrimination, women in medicine have unique personal problems which have no easy solutions. The training period of medical school and residency cuts directly across the childbearing years. This results in women physicians having fewer children, and at a later age, than non-physician women. Only 60-70% of married women physicians have children, compared to 90% of their married male counterparts.

Additional information for and about women in medicine can be obtained from the American Medical Women's Association (AMWA), 801 N. Fairfax, Suite 400, Alexandria, VA 22314. This organization also provides student members with educational loans, scholarships, awards, a bed-and-breakfast program, and a bimonthly journal. Another source of information is the Department of Women in Medicine, American Medical Association, 515 N. State St., Chicago, IL 60610. This section of the AMA serves as an information resource on issues relating to women physicians. Many individual specialties also have separate societies for women physicians. You can locate them through the main specialty society, AMWA, or the AMA.

## Marriage, Pregnancy, & Children

The problems associated with adjusting to marriage and having children during medical training were once thought to be solely a woman's concern. Not any longer. While women do have unique biological concerns regarding pregnancy, both men and women physicians are now more frequently basing career decisions, including choosing a residency, on how they will affect their family. The major concerns include maintaining the family relationship, pregnancy, and childcare.

## Marriage

Half of all medical students marry during medical school or residency training and more than 60% divorce within ten years after completing residency. (At least one study showed that psychiatrists have the highest rate of divorce—50%, followed by surgeons—33%.) Resident's marriages are at particular risk for work-related difficulties, since they work longer hours, have more difficulty "winding down" after work, are sleep deprived, and are often too tired to participate in social or leisure-time activities. One key to success is for both partners to recognize that, at least during residency, theirs will not be the idyllic marriage balancing a thriving career with a loving family life. Ultimately, however, residents with successful marriages cope better, remain more productive, and are happier than those whose marriages are foundering.

More than three-fourths of medical students' domestic partners play a significant role in deciding to which residency programs they apply, where they accept interviews, and how they finally rank the programs. Partners influence these decisions more than medical school faculty or residents, other family members, or classmates. Many partners travel to interview sites and make job inquiries while there. Ultimately, while nearly 60% of male and female medical students try to satisfy both their own and their partner's needs when selecting programs, nearly 33% of male and 20% of female medical students make their final selections based primarily on their own needs.

Marriages and relationships take effort to maintain, and up to 70% of medical marriages are dysfunctional. In part, it is because physicians often hold a position of unquestioned authority at work, and it can be difficult to relinquish this role at home. Residents don't have much personal time, and those in relationships wage a constant tug-of-war between their personal and professional lives. Does this mean that your partnership is doomed? No! All new professionals have the same stresses. The relationships that work are those in which both partners give each other emotional support for their careers. The key is to lend your partner as much support for his or her career as you deserve for your own.

Dual-physician marriages have their own difficulties. Both men and women physicians married to other physicians earn less money individually, and less often feel that their careers take precedence over their spouse's. However, they feel just as successful as other physicians in achieving their career and family goals, and benefit from more frequent enjoyment from shared work interests.

Balancing personal and professional goals, and the responsibilities accompanying each, can be a major challenge for both men and women—although women have more stressors. Significant social expectations on women physicians apart from their medical careers can create tension between their private and professional lives. This contributes to the fact that only 66% of women physicians marry, compared to 90% of both non-physician women and male physicians. In addition, since up to 70% of married women physicians are married to other physicians, the complications mount.

Compared with women physicians partnered with non-physicians (usually other professionals), the women in physician-physician relationships are more likely to bear the primary responsibility of caring for their children and home. Many do this by working fewer hours and subordinating their career to that of their partner. As many as half of all women physicians change their career plans because of marriage or family responsibilities. The best partnerships, regardless of the professions of the individuals, are those that are mutually supportive.

In the end, however, marriage enhances well-being. Married men and women are generally happier and less stressed than single people. Men benefit more from marriage than do women. However, both show decreased stress, which can help to enhance physicians' lives—especially during residency.

## Pregnancy & Family Leave

The most stressful personal situations that residents must deal with are pregnancy and child rearing. Increasing numbers of women are having children during their medical training. Before 1950, of women physicians having children, 24% had them during medical training. Between 1950 and 1989, 42% of them had their children during their training. Approximately 7,500 current women residents will become pregnant at least once during their training. (More than half of all women physicians with children have their first child during residency.) Many more residents will experience fatherhood.

Family leave (previously called maternity leave or parental leave) has lengthened over time, although women have become progressively less pleased with the amount of time off they are given for pregnancy and childbirth. These policies have been problematic for at least two reasons. First, women residents who have been pregnant feel that the leave, if less than six weeks long, is inadequate. Second, since these policies only apply to a subset of residents (parents, usually mothers), extended leave can wreak havoc on schedules and on the baseline educational requirements that must be met for Board certification.

The major specialty boards have policies on the amount of leave permitted during training (Figure 13.4). It should be noted, however, that since most programs actually deal with pregnancies on an ad hoc basis, how individual programs interpret the requirements may vary. Longer pregnancy leaves, greater flexibility in residency programs, and increased availability of childcare for medical students and residents will be mandatory as women become an even greater presence in medicine.

The Federal Family and Medical Leave Act, which took effect in August 1993, applies to most residents. It requires employers having 50 or more workers to grant up to 12 weeks of unpaid leave each year to new

### FIGURE 13.4

### *Amount of Time Allowed for Maternity/Family Leave by Medical Specialties*

| Specialty | Amount of Time |
|---|---|
| Allergy/Immunology | Discretion of program director |
| Anesthesiology | Twenty days/year |
| Dermatology | Six weeks/year |
| Emergency Medicine | Six weeks/year |
| Family Practice | One month/year |
| Internal Medicine | Discretion of program director |
| Neurological Surgery | No policy |
| Nuclear Medicine | Six weeks/year |
| Obstetrics/Gynecology | Six weeks/year |
| Ophthalmology | Two months/36-month program |
| Orthopedic Surgery | Discretion of program director |
| Otolaryngology | Six weeks/year |
| Pathology | Discretion of program director |
| Pediatrics | Three months/residency program |
| Physical Med/Rehab | Six weeks/year |
| Plastic Surgery | Four weeks/year |
| Preventive Medicine | Four weeks/year |
| Psychiatry | One month/year |
| Radiology | Six weeks/year |
| Surgery | Four weeks/year |
| Thoracic Surgery | No policy |
| Urology | No policy |

fathers and mothers (including adoptive and foster parents) after they have worked at the job for one year. The same amount of leave time must be permitted for employees to seek medical care themselves, or for them to care for a spouse, a child, or a parent with a serious health condition. Sick leave, vacation, or personal leave time can be incorporated into this time period so it may not all be unpaid. At the approximately three-fourths of teaching hospitals having written parental leave policies, maternity leave averages 64 days (range 21 to 180 days), but paternity leave averages only 46 days (range 1 to 120 days). At many institutions, much of this leave time is unpaid.

As evidenced by the relative sparsity of paternity leave policies (with at least one hospital generously offering just one day's leave), male residents may have more difficulty than women getting time off to fulfill their parental responsibilities around the time of birth. More male residents will, of course, become parents than will women residents. ("Of course," because there are more male residents, with most of their marriages being to non-physicians.)

The 1978 Pregnancy Discrimination Amendments to the Civil Rights Act of 1964 state that women affected by pregnancy, childbirth, or related medical conditions are to be treated the same as disabled employees for all employment-related purposes, including being covered by fringe-benefit programs. A number of states also have laws governing the rights of pregnant employees.

Most women physicians who have been pregnant during their residency training report inequitable treatment during pregnancy, ranging from unconscious slights to actual harassment. To lessen stress, some women physicians suggest trying to plan pregnancies for the time between the second and third year or during the fourth year of medical school, during the senior year of residency (not a surgical residency), during a year off, or after residency. (Of course, pregnancies often cannot be "planned.") Also, give your (hopefully supportive) colleagues adequate notice that you will be on leave.

Pregnant residents usually have lifestyles that they would not recommend to their patients—long hours, rigorous physical activity, poor eating and sleeping habits, and exposure to disease. Fortunately, studies have shown that these stressors have had little effect on the success of their pregnancies, although there appears to be a higher-than-expected incidence of preeclampsia and preterm labor (but not preterm delivery). Additionally, female resident physicians have the same number of induced abortions per pregnancy as their non-physician counterparts (Figure 13.5).

FIGURE 13.5

### Women Physicians' Pregnancy Complications

| Complication | % Women Physicians | % Physicians' Wives |
|---|---|---|
| Preterm labor requiring bed rest | 11.3 | 6.0 |
| Preeclampsia or eclampsia | 8.8 | 3.5 |
| Premature ruptured membranes | 6.4 | 6.7 |
| Placenta previa | 0.8 | 1.2 |
| Placental abruption | 0.4 | 0.7 |
| Miscarriages | 13.8 | 11.8 |

Adapted from: Klebanoff MA, Shiono PH, Rhoads GG. Outcomes of pregnancy in a national sample of resident physicians. *N Engl J Med.* 1990;323(15):1040-45.

According to an AMA review, pregnant residents should take breaks every few hours; take a longer "meal" break every four hours; maintain adequate hydration; regularly vary their work positions with sitting, standing, and walking; and minimize heavy lifting, especially if associated with bending.

Up to one-third of women who were pregnant during their residency training would counsel others to avoid the experience. They found that the farther along they were in their residency, the easier the pregnancy was to manage, since their work schedules were more flexible and coworkers were more supportive.

If you are considering pregnancy during your training, you may want to either look for large training programs that might have more flexibility to modify schedules for pregnancy leave, or investigate training programs that clearly state their maternity leave policies in their application material. (With the increasing sensitivity about these issues, it is becoming more common for these policies to be titled "parental," "family," or "maternity/paternity/adoption" leave, rather than "maternity" leave.) The AMA's *Fellowship and Residency Electronic Interactive Database Access (FREIDA)* program includes a question about maternity and paternity leave for each program.

## Children

Childcare can be an enormous burden for residents, especially if both parents work. Women carry most of the child-rearing burdens in our society, and cannot be both residents and parents without some help. Some resources containing helpful tips for men and women are listed under "Parenting" in the *Annotated Bibliography*.

Childcare facilities, although relatively common in the business world, have yet to appear in the medical field on a regular basis. Even where hospitals offer childcare, it is often not available to residents' children.

It is very difficult to find routine childcare services that can accommodate a resident's extremely long (and sometimes unexpectedly longer) hours. Start searching for childcare during pregnancy. Consider a nanny service, live-in childcare, a regular baby-sitter, or a day care center. Make sure that you have a back-up plan in case something unexpected happens at the hospital.

## Couples Matching

Resistance to matching couples at the same institution seems to have faded with the reality of nearly 4,000 new physician-physician couples each year. However, matching couples in the same training program, which occurs much more rarely, may still pose a problem. This may be due to the faculty's concerns about the effect upon both the individual residents and the esprit de corps of the entire program if there is any strife between, or even a breakup of, the couple. This concern is not at all assuaged by the marginal commitment to each other shown by some interviewing couples.

Using the NRMP Couples Match often lessens the strain in two-physician (medical student) marriages/relationships. Rather than being more difficult than individual matches, as might be expected, couples who match through the NRMP PGY-1 Couples Match actually have about the same match rate as do individuals going through the regular NRMP Match. Part-time, also described as "Shared-Schedule," positions are also available in some programs (see below).

In most cases, however, problems revolve around the process of successfully matching as a couple. This is particularly troublesome when both partners do not use the NRMP Match, are from different medical schools, or are in different years of training. The latter is the only problem that will be addressed here. The others will be discussed in Chapter 22.

If you and your partner are in different years of medical school training, there are three viable options for you.

1. The more senior partner goes through the Match for his or her specialty. The junior partner can then concentrate his or her efforts on the geographic area compatible with their partner's Match results. This, however, may mean separation for one or more years and may be unacceptable.

2. The senior partner goes through the Match and then the junior partner transfers to a medical school in the same geographic area to complete his or her medical school training. (Some schools, especially private schools relying on income from tuition, make transferring out very difficult.)

3. The senior partner limits selections to the geographic area of the junior partner's medical school and matches into a less desirable spot if necessary. Both partners can then attempt to match again, with the senior partner seeking an advanced position, when the junior partner graduates. In the past, this option was accomplished by matching into a "preliminary" or "transitional" year—both of which are disappearing as residency funding tightens.

There is no question that the whole Match process causes a great deal of stress among physician couples. And, if programs are not chosen with care, the stress does not end there. One thing that couples must inquire about in detail is how flexible the programs will be in scheduling both on-call and vacation time. With both partners in training, flexible scheduling may be needed if you are to see each other at all. Absence may make the heart grow fonder, but in excess it can devastate a relationship. Check for scheduling flexibility before you rank a program.

## Part-Time (Shared-Schedule) Positions

In many ways, physicians seeking part-time residency training face similar problems to those encountered by couples trying to match. Part-time positions came into their own in the late 1970s, when changes in attitudes caused federal law (now lapsed) to require most programs to offer positions to physicians who were only willing to commit limited time to residency training.

A trainee's need for a part-time residency position often results from other pressing needs, including family considerations, the simultaneous pursuit of another profession or training program, and significant involvement in outside personal interests. Individuals in this type of program spend less time in any one year working, but will, by the time they finish their longer program, spend as much or more total time in training than do full-time residents. (See also Chapter 10.)

Usually, two physicians, both entering the same year of training, agree to split one residency position. According to the now-defunct law, each was to receive no less than one-half of a normal resident's pay for no more than two-thirds of a normal resident's workload. The individual method by which a split position is achieved varies greatly from program to program. The keys to success in such a situation are:

1. You must find a flexible partner to pair with you, preferably before you begin to search out programs. This will often be a spouse, significant other, or good friend from school.

2. You must find a program willing to work with you in arranging a part-time position. *FREIDA* and the AMA's *Graduate Medical Education Directory-Supplement* list programs that have said they will accept shared positions. Of the 1,116 programs reporting the availability of part-time positions in 2000, more than half were in the five specialties of General Internal Medicine, Family Practice, Pediatrics, Psychiatry, and Child Psychiatry (Figure 10.8). The percentage of programs with shared-schedule/part-time positions varies widely among major specialties. Fewer than 1% of General Surgery programs offer part-time positions, while they are offered by 47% of Psychiatry programs, 23% of Internal Medicine programs, and 22% of Family Practice programs.

3. During the application process, you will have to work together closely and interview together. This will emphasize to the program that you are applying as a team. Many programs will, in fact, be unfamiliar with this type of arrangement.

4. Get an agreement *in writing* from each program about how their part-time position will work *before* you list it in the Match. Otherwise both you and the program will be going blindly into a nebulous arrangement from which it is unlikely that any party will emerge happy.

While the total number of part-time positions seems to be increasing, note that the number of such positions varies by geographic region. Only 8% of training programs in the South-Atlantic states (DE, FL, GA, MD, NC, SC, VA, WV) offer this option, while 14% of programs in the Mountain states (AZ, CO, ID, MT, NM, NV, UT, WY) and the West-North-Central states (IA, KS, MN, MO, ND, NE, SD) offer it. Only 1% of military programs and no programs in the U.S. Territories offer part-time positions.

Shared-schedule residencies do work, but the amount of preparation needed for them to work successfully is enormous. Getting a good partner, choosing the right program, and making certain that all parties detail everything up front are the keys to success.

# Gays, Lesbians, & Bisexuals

Gay, lesbian, and bisexual medical students and physicians are a largely invisible minority, although they are becoming more visible in the medical profession as our society changes. Maturing societal attitudes now acknowledge alternative lifestyles and many individuals feel more comfortable identifying themselves as gay, lesbian, or bisexual. Medical organizations of gay, lesbian, and bisexual physicians have thousands of dues-paying members, and membership is growing at the rate of 10% annually. The medical problems of this group, including AIDS, have forcefully gained the profession's attention. Yet, as mentioned in other sections, medical practitioners generally have conservative attitudes toward their life and work.

Organized medicine has not felt comfortable accepting gay, lesbian, and bisexual physicians, as exemplified by the difficulty that many national physician organizations have approving resolutions banning discrimination on the basis of sexual orientation. A 1996 study showed that about 10% of physicians would oppose openly gay and lesbian physicians seeking residency training in Obstetrics and Gynecology, Urology, and Pediatrics, and about 10% would not refer patients to them no matter what their specialty. About 4% would refuse gay or lesbians' admission to medical school and even oppose their training in Radiology.

While these numbers are an improvement over prior surveys in which 30% of physicians would refuse medical school admission based solely on an applicant being gay or lesbian, and 40% would discourage individuals from entering Pediatric or Psychiatric residencies on that basis alone, these numbers indicate a great deal of prejudice and fear among this highly educated population. This suggests that gay, lesbian, and bisexual medical students may not want to broadcast their sexual orientation when applying for residency positions.

As one medical student, Lydia Vaias, wrote in *JAMA*, "Interviews are uncomfortable, scary processes for everyone. They are particularly terrifying for lesbian and gay people, because we must grapple with telling who we are, without revealing an integral aspect of ourselves."

Gay and bisexual physicians may also encounter residency faculties' fears that they are among the estimated 5,000 HIV-infected physicians. This fear represents more than mere homophobia; it denotes concerns about having residents who need prolonged absences, have a disability, and have other problems with which residency directors do not want to deal if they can avoid them.

As with any applicant, demonstrating to interviewers that you are not "mainstream" may doom your application. Wearing triangle or rainbow jewelry or any other trapping of gay culture will most likely decrease the probability of your getting a residency position. If you feel, however, as some people do, that it is essential to demonstrate your sexual orientation to potential employers, be forewarned that it may cost you a residency position you desire. On the other hand, if this is the reason you don't get a position, you may not want it anyway.

Three national groups now lend assistance and support to gays, lesbians, and bisexuals in medicine: American Association of Physicians for Human Rights, 273 Church St., San Francisco, CA 94114; Gay and Lesbian Medical Association, 459 Futon St., Suite 107, San Francisco, CA 94102; and (for medical students): Lesbian, Gay & Bisexual People in Medicine, American Medical Student Association, 1902 Association Drive, Reston, VA 22091-1502. There are also a number of local groups in larger cities.

## Psychiatric Illness

Some medical students require psychiatric interventions, due either to pre-existing illnesses or to new conditions that appear during medical school. Why should this distinguish them from others needing medical treatments?

Some medical boards ask for all psychiatric records of physicians who have had psychiatric treatment and who are applying for or renewing their medical licenses. Since some state medical boards require at least educational licenses for residents, this includes those applying to residency positions.

One residency director (also a bioethicist), Norman Fost, M.D., showed the way to deal with this. He leaves this space blank when completing forms. Instead, he attaches a note stating, "All of our residents and faculty have emotional problems. Some are sensible enough to seek professional help. If I believed Dr. X's problems interfered with his/her ability to perform duties of the position he/she is applying for, I would tell you."

Perhaps your Dean of Students can treat these requests the same way.

## Underrepresented Minorities

The term "underrepresented minorities," based on government definitions of those groups who have fewer physicians than would be expected from the groups' population, refers to Blacks (African-Americans), Mexican-Americans (Chicanos), Native Americans/Alaskan Natives, and Puerto Ricans. Though there certainly are other minority groups facing many of the same problems, these groups contain the largest number of U.S. medical school graduates who appear to be underrepresented in residency programs—especially in the subspecialties. In recent years, they have comprised about 8.5% of all physicians in residency programs (Blacks 6%; Puerto Rican 1.5%; Mexican-American 1%; Native American/Native Alaskan <0.1%).

Underrepresented minority physicians are more likely to enter a generalist specialty (General Family Practice, General Internal Medicine, and General Pediatrics) than are other racial or ethnic groups. Among those entering generalist specialties, they are four times more likely to practice in socioeconomically deprived areas as are other physicians.

Although there has been an increase in the number of minority physicians in all specialties, relatively few of these specialists are on the faculties of medical schools. Approximately 4.9% of full-time medical school clinical faculty (excluding those individuals on faculty at the three predominantly Black schools and the three Puerto Rican schools) are minority physicians (Figure 13.6). The faculty at the six minority schools comprises less than 2% of all medical school faculty in the country.

FIGURE 13.6
### Minority Representation on Medical School Faculties in Various Clinical Specialties*

| Specialty | Native Amer | Black | Mexican Amer | Puerto Rican | Other Hispanic | % of Specialty's Faculty |
|---|---|---|---|---|---|---|
| Anesthesiology | <0.1% | 3.1% | 0.3% | 0.7% | 1.6% | 5.7% |
| Dermatology | 0.3 | 2.0 | 0.3 | 1.3 | 0.8 | 4.7 |
| Emergency Med | 0.2 | 4.1 | 0.6 | 1.9 | 1.1 | 7.9 |
| Family Practice | 0.5 | 5.2 | 1.4 | 1.2 | 1.4 | 9.7 |
| Internal Medicine | 0.1 | 2.7 | 0.3 | 0.8 | 1.8 | 5.7 |
| Neurology | 0.2 | 1.0 | 0.5 | 0.2 | 2.5 | 4.4 |
| Obstetrics/Gynecology | 0.1 | 5.8 | 0.4 | 1.4 | 2.2 | 9.9 |
| Ophthalmology | 0.1 | 1.8 | 0.4 | 0.4 | 1.5 | 4.4 |
| Orthopedic Surgery | 0.1 | 2.0 | 0.1 | 0.5 | 0.8 | 3.5 |
| Otolaryngology | 0.0 | 1.1 | 0.1 | 0.1 | 1.0 | 2.3 |
| Pathology-Clinical | 0.0 | 1.4 | 0.5 | 0.4 | 2.5 | 4.8 |
| Pediatrics | 0.1 | 3.1 | 0.6 | 1.3 | 2.2 | 7.3 |
| Physical Med/Rehab | 0.0 | 3.5 | 0.5 | 2.5 | 1.4 | 7.9 |
| Psychiatry | 0.2 | 3.2 | 0.5 | 0.7 | 2.4 | 7.0 |
| Public Health | 0.0 | 4.5 | 0.1 | 0.4 | 1.8 | 6.8 |
| Radiology | 0.1 | 2.1 | 0.2 | 0.7 | 1.9 | 5.0 |
| Surgery | 0.2 | 2.5 | 0.4 | 0.9 | 1.6 | 5.6 |

*Available information does not include all specialties.
Adapted from Association of American Medical Colleges: *AAMC Data Book.* Washington, DC: AAMC, 1999.

Minority faculty representation is important because these individuals provide role models for minority medical students. Their absence creates an enormous void that is hard for other faculty to fill. Because this absence is especially acute in many of the non-primary care specialties, many minority medical students feel considerable social pressure to enter primary care and "return to their communities." They are often are made to feel like traitors if they enter a subspecialty, since many of these physicians' services are not readily available to minority communities.

A higher percentage of minority medical students plan to enter Family Practice, Internal Medicine, Pediatrics, Psychiatry, Obstetrics and Gynecology, and General Surgery than their classmates. They do not plan to go into the smaller specialty and subspecialty areas in comparable numbers. Because role models are not available to show them alternative routes for their careers, they may feel that their options are more limited than the majority of medical students.

As Dr. Freeman Favors, a Black Emergency Physician, said, "Many minority students think to themselves, 'I don't see minorities in this specialty, so why try to get in?' " This becomes a self-fulfilling statement. It keeps many minority students from applying, so many specialties fail to accept more than a handful of minority residents. Dr. Favors wasn't intimidated and has done very well in his chosen field. He exhorts minority students to be courageous when setting their professional goals. He also suggests that minority students who desire to enter hard-to-match-with specialties look for regions of the country where their minority is under-represented. As he says, "They can be at a competitive advantage by being a 'rare gem' at such programs and institutions."

But no matter what specialty minority medical students want to enter, it appears that they do consistently worse in obtaining residency positions than other students, at least through the NRMP PGY-1 Match. Many reasons have been given for this. While racial and ethnic barriers appear to have fallen in some specialties, there still appears to be an "invisible quota system." This system is based upon many selection committees' reluctance to rank too many minority candidates for the Match. This may be because some faculty members still feel somewhat uncomfortable having more than one or two minority residents in a program. With the uncertainty of the Match, ranking many minority candidates could result in their having several such residents match with their program. This is probably equally true in those programs using the non-NRMP matching process. The result is that the programs with the highest percentage of minority residents and fellows are those in municipally owned hospitals (9.2%), in the Western U.S. (5.4%), that are major affiliates of universities (4.6%), with 700 or more beds (5.1%). The smallest number of minority residents and fellows as a percentage of total residents and fellows are in small hospitals (399 or fewer beds) that are university-owned (3.2%), Veterans' Administration (2.8%), or in the Southern U.S. (3.0%).

On the other hand, pressure is being put on medical schools to increase the number of both minority faculty and minority residents. This has taken the form of both "carrots and sticks." The "carrots" are the grants available to foster minority faculty's education and research, and the "sticks" are the embarrassing statistics published by the AMA, the AAMC, and the federal government about each school's and each specialty's minority representation. State governments that fund health-related positions are also looking at these numbers. If you are a minority student, this could work to your advantage. To get a good position, however, you may still have to be as good as or better than the competition—and be able to demonstrate that to the interviewers and selection committees. But, you are reading this book to learn how to do just that.

Of particular concern is one study that showed that 20% of Blacks and Hispanics (including Puerto Ricans) were not in a residency program three years after graduation from medical school. At present, it is unclear why this occurred, but these findings suggest that these physicians entered medical practice (probably in primary care areas) at a disadvantage when compared to their fully trained colleagues.

## Harassment

During their first year of residency, about one-third of underrepresented minority residents feel that they suffer ethnic discrimination. In most cases, this is expressed as racial or ethnic slurs, favoritism toward other groups, poor evaluations, and denied opportunities.

Minority woman physicians experience harassment based on their ethnicity at a rate six to nine times as frequent as do White women. Black woman physicians have the highest rate, with 35% of those less than 50 years old having experienced harassment during training and 32% of all Black woman physicians experiencing it in their practice. Among White women, 40% of Muslim women had experienced ethnic harassment, a rate four times higher than any other group of White woman physicians.

## Native Americans

Physicians identified as Native Americans make up considerably less than 0.5% of all U.S. physicians. One must be at least one-eighth Indian to be considered a Native American or an Alaskan Native. There are only about 35 Native American physicians per 100,000 Native Americans in the population. Most of these physicians practice in the West and the South. This is the lowest ratio of any ethnic group's physicians to their population in the United States. It is, therefore, unlikely that a Native American medical student will come across a role model either in his or her home environment or at medical school. Recent studies suggest that about half of all current Native American physicians are in primary care specialties. In 1995, only 0.4% of all new interns were either Native American or Alaskan Natives.

It is not always apparent that one is a Native American. Listing membership in the Association of American Indian Physicians on your application is an unobtrusive way of mentioning that you are a minority candidate. All other things being equal, this might just give you an edge. For more information about and for Native Americans in medicine, contact: Association of American Indian Physicians, Building D, 10015 S. Pennsylvania, Oklahoma City, OK 73159; telephone (405) 692-1202.

### Blacks (African-Americans)

The number of Black physicians in the United States has not changed appreciably over the past 70 years. Today, there are approximately 50 Black physicians per 100,000 Blacks in the population. Of these physicians, about 25% have graduated from one of the three predominantly Black medical schools: Meharry Medical College, Morehouse School of Medicine, and Howard University Medical School. In recent years, about 6% of new interns were Blacks.

Approximately 25% more Black physicians choose primary care specialties than does the general population of physicians. Most medical schools have at least some Black faculty members, albeit not in all specialties. There are usually role models available for Black medical students, either at the medical school or in the community.

Yet discrimination does exist within the medical fraternity. As you expand your horizons to search out the ideal training program, be aware that you may have to do more to prove yourself than other candidates. And unfortunately, this reality may also persist throughout your training, as well as afterwards. For more information, write: National Medical Association, 1012 Tenth Street N.W., Washington, DC 20001; telephone (202) 347-1895.

### Hispanics

A Hispanic applicant must know that all interviewers are not aware that the term "Hispanic" represents a diverse classification category. "Hispanic" includes persons of Cuban descent, Puerto Ricans, Mexican-Americans (Chicanos), and those of Latin American or Central American descent.

Federal government guidelines do not consider all of them minorities; in medicine, some are not minorities. Cuban-Americans, for example, are represented in medical schools to a greater extent, as a percentage of population, than nearly any other subgroup in the United States.

However, even including all Hispanic physicians, there are only about 129 Hispanic physicians in practice per 100,000 Hispanic population, compared to approximately 198 White physicians per 100,000 White population. Even among minority Hispanics, such as Puerto Ricans, there has been an increase in the number of physicians. But 61% of Puerto Rican physicians have graduated from the three medical schools in Puerto Rico. Partially due to language and cultural barriers, relatively few of these graduates apply to mainland training programs.

In recent years, only about 2% of new interns were Puerto Rican, 1.8% were Mexican-American, and 1.8% were "other Hispanics." As the national Hispanic population grows, however, fluency in both Spanish and English will become a definite plus for an applicant. If you have this skill, be certain to promote it in your application materials. For more information, write: Interamerican College of Physicians and Surgeons, 1612 K Street N.W., Suite 1000, Washington, DC 20006; telephone (202) 467-4756; or National Hispanic Medical Association, 1700 17th St., Suite 405, Washington, DC 20009.

## Physically Impaired

The subgroup of physically impaired medical students is unique. The individuals in this group are singular both among medical students for their tenacity and drive to overcome the obstacles to get where they are, and among the physically impaired, since they are able enough to complete medical school's clinical requirements.

There are currently about 3,000 practicing U.S. physicians with major physical disabilities. Of those medical students with known physical impairment (only about 0.25% of all medical students), approximately 25% have visual disabilities, 42% are neurologically or musculoskeletally impaired, 8% have an auditory disability, and 14% have learning disabilities. By 1995, more than one-third of all teaching hospitals had made accommodations under the Americans with Disabilities Act for disabled residents. While some residency programs may hesitate to take a physically impaired individual, this attitude is normally due to ignorance.

Educate these educators! Explain to them that you have been able to do what was necessary, with only "reasonable accommodations," in each of the clinical settings to which you were exposed. You may have to not only tell them in detail, but also show them. For, while federal legislation protects the individual from discriminatory questioning (such as being asked about the extent of your disability), it is permissible for interviewers to inquire about, and even to test, your ability to perform the job for which you are applying. Don't worry about this. If you did it in medical school, you can do it anywhere. Show your stuff!

As an example, after being denied admission to more than two dozen medical schools in the early 1990s, James B. Post IV, a quadriplegic since age 14, graduated in 1997 from Albert Einstein College of Medicine in the top 15% of his class. He planned to enter an Internal Medicine subspecialty. Upon graduating from medical school, he had little trouble getting a residency position. A physician's assistant, whom he pays for, assists him. Einstein had previously graduated a paraplegic who became a pathologist. In 1997, it was estimated that about ten quadriplegics were in U.S. medical schools.

In the past, a physician's disability usually influenced his or her specialty choice if it occurred before or during medical school. Severely handicapped individuals usually entered Physiatry, Psychiatry, Pathology, or Anesthesiology. Those with disabilities that occurred later tended to stay in their original specialties, if they could. Many severely handicapped medical students and physicians now use sophisticated medical assistive technology that helps them use necessary equipment or interpret clinical results. Two of the most common devices are rising electronic chairs that enable paralyzed practitioners to stand over an OR table and the "opticon" that converts EKG images into vibratory signals for the visually impaired.

Under the Americans with Disabilities Act of 1990, "disability" is defined as a physical or mental impairment that substantially limits one or more major life activities (e.g., limitations to caring for oneself, performing manual tasks, walking, seeing, hearing, speaking, breathing, learning, and working). Under the Act, persons are considered disabled if they have a record of such an impairment or are regarded as having such an impairment. The Act requires potential employers to make "reasonable accommodations" for disabled job applicants and workers, as long as the accommodations do not impose "undue hardships" on their business operation. If you are a disabled residency applicant, that applies to you. In addition, if you are not currently disabled, but become disabled once you are a resident, they must make reasonable accommodations for you.

While having a contagious disease (such as tuberculosis or HIV) is considered an impairment, current illegal- or excessive legal-drug use, alcoholism that interferes with performance, sex-related behavior and disorders, and certain behavioral disorders (including pyromania, kleptomania, and compulsive gambling) are not covered by the Act.

If you believe that your impairment will hinder you when taking the USMLE, be certain, well before the application deadline date, to contact the examining agency: National Board of Medical Examiners (NBME) or the Educational Commission for Foreign Medical Graduates (ECFMG) for Steps 1 and 2, and the state or territorial licensing authority for Step 3. They will advise you on the documentation necessary for them to arrange the special conditions for you to take the test. Special test accommodations that they can make include extra testing time, provision of a reader or recorder, extra rest breaks, visual aids, and enlarged-print examinations. If you test under these special conditions, all of your score reports and transcripts will include a note to that effect.

**One caveat** for those who do not think that they have a physical impairment that could keep them out of a training program. At least one-third of the Ophthalmology programs, all Aerospace Medicine programs, and a smattering of other programs test applicants for color vision and stereognosis. (This is perfectly legal if all applicants are screened and they can show that the examination is job related.) Some applicants, especially men, fail. You may want to find out whether you have this physical impairment prior to setting your heart on one of these specialties.

For more information about resources and referrals for physically impaired physicians, write: American Society of Handicapped Physicians, c/o Mr. Will Lambert, 105 Morris Dr., Bastrop, LA 71220; or Committee on Physically Challenged Physicians, Los Angeles County Medical Association, 1925 Wilshire Blvd., Los Angeles, CA 90057; or Equal Employment Opportunity Commission, Review and Appeals Division, 1801 L Street N.W., Washington, DC 20507.

## Osteopathic Physicians

As an Osteopathic physician, you have one of two different problems in getting a residency position, depending upon how you intend to approach your training: a limited number of Osteopathic residency positions, and the intransigence and constantly shifting rules of some Osteopathic licensing bodies.

If you want to do specialty training in an Osteopathic residency, your main problem will be that there are relatively few slots from which to choose. The increase in Osteopathic medical students now far outpaces the increase in students at M.D. medical schools. Between 1970 and 2000, the number of D.O.s doubled, the number of Osteopathic schools increased from nine to nineteen, and the number of graduates nearly *tripled*. There are now more than 2,000 D.O. graduates annually. The number of Osteopathic residency slots, however, barely increased. Those programs that do exist cannot accommodate the increasing percentage of young Osteopaths who want to pursue specialties other than primary care.

While the nearly 1,950 funded Osteopathic internships would be barely sufficient to meet the needs of Osteopathic graduates (if they all entered D.O. internships), the approximately 1,035 funded entry-level residency positions are far too few to accommodate the current number of Osteopathic graduates (Figure 22.9). This means that many Osteopathic graduates must look to the M.D. side of the profession for their training. The AOA's Osteopathic Matching Program and the military's matching program are the only ways to get an AOA-approved internship (see Chapter 22).

AOA-approved training provides three types of internships: transitional/rotating, specialty emphasis, and specialty track.

The *specialty emphasis* internship is intended for the student who has special interests in Anesthesiology, Emergency Medicine, Family Practice, Psychiatry, or Radiology. Similar to traditional rotating internships, it offers additional concentration within the specialty. However, completing a special emphasis internship is not credited towards the first year of a residency in the specialty.

*Specialty track internships* are considered the first year of a specialty residency program. They are only available in Internal Medicine, Obstetrics and Gynecology, Otolaryngology/Facial Plastic Surgery, Pediatrics, and Urological Surgery at institutions which have AOA-approved residencies in those specialties.

Osteopathic graduates say they "jump ship" to M.D. programs because they believe these programs provide better training, have higher salaries, and include specialty training unavailable in Osteopathic programs. That is not surprising since there are only 13 Osteopathic teaching hospitals with more than 300 beds in the United States. Osteopathic educators now see AOA-approved postgraduate programs becoming a haven for D.O.s interested in surgical or other non-Internal Medicine or non-Family Practice specialties. As one said, defending students who do M.D. residencies, "students do not see anything distinctive in what Osteopathic graduate medical education training programs have that would differentiate them from [M.D.] programs . . . these choices may be the result of enlightened decision making and not necessarily an indication of disloyalty." If you intend to pursue ACGME-approved (M.D.) training, as did nearly 2,500 of your fellow D.O.s (56% of all D.O.s in residency programs) in recent years, you will have to deal with both the American Osteopathic Association (AOA) and the programs.

About 10% of all residency programs in the United States have both AOA and ACGME (D.O. and M.D.) accreditation. About 10% of Osteopathic medical students plan on entering one of these positions. Another 40% plan on doing an M.D. residency program. Another 10% plan on entering a federal government-sponsored residency (that both M.D. and D.O. groups must recognize). Only about 36% plan on entering a residency approved by only the AOA.

The AOA, in its infinite wisdom, has made it very hard for you to pursue training at ACGME-approved programs. As a D.O., you may not be eligible to get a medical license in many states if you have not completed an AOA-approved internship. Some states may also require completion of an AOA-approved residency. If you want to do an AOA-approved residency, you will also need an AOA-approved internship. If you change your mind after you have completed an ACGME-approved internship and want to do an Osteopathic residency, they will not accept you. In addition, even though you will generally be eligible to take the AMA's specialty board examination upon successful completion of an ACGME-approved training program, you will not be allowed to take the AOA's specialty examination in the same field. (You may, however, take the COMLEX Level 3 examination, but you must request the application directly from the COMLEX.) This may mean that you will not be eligible for staff privileges in your specialty at some Osteopathic hospitals. The latter may not be important to you now, but things do change

One way of circumventing the AOA is to train in an ACGME-approved program that has also been approved by the AOA. For internships, the AOA will approve (or has already approved) most Transitional (or equivalent) programs in the military. Technically, they are also willing to give approval for other PGY-1-year ACGME-approved training. Don't count on this, however, since their track record is dismal.

Over the past 15 years, increasing numbers of ACGME (M.D.-approved) Internal Medicine and Family Practice programs have also become accredited by the American Osteopathic Association, so they are able to train both M.D.s and D.O.s in a manner so that both will be eligible for Board certification and licensure. This cooperation grew out of a need for more primary care residents, an increasing number of D.O. students without a corresponding increase in Osteopathic residency positions, and the M.D. programs' only alternatives—taking international medical graduates or having open positions. By 1997, 60 ACGME-accredited institutions had such dual-accredited programs, opening an additional 705 positions for Osteopathic graduates. This represents nearly one-third of all AOA internship positions.

The AOA is willing to consider approving ACGME-approved training programs on an individual basis. The "Catch 22" is that before the program can be considered, you must have been accepted into the program. In addition, the curriculum must meet the AOA's curriculum requirements and the individual must have special circumstances that necessitate not choosing an Osteopathic program, such as legal restrictions (e.g., military duty), personal or family health requirements, spousal employment restrictions, or financial or other hardships.

An application must be submitted to the AOA for approval. Documents that must accompany the application (obtained from the AOA) are: proof of acceptance into a residency program; documentation of the volume, variety, and scope of patients seen at the program; a written description of the program; a curriculum vita of the program director; and a substantial non-refundable fee. This application is sent to the Osteopathic specialty college or academy. Their recommendation is passed on to the AOA, which can then require an on-site review (the applicant [you] must pay for this). If the AOA approves the program, you must submit annual reports to the AOA. You must also provide "adequate documentation that similar training is not available within the Osteopathic profession."

Perhaps that is why many of the Osteopaths training at M.D. institutions are in federal programs. The military has many good training programs under the direction of either M.D.s or D.O.s, or both. Usually they are at very busy hospitals with adequate amounts of both resident responsibility and teaching from the staff. The AOA's procedures for approving ACGME-approved training are detailed in their pamphlet, *Protocol for Approval of Postdoctoral Training,* AOA Division of Postdoctoral Training, 142 Ontario St., Chicago, IL 60611.

More Osteopathic graduates are entering ACGME-approved training programs each year. Between 1993 to 1999 the number of D.O.s entering GY-1 positions in M.D. residency programs has grown 55.7%. However, you must recognize that, for whatever reason, ACGME-approved training in some specialties is almost completely off-limits to Osteopaths (Figure 13.7). Chief among these are Diagnostic Radiology, General Surgery, and various surgical specialties, such as Colon and Rectal Surgery, Neurosurgery, Otolaryngology, Thoracic Surgery, and Urology. Even in the military, it is nearly impossible for an Osteopathic medical school graduate to obtain a position in, and be allowed to finish, a Surgical residency program. This is controlled by the "powers" granting accreditation to residency programs. It may change in the future, but don't hold your breath.

FIGURE 13.7

## *Osteopathic Graduates in ACGME-Approved Programs*

| Specialty | Number in Training* | % of all Available M.D. Positions# |
|---|---|---|
| Allergy/Immunology | 5 | 1% |
| Anesthesiology | 216 | 4 |
| Cardiovascular Disease | 54 | 2 |
| Child/Adolescent Psychiatry | 17 | 2 |
| Colon & Rectal Surgery | 0 | 0 |
| Critical Care Medicine | 7 | 3 |
| Dermatology | 11 | 1 |
| Emergency Medicine | 118 | 5 |
| Endocrinology | 9 | 2 |
| Family Practice | 534 | 6 |
| Gastroenterology | 18 | 4 |
| Geriatrics | 8 | 2 |
| Hematology/Oncology | 20 | 5 |
| Infectious Diseases | 15 | 2 |
| Internal Medicine | 451 | 2 |
| Internal Med–Pediatrics | 19 | 1 |
| Nephrology | 12 | 2 |
| Neurological Surgery | 3 | <1 |
| Neurology | 58 | 4 |
| Nuclear Medicine | 3 | 1 |
| Obstetrics & Gynecology | 89 | 2 |
| Ophthalmology | 14 | 1 |
| Orthopedic Surgery | 25 | 1 |
| Otolaryngology | 7 | <1 |
| Pathology | 49 | 2 |
| Pediatrics | 128 | 2 |
| Pediatric Surgery | 1 | 2 |
| Physical Med/Rehabilitation | 93 | 8 |
| Plastic Surgery | 6 | 1 |
| Prevent Med/Pub Hlth (all) | 41 | 6 |
| Psychiatry | 161 | 3 |
| Pulmonary Diseases | 14 | 1 |
| Radiation Oncology | 8 | 1 |
| Radiology, Diagnostic | 11 | <1 |
| Rheumatology | 10 | 2 |
| Surgery | 36 | <1 |
| Thoracic Surgery | 7 | 2 |
| Urology | 6 | <1 |

Adapted from: *Ross-Lee B, Weiser MA, Kiss L. The outlook for osteopathic medical specialists within a reformed healthcare system. *JAOA.* 1994;94(7):564-65; and #Appendix II, Table 2. *JAMA.* 1995;274(9):757.

If you apply to ACGME-approved programs, make certain that you explain, in detail, exactly what your COMLEX scores mean (unless you took the USMLE—a smart move), what your curriculum consists of, and what the grading scale on your transcript signifies. Remember that these may be significantly different from the scores, curricula, and grading scales seen in applications from M.D. students.

Also, be careful about your Dean's letter. While most Deans of Osteopathic medical schools send out respectable letters which are comparable to those sent out by M.D. Deans, some send out almost cursory statements. One wonders if these are sent only to ACGME-approved programs, in an attempt to "keep you in the fold?"

While you will encounter problems when crossing over to enter ACGME-approved programs, if that is the training that will meet your future needs, by all means, go for it!

## Common Questions

The following are some common questions Osteopathic medical students ask:

*As an Osteopathic medical student or graduate, can I participate in the National Residency Matching Program (NRMP)?* Yes. You must request your own NRMP Independent Applicant Packet and enter the Match as an "Independent Applicant." For additional information, see Chapter 22, *NRMP and Other Matches.* To apply to most programs, you must now also participate in the Electronic Residency Application Service (ERAS) (see Chapter 12). The Dean's office at Osteopathic medical schools has materials to allow their students and graduates to participate.

*Should I take the USMLE or just the Osteopathic licensing exam?* Taking the USMLE is useful, although not required. The main reasons to take the USMLE are that (1) residency directors at M.D. programs can more easily judge your qualifications for their program against other applicants; and (2) some states may not be willing to license you based on the Osteopathic exam. Some D.O state licensing boards may not recognize the USMLE (Figure 7.9). If you only take the Osteopathic licensing exam and apply for an M.D. residency, be certain to explain how the test is scored. If possible, send them copies of the official information sheet that comes with your exam results. Also, attach a small "cheat sheet" to summarize your performance.

*How much discrimination against D.O.s is there among M.D. residency directors?* To deny that many M.D. residency programs discriminate against D.O.s would be foolish. Many residency directors do not understand that Osteopathic training parallels that in M.D. schools. This discrimination, however, varies greatly by the area of the country and the specialty. Where many D.O.s practice and Osteopathic medical schools have been established, there is minimal discrimination—and what there is has been rapidly diminishing. Where there are few D.O.s, ignorance abounds. As to specialties, General Surgery and its subspecialties remain the major area that continues to reject virtually all D.O. residency applicants.

## Older Applicants

Many students now enter medicine either after they have raised a family or as a second career. In the last decade, the number of students over 28 years old entering medical school has doubled. This group now comprises more than 12% of all first-year students, with more than half being at least 31 years old. Older students may have some unique problems in medical school and they may face some new obstacles when applying for residency positions.

First, because older students may have more debts and more financial responsibilities than younger students, they may be tempted to jump into the most lucrative practice they can in the shortest amount of time. Many may decide to bypass specialties in which they have a real interest but whose training takes longer. Bad move! If you have invested the time, lost income, and strife to go through medical school, go for the goal you really want. Apply to the specialty that most interests you. The extra year or two of training will pay you back immeasurably in the satisfaction you (and your family) have in your work during your career.

The second difficulty older applicants face is the negative attitude of some residency faculty members. They may perceive the older applicant as possessing maturity, but not enough stamina and energy to complete a demanding residency. Spending time with the program faculty, either in a clinical setting on a formal rotation or in educational rounds may overcome their hesitation. During your interviews, describe your high energy level within the context of other answers. One example might be, "I stayed by her bedside all night in the ICU, monitoring her status and adjusting her medications. It was exhilarating." Finally, many older applicants come to medicine after other life experiences to truly serve humanity. Many faculty will respond positively to a heartfelt description of why you made such a difficult life decision. Tell them.

Physicians who are making a mid-career switch—changing specialties— make up another subgroup of older applicants. The most common reasons physicians give for changing specialties, either during residency or after they are in practice, are: (1) they become enlightened, or (2) they become disillusioned with their prior specialty.

While about 40% of those who change specialties are generalists, 60% are specialists. Of those who change specialties late in their career (40 to 69 years old), the most common profile is a woman international medical graduate with a hospital-based practice in subspecialty Internal Medicine, Emergency Medicine (probably not residency-trained with this profile), subspecialty Pediatrics, or Pathology.

Some physicians are forced to change specialties due to physical disabilities. Others want to change specialties, often to a primary care specialty, to find a job where they want to live. Residency directors may be reluctant to warmly accept these applicants unless they can adequately demonstrate that they have come to terms with making the specialty change. Programs are not looking for applicants who do not really want to be in their residency.

The first question residency directors ask is, "Are you seeking to enter our specialty or simply running away from the one you are in?" That is a darn good question—one you need to ask yourself before starting the process. Why do you really want to do this? At the least, it will probably cost you extra time, decrease your income, and alter your lifestyle or even where you live.

However, if your extensive qualifications are used as a reason not to hire you as a resident, note that a New York Federal District Court ruled that an employer declining to offer a position on the grounds that the candidate is "overqualified" may be violating the Age Discrimination in Employment Act. According to the court, the term "overqualified" may simply be a code word for too old.

Physicians face multiple problems in making such a change. The most obvious problem for those going back to residency after being in practice is the resultant change in lifestyle. Going from a practicing physician's salary to a resident's salary can be a rude experience for both the physician and his or her family. Ego damage can also be a problem. The shift from the role of omnipotent attending to lowly resident can be quite a blow—especially when some of the residency faculty are younger than you (or sometimes, your children).

Occasionally, physicians who have left clinical practice for administration or the laboratory decide to reenter the clinical world. This may be a daunting step. As one returnee noted, "My greatest fear was my ignorance—the amalgam of what I had forgotten combined with what had been added to the realm of practice since I had last been there." The key is to choose a supportive program that will provide a curriculum tailored to your individual needs. This may be harder to find than you assume.

The specialties that most commonly receive trainees who previously were in other specialties are Anesthesiology (sometimes called "the Foreign Legion of Medicine" for all the escapees from other specialties in its ranks), Diagnostic Radiology, Emergency Medicine, Family Practice, Internal Medicine, and Neurology. Practitioners most commonly leave Internal Medicine for other specialties.

The keys to successfully making a mid-career switch are to adequately prepare yourself and your family for the changes, to carefully investigate what you are getting into, and to make advance contacts with potential residency directors. If you plan to take training in the town where you practice, attend some teaching conferences and make arrangements to observe or participate clinically with some of the attendings. Knowledgeable residency directors will see an applicant who comes to residency training with prior clinical experience as a real bonus—if you can show them that you know what you are getting into and that you want to be there.

## Military/Public Health Service

Two basic questions come up when discussing your involvement in military residencies. The first is: why should you get drawn into this system? Second, how is playing this game different from competing in the normal application and matching processes?

There are several reasons why you may want to get a military residency. If you are in the School of Medicine of the Uniform Services University of the Health Sciences (USUHS), you are obligated to do a military residency. The military is also obligated to find you a first-year training slot. You have saved a great deal of money, and will pay it back with the years you commit to the service. If you have enrolled in the Health Professions Scholarship Program, you owe the military one year for each year you are funded, with a two-year minimum obligation. You have, of course, saved a large debt by obligating yourself to military service. In addition, if you train in a military residency, you can expect a higher rate of compensation than if you were in a civilian residency. But you don't get something for nothing. Your colleagues will normally make up the difference after they get out in practice, although they will also usually be saddled with a large educational debt that you do not have.

Military medicine is changing rapidly as the armed forces are downsized and more dependent medical care is being outsourced to the civilian sector. It is now thought that operations other than war, such as disaster relief, will be the major operations for future military physicians. Battlefield medicine is going "high tech," however, with many cutting-edge developments to assist military physicians in the field.

As noted above, Osteopathic medical students might want to consider military residency training. The American Osteopathic Association is usually willing to recognize as valid any residency that is done in the military. This provides Osteopathic graduates a chance at what may be a more intense and varied residency experience than they could obtain in the civilian world. Additionally, successful completion of a military residency generally allows the Osteopathic physician to apply for both M.D. and Osteopathic specialty boards. Make sure, however, that the individual program has been approved by the AOA *before* you start your training.

Finally, if you have your heart set on entering the specialty of Aerospace Medicine, you will normally need to join the Air Force or Navy to get a residency position. And you usually will not be able to enter the residency either directly from school or even after your internship. Such programs routinely require applicants to have some experience, as well as having passed short courses in Aerospace Medicine offered through the military. One bright note. There is a single civilian residency program in Aerospace Medicine at Wright State University School of Medicine, Dayton, Ohio. If, however, you are interested in training for Hyperbaric and Undersea Medicine, you will normally have to join the Navy.

If you want to do a military residency, how do you obtain a position? All U.S. Army residency programs (all specialties) go through the Electronic Residency Application Service (ERAS). (See Chapter 12 for more information about ERAS.) According to the U.S. Army Surgeon General, Ronald R. Blank, the Army, Navy, and Air Force fill their first-year residency positions with graduates of the Uniformed Services University of the Health Sciences, those in medical school with an individual military commitment (often through HPSP), and those in the Reserve Officers' Training Corps. Only individuals on active military duty can participate in Armed Forces residency programs.

As for matching with programs, neither the selection system that military training programs use nor the timing of their selections is similar to civilian programs. The military's selection system is similar to the NRMP Match in that both applicants and programs send in rank lists. However, representatives of the teaching hospitals who meet and exchange information about the candidates make the selections, rather than having it done impartially by computer. Priority is given to those on active duty at the time of selection and to graduates of the F. Edward Hebert School of Medicine, Uniformed Services University of the Health Sciences (military medical school) in Bethesda, Maryland. The selections are then finalized. There are generally many more applicants for military residency positions than there are available slots.

The military match occurs early in the senior year. Therefore, competing in the military match means you have to make career decisions very early. Finding out about military training programs is often more difficult than getting information about civilian programs. Your best sources of information, aside from the "Green Book" or the *FREIDA* system, are military physicians and your military branch's Medical Personnel Counselor. These latter individuals vary greatly in quality and interest. Be certain to cross-check any information they give you.

Early planning and preparation are very important. To get into the specialty and the military residency program you think is right, you should do your Active Duty for Training (subinternship) in that specialty and at that site. The experience of those who have applied to military residencies suggests that this is the best way to get into a good military program. You are highly encouraged to do these rotations during your third year of medical school. If this is not possible, the rotations should be scheduled immediately following your third year. Arranging for this rotation can often take six months or more. Your activities during this subinternship are not much different than those described for a civilian subinternship. Be sure that the residency director and department chairman know who you are and are impressed with the job that you do.

You must submit applications to residency programs the summer before your senior year. Interviews start shortly thereafter. Health Professions Scholarship Program (HPSP) students should also plan to interview at some civilian programs and enter the NRMP PGY-1 Match. There is about a 20% chance that you will not match with the military. Therefore, you will need to apply to civilian programs as a backup. If you do match with the military, you will be able to drop out of the NRMP PGY-1 Match. But your money won't be refunded.

One important note. If you owe an obligation to serve in the military or PHS, but either did not match with a military program or there is no military program in your specialty (e.g., the Air Force does not have a program in Neurosurgery), you will need a civilian residency. No civilian program will want you as a resident, however, if they cannot be assured that you will be around for the duration of the program. The Navy, for example, has had a gloomy record of pulling their people out of training after the PGY-1 year to go on sea duty.

Therefore, civilian programs will want to see a *written commitment* from the service allowing you to complete your training before going on active duty. There should be no difficulty in obtaining this before it is time for the civilian training programs to make up their rank lists for the Match. The military services also sponsor some physicians during their civilian training programs. Residents in this program receive officer's pay, some benefits, and a salary bonus. The military obligation is equal to the time sponsored with a minimum of two years.

At present, physicians who do a military residency owe the service one year for every year of residency training, with a minimum of two years. However, this could change at any time. Make certain that you check this out before you sign on the dotted line.

For those of you who have participated in the National Health Service Corps' Scholarship Program, there is really no significant option of doing a Public Health Service (PHS) residency, and there are only limited spots available in military residency programs. Therefore, almost all PHS Scholars must go through the normal process of matching with civilian programs. However, if you plan to apply to anything other than a one-year program (such as a Transitional year or a single Preliminary Medicine or Surgery year), you must also have a waiver *in writing* from the PHS to complete the residency training before the programs will consider you seriously. Anyone who receives these scholarships and then neglects to serve will owe the government treble damages—and they know how to collect.

For more information about and for physicians in military and federal service, contact: Association of Military Surgeons of the U.S., 9320 Old Georgetown Rd., Bethesda, MD 20814 (310-897-8800, fax 301-530-5446); or Society of Air Force Physicians, HQ USAF/SGPC, Bolling Air Force Base, Washington, DC 20332; or Uniformed Services Academy of Family Physicians, 2315 Westwood Ave., P.O. Box 11086, Richmond, VA 23230; or Federal Physicians Association, 1707 L Street N.W., #400, Washington, DC 20036.

# 14

# International Medical Graduates

*If you really want to do something, you'll find a way;*
*if you don't, you'll find an excuse.*

– Anonymous

International medical graduates (IMGs), often referred to as foreign medical graduates (FMGs), include all those who have graduated from any of the approximately 1,400 medical schools outside the United States, its possessions, and Canada. IMGs functionally break down into three subgroups:

1. **U.S. IMGs (USIMGs).** Those individuals who are currently citizens or permanent residents of the United States, but who received their medical degree outside the United States, Puerto Rico, or Canada. Most IMG physicians who get U.S. residency slots are in this category.

2. **Foreign National IMGs (FNIMGs).** Individuals who are not U.S. citizens and who received their medical degree from a medical school not approved by the LCME, usually located outside the United States, Puerto Rico, or Canada.

3. **Exchange Visitor IMGs (EVIMGs).** The largest subset of FNIMGs applying for residency slots, these individuals are in the United States only temporarily as Exchange Visitors (with J-1, or occasionally H-type visas) to study, teach, or do research.

Each group has unique problems in terms of acquiring U.S. residency positions. But since EVIMGs and FNIMGs have such similar problems, they will be discussed together. (Note that foreign nationals who graduate from U. S., Canadian, or Puerto Rican medical schools are not considered IMGs.) See also *The International Medical Graduate's Guide to U.S. Medicine: Negotiating the Maze* by Louise B. Ball (Galen Press, 1995).

By 1998, more than 176,000 (or about 23% of) physicians practicing medicine in the United States were trained outside the United States, Puerto Rico, or Canada. Their practices tend to be medical, rather than surgical (Figure 14.1). In 1998, about 83% of IMGs worked in clinical care, with 61% in office-based practices (nearly one-quarter of all office-based U.S. physicians). Most IMGs work in New York (17%), California (11%), Florida (8%), New Jersey (6%), or Illinois (6%).

IMGs account for nearly 24% of physicians in residency training, but nearly 37% of PGY-1s. More than one-third of IMG residents come from India, Pakistan, or China. Twenty-three percent of all IMG residents are U.S. citizens and another 39% are permanent U.S. residents. About 40% of IMGs train in New York or California, with almost half training in Internal Medicine or a Medicine specialty. Nearly 28% of all primary care residency positions are filled by IMGs. About 33% of IMGs pursue post-residency fellowships, while only about 24% of U.S. medical graduates do so.

## The Negative Image

This large number of IMGs continues to practice and train despite a lot of negative press. In their 1990-91 *Annual Report*, the Educational Commission for Foreign Medical Graduates (ECFMG) revealed that IMGs' passing scores on the old FMGEMS examination were stunningly lower than would be expected of U.S. medical students or graduates. This negative image was reinforced by a scandal in the mid-1980s implicating two Caribbean medical schools (since closed) in counterfeit diploma scams. As late as 1992, however, the U.S. Government Accounting Office found a school in the Dominican Republic again granting "worthless" medical degrees. While this school has closed, another school, Universidad Federico Henriquez y Carvajal, was immediately opened at the same location with the same leadership.

These incidents have led the ECFMG to establish a special telephone line on which residency directors, among others, can quickly verify ECFMG certification. They also led three jurisdictions (Pennsylvania, Puerto Rico, and Texas) to ban international medical students from taking clinical clerkships in their hospitals. Six other states (California, Florida, Massachusetts, New Jersey, New York, Texas) regulate international medical students in clinical clerkships. New York reportedly has the toughest regulations (and most expensive process) to certify non-U.S. medical schools to send their students for clerkships: currently there are only two schools whose students may spend more than 12 weeks in New York doing clerkships. In addition, AAMC rules preclude U.S. medical schools from "co-mingling" their students with students from non-U.S. schools during

FIGURE 14.1

### *IMGs Practicing Medicine in Various Specialties*

| | Number of IMGs | % of All Physicians in Specialty | % of all IMGs |
|---|---|---|---|
| Nuclear Medicine | 492 | 34% | 0.3% |
| Pathology | 5,798 | 32 | 3.3 |
| Internal Medicine | 40,834 | 32 | 23.1 |
| Physical Med/Rehab | 1,797 | 31 | 1.0 |
| Psychiatry | 11,677 | 30 | 6.6 |
| Anesthesiology | 9,853 | 29 | 5.6 |
| Pediatrics | 16,087 | 29 | 9.1 |
| Cardiovascular Disease | 5,417 | 28 | 3.1 |
| Neurology | 3,291 | 28 | 1.9 |
| Pulmonary Disease | 1,729 | 26 | 1.0 |
| Child Psychiatry | 1, 358 | 24 | 0.8 |
| Gastroenterology | 2,287 | 24 | 1.3 |
| Thoracic Surgery | 534 | 24 | 0.1 |
| Allergy & Immunology | 883 | 23 | 0.5 |
| Colon & Rectal Surgery | 236 | 23 | 0.1 |
| General/Family Practice | 16,896 | 21 | 9.5 |
| General Surgery | 8,324 | 20 | 4.7 |
| Radiation Oncology | 782 | 20 | 0.4 |
| Medical Genetics | 44 | 18% | <0.1% |
| Obstetrics/Gynecology | 7,169 | 18 | 4.1 |
| Urology | 1,786 | 18 | 1.0 |
| Neurological Surgery | 732 | 15 | 0.4 |
| Occupational Medicine | 413 | 14 | 0.2 |
| Plastic Surgery | 832 | 14 | 0.5 |
| Radiology (All) | 3,915 | 14 | 1.5 |
| Gen. Preventive Med | 200 | 13 | 0.1 |
| Public Health | 203 | 12 | 0.1 |
| Emergency Medicine | 2,267 | 11 | 1.3 |
| Otolaryngology | 1,046 | 11 | 0.6 |
| Aerospace Medicine | 48 | 8 | <0.1 |
| Ophthalmology | 1,465 | 8 | 0.8 |
| Orthopedic Surgery | 1,854 | 8 | 1.0 |
| Dermatology | 637 | 7 | 2.2 |

Adapted from: American Medical Association. *Physician Characteristics and Distribution in the U.S., 1999.* Chicago, IL: AMA, 1999, Tables A-6 and A-7.

required clerkships. (Some hospitals have gotten around this by using "separate-but-equal" ward teams.) These restrictions, however, attack the mechanism through which foreign-trained medical students demonstrate their clinical competence and, subsequently, get residency slots and become licensed. (Twenty-four licensing boards evaluate the quality of a clinical clerkship in deciding whether to grant a license to an IMG.)

## Licensing, Funding, & Residency Positions

There are thousands of IMGs in the United States who have not been able to obtain a license to practice medicine. In many cases, this is because residency programs will not accept them for training, and all jurisdictions in the United States require *at least one year of postgraduate training in the U.S. or Canada for licensure* (Figure 7.8). Fifteen jurisdictions require IMGs to have at least two years of training and twenty-nine require three or more years. This exceeds what most jurisdictions require from U.S. graduates. In addition, five licensing boards (Alabama, Maryland, Ohio, Puerto Rico, Virginia) maintain lists of state-approved foreign medical schools whose graduates are eligible for a medical license.

Residency programs, especially those that train large numbers of international medical graduates, are also concerned about changes in Medicare laws that severely restrict the programs' and hospitals' reimbursement for training non-U.S.-medical-school graduates. These residency programs often operate on a shoestring as it is; threatening to restrict their funds even further has already had the desired effect of closing down many training opportunities for international medical graduates. As this book goes to press, the Council on Graduate Medical Education is re-examining its position that the number of first-year residency positions be limited to 110% of U.S. M.D. and D.O. graduates and that 50% of all physicians entering practice must be in primary care. They believe, in part, that the Clinical Skills Assessment (see below) will markedly decrease the number of IMGs entering the workforce. Discrimination? Read on.

Section 102 of the 1992 Federal Health Professions Education Extension Amendments (PL 102-408) states:

> Graduates of Foreign Medical Schools.–The Secretary [of Health and Human Services] may make an award of a grant, cooperative agreement, or contract under this title to an entity [including a medical school] that provides graduate training in the health professions only if the entity agrees that, in considering applications for admissions to a program of such training, the entity will not refuse to consider an application solely on the basis that the application is submitted by a graduate of a foreign medical school.

How much sway this law holds over residency directors is unknown, since most are probably not aware of it. Studies show that some residency programs discriminate against IMGs as early as when they send out application materials. As residency positions decrease, however, enterprising IMGs will certainly begin making them aware of the law.

What does sway residency directors, however, is the past performance of IMGs in residency programs. For example, IMGs, especially those who contract with residencies outside a matching program, have a higher attrition rate than U.S. graduates. Also, IMGs pass some specialty board examinations, such as Internal Medicine's, only about two-thirds as often on their first try as do U.S. graduates. Since residency programs are judged, in part, on their graduates' pass rates, this is important to residency directors.

At least one state medical society (New York) has developed a program to assist IMGs trying to puzzle through the maze of obtaining residency positions within the state. They hold an annual IMG Information Forum. The Forum includes informational talks, question-answer sessions, and sessions in which residency program representatives get to meet prospective IMG applicants. For information about this program, contact: Membership Support Services, Medical Society of New York, 420 Lakeville Rd., Lake Success, NY 11042.

Despite all the unfavorable press and the tough requirements, the number of IMGs in U.S. residency positions increased from 12,259 in 1989 to 25,415 in 1998. The number of IMGs in first-year residency positions increased over this same period from 2,689 to 5,134. USIMGs (U.S. natives and permanent residents) make up about 15% of first-year residents, but 62% of all first-year IMG residents. In the 1999 NRMP Match, IMGs made up a large proportion of those entering some specialties (Figure 14.2).

The American Medical Association has formed a Department of International Medical Graduates. It is designed to tackle licensure, discrimination, and visa issues on behalf of IMGs. For information, contact: AMA International Graduate Services, 515 N. State St., Chicago, IL 60610.

## ECFMG Certification

International medical school graduates must get ECFMG certification to be eligible for: (1) acceptance into an Accreditation Council for Graduate Medical Education (ACGME) -accredited residency or fellowship training position in the United States; (2) a visa for entry into the United States as a medical trainee; (3) a medical license in most states; and (4) an application to take the USMLE Step 3 examination. (Fifth-Pathway students do not need an ECFMG Certificate.) The ECFMG issues about 4,500 new Certificates each year.

FIGURE 14.2

## Types of Applicants (Percentages) Filling PGY-1 and Advanced Positions in Specialties through NRMP Match[1]

| Specialty | % Filled by U.S. Senior Students | % Filled by Osteopaths & U.S. Grad Physicians | % Filled by IMGs, Fifth-Pathway, & Can. Grads | % Total Positions Filled thru NRMP |
|---|---|---|---|---|
| Anesthesiology[2] | 42% | 2% | 33% | 77% |
| Emergency Medicine | 78 | 15 | 4 | 96 |
| Family Practice | 62 | 8 | 13 | 83 |
| Internal Medicine | 60 | 5 | 30 | 95 |
| Obstetrics/Gynecology | 80 | 7 | 6 | 93 |
| Orthopedic Surgery | 90 | 7 | 2 | 99 |
| Pathology[2] | 42 | 3 | 36 | 82 |
| Pediatrics | 83 | 6 | 10 | 99 |
| Psychiatry | 53 | 7 | 35 | 94 |
| Radiology, Diagnostic[2] | 78 | 6 | 9 | 93 |
| Surgery, General | 83 | 7 | 6 | 96 |
| Transitional | 76 | 4 | 14 | 94 |
| Osteopaths Unmatched[3] | — | 32 | — | — |
| 5th Pathway Unmatched[3] | — | — | 46 | — |
| U.S. IMGs Unmatched[3] | — | — | 53 | — |
| FNIMGs Unmatched[3] | — | — | 68 | — |
| **Total Unmatched[3]** | **6%** | **39%** | **65%** | — |

[1]Numbers in the columns for percent of graduates matching within a specialty may not add up to total percentage matched due to rounding.

[2]A significant number of entry-level positions (PGY-1 or above) are offered outside the Match.

[3]The percentage is of those going through the entire NRMP process. Between 8% (U.S. Seniors) and 46% (Canadians) of the candidates withdrew before the Match or did not submit a Rank Order List.

Derived from: National Residency Matching Program. *1999 NRMP Match Data.* Washington, DC:NRMP, 1999 (April).

Note, however, that fourteen states have requirements in addition to an ECFMG Certificate for IMGs to be appointed to a residency position. These states are California, Connecticut, Iowa, Kansas, Kentucky, Louisiana, Michigan, Minnesota, Nevada, New Jersey, New Mexico, Pennsylvania, Texas, and Vermont.

This is how you get that certification (Figure 14.3). To qualify for an ECFMG Certificate, you must be either a student attending a medical school listed in the current edition of the *World Directory of Medical Schools* published by the World Health Organization, *or a graduate* of a medical school which was listed in this directory at the time of your graduation. If you have graduated, you must also document completion of the educational requirements to practice medicine in the country in which you received your medical education. This must include at least four years of medical

FIGURE 14.3

**Requirements to Practice Medicine, Do Post-Graduate Training, or be a Clinical Research Fellow in the United States (Patient Contact)**

| | ECFMG English Test | USMLE | CSA Exam | ECFMG Certification | Applicable Visas |
|---|---|---|---|---|---|
| **Foreign National:** Graduate of LCME-accredited U.S., Canadian, or Puerto Rican Medical School (EVIMG). | ✔ | | | | ✔ |
| **American Citizen:** Graduate of Foreign Medical School (USIMG)* | ✔ | ✔ | ✔ | ✔ | |
| **Foreign National:** Graduate of Foreign Medical School (FNIMG) | ✔ | ✔ | ✔ | ✔ | ✔ |

*An alternative for US citizen/permanent resident IMGs is to take the Fifth-Pathway Program. In that case, they do not need to get an ECFMG Certificate, so do not need to take the English-language test or the CSA exam.

study for which credit was received. Foreign nationals must also have an unrestricted license or certificate to practice medicine in their own country. The specific credentials accepted for each country are listed in the *Information Booklet, ECFMG Certification and Application*, available from the ECFMG, 3624 Market St., 4th Floor, Philadelphia, PA 19104-2685, USA. Those licensed only in stomatology, as Licensed Medical Practitioners, or as Assistant Medical Practitioners are not eligible for an ECFMG Certificate.

You must submit an application and the required documentation to the ECFMG. Processing this application may take several months since education credentials will be checked with your medical school. To speed up the processing on all paperwork, always use the same (formal) name that is on your medical school diploma. Once the ECFMG has assigned you a number, also use that on any correspondence with the ECFMG, licensing bodies, and residency programs.

United States Licensing Examination (USMLE) application and ECFMG materials can be obtained from the ECFMG. You must request these materials in writing; do not telephone or fax for this information. The information/application booklet includes the application requirements, sample questions from the English tests (see below), the acceptable medical credentials for each country, and a list of available ECFMG test centers. If you receive approval to take the exam, you will receive a receipt showing the date of the exam, examination center address, and cost of the examination. About four weeks before the exam, an official admission permit that includes the time and location of the test will be sent out. All IMGs must pass Step 1 and Step 2 of the USMLE to meet the medical science examination requirement for ECFMG certification. (If you passed one part of the National Boards, FLEX, or FMGEMS, you must now, for the other part, take the equivalent USMLE Step. For more information about the USMLE, see Chapter 7.)

The ECFMG administers the USMLE to IMGs at more than one hundred locations throughout the world, and at about fifty centers in the United States and Canada. Applicants may list two choices of test centers when they apply to take the examinations. The ECFMG gives Step 1 in June and September. They give Step 2 in March and August or September. Both tests last two days. There is no limit to the number of times an applicant can take either Step. Once a Step is passed, however, it may not be repeated for seven years. Applicants therefore have seven years to pass the other Step, or they must begin the process over again.

While there are rumors to the contrary, the USMLE Steps 1 and 2 are scored identically for all examinees whether they are IMGs or U.S. or Canadian graduates. It does usually cost more to take these exams outside the United States or Canada, however. The current charges and testing cities with Sylvan Technology Centers can be found on the ECFMG website (www.ecfmg.org).

To apply to take Step 3, an applicant must have obtained an M.D. degree or equivalent, successfully passed Steps 1 and 2, obtained an ECFMG Certificate or completed a Fifth-Pathway program, and met any other specific requirements imposed by the state licensing board administering the test. Information about specific state requirements is available from individual state boards, or The Federation of State Medical Boards of the United States, Inc., 400 Fuller Wiser Rd., Suite 300, Euless, TX 76039, USA; telephone (817) 735-80722.

In the past, individuals with the best chance of passing the old ECFMG examination of medical knowledge (a trend that will probably continue) were younger than thirty years old, male, native English speakers, FNIMGs, and educated in countries with low infant mortality rates and high per capita incomes. Those with the least chance of passing the ECFMG examination were those over forty years of age, female, non-native English speakers, those taking the test more than ten years after medical school, USIMGs, and those educated in countries with medium to high infant mortality rates and medium per capita income. Women comprise only 30% of all IMGs in U.S. residencies.

In recent years, the citizenship of individuals receiving the highest number of ECFMG Certificates was: India (17%), U.S. (9%), Pakistan (9%), Philippines (8%), Syria (4%), and Australia, Egypt, Germany, Israel, Lebanon, Nigeria, Poland, United Kingdom, and the former USSR (all 2%).

## ECFMG English Language Examinations

*All IMGs must also pass an English proficiency examination* for ECFMG certification, even if they are U.S. citizens or native English speakers. As of March 1999, the ECFMG is only using the Test of English as a Foreign Language (TOEFL) developed by the Educational Testing Service. (Those who previously passed the ECFMG English test need to take TOEFL if their English Language Examination Certificate lapses.)

The TOEFL can be taken using either a computer-based administration or a paper-based, Friday or Saturday, administration (formerly called the "special" or "international" TOEFL). It is administered at 180 worldwide sites, and most have the computer-based test available. A booklet describing the test in more detail is available through the TOEFL website (www.toefl.org) or by mail from: Educational Testing Service (ETS), Rosedale Rd., Princeton, NJ 08541 USA; telephone (609) 921-9000; fax 609-734-5410.

The computerized version has four sections: listening, structure, reading, and writing. There are a variety of question types. All examinees must compose an essay, either by typing it or handwriting it. One benefit of the computerized test is that immediately following the test, examinees have the option of viewing their unofficial scores on the computer for all sections, except for the writing section. If the essay was typed, results come in about two weeks. If handwritten, the results take five weeks. The test lasts 3½ to 4 hours. The benefit of the computerized test is that it is taken in an individual test station, can be canceled if necessary, and there is a wide range of dates and times to take the test. Study materials include tutorials with practice questions that are available on CD-ROM or can be downloaded from the website.

For the paper-based TOEFL, examinees work with a test booklet and answer sheet. All questions are multiple choice. They choose from one of four possible answers for each question. The test has three sections: Listening Comprehension, Structure and Written Expression, and Reading Comprehension. The test lasts 3 hours. This test is taken in a group setting, has a limited number of test dates to choose from, and may not be canceled once scheduled. A test preparation kit with practice tests is available from the ETS.

The pass rate for the old ECFMG English test hovered around 60%, and TOEFL should be about the same. (Since native English speakers must also take the test, the pass rate for non-native English speakers is really much lower.) Those who pass the exam get an ECFMG English Language Examination Certificate, which must be renewed every two years until the Certificate is validated as permanent. If the candidate enters an ACGME-approved training program during this time, the English Proficiency Certificate is considered permanent and the Certificate may be returned to the ECFMG with a "Request for Permanent Validation of Standard ECFMG Certificate" (Form 246), for permanent revalidation. (The CSA results are simultaneously validated as permanent.) A letter must accompany it from the program director stating the date on which the residency began and the field or specialty.

Even if your ability to read and write English is excellent, and if you are a native English speaker but not familiar with American idioms, your chances of obtaining the residency you want (or any residency in the United States) may be improved if you take a *conversational* English course. Unlike the standard English course, this type of course prepares people to verbally communicate—to speak American-English. It is a skill you will need as a resident and, later, as a practicing physician.

## Clinical Skills Assessment (CSA Exam)

### What is the CSA?

The Clinical Skills Assessment (CSA) is a test of the clinical and communication skills (especially a proficiency in spoken English) that U.S. medical school graduates are expected to have. All applicants for an ECFMG Certificate who had not received it by June 30, 1998 must take the CSA as the *last step* in their ECFMG Certification process.

New ECFMG Certificates indicate the date the CSA was passed, the duration of its validity for entry into U.S. graduate medical education, and how long the English-language test is valid. A passing score on the CSA is valid for three years from the exam date. If the CSA date expires before a physician begins a residency in the United States, the applicant must re-pass the exam.

Ninety percent of LCME-accredited medical schools in the United States and Canada use Standardized Patients (SPs) for instruction. About 70% of these same institutions use them for evaluation—usually in the form of an OSCE (objective, structured clinical examination). Standardized Patients are also incorporated into the Medical Council of Canada's (MCC) medical licensure examination for Canadian and foreign medical graduates.

The NBME plans to eventually include a Standardized Patient Test (SPT) of clinical skills, analogous to the CSA, as part of the USMLE.

The CSA is currently given throughout the year, seven days a week at: ECFMG, 3624 Market St., CSA Center: 3rd Floor, Philadelphia, PA 19104, USA.

## How does the test work?

The examination consists of eleven standardized patient (SP) encounters, ten of which are scored; one case is used for research. The test cases are those that you commonly encounter in a doctor's office and in an emergency department in the United States or Canada. They include areas from Internal Medicine, Surgery, OB/GYN, Pediatrics, Psychiatry and Family Medicine. They cover clinical areas such as cardiovascular, respiratory, gastrointestinal, nutrition, genitourinary neurology/psychiatry, otolaryngology, and orthopedics. The SPs are a balance of genders, ages, and ethnicities. (All SPs are adults, although they may present as parents of a child with a problem.) On any test day, the set of cases will differ from the combination presented the day before or the following day, but each set of eleven cases will have comparable degrees of difficulty.

The SPs are non-medical people who are trained to portray a patient with a particular medical problem. They are also trained to document (using checklists) an examinee's history-taking, physical exam, and communication skills. They respond to candidates' questions with standardized answers for the case and demonstrate appropriate physical findings during the physical examination. (Some physical findings may be real; others may be simulated. Accept all as real.) Candidates interact with the SPs as they would with a real patient, but no treatment is performed. Examinees have fifteen minutes to perform a focused history and physical on each SP. After each case, examinees have ten minutes to write a patient note. The examination itself takes approximately five hours. Including orientation, registration, and breaks, the testing period lasts approximately eight hours.

A typical (morning session) day goes from 8:30 A.M. to 3:30 P.M. with two breaks—a 30-minute lunch break after fourth case and a 15-minute coffee break after seventh case. The ECFMG provides lunch and coffee/tea. On the day of the examination, you are requested to be there no more than 30 minutes before 8:30 A.M. and the examination begins by issuing a card with the photograph of yourself and a number assigned to you, after checking one of your photo IDs and the admission permit. The sessions begin with an on-site orientation.

The test rooms are a series of doctors' offices, equipped with standard examination tables, commonly-used diagnostic instruments (blood pressure cuffs, otoscopes, and ophthalmoscopes), latex gloves, sinks, and paper towels. Part of the orientation room simulates the test examination rooms. At the end of orientation, there is time to familiarize yourself with the equipment.

Once inside the testing area, each candidate stands in front of a doorway and awaits the announcement, "examinees, you can begin your work now." At that point, uncover the patient information posted outside the room. This information usually includes the patient's name, age, occupation, the reason for their visit, the site at which you are working, (i.e., doctor's office, emergency department), and vital signs (pulse, BP, temperature, and respiratory rate). *Accept these vital signs as accurate* and, to save time, do not repeat them unless you feel the case specifically requires it.

Examinees interact with each SP for fifteen minutes. They then have ten minutes to write their patient note. When you do the physical examination, preserve the patient's privacy; e.g., inform the patient when you want to remove the gown, and drape the patient appropriately. Also pay attention to personal hygiene, such as washing your hands before or after the examination. Be very polite and courteous to the SPs and be gentle— they are both "patients" and evaluators. One way is to warm your hands and stethoscope before placing it on the patient.

If breast, genital, or rectal examinations are essential for the patient's evaluation, list them in the diagnostic work-up part of the write-up. These areas may be exposed, if necessary, as part of the physical examination, such as for cardiac auscultation. Be sure to ask about a drug, sexual, and social history—since they will be relevant in many of these cases.

Some prior examinees suggest the best way to manage time during each encounter is to divide the fifteen minutes into three parts. Spend seven to eight minutes for the history—where you get most of your information, four to five minutes for a *focused* physical exam, and two to three minutes to clear up any questionable items. They also suggest mimicking the American accent (if you can), since it may improve your communication score.

When the candidate has been inside with the SP for ten minutes, there will be a cue saying "examinees, you have five more minutes to finish the encounter." This is so that the examinee can speed up their encounter, if necessary. At the end of the encounter, there is another cue saying "examinees, please stop your work." If examinees finish their history taking and physical examination before the allocated fifteen minutes, they may leave the room. Once they leave they cannot return, since the SP will immediately begin to complete the performance questionnaire.

When writing the patient note, make your writing legible (print if necessary) and do not write beyond the margins or it won't be scanned into the computer. The test center has pages for your write-ups containing three sections: (1) history—note significant positives and negatives, (2) physical findings, (3) two columns for differential diagnosis and for diagnostic work-up. List at least three and no more than five items in each column. Which tests to order? Those that rule in or out the differential diagnoses listed. Order only specific tests. The only test groups permitted are complete blood counts (CBC), urinalysis, electrolytes, and arterial blood gas. Treatment (therapeutics), such as hospitalization, consultations, or referrals, should *not* be included in this list. Standard abbreviations can be used and there is a list of them in the *Candidate Orientation Manual*. If you don't know these abbreviations, however, write it all out.

### Who is eligible to take it?

To take the CSA, registrants must first:

1. Pass the USMLE Step 1. (Step 2 is not required to take the CSA. Step 3 is not required for either the CSA or an ECFMG Certification, since it is taken during or after residency.)

2. Pass the English language proficiency test (usually TOEFL).

3. Be a medical student officially enrolled in a medical school listed in the current edition of the *World Directory of Medical Schools* published by the World Health Organization and be within six months of completion of the full didactic curriculum. — *or* — Be a graduate of a medical school that was listed in the *World Directory of Medical Schools* at the time of graduation. Graduates must have credit for at least four academic years of attendance at the medical school.

Those IMGs holding ECFMG Certificates issued before the CSA was given may, but are not required, to take the exam. (The ECFMG suggests that this will make them more desirable to residency programs, but that is uncertain.)

### How do you register for it and arrange a test date?

The official four-page application (Form 716) comes with the ECFMG *Information Booklet*. To register for the CSA, the application form must be completed in full and sent to ECFMG in the envelope provided. They will only accept the official application form. Applicants must also document the completion of all requirements for, and receipt of, the final medical diploma. Once the completed application form and payment are received at ECFMG, and the applicant is determined to be eligible to take the CSA, notification of registration and information about scheduling the CSA will be sent to the applicant.

Since the CSA is offered daily throughout the year except for major U.S. holidays, there is no deadline for submitting the application form to register for the test. Register for the test well in advance. At present, it takes about six to twelve weeks to receive the informational materials after you send your application materials and payment. It is best to register first and receive the notification to schedule the CSA; then start studying. Once a completed application form and payment ($1,200) is received from qualified applicants, ECFMG sends a:

- Notification of Registration.
- *Candidate Orientation Manual.*
- *Candidate Orientation Video* (17 minutes).
- Letter to immigration officials asking that they help obtain visas for test candidates living outside the United States.
- Booklet with information about hotels in, and travel to and around, Philadelphia.

To avoid forfeiting the registration fee, candidates must schedule their CSA test date within four months and take the CSA within one year of receiving their registration notification. To schedule a test date after you have registered, contact the CSA Scheduling Program. This can be done in either of two ways. You may telephone 1-215-970-1982 (Monday through Friday, 0800-2400 EST) to have an operator assist you with scheduling, or do it through the CSA Scheduling Program on the Internet. You will need to give your name, ECFMG identification number, and date of birth as it appears on your Notification of Registration. Have several preferred dates in mind, all within one year from your Notification of Registration. A written confirmation (admission permit) will be mailed to you the next business day. The admission permit confirms the date, time, and location of the exam. Applicants must present this admission permit at the Clinical Skills Assessment Center.

Once scheduled, a CSA test date cannot be rescheduled or canceled without forfeiting the examination fee. Failure to appear on the test date also results in forfeiture. In these cases, candidates must submit a new application with the full examination fee. Those who fail the CSA may reapply as often as they wish, three months after their last exam, and pay the entire $1,200 registration fee each time.

## What is the process when I get to the test site?

Test sessions may be held in the morning or the afternoon. Yours is specified on your admission permit. If you have a morning session, arrive between 8:00 A.M. and 8:30 A.M. on the assigned day; registration begins promptly at 8:30 A.M. Arrive for afternoon sessions between 3:00 P.M. and 3:30 P.M.; registration begins promptly at 3:30 P.M. If you are coming from a different time zone, it is best to get to the Philadelphia area several days in advance. On the exam day, present valid photo identification and your admission permit at the CSA Center.

Limit the personal items you bring, since there is only a small amount of unsecured storage space (ergo, no luggage). There is also no waiting area for anyone accompanying you. Wear comfortable, professional clothing and a white laboratory or clinic coat. Bring your stethoscope.

After registering, there is a live orientation using visual material and live demonstrations to familiarize you with the equipment in each exam room and the nature of typical encounters. You also sign a confidentiality agreement and complete a demographic questionnaire.

There are vending machines available for snacks. The one thing you cannot do during breaks, or at any time, is discuss the cases with your fellow candidates. Conversation among candidates in languages other than English about any subject is strictly prohibited at all times during these breaks. To maintain security and quality assurance, each examination room in the CSA Center is equipped with video cameras and microphones to record every encounter.

## Who passes?

As of December 1999, 97% of those taking the CSA passed. The failures were primarily for issues related to communication. The high pass rate was thought to be due to candidate self-selection. In the initial one and a half years of the test's administration, there has been a much higher percentage of U.S. citizen IMGs taking the test than had applied previously for ECFMG Certificates. Also, as the ECFMG suggests, potential applicants were screening themselves before applying by taking the Test of Spoken English. (This test, given around the world, examines whether individuals can speak and understand the language in oral form. It is a separate test from the TOEFL. They recommend a score of at least 35 on this test to have a chance of passing the CSA.) The high cost of the test and travel also contributed to the small numbers of non-U.S.-citizen IMGs taking the test.

In the 1999 Match, 64% of applicants who passed the CSA matched with residency positions, as opposed to about 32% of ECGMG Certificate holders without the CSA. This, however, may be that the group included more Americans and better English speakers.

## How is it scored?

This test is standards-based (criterion-referenced), meaning that a specific score is required to pass—it is not graded on "a curve." The examinees that meet the preset criteria pass; those who don't, fail. The ECFMG is planning on revising the test criteria in the future to make passing somewhat more difficult.

All scores are averaged over the ten cases. For each case, the following skills are being assessed:

### Integrated Clinical Encounter (ICE) Score
### (Combines DG and PN scores)

- *Data Gathering (DG)*
  The DG score for a particular encounter is the percentage of checklist items the candidate completed, such as obtaining relevant information or correctly performing the physical examination maneuvers.

- *Patient Note (PN)*
  After you leave the exam, trained health care professionals rate your written notes on the organization, quality of information, interpretation of data, egregious/dangerous actions, and legibility.

### Communication (COM) Score
### (Combines the IPS and ENG ratings)

- *Interpersonal Skills (IPS)*
  Candidates are rated for interviewing ability, counseling and delivering information, rapport, and personal manner.

- *Spoken English Proficiency (ENG)*
  These criteria include pronunciation, grammar, and the amount of effort required by the SPs to understand the examinee. They rate the overall comprehensibility as "low," "medium," "high," and "very high."

Scores are normally mailed within six to eight weeks after the examination. Examinees who pass both the Communication and Integrated Clinical Encounter components receive a "PASS" score. Substandard performance on *either* the Communication or the Integrated Clinical Encounter component results in a "FAIL" score. The CSA results are not provided by telephone, facsimile, or telex.

## How do you prepare for it?

A good clinical education and proficiency in speaking and understanding spoken English is essential to pass the CSA. However, since, as with all exams, it is an artificial situation, some additional preparation might be useful. The first source of information is the *Candidate Orientation Manual* and *Candidate Orientation Video* that the ECFMG sends registrants once they select a date. Much of the Manual's information is also available on-line at www.ecfmg.org/cs_cont.htm.

The ECFMG recommends preparing by seeing actual patients in real clinical settings, particularly under the supervision of competent clinical teachers. For those who are not comfortable with spoken English, these encounters should ideally be in English. It also helps to practice what you will say and how you will act with patient simulators. Practice with colleagues or teachers who can role-play patients with realistic, common complaints.

Several professional preparation courses exist, and one book comes highly recommended: *Mastering the OSCE/CSA* by Jo-Ann Reteguiz and Beverly Cornel-Avendano (McGraw-Hill, 1999). General history/physical examination books should also prove useful.

Finally, if you need technical information about the CSA, contact the ECFMG Applicant Information Services, telephone 1-215-823-2282.

## Tips For All IMGs

Several hints have been passed on to me from IMGs who used previous editions of this book. Some of the most useful were from Bill Groves, M.D., currently a resident at his first-choice program. He writes:

> If you are in an interview and cannot remember anything at all, and your English is deteriorating rapidly [even if you are native English speaker, as is Dr. Groves], remember how many babies you have delivered, how many times you did CPR, and how many times you were alone. Your education may at times have lacked quality, machinery, or medications, but it did not lack vitality.

> If the program apologizes for having IMGs and the resident apologizing is from Bangladesh, there is a double standard here, and no doubt friction between the residents and administration.

> If a program director calls you and says that all the competing programs are dropping out of the Match, that all of his slots will be filled by early February, and that you need to sign onto one of his remaining two slots immediately, don't do anything precipitously. Call the Match to check on his story—it is probably untrue. Yet you might want to take his interest as a compliment and consider the offer.

> It may seem unfair that American graduates can take clerkships right up until they begin residency, while you are barred from any contact [with patients, which may represent a year of decay of your clinical skills]. Do not doubt, however, that the law applies to you and will be

enforced. Your temporary license may depend upon adhering to state requirements. If necessary, work temporarily in another state, and write the AMA for information and help.

What Dr. Groves did not mention is that there may be an even greater image problem for USIMGs than for FNIMGs. While foreign-born physicians have a reason for training outside the United States, it is often assumed that USIMGs could not measure up to U.S. standards and so had to leave the country. While this may be true for some, the fact remains that many qualified applicants are rejected from U.S. schools simply because there are not enough positions. USIMGs, at least, do not have to broach the language or cultural barriers faced by their foreign-born counterparts.

## Non-U.S./Non-Canadian Citizens (FNIMGs)

International medical graduates who are not U.S. citizens generally encounter the biggest problems in obtaining residency training positions. Many programs just will not accept such applicants. Often, they will not state this plainly for fear of legal reprisal, although some programs have lately begun stating in their program information that they will only accept graduates of U.S. medical schools as applicants. However, Sec 102 of the Health Professions Education Extension Amendments of 1992, quoted above, may help. While it is unclear how much effect this law will have, it certainly is ammunition.

While selection committees have some problems evaluating an IMG's credentials, the problem is not as grave as it was in the past. The USMLE has provided an even playing field to assess all medical school graduates' level of knowledge. Apples can now be compared directly with other apples (if you don't mind being an "apple").

Some U.S. residency programs actually prefer international graduates. Though this may seem paradoxical, they feel that way for a very good reason. The medical system views residencies with a high percentage of international medical graduates as inferior—even if their training is just as good as any other program. This message is clearly sent to U.S. graduates. Therefore, only the poorest U.S. students apply to such programs. This, according to the directors of some of these programs, is in direct contradistinction to the high quality of international medical graduates who are applying to their programs.

As an FNIMG, the best way to get a residency position is to apply to a program that has a relationship with your medical school. Some of these programs have drawn excellent graduates from one or two specific foreign medical schools over the years. They have developed good contacts within the schools and are not afraid, as are many other programs, of encountering forged documents, inflated grades, or poor quality instruction.

Some international graduates are forced to take residency slots that are unfunded. In some cases they are called externships; in others they actually count toward completion of a residency. It is not unusual to see offers of payment for a residency slot from either the applicants themselves or third-parties acting on their behalf. Proposals of $25,000 or more per year (plus any cost for salary, benefits, and allowances) have been offered for competitive positions. There is concern, however, that many of the individuals filling these positions are not treated as equals, do not get similar responsibilities, or do not end up with training equivalent to that of other residents in the same program.

A good method for evaluating whether you, as an IMG, have a reasonable chance of getting accepted into a program in a particular specialty, is to check the charts in the annual "Medical Education Issue" of *JAMA*, or Figures 14.1 and 14.2, to see how many foreign-trained residents are currently training in or entering that specialty. In addition, check with your school to see if there are any particular programs in the United States with which they have a working relationship.

Even if you get a residency position, you have to worry about your visa. About one-third of all IMG residents hold J-1 visas. (Another 8% hold H-type visas.) J-1 visas are limited to the time typically required to complete the advanced medical education program. This means the time required for board certification by the American Board of Medical Specialists for a specialty and subspecialty. The limit, reiterated in June 1999, is seven years. This limitation mostly affects individuals who extend their program to include research or chief resident years and then want to do a fellowship.

This same statement added that IMGs on Exchange-Visitor visas may participate only in ACGME-accredited programs, thus disallowing participation in a number of specialty programs, including Pediatric Emergency Medicine, Trauma fellowships, and a number of subspecialty areas in Obstetrics and Gynecology, Ophthalmology, and other specialties. The INS also restated the ban on moonlighting for these residents and the necessity of getting a letter from their home country confirming that the individual needs to have U.S. medical training before a J-1 visa is granted.

The ECFMG usually issues J-1 visas for physicians in training. On this visa, although you can leave the United States at any time, you must have proper documentation to reenter the United States (a valid J-1 visa stamp in the passport and either a duplicate copy of the IAP-66 or the pink copy of the current IAP-66 endorsed by the ECFMG). If you have questions about this, check with the ECFMG.

J-1 visas normally require the holder to return to their *home country* for a minimum of two years after training. This requirement also extends to relatives holding J-2 dependent visas. Occasionally, exceptions are made if the home country writes a "no objection" letter, the IMG qualifies for a hardship or asylum waiver, or a U.S. government agency requests a waiver because they have a need for the individual. Visas and the laws governing them, however, constantly change.

While it is easier to obtain a visa to be a "Research Scholar" or "Professor," those entering the United States as an Exchange Visitor with these designations are not allowed to transfer into a residency program for at least 12 months after arriving.

For an overview of the situation, see *The International Medical Graduates' Guide to U.S. Medicine—Negotiating the Maze* (L. B. Ball, Galen Press, 1995). For current specific information about visas for IMG residents, contact: Exchange Visitor Department, ECFMG, 3624 Market St., Philadelphia, PA 19104-2685, USA. The bottom line, though, is that the United States is tightening up on letting international medical graduates in the door. They perceive that there already is a doctor glut—and they don't want you to make it worse.

## U.S. International Medical Graduates (USIMGs)

Most of the same problems described above also exist for U.S. citizens who have taken their medical school training outside the United States.

What you have going for you is that you are a native English speaker, so there should be no trouble with passing the difficult ECFMG English test. What you have going against you is that you did not have the experience of going to a U.S. medical school. In 1999, 52% of IMGs in U.S. residency training programs were U.S. citizens or permanent U.S. residents. (Only 9%, however, were native U.S. citizens.) This is an increase from 1988, when USIMGs made up only 41% of IMGs in U.S. residencies. Of the 1,867 USIMGs who completed the NRMP PGY-1 Match process in 1999, only 889 (48%) obtained a residency position. This is higher than the rate for foreign-born IMGs (32%).

The best advice for getting into a residency is to do everything possible to transfer into a U.S. medical school prior to graduation, although this is getting progressively more difficult each year. To accomplish this, you will have to do very well in your studies in the first two or three years of medical school, in addition to performing well on Step 1, and possibly Step 2, of the United States Medical Licensing Examination (USMLE) as administered through the Educational Commission for Foreign Medical Graduates (ECFMG). Doing well on the USMLE will be an impressive accomplishment, since USIMGs have consistently done worse on licensing examinations than their foreign-born counterparts. Perhaps FNIMGs take the test more seriously—you should too. Study!

In recent years, most students who have successfully transferred to U.S. schools had high GPAs after competing at least two years of medical school, did very well on the USMLE, and transferred to schools in states where they were official residents or to private schools. (Note that you cannot "transfer" once you have received your medical degree.)

No one keeps a master list of which schools will accept transfer students from non-U.S. medical schools, although Deans of Students at international schools with large numbers of U.S. citizens do keep lists of U.S. medical schools that have accepted their students. To locate a school which might accept you:

1. Contact U.S. medical schools directly to inquire about their willingness to take USIMGs. Do not be "picky" about their location.

2. Mail inquiry letters to the admissions offices of all U.S. medical schools. For any school where you have any kind of "tie" (such as birthplace, undergraduate school, long residence, parents' residence, etc.), specifically mention that.

3. If you have to limit the number of letters sent, concentrate on the non-Ivy League private schools. State schools will often accept only students who are considered residents.

4. Also write to Osteopathic medical schools. They often will be more flexible than M.D. schools.

## Fifth-Pathway Program

If you cannot transfer to a school in the United States, you may be eligible to enter a *Fifth-Pathway Program* (a year of supervised clinical training). The Fifth-Pathway route allows students in countries that require a year of internship or of social service before granting the M.D. degree (such as Mexico), to qualify for their M.D. and medical license by taking a year of supervised clinical training at a U.S. medical school. Finishing this program is a route to medical licensure without getting an ECFMG Certificate with its attendant requirements, such as the English language test and CSA exam. To qualify for this program, students *must be U.S. citizen/permanent residents* and have:

1. Completed their undergraduate premedical studies at a U.S. college or university with grades and scores acceptable for entrance into a U.S. medical school.

2. Completed all formal requirements except the internship/social service at a foreign medical school listed in the *World Directory of Medical Schools.*

3. Passed USMLE Step 1.

4. *Not* completed their internship/social service requirement.

5. *Not* received their M.D. degree.

6. *Not* met the ECFMG's certification requirements.

Four U.S. medical schools list themselves as accepting Fifth-Pathway students. However, only the New York Medical College (NYMC), Valhala, New York and Brown University in Rhode Island actually accept students for this program. (Brown University accepts only Rhode Island residents, so very few people are eligible each year.) NYMC's contact information is: telephone (914) 594-4489; fax (914) 594-4325; web address www. nymc. edu/depthome/fifth.htm)

The NYMC program charges a $50 application fee, and a non-refundable $500 reservation fee once the student is accepted. To receive an application, complete the short screening pre-application form on their website. If you qualify, they will send an application.

Tuition varies—for year 2000, it is $20,000. NYMC now has at least eight hospitals in New York, New Jersey, and Connecticut participating. Priority is given to students from Mexican medical schools, since New York State recognizes these schools. Students from the Simmelweiss Medical School in Hungary have also gone through NYMC's program, but must be placed in hospitals outside New York.

NYMC's Fifth-Pathway program lasts 12 months, with starting dates in January and July. The clinical programs vary among the participating hospitals. From this springboard, USIMGs are usually able to leap into residency slots much more easily. They may apply to residencies through the Match as an Independent Candidate. The school assists students by allowing time to study for USMLE Step 2 and to go for residency interviews.

There is a problem, however. Eight jurisdictions (Alaska, Guam, Indiana, Michigan, Utah, Vermont) do not accept a Fifth-Pathway certificate as part of an application for licensure. Twenty-three other states and the District of Columbia require that the Fifth-Pathway graduates either complete the USMLE or have an ECFMG Certificate. Mississippi and South Carolina accept Fifth-Pathway only if the applicant also is certified by an ABMS Board (in other words, has completed both residency and board certification). Other jurisdictions leave acceptance of the Fifth-Pathway certificate to the licensing board's discretion, with only thirteen jurisdictions accepting it unconditionally.

This can lead to horror stories, as one physician related:

I had been accepted in an Orthopedic Surgery residency in my home state after finishing the Fifth-Pathway program. I was ecstatic! However, the residency was notified that the state's Board of Medical Examiners had decided not to accept the Fifth-Pathway route to licensure. Since residents were required to be licensed, I could not take the position and had to sit out a year until I could reapply somewhere else.

One state, Louisiana, may count the Fifth-Pathway as one year of the three years that they require for IMG licensure. For more information about the Fifth-Pathway program, contact: Licensure and Certification Section, American Medical Association, 515 N. State St., Chicago, IL 60610.

USIMGs will also feel the impact of restrictions now being imposed upon all international medical graduates. Getting into a residency will become harder and harder as time passes and the laws become more strict. In the future, it will take more than just excellent grades and good examination scores for you to get any position at all, let alone in the specialty that you desire.

## Only In Florida

Florida is the only state that allows physicians who were licensed in other countries to get a license without either getting an ECFMG Certificate or taking the USMLE. In May 1999, they began giving the Florida Medical Licensure Exam twice a year. It has both a basic and a clinical sciences component. However, of the 264 physicians who took the first exam, only 4% passed. The state has agreed to reduce the basic science component and increase the clinical component for future test administrations.

Florida also has given a unique Florida Physician Assistant Licensure Exam since 1995, allowing licensed physicians to bypass the national exam (for which they are not eligible) and to become PAs. The pass rate has been dismal. The state has agreed to ensure that their test is similar to the Physician Assistant National Certification Exam.

## Canadian Citizens

Canadian citizens are not IMGs. But the United States has a somewhat schizophrenic attitude toward Canadian medical school graduates. While the same association that accredits U.S. schools accredits Canadian medical schools and there is no question that their training is excellent, there is still ambivalence in many sectors about considering Canadian applicants for residency positions. In part, this stems from the dissimilarity of the entire

Canadian educational system and the resultant difficulties in comparing Canadian applicants with those from U.S. schools. This can be at least partially remedied by including as much explanation as possible about your training, grades, honors, etc., with your application materials.

However, aside from the problem of comparing applicants, there also is concern about the lack of reimbursement in the future if Canadians are taken into residency training programs. Some state monies have already been withdrawn from programs that have Canadian trainees. Therefore, it is wise for any Canadian considering training at a U.S. program to first check to see if the program will seriously consider Canadian applicants.

Even if you want to eventually practice medicine in the United States, it may not be as important as it seems to do a U.S. residency. That is because thirty-seven U.S. states and territories will issue a medical license by endorsement to graduates of accredited Canadian medical schools who hold a Licentiate of the Medical Council of Canada. Those that don't are Delaware, Florida, Georgia, Guam, Hawaii, Idaho, Louisiana, Michigan, Mississippi, Missouri, Montana, New Jersey, North Carolina, South Carolina, Utah, Vermont, and the Virgin Islands.

Nevertheless, increasing numbers of Canadian medical school graduates now seek residency training in the United States. Their medical education system forces specialty decisions earlier than in the past, they have reduced the number of residency positions, and Canadian provinces now make it very difficult for physicians to change specialties, or even to get licensed in their own specialty in another province.

The Canadian government forcefully discourages Canadian graduates from taking U.S. residencies. Canadians wishing to enter a U.S. residency program must now get letters of support from their Dean, Province, and Health-Welfare Canada. For the most part, Canadian officials balk at providing these letters. For more information, contact: Health Human Resources Unit, Health Services System Division, Health & Social Program Branch, Health-Welfare Canada, Jeane Marie Bldg., Room 672, Ottawa, Ontario, Canada, K1A 1B4; telephone (613) 954-8671; fax (613) 957-1406.

Finally, to be seriously considered as an applicant, it will be necessary to get an immigration card approving your working in the United States before you apply. Otherwise, even if you match with a program, you may not be able to work there. Without an immigration card, no program will consider you.

# 15

# Preparing For The Interview

*Every new answer raises a new question.*

– Folk Saying

No matter how irrational it may seem, the ten- to thirty-minute interviews that you will have at the residency programs will count for more, in most cases, toward getting you into the program than the total weight of your previous 3½ years of medical school. That's not just my personal belief. Several recent studies have shown this to be true. And it is not only the most important part of the resident-selection process, but also the most costly and most time-consuming. So now that you are preparing to go for interviews, put your best effort toward doing a good job. This is where it all comes together!

## The Mock Interview

How well will you do when you are actually sitting in the hot seat being interviewed for that residency slot you want above all others? Do not wait until you sit in the real chair to find out! When you think that you are prepared to go out on the interview circuit, arrange for a mock interview. This practice instills confidence and stifles anxiety, makes you calmer and more organized, and helps you sound better during the real thing.

### What Is A Mock Interview?

A mock interview is to an interview what near-drowning is to drowning. In both cases, you think that you are going to die, but in the former, you end up out of danger. Your mock interview should closely imitate the actual interview process. You must prepare for it in exactly the same way that you will prepare for your real interviews. Dress the same, carry identical materials with you, and go over your interview answers just as you will before interviews at the residency programs. If you don't feel anxiety, you're not doing it correctly. This interview must be as realistic as possible so that you will get the most accurate and useful feedback.

Who should conduct the mock interview? Ideally, your mentor and a specialty adviser, if you have one, since they are probably used to interviewing residency applicants. If not, the Dean of Students or another faculty member in the specialty with interviewing experience and your mentor should interview you. Tell them, if they do not know, that you want the mock interview to be as realistic as possible. You want them to ask you the "difficult" questions and treat you in the same manner they would treat any candidate—not as someone they already know. Then you want feedback: on the way you presented yourself, the manner in which you were dressed, how you handled the questions, and an overall assessment of areas to be improved upon before you hit the interview trail.

One useful technique for self-critique is to audio- or videotape the interview. Would you hire the person you hear or see? What seems wrong with the applicant (you)? How can you improve your interview performance next time? As with all other parts of the application process, this takes a little extra effort. Experience has shown that it pays off in a big way.

Besides the formal mock interview, it also helps to go over interview elements in your mind during those odd times when you are commuting, awaiting others, or holding retractors. Review potential questions and situations, as well as those from previous interviews. One way to remember some of the areas you want to review, before embarking on the real interview, is to use the mnemonic, "SHOWTIME."

The "SHOW" part should not be recited as a litany, but rather used when questions arise in any of these areas. Two things you probably want to memorize, or at least get them down pat enough so that they sound smooth, are your opening introduction to the interviewer and a two- or three-sentence summation of your message (your strengths and desire to come to the program).

The "TIME" elements are how you convey your message. Practice both.

- **Self:** What do you know about yourself? Have you adequately assessed your own knowledge, skills, and desires?

- **History:** How did you decide to enter this specialty and this program? Which aspects of your personal history can help you relate to an interviewer in this specialty, and this interviewer in particular?

- **Originality:** What makes you unique? What have you accomplished, experienced, or set as a personal goal that sets you apart from the crowd?
- **World View:** What do you believe in? Why are you striving for this particular goal? What will it mean in your life? How does this program fit into these goals?

---

- **Tell:** How are you presenting yourself—from the moment you first interact with hospital and residency personnel? Remember that the impression you make begins at the beginning and extends through every contact. For the interview itself, practice effective verbal communication, including looking alert and interested, appearing organized, and listening carefully.
- **Illustrate:** Also practice non-verbal communication, including maintaining eye contact, sitting forward, gesturing effectively, and smiling—when appropriate. This is vital, since more than half of the message may be delivered through non-verbal cues.
- **Manage:** Use well-placed questions and time-awareness to manage the interview. Be sure to get your key message across while fully (but not endlessly) answering the interviewer's questions.
- **Engage:** Throughout the interview, try to discuss those areas about which you are enthusiastic so that your conversation is animated and stimulating for the interviewer. If you enjoyed the interview, it is likely that the interviewer did also.

Give the right non-verbal signals. Use a strong handshake to communicate energy and drive. Maintain eye contact. For successful eye contact, you must hold the interviewer's gaze for three to five seconds or until a thought or sentence is complete. Don't glance around the room, signaling that you are bored. Avoid nervous mannerisms such as doodling or tapping your fingers. Smile often. Avoid slouching and other forms of bad posture that make you seem to lack confidence. Send a positive message. For example, lean forward in the chair to show interest and alertness.

Don't sweat over past interviews, just think about how they could have gone better. This frequent review will keep you prepared to face the next interview without needing too much last-minute preparation.

# Timing

Students always have many questions about the timing of the actual interviews. Because there is very little information or guidance offered to applicants, they must wallow through the morass of scheduling, traveling, and interviewing on their own. The most common question is whether to do an interview close to home or at the bottom-choice program first as a trial interview, thereby getting an idea of the interview process. Neither of these is advisable.

As discussed above, you should learn how to go through the interview process by participating in a mock interview with your mentor and specialty adviser prior to embarking on your first trip. If you can avoid it, do not waste any real interviews on "practice." The programs that you consider weak based upon their written material may surprise you with their strengths when you visit them.

## Ratings Inflate As The "Season" Goes On

A number of studies on interviewing show that programs' ratings of applicants become more favorable as the "season" progresses. (Although one emergency medicine study showed no relationship between the date interviewed and the match list position, this may not hold true for all specialties—or even all programs within a single specialty.)

Just as the requirements to get an interview slot are easier when the composition of the entire applicant pool is uncertain, interviewers' evaluations tend to be lower for the candidates interviewed early. This is, in part, because early interviewees are being compared to a hypothetical "best applicant" rather than the available applicant pool. As reality sinks in, interviewers tend to raise their ratings to more accurately reflect a candidate's true position in comparison with his or her cohorts. This suggests that it is better for you to interview in the second half, if not near the end, of the interview season.

## Last Interviewed Are Remembered Best

Unless you are among the last applicants interviewed, the impression you make will tend to fade as faculty members interview other applicants. When they make their selection decisions, the faculty will best remember those individuals who are interviewed last.

The difference in the rate of selection between candidates interviewed in the second half of the season and those interviewed in the first half is only a few percentage points. But don't you want those points to work for you rather than against you? If so, plan to interview late. In fact, if you can manage it, schedule your interview on or near the last available date that each program offers. This can often be done easily if you get your materials to the program early. You will be offered an interview when there is still a wide choice of available dates. Scheduling your interviews at the end of multiple programs' interview schedules may not be as difficult as you might imagine, since various programs end their interviewing at different times.

After you schedule your interviews, send each program a letter confirming your interview date, time, and location. Keep a copy for your records and take it with you as a reminder on your interview trip.

## Not My Top Choice

What should you do when your "bottom" program offers you an invitation to interview and you have yet to hear from your "top" programs? As they say, "A bird in the hand . . ."

Schedule interviews at those programs that offer you an interview and where you would actually be willing to go as a resident. This should logically be all the programs to which you apply—unless you get additional information after you submit your application. Do this for three reasons:

1. You may find that one or more of these "bottom" programs actually perfectly meets your needs when you visit.

2. You may not hear from any other programs, so you need to make certain that you have an opportunity to train in the specialty that you have chosen.

3. Residency programs know that applicants will face this dilemma and expect a certain percentage of applicants, especially late in the interview season, to cancel their interviews.

Hopefully, you will eventually interview at some of your top choice programs, but you may not like them as well as the programs where you have already interviewed.

## Time Off—Arranging The Senior Schedule

You must have the necessary time off to go to interviews. The average senior medical student spends eighteen days away from school on the interview circuit. However, over one-fourth spend more than twenty-one days on the road. This requires a little advance planning.

When should you go for interviews? If you are applying to a specialty that has a second-year Match right out of medical school, such as Neurology, Urology, Neurosurgery, Otolaryngology, or Ophthalmology, you will interview from September through December. If you are applying to programs through the standard NRMP PGY-1 Match (most of you will be in this group), interview season generally runs from November through early February. Some programs only interview during a portion, often the mid- to latter parts, of these time periods.

There are two ways to arrange for time off to interview; you can either take vacation time or take an elective or research block that will allow you to obtain the time off you need. While attractive, this latter option must be investigated carefully. If you make a mistake, and cannot get the time off once you are on such a rotation, you may miss some important interviews. You cannot afford this. If possible, talk with the faculty member responsible for the rotation ahead of time. Find out if you will be able to have days off for interviews. If you know the specific dates or blocks of time, write them down, give the faculty member a copy and have him or her sign the copy that you keep. This way a faulty memory at the last minute will play no part in determining your future.

By the way, if you have followed the schema proposed in this book, you should have plenty of vacation time available. While the interview circuit is usually no holiday (though it can be, see the next section), taking vacation time at this point may ease some of the pressures which can exist if you are trying to sandwich interviews among other responsibilities.

## Wait-Listed?

If you get a letter from a residency program saying that you are "wait-listed" for an interview, do not despair. Residency programs sometimes send such letters when they think that there is little chance that an applicant really is serious—such as someone from the other end of the country.

Write a short note thanking them and saying that you are still interested. One applicant who did that almost immediately got a letter back from the program that was her top choice offering her an interview. She later matched with that program.

## Travel Arrangements

The extensive traveling that you undertake during the interview process may be the most that you have ever done. It may be your first real chance to see many other parts of the country. It will also be a rude introduction to the frequent delays, cancellations, and sardine-can-like accommodations of our nation's air travel system.

Simply traveling to many parts of the country, packing and unpacking in hotels, and finding your way around strange cities will be very tiring—

not to mention costly. More than 60% of all senior medical students find the cost of interviewing burdensome—the average student spends more than $1,600 on travel. There are, however, some methods to decrease your fatigue and make traveling the interview circuit more tolerable, if not actually pleasant.

## Clustering Interviews

The first method to consider is the possibility of clustering your interviews. This can be done either chronologically (to use available blocks of time) or geographically.

It is not unusual for some applicants to fly back and forth across the country several times, as well as to make many side trips, for interviews. Clustering interviews geographically, however, saves both time and the considerable effort which is involved in traveling great distances. It also, of course, saves money. Clustering reduces your interviewing costs by lessening your time away from home (usually spent in hotels) and the amount of traveling you do. These costs, aside from the clothes you bought for the interview, can run anywhere from nothing to $5,000 or more. It will depend upon the geographical range in which you evaluate programs, the level of your accommodations, and your savvy in clustering interviews to use available transportation in the least expensive manner possible.

To cluster interviews, it is essential that you have both luck and flexibility. The harder you work on the problem, the luckier you will become. Flexibility results from getting your materials to programs early. This will allow you a maximum number of interview dates to choose from. Luck is involved with being offered interviews at the right programs in time for you to arrange clusters. Work with the residency secretaries to try to arrange these clusters of interviews. Most of the time they understand your situation and are willing to try to help you out.

Some obsessive-compulsive individuals will try to schedule multiple interviews day after day for a period of time. This is very dangerous. Not only will these individuals become stressed out, but they will also have very little flexibility if they encounter transportation delays. Remember, bad weather shuts down many of the nation's major airports during the interview season. In addition, they will have too little time to digest the information obtained from one interview before getting involved in the next one.

One method some applicants have used to obtain additional insight into the program at which they just interviewed is to informally drop by the hospital that evening or the next morning to talk with some residents. This practice provides an opportunity to get a better perspective on the information gained in the midst of hectic interviewing. Some applicants also take some time to get a feel for the community in which the program is based while they are there. But if you are going to do this, you need a little extra breathing time. Take that time, even if you are clustering your interviews chronologically.

## Special Fares

Another way to save money is by using special fares available from airlines, railroads, and bus companies. Often these allow you unlimited travel during a specified period of time. With the deregulation of the travel industry and its resultant fierce competition, the rates, rules, and special offers change with dizzying frequency. Shop around and use several travel agents, if necessary, until you are satisfied that you are getting the best possible value for your money. Don't forget to tell them that you are a medical student. "Medical" indicates that you may generate very good business in the future. "Student" may entitle you to special rates on some carriers. Remember, the only people paying full fare for transportation, especially air travel, are those having someone else pay for their trip. And the savings can be astronomical. Frequent-flyer programs can also save you money by supplying you with free car rentals, free airline tickets, and free or reduced-cost hotel accommodations.

While getting cheap airline fares has become more complicated in the past few years, there are some specific strategies you can use. Once you know which cities you will visit for interviews, learn what the standard 21-day advance-purchase fare costs. Then, if you find a fare that is 45% to 50% less, book it immediately. These discounts are usually available only for limited times and there may be only a few seats available at that rate. You can also save up to 70% off the price of the airfares charged by major airlines by flying one of the no-frills, low-cost carriers.

The cheapest airline fares may be to a lesser-used airport or an adjacent city, from which you will have to rent a car or arrange other transportation. The difference can reduce ticket prices by a third or more. The best airline deals may be found on the Internet. Many airlines post their best fares there, although they may only equal an advance-fare purchase price. You may also want to bid for tickets at one of the on-line auctions or contact one of the special discount agencies available through the AAMC, AMSA, or similar groups. They can sometimes be found listed in *The New Physician*. Although the rules change constantly, many airlines have special one-price passes allowing travel in certain areas of the United States or in North America during a limited time period. Check the airline websites or with your travel agent for up-to-date information.

If you buy a discount restricted ticket (as you probably want to do), unless you pay a $35-$50 change fee, you will not get a lower fare, even if it is later advertised. Still, it may be worth it.

In recent years, the National Organization of Student Representatives, coordinated by the Association of American Medical Colleges, has arranged special airfares for students who were going on interviews. If your Dean of Students doesn't know anything about this, give the AAMC a call at (202) 828-0682. Deregulation has somewhat disrupted this program, but the AAMC still tries to negotiate contracts with the airlines each year. It doesn't hurt to give them a call.

If you must rent a car, the average daily rate varies depending upon which of the four types of basic rates you choose. The pricing packages are (1) a daily rate with a mileage charge; (2) a daily rate with a limited number of free miles per day; (3) a daily rate with unlimited mileage; and (4) a rate that has free mileage over an extended period. Rates vary according to the size and style of vehicle, and additional fees (such as drop-off fees) can increase these rates. Special promotional rates are often available, especially over weekends, but should be specifically requested in advance.

You can often improve on that by checking several different rental agencies. Local car rental agencies and those not located at the airport (but who will pick you up at the airport) often have much lower rates than the national companies. You can get their telephone numbers from the phone books at your library or off their websites. If you do drive to your interview, check ahead to find out where to park. At many medical centers, visitor parking can be almost impossible to find.

## Surviving Air Travel

Most residency applicants fly to many interviews. As a business traveler, unlike flying for pleasure, you must do everything possible to save time and fly comfortably. Figure 15.1 lists suggestions gleaned from thousands of business travelers on how to do this.

## Cheap Housing

The National Organization of Student Representatives also runs the Housing Extension Network to help applicants to residencies eliminate some housing costs on the road. Each year they ask the medical school representative to find ten students willing to volunteer the use of their homes to students from other schools interviewing for residencies at their institution. If there are at least eight participants, a school is listed in the directory that is sent out each Fall. One copy goes to the student representative and one to the Student Affairs Office. Students from participating

## FIGURE 15.1

### *Air Travel Made Easier*

- Take early morning or late-night flights. Late in the day, delays are common. (Late-night flights may also be less expensive.)

- Go a day before you must arrive—or at least not on the last flight of the day to your destination. Residency interviews occur during the worst travel weather of the year and your flight may get canceled or badly delayed.

- You may also get "bumped" from your flight, meaning there is no room for you even though you have a confirmed reservation. If you arrive on time and are bumped, but the airline can get to your destination within an hour of the scheduled time, the airline must pay you the one-way cost of your ticket up to $200. If they cannot get you there within two hours of the scheduled time, the compensation is doubled, up to $400. In some cases, they also throw in free tickets—so getting bumped may be a good deal if you have some time to spare.

- Keep your travel agent's telephone number handy. (Many have 800 or 888 numbers.) If your flight is canceled, call the agent to rebook you, rather than standing in line with the angry masses.

- Have a copy of that month's *Official Airline Guide* (or a copy of the relevant pages) to help reschedule flights if necessary. Your library or some of the more-traveled faculty may have a copy.

- If you arrive at the airport early, try to get on an earlier flight.

- Board the plane as soon as possible. It is easier to find storage space for your carry-on bags, as well as a pillow and a blanket.

- Sit in the front of the plane to be one of the first off the plane.

- Get an aisle seat. You can get to the bathroom easier and get off the plane faster. (You may, however, be disturbed by the "inside" passengers climbing over you to get out.)

- If you are right-handed, sit on the right side of the plane. That way, people passing you in the aisle won't jiggle your arm when you work or eat. If you plan to sleep on the plane, get a window seat so other passengers won't crawl over you to get out. Ask for a seat in the exit row to get more legroom. On some planes, though, those seat backs don't recline.

- Carry foam ear plugs if you want to sleep on the plane or if you fly on a small (usually commuter) plane. Carry eyeshades if you want to sleep.

- Join the airlines' frequent flier clubs. You may be able to board earlier and get special perquisites. Use one airline and its affiliated hotel and car rental companies as much as possible to maximize benefits.

- If you will fly a lot on one airline, consider joining their airport club. The relaxation between flights may be worth the cost of a one-year membership.

- Join hotel and car rental clubs if you will be using them frequently.

**FIGURE 15.1 (continued)**

- Don't check luggage, if at all possible. Use a carry-on bag with wheels and, if necessary, a garment bag that clips onto it.

- If your checked bags are damaged or lost, reimbursement is only up to $1,250. Keep a list of what is in your bag, file a claim with the airline's baggage claim department on arrival, and keep your baggage claim receipts. They will normally get your bag to you (if you stay in the same city) by the next day.

- Dress comfortably. Unless you will go directly to your interview, carry your interview clothes and dress casually for the flight.

- Pack a snack and a small bottle of water. Many airlines no longer offer meals, and flight delays often prevent travelers from eating between flights.

- Order special meals, such as vegetarian, weight-watcher, or kosher, if meals are served on the flights. They are usually fresher than other meals.

- Do exercises on the airplane:
  - *Neck Stretches*: Flex and extend your neck 5 times anteriorly-posteriorly to and away from the chest and 5 times laterally toward the shoulders. Then rotate your head from side to side 5 times, holding it at full rotation for 3 to 5 seconds.
  - *Shoulder Stretch*: Link fingers and hold them in front of your chest. Lift them above your head, breathing in while stretching toward the ceiling and hold your breath and position for 3 seconds. Bring your arms behind your head while breathing out. Hold your breath and position for 3 seconds.
  - *Arm Isometrics*: Push down on the armrest for the count of 5 and then pull up on the armrest for the count of 5. Repeat 5 times.
  - *Lower-Back Stretch*: Clasp your knee with both hands, pull it to your chest, and hold it there for the count of 5. Repeat with other leg.
  - *Leg/Foot Stretch*: With your shoes off, press firmly with your palms on both knees. Dorsiflex your foot so your heels are touching the floor and your toes are raised as high as possible. Then plantar flex so that your toes touch the floor and the heels are raised. Repeat quickly 8 times.

- Use the airplane restroom before landing. This may save up to 20 minutes on the ground if you are first to the taxis or car rental counters.

- Shuttle/taxi/train/rental car: Ask the residency program you are visiting for the best and cheapest (they may be different) way to get from the airport to the hospital. Trains will usually be the cheapest and fastest transportation method—but may not be the safest method at certain times of the day. Also, you may have to lug your baggage a distance to get to the train. A useful alternative is an airport shuttle. Remember to get the cheaper round-trip fare. Taxis are for those who don't have to watch their budget and cars are for special situations or for additional sightseeing in the area.

- Use a skycap to avoid taxi lines. A small tip can save lots of time.

schools may use this service to contact student-housers at other participating schools when they go there to interview. If you have trouble finding out about this service, call the Association of American Medical Colleges at (202) 828-0682.

The American Medical Women's Association runs a "Bed and Breakfast Program" for its student members traveling to residency interviews (and also for physician members going to job interviews or conferences). When a member calls the AMWA office with her trip details, they supply a list of volunteer hosts in the city to which the member is traveling so she can call to make appropriate arrangements. This seems more personal and, of course, much cheaper than typical out-of-town accommodations. For further information, write AMWA, 801 N. Fairfax St., Suite 400, Alexandria, VA 22314-1767, or call (703) 838-0500, fax (703) 549-3864.

The American Medical Student Association has the "Mi Casa, Su Casa" program for its members. Once you know when you will travel to a specific location, call AMSA membership services at (800) 767-2266 to find out if there is a local AMSA host.

Another source for information about inexpensive housing is the residency program at which you are interviewing. If such information is not included in the material they send, call the residency's secretary and ask about good, inexpensive, and *safe* housing near the hospital. You will not be the first one to ask, and the program probably has a list of good places to stay. They may have a special deal with special rates for applicants at local hotels. Some programs even offer housing in a resident's or faculty member's home to applicants who request it. This is especially true if your host is an alumnus of your medical school.

If you decide to go it alone, make sure the location will allow you to make the interview on time. Check out their security in advance—especially if it is in a crime-prone area, as are many locations around large teaching hospitals. If the establishment offers free services, such as breakfast, take advantage of them.

Get enough sleep. Before turning in, make sure that the curtains are tightly closed—and bring along some clothespins to keep them closed. Use a sleep mask for added darkness and a pair of soft earplugs for quiet. (Make sure to test the mask and earplugs at home to become used to them—and to be sure you can still hear your alarm clock.) Check the alarm clock (bringing yours is even better) to make sure that it works. Then go to bed in time to get enough sleep and still get to the interview a little early (to reduce your stress).

During your personal time, take advantage of the local area, including the museums, sporting and cultural events, or shopping. To avoid the common feelings of isolation, stay in touch with friends and family via phone or E-mail. You might want to invest in a long-distance pager or cell phone for a few months, so people can contact you, if necessary. Also, exercise as you would at home. Check with your hosts or the hotel about nearby, safe exercise areas.

### Simultaneous Vacationing

As mentioned, the interview circuit is no picnic. But in some situations, you can turn it into a real vacation. If you try to chronologically cluster interviews, but there is a break in your interview schedule, see if there are places for you to vacation in the surrounding area. This can give you a relaxing break in the action—a needed rest period at a relatively low cost, since you are already nearby. If you have a spouse or significant other, he or she might want to meet you at this spot. A friendly face is sometimes a very welcome sight and helps to bolster the spirits. And having someone to talk to and to share your experiences with may add to the relief. Given the stresses of medical school and the anticipated heavy work schedule to come, you and (if you have one) your spouse or significant other probably need a vacation anyway!

## Updating Information About The Programs

As the time for your interviews draws near, recontact the programs where you will be interviewing to request any new or updated information and re-check their websites. The material that you were initially sent was prepared the previous spring or earlier. Many things could have changed at the program. Some might even affect whether you still go to that institution for an interview. Other changes may affect your final program rankings.

The best time to ask about any changes in the program is when you arrange a date for your interview. If there is new written material, ask them to send you a copy. If it has not yet been printed, ask for as much information about the changes as possible.

Undoubtedly, you will be a more appealing candidate to the interviewers if you know up-to-date information about their program. If you don't, they will wonder why. So be sure to get the latest available information on the program before you leave for your interviews. Ask about changes once again when you are at the program—of the program director, the residency secretary, and the current residents.

## Communicating With The Programs

Once you send your initial application packet, you will mostly communicate with programs by telephone.

The first time you should call the programs is about a month after you have requested that your material be sent to them. Find out if it has all arrived. If not, what is missing?

How you communicate with a program is very important. It is amazing that the nicest, most sophisticated individuals often have a terrible telephone "presence." Your voice over the telephone and your attitude on it will make a big impression on a program. Don't think that you can behave any way you want to on the telephone because you are *only* talking to the residency secretary! And don't express your extreme annoyance at being put on hold in rather crude terms.

As in many businesses, a secretary who interacts with applicants often has a major impact on who is selected—both for interviews and for final positions. Many residency directors ask their secretaries for input. And most take this input very seriously. Polish your telephone technique. Polish up those residency secretaries. They can be either your allies or your enemies. Make them think of you as a nice person, the kind that they want as a resident in *their* program.

E-mail is the modern way to communicate, and this also goes for residency programs. Increasingly, programs notify applicants via E-mail when they are selected for interviews. They also request that specific questions be forwarded either to the residency directors or their assistants via E-mail. As with other correspondence, be certain that your E-mail messages to the programs are coherent, spell-checked, and grammatically correct. One way of improving your E-mail is to write them on a word processor and then paste the messages into your correspondence.

# 16

# Looking The Part:
# Interview Attire

*In your town, your reputation counts; in another, your clothes do.*
— Talmud, Shabboth

*I base most of my fashion sense on what doesn't itch.*
— Gilda Radner

The key here is to do what others do—but better. Yes, there is a "uniform" to wear. It is conservative, tasteful, and neat. It looks like upper-middle-class success. And it works. Of course, you wore jeans and sweatshirts during your first two years of medical school. Maybe you wore less as an undergraduate. You love to hang around the wards dressed in a wrinkled scrub suit, looking just like the residents. Don't imitate their sloppy dress; residents already have their training slots. Now is the time for you to shine—both literally and figuratively.

One interviewee, medical student Scott Fishman, described this uniform as "remarkably drab . . . a ridiculous costume . . . a rite of passage." He went on to say that, "sitting there waiting for our turns outside the interviewer's office, we all look like we are going to a funeral." Perhaps. But better to wear the uniform and appear to go to a funeral than not wear it and attend your own.

No, you don't have to go out and spend lots of money you don't have on clothes you can't afford. Just do what you can to get into the uniform. Ideally, interviewers should not be aware of your clothes; you want them to remember you, not what you wore. The proper dress for residency interviews is essentially identical, no matter where in the country you are applying. Appropriate dress can help you a little. The wrong outfit will destroy you.

401

Remember that in the first seven seconds, interviewers make decisions based on your visual cues: your clothes, grooming, walk, stance, etc. After that, they begin evaluating you through your verbal skills.

# Men

### The Suit
A *suit* is the standard dress for an interview. It should be solid or pinstripe, navy or gray. "The men who run America," says John T. Molloy, author of *Dress for Success*, "run it blue, gray, and dull." Do not wear a suit with bright or avant-garde colors or designs. "If you try to spruce up the look," Mr. Molloy continues, "you're in trouble."

The suit need be neither expensive nor in the latest style, but it should be well-cut and well-tailored. If you either don't have or cannot afford a suit, wear a navy-blue sport jacket with matching pants. If you don't have these either, it is time you visited a clothing store. Charge the bill to your future. Serious and solid is the image you are looking for in your outfit. And *before* you show up at your first interview, make sure that your clothes fit well. Few things distract an interviewer more than an applicant fidgeting with his tight collar.

### The Shirt
Wear either a white or pale-blue solid-color *shirt*. Long sleeves are in order if you plan to remove your jacket. Avoid stripes, loud colors, or any weird designs. Shirttails should be long enough to keep the shirt tucked in, even when you raise your arms. With the top button fastened, your collar should fit snugly, but not so tightly that your eyes bulge.

### The Tie
Wear a *tie*—even if you are a laid-back individual. An open-neck shirt and gold chain just won't cut it. Your tie should be solid, have repeating stripes (rep), small polka dots, or repeating small insignias (club). Avoid gaudy, bright colors, large patterns, and black. The "power colors" are red and navy. Knot the tie so its tip meets the belt and put the back of the tie through the label, so the ends stay together. Do not wear a bow tie. It gives the impression that you're odd, like showing the world that you're odd, and are out of touch with this decade.

### The Shoes & Socks
Wear black or very dark brown conservatively designed *shoes*. Make sure that they are in good repair and shined. Dirty shoes are male applicants' most common clothing error. Also make sure that there are no holes in

your soles, and if there are, be sure to keep your feet flat on the floor. Wear calf-length plain socks that match your suit.

If you wear an *undershirt*, a crew neck looks best, since it doesn't show through a shirt. A plain, dark leather *belt* with a small square buckle works well. If you wear *suspenders*, be sure that they button to your pants. If you carry a *wallet*, make sure that it does not bulge out of your pocket.

## Accessories

The key here is sedate. Limit *jewelry* to a watch and wedding band (only if you are married). If you wear a watch, avoid anything unusual such as a dive watch or one with a picture of Mickey Mouse on the front. No lapel pins, no ID bracelets, no tie clasps, and—definitely—*NO EARRINGS!* No matter what the protestations, that little flash of gold will cost you big points. Save it for later. Inappropriate or too much jewelry will elicit very strong negative responses.

If you wear *glasses*, make sure that they are in standard frames. No initials on the lenses or unusual colors. It's best not to wear tinted or photo-gray lenses, since they tend to place a barrier between you and the interviewer. Also, keep the lenses clean.

The *pen* and *pencil* you carry should look classy. They do not have to be gold, but they should not look like you got them from hospital stores or the local drug rep. And don't stick them in a shirt-pocket protector. To look the part of a serious candidate and have a convenient place to make notes and store papers, carry a small, folding, zippered, leather-covered *note pad* with the materials you need.

## Grooming

As for *personal grooming*, be neat, squeaky clean, and conservative. Your *hair* should be short. If it's shorter than you like it, it's probably close to the right length. Ask your mentor (if he or she is over 35 years old), a parent, or close (older) friend to advise you on this. Definitely, no ponytails, punk, or otherwise unusual haircuts. Make sure all hair has been very recently trimmed and washed. Invest in a good haircut about one week before the interview; haircuts look best after one week. If you wear facial hair, avoid goatees and handlebar mustaches which have strong negative connotations. Keep any tattoos covered. Trim and manicure your *nails*. Remember, you are about to be a physician, putting your hands on, and in, patients.

The *odor* the interviewer perceives should only be that of deodorant or nervousness. Avoid after-shave; you are not going on a date. If you are concerned about your breath, carry breath mints. And, above all, no alcohol within 24 hours of the interview. There are enough perceived and anticipated problems with drug abuse among housestaff. You do not have to show the interviewers that you could be part of the problem.

The bottom line is that you want to look as much like a successful upper-middle-class physician as possible. Wear the garments symbolizing the successful individual in our society. You certainly did it to get into medical school. It's time to do it again. There is no need to flaunt your lifestyle in your dress. Leave your personal preferences out of this. They can only harm you.

# Women

### The Suit
Although styles are changing in the workplace, the standard dress for a woman going to an interview is still the *suit*. In this case, it is a skirted suit. A good skirted suit suggests that you are an upper-middle-class professional—just the image you want to project. Don't be led down the path to destruction by following fads or fashion. The classic suit is the uniform of success. Find out what woman accountants or lawyers who work for large firms wear. This will be the "classic" style.

In purchasing a suit, choose wool, linen, or a synthetic that simulates either. The fabric should be solid, tweed, or plaid. For solid suits, the three best colors are gray (a couple of shades lighter than charcoal), medium-range blue, and dark maroon. Stay away from bold, flashy patterns. The skirt should extend to just below the knee (no miniskirts!) and the matching jacket should be a blazer cut with long sleeves.

Two alternatives to the suit are a tailored dress or a skirt worn with a jacket. Neither is as powerful as the suit, but if you do not feel comfortable in a suit, these are two reasonable substitutes.

### The Blouse
Your *blouse* should be simply cut, neither too frilly nor with excess lace. The neckline must not be too low. If it is equivalent to a man's shirt with one button open, it will be acceptable. The blouse should be cotton, silk, or a look-alike synthetic. In general, it should be in a complementary solid color to the suit. Usually it will be white, cream, or pastel—not red or fuchsia.

### The Shoes
*Shoes* should be simple pumps, closed at the toe and heel—and not brand new. They should be in a dark or neutral color that is compatible with your suit. The heels should not be more than 1½ inches high. Do not wear boots. Most residency applicants will be doing a lot of walking around the hospital; be sure that you will survive in the shoes you wear.

## Accessories

Although a *scarf* is not as essential as a man's tie, it can be eye-catching if used properly. Wear silk or a look-alike synthetic and tie it in an ascot, necktie, or scout style. If worn, a scarf must have simple lines and no frills to detract from the center of attention—your face. *Hosiery* should be skin-colored.

As with men, the less *jewelry* that you wear the better. Aside from a simple watch and wedding ring (if married), be careful about what other ornaments you wear. While a brooch or a simple necklace is often very suitable, multiple rings, bracelets, or anything ornate or gaudy is not. The appropriate watch is plain gold or silver. Only wear nose rings for religious reasons. If you need to wear an *overcoat*, make sure that it is long enough to cover the bottom of your skirt. Multiple coat styles are acceptable; furs are not. If you wear *gloves*, make them leather. They should match your coat in color.

*Do not carry a purse.* Carry a leather zippered case, attaché case, or leather-bound zippered notebook with any necessities. This connotes power and authority. Put everything that you need in it, but do not overstuff it or keep it sloppy—you may have to open it during an interview. Some students have written that using the zippered notebook is less awkward when carried to lunch, labs, or on ward tours. If using an attaché case, include a small leather-covered notepad. Avoid the drug company *pens* you use on the wards.

## Grooming

As for the more *personal items*, such as hair, makeup, and perfume, just remember that you are going on a job interview, not on a date. If the interviewer is aware that you are wearing *perfume*, you are wearing too much. Similarly with *makeup*—it works best when it is not obvious. Be especially careful to avoid obvious eye shadow or eyeliner. *Nails* should be well manicured. Your *hair* should be clean and conservative in appearance. If it is long, it is often a good idea to put it up to keep it from looking sloppy. Many consultants recommend that women should not have hairstyles that cover either eye and should be pulled away from the jaw line and ears so they will look more serious.

The bottom line is that you dress for the interview in a uniform. Although there is considerable variation allowed, for maximum success, applicants should adhere to the standard style. As one woman physician who did very well in her resident interviews said about the wardrobe, "sophistication and maturity are the keys to success."

## Clothing As Camouflage

Clothes can hide real or perceived problems. For those "Doogie Howser" types who think they look too young to be taken seriously, dressing conservatively will age you a bit. Wearing glasses, even if you normally wear contacts, also helps.

Some people are self-conscious about their weight. Clothes can help disguise those extra pounds. Both men and women can wear suit jackets slightly longer than normal, and women can wear a loose jacket over a business dress or flared skirt. The key is to be certain that your clothes fit well. Even thin people look heavy if their buttons are popping out or their collar is too tight.

## Wear The "Uniform" Stylishly

Now that you have acquired the uniform, make sure that you get the most out of it. Your clothes must appear neat, clean, and pressed. Do *not* travel in your clothes and show up five minutes before the interview looking like a Raggedy Anne doll that has gone through the washer. If possible, arrive at the interview city the night before, having traveled in your normal attire. You will get a good night's sleep and put on your freshly pressed uniform the next morning to go to the interview. Be sure to have the appropriate garments, such as overcoat, umbrella, etc., to protect your uniform in case of inclement weather. When you get to the interview site, slip into the restroom and give yourself a last-minute inspection.

Once you dress correctly for your interview, forget about your clothes. They should be a natural part of you. Think of these clothes like new hiking boots. You don't want to go 20 miles in a new pair without breaking them in first. If you aren't comfortable in these fancy duds, wear them a few times before you hit the interview trail.

## How To Pack For The Interview Trip

In packing for interviews, the motto should be "less is more." That will often be the only way to get all the necessities into the allowable size and number of bags. Two simple techniques for doing this are to either limit the time you have to pack to 20 minutes per city you will visit, or to put out everything you want for your trip—and then put half of it away.

Sophisticated travelers decrease the amount they carry by making sure that all their clothes go with everything else, by packing clothes that can serve more than one function, and by avoiding the tendency to pack for each potential "what if?" that could happen on the trip. Wear the bulky items. You can always stow a heavy coat in the overhead bin.

Packing lists ease pre-trip anxieties. Once you make a decision about what to take with you on one trip, use the same packing list for subsequent trips. That way you won't forget anything. Keep the list with you to serve as a record of your belongings in case your bags are lost.

## How To Pack A Suitcase

Whether you use a large suitcase or a smaller carry-on, the goal is for your clothes to arrive intact and as pristine as possible. To accomplish this, place trousers, skirts, dresses, shirts, blouses and jackets (all zipped or buttoned, and folded along their natural seams) in the suitcase, alternating side to side. If first placed in a plastic cleaner's bag, suits, skirts, and dresses will often remain more pristine.

Only after all items are laying partially in the suitcase should the remainder lying outside the suitcase be folded in, one garment over the other (Figure 16.1). Each item will then cushion the others and help prevent creases. Pack shoes, stuffed with toiletries, rolled-up socks, belts, etc., along the hinged side of the bag. Finally, stuff rolled T-shirts, under-garments, sleepwear, and sweaters in any available space to cushion the contents and keep them from shifting. The result should be neat and clean clothing.

On multi-day trips, where you won't unpack and stay at the same location, put the items you will wear together on the same layer, so you can simply reach in and pull them all out together. To reduce the stress of residency interview trips, take along a memento of home, such as a family picture, a favorite book, or even a pillow (if you are not traveling by air).

## What To Do If Your Suitcase Doesn't Show Up

### Use Carry-on, if Possible

A danger when flying is that your checked baggage won't show up—at least not in time to do you any good. The fact that it appears back at your home the day after the interview is little consolation for being forced to dress in "low camp" style for the interview at your most desired program. The solution, especially if you are only going to be away from home for one or two days, is to use the combination of a carry-on suit bag and an under-the-seat bag. This often suffices very well, saves you time retrieving your bags at the airport, and alleviates any worry about your uniform not showing up.

It is *essential* to carry interview schedules, airline tickets, travelers checks, credit cards, drivers license, jewelry, hotel and automobile confir-mations, airline schedules, medications, and the telephone numbers and addresses for your travel agent and your interviews with you. (I have seen

## FIGURE 16.1

### *Packing a Suitcase*

Before packing, every garment should be buttoned, zippered, belted, and folded along natural creases.

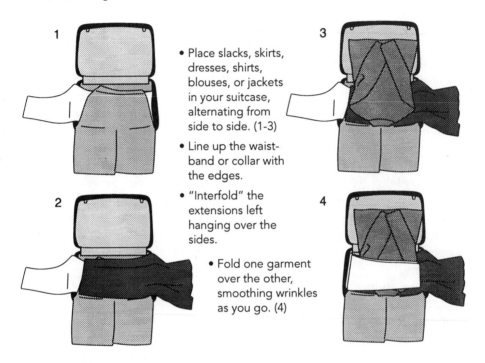

• Place slacks, skirts, dresses, shirts, blouses, or jackets in your suitcase, alternating from side to side. (1-3)

• Line up the waist-band or collar with the edges.

• "Interfold" the extensions left hanging over the sides.

  • Fold one garment over the other, smoothing wrinkles as you go. (4)

**Each item will cushion the other, helping to prevent creases.**

more than one distraught applicant whose bag containing his interview materials, not to mention his clothes, had been lost.)

Be careful when choosing your carry-on bags. Each airline, and even each plane or configuration of seats on a particular airline, has different allowable space and different rules for carry-ons. It is wise to check with a travel agent or the airline to avoid arriving with one bag too many. Typically, airlines allow each traveler two carry-ons, not counting purses, umbrellas, coats, cameras and books. The typical maximum size for under-seat bags is 9" x 14" x 22", and for overhead compartments it is 10" x 14" x 24". If possible, get a carry-on with wheels and a garment bag that attaches to it. (Many coach flights, however, will no longer accommodate garment bags.) If you can roll it, your back will thank you.

### Honesty Works (The Sympathy & Uniqueness Votes)

Okay, so you weren't able to use the carry-on method—and now your baggage is somewhere between here and Outer Mongolia. You have an interview in three hours and are wearing hand-me-downs from a back-woods orphanage. What should you do?

First, don't panic. Any faculty member who will be interviewing you has undoubtedly had a great deal of airline travel experience. And anyone with that amount of experience has also had his or her bags misplaced by the airlines—more than once. However, you need to make some show of good faith. First, badger the airline representatives. If you present a good enough sob story, they might front you money for a decent shirt and tie (or blouse and scarf). You will need at least this much. Then, when you get to the interview, apologize to everyone you meet for your appearance. The "airline-lost-my-luggage" story never fails to both get the sympathy (or empathy) vote and to keep that applicant in the interviewers' minds. A good story and a good attitude may actually win you some points.

### Tax Tip

Since you may have just spent substantial sums on clothes, travel and transportation, you may be asking yourself whether these expenses are tax deductible. The answer is yes and no.

Most applicants are medical students who have no substantial income. Without income, they pay no taxes, so there are no deductions. In any event, students will be applying for their first job in medicine, so Uncle Sam would not allow the deductions anyway.

If, however, you are already working as a physician and are now applying for a residency or fellowship position, keep a careful record of your expenses (including postage, copying, telephone calls, travel, and lodging). These may be deductible as job search expenses if you itemize your income tax return.

# FEEDBACK FORM*

Much of the most valuable information in this book comes from students like yourself. Please share your experiences. I would like to pass on the following information or experience for inclusion in the next edition of this book:

_____

_____

_____

_____

_____

_____

_____

_____

_____

Name (please print)

_____

Address

_____

_____

E-mail (optional)

**\*Please return to:**
Kenneth V. Iserson, M.D., Galen Press, Ltd.
P.O. Box 64400, Tucson, Arizona 85728-4400 USA

or E-mail: info@galenpress.com

# 17

# The Visit

*Hiring decisions are made in the first 30 seconds of the interview—*
*the balance of the time is used to justify the decision.*
– An axiom in the personnel field

*Illusions are comforting; just don't rely on them.*
– Folk Saying

Okay, so you have your interviews set up and you are ready to go and "knock their socks off." Remember that it is not only your interview performance, but also how you conduct yourself throughout your entire time at a program that will determine whether the faculty ranks you highly. So, here are some last minute tips to help you smooth out any remaining rough spots in the way you will present yourself.

## Timeliness

To mangle an old saying, "Timeliness is next to Godliness." You will make a major impact on all interviewers, a significantly *negative* impact, if you are late for your appointments. Excuses are fine for your mother, your spouse, and sometimes your friends and teachers. But they work poorly on prospective employers. Faculty's time is valuable, and they have set some of it aside to interview you. Don't waste their time, or yours, by being late.

Of course, unavoidable delays do occur. Unexpected bad weather and transportation breakdowns are the two most common causes (especially during the interview season—with the worst weather of the year). If you run into difficulties that will cause you to be late, have the courtesy to call ahead. Even if you only think that you *might* be delayed due to these or other valid factors, let the program know early. They will then be able to reschedule people and, possibly, to work you in at a later time or on a later date. Do not leave them wondering what happened to you. Even if you do not care about that program, leaving them hanging is extremely discourteous and unprofessional, and it may cost you a position at another program. Remember that many academics know each other—and they do talk about applicants when they get together. *The key then is to show up on time, ready for action!*

## Confirm Your Interview

Although you are expected to be on time and at the correct location, either you or the program may have made a scheduling error. It is very embarrassing for an applicant to show up on the wrong day for a scheduled interview because of a communication error.

Occasionally there is a disaster at the residency program that mandates that interviews be postponed or rescheduled. Mistakes happen, especially when there are dozens or hundreds of individuals interviewing at the same program during a short time period. And since you may very well be on the road, there may be no way to contact you about such a situation. The professional way to avoid complications is to call ahead to confirm your interview a day or two before traveling to the program. That way you stand little chance of making a wasted trip or being embarrassed by a scheduling mistake.

## Know The Schedule

If you can get your interview schedule for each program before you arrive, so much the better. Have them fax or E-mail it to you. You will then know how to pace yourself throughout the visit. You will also be able to plan specific activities for any "free-time" blocks. These periods can be used to visit the library, the wards, the other teaching hospitals in the program if they are nearby, and the cafeteria. Since this could be the food you eat for the next several years—how bad is it?

If you cannot get your entire schedule, at least find out what time you begin. Recheck your information the afternoon before to make certain that it is correct. You cannot afford to be late. It usually helps if you are early. Even if you have never been early for anything in your life, this would be an excellent time to start.

Once you get started on your interviews, it is up to the interviewers themselves, and the residency secretary, to keep everyone on schedule. Many interviewers have a bad habit of running over their allotted time. Do not let this make you uncomfortable. However, when you get to the next appointment late, apologize immediately and explain that you just got out of your last interview with Dr. X. If it happens to you, it has happened to others—and faculty members will understand and not count it against you. They probably are already aware of their colleagues' foibles.

## Leave Some Time Flexible

Now that you have gotten the interview and have worked hard to make a good impression, do not ruin it all by running out early. Would you leave a fancy dinner party before dessert? Of course not. Scheduling departing flights out of town without giving yourself enough flexibility to "eat dessert" is the same situation. If you book yourself too tightly, you will not allow yourself any leeway in case your interviews run overtime. When they do, it will usually be because one or more of the faculty has an extra interest in your candidacy. This is a golden opportunity; don't blow it.

Also, you may find you have a greater interest in a program than you initially thought you would. In that case, you may want to investigate that program's finer points while you are there. You will need some extra time to do this. Remain a little flexible.

# Attitude

*SMILE!* It doesn't cost you anything. Of course you are prepared to be on your best behavior with interviewers. But astute program directors are just as interested in how you act outside the formal interview setting as in how you do in it. This tells them more about how you will act during day-to-day program activities, how you will interact with your peers, and whether you will be able to get along with the ancillary medical staff.

Be pleasant to everyone, and be pleasant at all times. This does not mean you must fawn over the residents and bow down to the secretaries. It does mean, at the least, that you should not ignore them. They are real people. Treat them as the friendly individuals they probably are. Be pleasant and try to interact with them warmly. This also holds true for other applicants. If the other applicants like you, this is often seen as a very positive point in your favor. When applicants are observed as a group, those who get along with others can be clearly identified. And working well with a team is a key ingredient in being a successful resident.

The bottom line, then, is that input from sources other than the interviewers is often very important. You should consider yourself under observation the entire time you interact with the program. The show doesn't stop until you walk out the hospital door at the end of the day, and it continues with every phone and written contact you make with the program.

One point worthy of mention is that reviewing your own medical school file may help you prepare for these interactions. The narrative part of your file usually contains a wealth of information from faculty and residents concerning how others perceive you. Take time to read through it before your interviews. Insights that you gain could lead to more positive interactions with the interviewers, as well as improvements in all of your personal relations.

## Uniqueness

Interviewers, like all individuals, receive only a small portion of the information sent to them. There is a great deal of "noise" between the sender's encoded message and the receiver's decoding of that message (Figure 17.1). Receivers take this information and change it to fit their preconceived ideas. It is from this information that they make decisions. As a residency applicant, you battle three communication devils.

### Selective Exposure

People are constantly exposed to a tremendous amount of stimuli. They really notice only exceptional deviations from normal patterns. These deviations can either be positive (beneficial to you) or negative (counterproductive to you). It is essential that you be noticed—and noticed positively.

FIGURE 17.1

*Elements in the Communication Process*

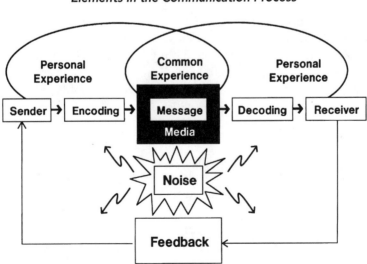

## Selective Distortion

People tend to interpret data in ways that support, rather than challenge, their preconceptions. These preconceptions of you will, most likely, be based upon the written material that you have supplied to the program. It is your job to add to the positive feeling you have already worked so hard to create.

## Selective Retention

People forget much of what they learn. And they forget it quickly. Your job is to make sure that they remember you.

# Knowledge

## About The Specialty

You have worked hard to get interviews for a position in your chosen specialty. Be certain you know a great deal about that specialty before you arrive at the programs. This does not mean medical knowledge; you will acquire that during your training. It means that you should know about the specialty's culture.

- What do the practitioners in the field really do?
- What types of procedures do they perform?
- What level of reimbursement should they expect?
- How do other specialists perceive them?
- Do they have opportunities for subspecialty training?
- What are the requirements to take the specialty's board examination?
- What is the outlook for the specialty in the future?

These are the types of questions that you should have asked yourself while making an informed decision about which specialty you wanted to enter. Faculty members want to know that you have made the effort to learn about their specialty before you commit your entire professional life to it.

If you do not have this information, you may not have fully thought out your decision, and could later be very unhappy. Unhappiness is bad for both the resident and the faculty. It leads to depression, anger, and poor performance. It can also cause a resident to drop out of a program before graduation. Therefore, demonstrate that you have seriously thought about your career choice. Know about the specialty. Read the specialty journals and newsletters concerning pending changes within the field. The latter, if you can get copies, are the most current. Read the editorials to know about the specialty's "hot topics." The more you know about a specialty, the more committed to it you will appear. And commitment is one of the most important qualities interviewers seek.

### About The Program
Just as you must know the basic information about your chosen specialty, you also need to know about each program you visit.

You initially received a lot of information in the program's packet. If you were as careful as you should have been, you also have received additional written or oral information which updated the packet. Review this information before going into the interview. No matter whether this is the first program at which you are interviewing or the twentieth, it is a major *faux pas* to confuse basics about the program where you are currently interviewing with information from another program. Be sure that you have the facts about the current program firmly in your mind before you set out in the morning. If you, like most people, have a little trouble keeping the details straight, write yourself some notes for reference.

Another way to get additional information about a program is to run a MEDLINE search on the faculty. Looking at articles that the faculty have published will give you an idea of their medical interests. It may also provide some insight into questions they might ask you or subjects they might like to discuss. In any case, the more you know about a specific program before going into the interview setting, the better the chance that you will leave highly regarded and be well-remembered.

Many programs use more than one hospital for training. If possible, see them all, even if you are only scheduled for interviews at one or two of them. They may not want to show you the other institution(s) for a very good reason—you would not rank the program if you saw them!

## Talk To Residents For The Real Story

If you haven't talked to the current residents, assume that you really do not know very much about the program. Be very wary of any program that not only does not give you the opportunity, but also does not insist that you talk to some of its residents. Residents often see things quite differently than the attending physicians. And their perspectives, while not necessarily the same as those you might have in the same situation, may be much closer to yours than those of the faculty. These talks are usually informal, and because of limitations on the residents' time, may occur in group settings. Nevertheless, the residents' opinions, viewpoints, and insights about the program should strongly influence how you will rate it for each of the factors on your "Must/Want" Analysis.

If there is a senior medical student on rotation in the department while you are there, try to talk to him or her. You cannot afford to miss this valuable perspective. One other source of information might be a graduate from your medical school who is currently training at that institution. Even if not in the same program to which you are applying, he or she will have intimate knowledge of the institution, and may even know something about your prospective department. Graduates from your *alma mater* may also feel some loyalty to you—and give you otherwise "forgotten" information. You will probably be able to locate such graduates through either your Dean of Students or your school's Alumni Office.

## Basic Rules

Once you actually get to the interview site there are some very basic things that you need to do, aside from answering any questions in a satisfactory manner. In fact, questions and answers may, in some cases, be merely window dressing for the actual interview process.

The "behavioral interview" is becoming more common as laws limit to an ever greater extent the questions that interviewers can ask. Behavioral interviewers are much more interested in whether you look and act like you would fit into a job rather than whether you can answer any specific questions. They look for communication skills, physical presence, motivation, truthfulness, and how suited each applicant is to be a resident in their program.

All good interviewers look for small, but important, details. Some of these are discussed below.

### Show Enthusiasm For This Program

It is important to show your enthusiasm for the specialty. But being enthusiastic about entering the training program *at which you are currently interviewing* makes interviewers rate you even more highly. Base your eagerness on the strong points that you gleaned from the program's packet of information. Generally the areas of which the program is most proud are included in their packet. So basing your interest on these areas will get the best results.

An amazing number of applicants arrive at programs with the attitude that either: (1) they are browsing and will not reveal that they really *want* a position at the program; or (2) the attitude toward the program that they demonstrate while interviewing will not influence their selection as a potential resident. Both approaches are wrong. Show enthusiasm! If you cannot work up any enthusiasm for a program, perhaps you should not be interviewing there. Also, if you can't garner enthusiasm for the program and specialty now, you won't be able to do it during your third 30-hour on-call stint in a week.

## Know How To Pronounce Your Interviewers' Names

How do you say Dr. Llnoyphthg? You don't know? How could that be when he will be interviewing you in five minutes? It may seem petty, especially with some of the difficult or unique pronunciations of names in the medical world, to expect you to know how to pronounce, on the first try, all the names of the people that you will meet. But it is expected. So you should know how. Remember that above all else, a person's name is a unique part of him or her. Mispronouncing an interviewer's name can, even if sub-consciously, leave a negative impression of an applicant.

At the start of the day, ask the residency secretary how to pronounce any difficult or unusual names among those listed on your interview schedule. As she tells you, write each down phonetically so you will be able to repeat it correctly when necessary. If this is not possible, listen carefully when the individual introduces him or herself to you. If it is a difficult name, repeat it and ask if you said it right. Don't slip up on this simple point of etiquette.

## Enter & Depart In A Polite, Assured Manner

Look confident! Walk into the interview with your head up, shoulders squared, looking poised. Pause briefly as you enter the room to assert your strong presence. If you slink into an interview like a scared rabbit, how are you going to look to an interviewer? Certainly not like one of the people likely to get a spot in their residency program. Remember that initial impressions are very important. In the first minute, interviewers determine whether applicants meet their expectations. Let your body send a message of confidence, calmness, and control.

Greet interviewers with a firm, but not bone-crushing, handshake. This goes for both men and women. The dainty dead-fish handshake used by many women, as well as some men in the past, connotes only meekness and a lack of authority. Avoid it like the plague. Extend your hand to the other person with the thumb up and out. Make sure that the web between your thumb and index finger meets the other person's web. Try to shake hands from the elbow, not the shoulder or wrist. It is also desirable to have reasonably dry hands. If your palms have a tendency to sweat when you get nervous, dry them off just before meeting each interviewer. One solution to sweaty palms is to sit, before interviews, with your palms exposed to the air rather than stuffed in a pocket or lying face down in your lap.

Also greet the interviewer with an enthusiastic voice and manner. When you begin speaking to an individual, the actual words you speak are much less important than the manner in which you say them. The first thing interviewers notice is your tone of voice. You will also be judged by your enthusiasm, facial expressions, gestures, and posture. Therefore, try to act as if you are really pleased to have an opportunity to talk with the faculty and residents. Practice this with some critical observers at home. You must not sound forced or pretentious. If you do, you will do yourself more harm than good. Sincere enthusiasm will greatly enhance your entire visit.

During the interview, sit comfortably straight, leaning slightly forward in the chair. This demonstrates your interest through nonverbal cues. You can prove this to yourself. Have a friend (trying to keep a neutral expression in both instances) first face you, sitting forward in a chair. Then have the individual lean back in a relaxed posture. If you were the interviewer, which candidate would interest you more?

Other negative body-language traits include resting your head on your hand, tilting your head to one side (the coy look), and fiddling with your beard, hair, mustache, or earrings. Keep your head upright and your hands away from your head. Likewise, don't fiddle with your clothes, pen, or anything else.

Look your interviewer in the eyes. Applicants who look away when they answer questions suggest either that there is something less than honest about their answers or that they are afraid of the situation. Those who look away when the interviewer is talking (a true kiss of death) indicate that they do not care about what the interviewer is saying. Obviously, neither situation is favorable. Always try to look an interviewer in the eyes. Some experienced interviewers suggest looking at a person first in one eye, then the other. The recipient gets the feeling that the listener is listening intently; the listener avoids a glazed look some people get when they look at a person only in one eye (a common behavior). If you plan to try this, practice ahead of time; the first few times you do this you may be distracted and not hear what the speaker is saying.

Acknowledge what the interviewer is saying by nodding, and with brief verbal phrases such as "I see," "Of course," or "Yes." Try not to use expressions such as "wow," "right on," or "groovy," which connote something other than professionalism. It helps to vary the expression you use so you don't sound wooden or monotonous.

Your exit from the interview must also be graceful and enthusiastic. As speech writers know, the last thing heard will be remembered best. Shake your interviewer's hand and say again how glad you are to have had a chance to talk with him or her. Offer to provide any other information he or she might desire about you. You will rarely, if ever, be taken up on this offer. State that you look forward to working with him or her. This should take less than fifteen seconds and appear very smooth. It would not hurt to practice this one little segment so you don't appear awkward. As you can see from some television interviews, even the best speakers and the most intelligent individuals often look like dolts when terminating an interview. Don't let this be your downfall.

### You Are Not Selling A Medical Student—You Are Selling A Promise

Forget that you are a medical student. In the interview scenario, you are the promise of a bright future. You will be the specialty's finest clinician, a noted researcher, a diligent healer of indigent patients, a solid member of the medical community. You will achieve this because you are an extremely hard worker who is compulsive, intelligent, responsive to teaching, happy in your work, and no trouble to the faculty.

That is the promise you are selling. To get into your chosen program, you must project the ability to make this promise a reality. How can you make a contribution to this program? You are the salesman. You are the product. Go forth and sell.

## Materials For The Interview

Although it may seem rather silly to detail what you need to take with you to interviews, it is surprising how many applicants seem to forget some of the necessary basic materials. In addition to the basics, two forms, the *Interview Notes*, Figure 17.2, and your "*Must/Want*" Analysis (see Figure 10.1 for a blank copy) are suggested as part of your standard interview equipment. These will aid you later when you evaluate each program and write your follow-up letters.

### General Materials

The first two items that you need to bring with you are the *directions to the interview site and the telephone numbers* with which to contact the program if you get lost or are delayed. Next, carry along whatever *information you have received from the program*. Not only should you review it immediately prior to setting out for the interview in the morning, but you may also want to consult it during the interview day to refresh your memory or recheck questionable points brought up in conversation.

Of course, you should have a *list of questions* that you want to ask at each program (see Chapter 19), as well as a pad of *paper* and a *pen* to record the answers. Test your pens to make sure that they work. Bring a *photograph* of yourself to give to the residency secretary when you arrive. Finally, if you have any additional credentials or paperwork that will be vital for the program to have, such as a written military deferment for training, be certain that you bring these with you.

Finally, bring *something to read*, be it a specialty journal, a news magazine, or newspaper. At most programs, you will spend a lot of time waiting. If you have something to occupy your mind, it will make you more alert and less cranky.

## Interview Notes

The Interview Notes form (Figure 17.2) is designed to give you an organized method for remembering key information obtained during interviews. It will also act as a reminder when you want to send follow-up notes or materials to individual interviewers. Write the phonetic spelling of the interviewers' names on this form. The *Companion Disk for Getting Into A Residency* will print out blank Interview Notes forms.

Some students have written that they took the elements from the "Must/Want" Analysis that were key to their decision making and abstracted the information onto a separate form. They used that form to take notes during the interview day. If this serves your needs, go for it.

## Your "Must/Want" Analysis As An Interview Checklist

The "Must/Want" Analysis you previously completed (see Figure 10.1) can now act as an interview checklist (example, Figure 17.3). Its use both simplifies your evaluation of each program and helps you discriminate among them. The factors that compose your personal "Must/Want" Analysis and the weights you assigned to each one will remain constant for all the programs you visit.

Immediately following your visit to each program, score on a 1 to 10 scale (10 is perfect) how well the program does in each category. Even if you have previously given some items "Scores" based on written materials, those "Scores" should be considered tentative until confirmed during the site visit. Then multiply the "Weights" by the "Scores" for each factor to obtain the factor "Total." Adding the values in the "Total" column will give you your personal ranking for the program ("Program Evaluation Score").

FIGURE 17.2
**Interview Notes**

Program _____

Address _____

_____

Secretary _____

Telephone _____

INTERVIEWER                    NOTES

1._____    _____

_____    _____

_____

2._____    _____

_____    _____

_____

3._____    _____

_____    _____

_____

4._____    _____

_____    _____

_____

5._____    _____

_____    _____

_____

6._____    _____

_____    _____

_____

OTHER NOTES

_____

_____

_____

_____

_____

FIGURE 17.3

## *"Must/Want" Analysis as an Interview Checklist–An Example*

PROGRAM  #2–Mako General Hospital          DATE INTERVIEWED:  January 30

| Clinical Experience | WEIGHT | X SCORE | = TOTAL |
|---|---|---|---|
| On-Call Schedule | 5 | 6 | 30 |
| Patient Population | 2 | 5 | 10 |
| Responsibility | 14 | 8 | 112 |
| Setting | 7 | 8 | 56 |
| Volume | 10 | 8 | 80 |
| **Geographic Location** | | | |
| Part of Country | 1 | 2 | 2 |
| Specific City | 1 | 1 | 1 |
| **Reputation** | | | |
| Program Age and Stability | 2 | 5 | 10 |
| **Faculty** | | | |
| Availability | 5 | 4 | 20 |
| Interest | 7 | 7 | 49 |
| Stability | 3 | 3 | 9 |
| **Curriculum** | | | |
| Number of Conferences | 1 | 7 | 7 |
| Special Training | 6 | 9 | 54 |
| Types of Conferences | 2 | 5 | 10 |
| **Esprit de Corps** | 8 | 7 | 56 |
| **Research Opportunities/Training** | | | |
| Knowledge | 5 | 3 | 15 |
| Materials | 2 | 8 | 16 |
| Time | 7 | 8 | 56 |
| **Facilities** | | | |
| Clinical Laboratory Support | 1 | 2 | 2 |
| Library/Media | 2 | 6 | 12 |
| Safety/Security | 3 | 5 | 15 |
| No Restrictive Covenant | MUST | Yes | OK |
| **Benefits: Health Benefits** | | | |
| Health Insurance | MUST | Yes | OK |
| Hospitalization | MUST | Yes | OK |

FIGURE 17.3 (continued)

|  | WEIGHT | X   SCORE | =   TOTAL |
|---|---|---|---|
| **Benefits: Non-Health Benefits** |  |  |  |
| Childcare | MUST | Yes | OK |
| Disability Insurance | MUST | Yes | OK |
| Educational Leave: Funding Available | 1 | 8 | 8 |
| Time Off | 2 | 9 | 18 |
| Liability Insurance | MUST | Yes | OK |
| Vacation | 1 | 7 | 7 |
| **Moonlighting** | 2 | 2 | 4 |

TOTAL OF ALL WEIGHTS  =  __100__

**PROGRAM EVALUATION SCORE = 659**

This "Program Evaluation Score" can later be compared to similar scores which you will calculate after you visit other programs. In some cases, of course, your ratings may suffer from the same problem that interviewers face; early ratings will tend to be lower because they are compared to an ideal, whereas later ratings will tend to be higher since they are being scored in comparison to programs you have already visited. If this is taken into account, you should have no difficulty in correctly interpreting the scores.

The numbers in Figure 17.3 are based on the "Weights" given by our hypothetical applicant from Chapter 10. If you compare Figure 17.3 with Figure 10.10, you will note that some of the "Scores" (in boldface) and "Totals" for this program have been changed based on information obtained during the site visit and interviews. The applicant now has a more complete picture of this program; its "Program Evaluation Score" is now 659.

## Behavior At Lunch

Applicants often go to lunch with the program's residents or faculty members. Several rules apply to this experience, as well as to any business lunch—for that is exactly what it is.

*Stay away from alcohol!* You need to be on your toes, not under the table. Even if you don't lose your wits after imbibing alcohol, your afternoon interviewers may be teetotalers, and thus discount you as a viable candidate if you have been drinking.

*Do not eat too much*. The postprandial tide is a very effective soporific. You don't want to sleep through the afternoon's activities, do you?

*Use good table manners*. If you have never learned them before, now would be an excellent opportunity. You will need to know how to eat in a reasonably civilized manner throughout your medical career. Start this behavior at the interview lunch. Common errors in table manners that cost people jobs include: holding your fork like a knife, talking with your mouth full, not putting the napkin in your lap, not breaking bread before you eat it, and pushing food onto the fork with your thumb. Even in the hospital cafeteria, some table manners are necessary. If you need help, ask a civilized friend.

Pitfalls abound during meals. For example, a tale is told of Admiral Rickover, the father of the U.S. nuclear submarine service, who personally interviewed every officer applying to be a sub captain. If a person salted his food without tasting it, he was eliminated as too rash a decision-maker. Be wary.

If you go to a restaurant, don't order the most expensive items. Also, order food that is easy to eat. Avoid any food that you cannot control. If you aren't skilled at twirling pasta, don't order it—it will be too messy. Shellfish that requires squeezing and digging, ribs, corn on the cob, and fried chicken are all too difficult to eat daintily. Also, avoid foods that can cause accidents and embarrassment. Soups, creamy dressings, desserts, and greasy hand-held foods, such as tacos, can easily end up on your brand-new clothes. Onions and garlic can make even the most stalwart interviewer want to avoid you.

Never eat all the bread in the basket. If it is in front of you, pass it around before you take any; same with the butter. Once you get it, tear your roll gently; don't saw it with a knife. And don't butter all your bread at once. You also don't want to blow on the soup; you may splatter it on others. Only cut and take one bite of food at a time—and always use your knife (not the fork) to cut your food. In a fancy restaurant with lots of cutlery, use the outer silverware first, reserving those above your plate for dessert.

Sit up straight in the chair without hovering over your plate or leaning backward on the chair's back two legs. Keep elbows off the table and, as your mother said, never talk with food in your mouth. If you are asked a question just as you are about to put something in your mouth, go ahead and eat it, and think about your answer while you chew. To acknowledge the question, look at the person and nod. If you feel a bit of food between your teeth, swish silently and unobtrusively. If you notice someone else with food in his or her teeth, mention it unobtrusively. Don't do as one interviewee did at a Chinese restaurant. She popped an entire fortune cookie into her mouth, then removed the fortune and read it to her dining companions!

Don't share another person's appetizer or dessert unless invited to do so—and then ask the waiter to split it for you. As for the napkin, rest it in your lap, never use it as a bib. When you finish your meal, don't place your napkin in the center of a dirty plate—put it next to the plate.

As for the conversation, generally avoid religion, politics, and sexual preferences. The best advice is to use lunch to ward off true hypoglycemia. Consider that mealtime is simply another part of your interview. Do your real eating after you have left the program for the day and can relax.

# 18

# The Perfect Applicant

*How do you make silk purses out of a sow's ear? Start with silk sows.*
— Samuel P. Martin III, M.D.

*Perfection is in the eye of the beholder.*
— Proverb

By now, as you prepare to go for your first interviews, you are probably wondering just what residency directors are looking for in an applicant. There is no absolute answer, but here are some program directors' thoughts on the subject.

The *fundamental rule is that there is no perfect applicant.* Although program directors constantly search for the beast known as the "perfect applicant," they know that this hunt is very similar to the quest for the Holy Grail, a fruitless endeavor. And yet, just as with the Holy Grail, the search continues.

As an applicant, you are probably paranoid enough to want to compare yourself against the perceived ideal of residency selection committees and program directors. While the ideal candidate varies from specialty to specialty and from program to program, there are some basics that seem to hold true for all.

A residency director in a competitive specialty once told me that his perfect applicant would be "a minority woman who graduated from Harvard Medical School at the top of her class, got honors in all her required third-year clinical rotations, had been elected to AOA, had a Ph.D. with a record of significant research and funding, scored in the 99th percentile on USMLE Steps 1 and 2, acquired superior reference letters from top colleagues in our specialty with whom she had worked closely and who said they wanted her in their program, had a dynamite personality, and had the energy of a thirteen-year-old."

"Why," I asked, "are you looking for these criteria?"

He explained that women and minorities are generally under-represented in medicine and, if possible, he wanted to help correct this. Election to AOA, top class ranking at a good medical school, and high U.S. Medical Licensing Exam (USMLE) scores were the only standard criteria across all medical schools he could use to measure candidates. "Of course the USMLE Step 1 has little to do with clinical medicine, but what else is there?" he asked, rather frustrated.

The answer is that excellent performance in third-year clinical clerkships is another, although less accurate, measure of performance. Since medical schools vary so much in their grading schemes (many do not have grading systems discriminating enough to obtain class ranks), it is often very difficult to know what a particular grade means. The courses also frequently vary in their levels of difficulty and intensity. The closest thing to uniformity among medical schools comes in the third-year required clinical clerkships. Excellent grades in these courses usually suggest at least a modicum of clinical knowledge and ability.

Letters from colleagues in the field, especially those who have worked with the applicant, who want the applicant in their own program and who are available to honestly answer questions over the telephone are often the most significant part of an application package. Unlike the typical Dean's letter where every student appears to "walk on water," this is the closest thing to an honest appraisal one can get.

"But why include the other criteria?" I asked.

"No matter how good an applicant is," he continued, "he or she has to fit in with our program's residents and faculty. This is where our opportunity to talk with and interview the applicant comes in. And, because our program is so intensive, we need people with a great deal of energy and enthusiasm. The Ph.D. and research are there to be certain that I never get an applicant who meets all the criteria. If I did, I would probably be disappointed."

I asked him if he had ever met anyone, applicant or not, who met these criteria. Smiling, he replied that of course he hadn't, but he could still look for her.

What this residency director is seeking in applicants is little different from what the vast majority of program directors seek when deciding whom to interview. One survey showed that the most common traits that program directors look for include: grades in required and elective rotations in the specialty, grades in other clerkships, class rank, USMLE Step 2 scores, and AOA membership (Figure 18.1).

FIGURE 18.1

## Relative Importance Among Various Specialties of Academic Criteria When Selecting Residents

| | Ortho-ped | Gen Surg | OB/ Gyn | Ophth-amal | Peds | Fam Med | Int Med | Emer Med | Psych | PM&R | Path | Rad-Onc | DX Rad | Anesth |
|---|---|---|---|---|---|---|---|---|---|---|---|---|---|---|
| Grades in required clerkships | 2 | 1 | 1 | 1 | 1 | 1 | 1 | 2 | 1 | 2 | 8 | 4 | 3 | 1 |
| Number of honors grades | 4 | 4 | 2 | 2 | 3 | 3 | 3 | 3 | 2 | 5 | 6 | 2 | 2 | 7 |
| Sr. specialty elective grades | 1 | 8 | 9 | 5 | 2 | 2 | 6 | 1 | 3 | 1 | 3 | 1 | 10 | 2 |
| Class rank | 5 | 2 | 5 | 3 | 4 | 6 | 5 | 4 | 7 | 10 | 2 | 5 | 1 | 2 |
| AOA honorary membership | 5 | 2 | 7 | 3 | 7 | 7 | 4 | 6 | 9 | 10 | 5 | 7 | 4 | 9 |
| USMLE Step 2 score | 7 | 7 | 4 | 6 | 8 | 4 | 2 | 7 | 8 | 5 | 9 | 8 | 8 | 6 |
| Med. sch. academic awards | 8 | 6 | 6 | 8 | 5 | 8 | 7 | 5 | 6 | 10 | 3 | 8 | 6 | 5 |
| USMLE Step 1 score | 3 | 5 | 3 | 7 | 9 | 9 | 8 | 9 | 11 | 5 | 10 | 10 | 5 | 4 |
| Med. school's reputation | 8 | 10 | 8 | 9 | 10 | 10 | 9 | 8 | 4 | 8 | 7 | 10 | 7 | 9 |
| Other senior elective grades | 10 | 12 | 11 | 10 | 5 | 5 | 10 | 9 | 10 | 3 | 11 | 5 | 11 | 7 |
| Published med. sch. research | 12 | 9 | 10 | 11 | 12 | 12 | 11 | 11 | 5 | 4 | 1 | 2 | 9 | 11 |
| Grades in preclinical courses | 11 | 11 | 12 | 12 | 11 | 11 | 12 | 12 | 12 | 9 | 12 | 12 | 11 | 12 |

*Criteria with identical numbers were considered by the residency directors to be equivalent.

Adapted from: Wagoner NE, Suriano JR: Program directors' responses to a survey on variables used to select residents in a time of change. Acad Med. 1999;74(1): 51-58.

The importance of various criteria may vary, however, among specialties. Figure 18.2 shows the importance given to the same criteria by residency directors in Family Practice and Obstetrics and Gynecology. Based on similar studies, the Family Practice criteria seem to mirror those of Internal Medicine, Pediatrics, and Psychiatry, while the Obstetrics and Gynecology criteria reflect those of other surgical specialties.

Most program directors have a good idea of what they are looking for in a resident. If they really know what they're doing, they have written these criteria down (it is an ACGME rule to do this), discussed them with the rest of the department, and given a copy to all interviewers. As an applicant, you should be able to determine what programs are seeking based on what they highlight in their written materials, how their program is structured, and the institution(s) in which they reside. Make a list of the top three or four criteria you believe each program is seeking and stress, in the interviews, your qualities that match these criteria.

FIGURE 18.2

## *Importance of Information to Residency When Selecting Interviewees and Ranking Applicants*

### Selecting Interviewees*

|  | FP | OB/GYN |
|---|---|---|
| Dean's letter | 1 | 2 |
| Well-written personal statement | 2 | 6 |
| Transcript | 3 | 1 |
| Application form | 4 | 5 |
| USMLE scores | 5 | 3 |
| Letter from known/respected colleague | 6 | 4 |

### Ranking Candidates *

|  | FP | OB/GYN |
|---|---|---|
| Interview | 1 | 1 |
| Dean's letter | 2 | 3 |
| Well-written personal statement | 3 | 7 |
| Transcript | 4 | 2 |
| Application form | 5 | 6 |
| Letter from known/respected colleague | 6 | 5 |
| USMLE scores | 7 | 4 |

*1 is the most important factor and 7 is the least important factor among those listed.

Adapted from: Taylor CA, Weinstein L, Mayhew HE. The process of resident selection: a view from the residency director's desk. *Obstet Gynecol.* 1995;85:299-303.

What residency directors *really* want are residents who will perform well clinically in their program without causing the faculty too much agitation or grief. Among knowledgeable employers, the jargon for an applicant who will easily fit into the program, requires minimal coaching to do extremely well, and already has proven clinical skills and judgment is "plug and play."

No matter what criteria are used, the system is imperfect. The best that can be said about AOA election, high USMLE scores, clinical honors in medical school courses, high class rankings, and positive interviews by faculty is that individuals who meet these criteria usually do not perform dismally in training programs. Their performance is, in fact, usually above average. Similarly, those who performed near the bottom of their class in medical school continue to do the poorest in residency. Individuals who seem to fare the worst during residency are those who took leaves of absence or had academic difficulty during medical school, or who performed below average in their required clinical clerkships.

Residency directors have different levels of concerns about applicants, depending upon what they see and hear. Figure 18.3 shows how they feel about some common things they see in residency candidates' histories.

---

### FIGURE 18.3

#### *Items in Applicant's History that Worry Residency Directors*

**Very Concerned**
- Received disciplinary action in medical school.
- Treated for alcoholism.
- Received failure in a required clerkship.
- Took extended time to graduate for academic reasons.
- Has learning disability.
- Failed USMLE Step 1 prior to passing.
- Passed USMLE with minimal scores.

**Worrisome**
- Graduated in lower third of class.
- Received a failure in a preclinical course.
- Had mediocre preclinical grades but strong clinical evaluations.

**Concerned**
- Has family responsibilities.
- Did not participate in extracurricular activities in medical school.

---

Adapted from: Wagoner NE, Suriano JR: Program directors' response to a survey on variables used to select residents in a time of change. *Acad Med.* 1999;74(1):51-58.

Applicants and residency directors seem to place different values on applicant qualities. Some studies have shown that directors most admire personal characteristics, while students believe that their knowledge and skills are more important attributes in getting a residency position.

Regardless of studies or personal opinions, however, program directors will give up neither their search for the ideal resident nor their use of measurement criteria for applicants. Their job is still to weed through the morass of applications to cull out a group of potential residents. And since precious little else is available to help them make this decision, these are the criteria they will use and by which you will be measured.

# 19

# The Interview

*A job interview is like being on trial for your life.*
— Russian Proverb

*He who asks is a fool for a minute; he who doesn't is a fool forever.*
— Chinese Proverb

## Interview Truisms

Before beginning the interview, keep in mind some research-based information about the process. First, interviewers develop a stereotype of a good applicant and then try to match the candidates to it. By reading the program information carefully, you may get a hint of what they think the "perfect" applicant is. Also, see Chapter 18, The Perfect Applicant.

The typical residency faculty member is unskilled at employment interviews and makes many errors when evaluating applicants. A typical rating error is the "halo effect" in which they are overly influenced by a single favorable or unfavorable trait. Unfortunately, unfavorable information carries more weight than favorable information, so the halo effect is more likely to work against you than for you.

Related to this, if several outstanding or several poor candidates have been interviewed in succession, an average candidate who follows them will look better or worse than he or she is because of the comparison. You can't do much about these factors, but they are worth remembering as you head into the lion's den.

## Know Your Questions

It is important to know not only what questions you want to ask, but also what you are searching for in the replies. You will be looking for specific answers, e.g., the percentage of residency graduates that have passed the specialty's board examination on the first try, as well as observing the interviewers' attitudes toward the subjects you raise. Notice as well the their attitudes toward you as a person and toward residents in general. Are they friendly and open? Or haughty and cold? This could make a big difference in how you rank the program.

Know when to ask your questions. You will rarely run out of questions before you run out of opportunities to ask them. Most programs try to allow applicants the opportunity to have their questions answered fully. They gain as much, or more, information about you from your questions as they do from your answers to their questions. But wait for the proper time. Let the interviewers ask their questions first. Wait for them to ask if you have any questions of your own (Figure 19.1).

When you ask your own questions, do so in a courteous, diplomatic manner. More than one applicant has "gone down the tubes" by trying to cross-examine interviewers. Doing so is crass and demonstrates immaturity. Ask your questions in a way that expresses enthusiasm for a positive answer. Rather than the question, "What problems have you had with accreditation?" you might inquire, "There haven't been any accreditation problems, have there?" The first is accusatory, the second merely inquisitive. Get your information. But be nice about it.

Ask simple, straightforward, open-ended (requiring more than a "yes" or "no" answer) questions. Do not ask questions with multiple parts or that are too long to easily follow. If you ask these types of questions, you may not get the information you want, but you will probably make a negative impression on the interviewer.

## FIGURE 19.1

### *Typical Interview from the Interviewer's Viewpoint*

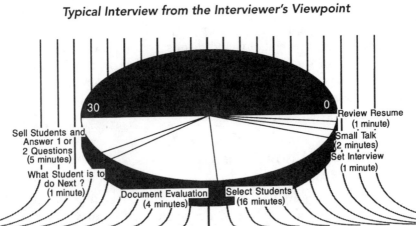

Finally, ask the right people the right questions. At the start of your interview day, ask the residency secretary which individuals you will meet with and what their positions are within the program. Ask the residency or department director about changes in the program or the current status of prior residents. Do not ask them about the call schedule or resident esprit de corps. These are questions to ask residents.

Prepare a typed list of your questions in advance so that you can easily refer to it (and read it) during your interviews. What are some of the questions you should ask, and what should you look for in the answers? The list below is divided into questions you should ask the faculty and those that you will want to ask residents. Some you may want to ask of both groups, especially Question 18, "Could you give me (show me) an example?"

# The List—To Ask Faculty

### 1. Where are your graduates?

This question is actually a two-parter. The first part asks, "Where are your graduates geographically?" Are they practicing in the vicinity of the program or spread throughout the United States? Are they primarily concentrated in major cities or in rural communities? This gives you a realistic perspective about the program's orientation. Training programs reflect the needs of the populations they serve. The places where residency graduates feel comfortable working reflect the training that they have received.

The second part of the question asks, "What types of jobs do your graduates have?" Are they working primarily in academic centers, in private communities, in group practices, in research, in administration, or in other specific areas? Or are they in many diverse areas of practice? Again, this is highly reflective of the scope and quality of the training that residents in a program receive.

Ask this question in a general manner. If either part is not answered, follow up with a more specific question designed to get the missing information. You might ask to see the map on which residencies often post the location of their graduates. If you locate a residency graduate in your home area, you can gain valuable insight into the program by talking with this individual.

### 2. How have your graduates done on the specialty's board exam?

Although the primary goal of residency training is to prepare you to practice in your chosen field, an important milepost during your career will be passing the specialty's board examination. In many cases, passing "the

Boards" determines the type and level of position you can fill. How have this program's residents done when they took their specialty board exams? If they have all passed, was this on the first try? This can be asked tactfully, as in "Did any of them have to take their Boards more than once?" Did they fare as well on the oral exams (you should already know if they have these in your chosen specialty) as they did on the written exams?

Residency directors should know this type of information. Although information on specific graduates is, of course, confidential, the cumulative data should be available to all residency applicants. If it isn't, then there may be a problem.

You also want to know how residents have done on the specialty's in-training examinations. These tests, usually given annually, mirror subsequent performance on specialty board exams. In addition, does the program have any conferences or special programs to help their residents prepare for the specialty's boards?

The information you glean from these questions indicates, in part, the amount of didactic teaching, reading time, and interaction with the faculty that you will receive at this program. As might be expected, graduates of high-volume, high-workload programs often have worse records on board examinations than do those from lower volume programs. However, this is not always true, so it is important to get the specifics from each program you visit.

### 3. Is there much faculty turnover?

Tread gently in this area—it may be very sensitive. But do tread. You need to know about faculty stability. It gives a strong indication about the staff's and, by extension, the entire program's esprit de corps. If there is a large or rapid turnover in faculty positions, it may indicate that all is not well, even if there is a pretty façade.

There are several ways to get this information. If the program sent you a list of instructors with its material, simply ask how many of these individuals will still be there in July. Otherwise, you can ask if any faculty have recently been added—"As replacements?" you ask not so naively—or if any of the current staff will be leaving in the near future. This last is the least favorable way to ask the question. If you hear from the residents, however, that either the residency director or the department director is planning to leave, ask about it. These are two changes that can markedly affect the program's tenor.

You might feel that faculty turnover is their business, not yours. Wrong! Would you make reservations at an expensive French restaurant for your birthday celebration if you thought that the chef/owner was going on vacation—and being replaced by the short-order cook from the greasy spoon next door? Don't go hungry. Ask before you commit to a reservation.

## 4. Are there non-clinical responsibilities?

Of course you will be doing clinical work, and you need to talk to the residents about this. But what other requirements are there? If you arrive at a program expecting nothing but clinical work and there are additional requirements, you may be upset. Find out about all your obligations ahead of time.

There are usually four categories of extra activities:

1. *Research*. Either development and implementation of a research project or participation in ongoing research may be required.

2. *Projects*. Development of or participation in projects, such as those designed around medical student education, or in specialty society activities may be strongly encouraged.

3. *Writing*. Written case reports, abstracts, and book reviews may be mandatory.

4. *Administration*. Either a specialty board or the program may require spending time as chief resident. This usually includes a number of administrative duties.

These extra activities may demand a considerable amount of your time during your residency training. They may also contribute greatly to your education. But to make a rational decision about which program to choose, you need to know what extra activities each program requires.

## 5. Is this program especially strong or well known in any special areas?

If you know of any special programs the residency program offers, either from their brochure, website, or from residents or other interviewees with whom you have talked, you may want to ask for more details. You also want to know about any other special programs, some of which may be too new to list in the brochures or which have not yet started. These will be extra perquisites of attending this program, and the interviewers will generally be thrilled that you asked. This allows them to show off their program to its best advantage.

Remember, when evaluating the interviewers' answers, that programs in which you do not plan to participate (such as an international electives program which won't fit in with caring for your three young children) is of no benefit to you. It may, though, demonstrate the program's educational direction, which is very useful to know.

## 6. What types of clinical sites are used?

Residency programs generally use a variety of clinical settings, including private, public and Veterans Administration hospitals, private-practice preceptors, or distant rotations for specialized training. Which types does this program offer—or require? Are there a wide variety of both outpatient and inpatient facilities appropriate for your education in this specialty? Or have the sites seemingly been chosen for reasons other than optimal resident education (for example, because they provide some resident funding)? Do the types of clinical facilities mimic the medical practice you envision yourself having?

Logistical questions associated with this are: Are any of these rotations out of town? Is housing (and, if distant, transportation) supplied? If the primary residency is in an urban center with good mass transit, you may want to ask if you will need a car for some rotations.

Since residents spend virtually all their time in clinical settings, this information is very important. Be aware that many older, poorer, and badly funded residency-associated hospitals and clinics don't have enough staff (you do the "scut" work), up-to-date working equipment (you make do using available materials), or the necessary variety of clinicians (you must refer interesting patients to other facilities) to provide you with the quality experience you need.

## 7. Are there elective opportunities?

Each of us has a unique view of what our professional lives will be like. Some may envision a life in private or group practice, while others believe their career will involve research, teaching, or foreign travel. Since residency program structures generally fit the generic physician entering the specialty, you may need specific educational opportunities to learn something about specific specialty areas—either to gain expertise or to find out if that is the direction you want to follow. Does this program allow sufficient time and flexibility to sample these different specialty environments?

Note that even if you don't think you may have interests outside the specialty's mainstream now, you will grow as a clinician over the years you spend in residency. Having the option to explore different tracks may become important to you.

## 8. Are there research opportunities?

Some applicants may envision careers in academia or research. If you are one of them, you will certainly want to enter a residency that can provide you with the resources and guidance to do research.

Start with the question "What research projects are the department's faculty and residents working on now?" That will give you a range of interests and level of activity. Then, if one of the projects interests you, focus on that. Will you have a mentor? Is that person funded for his or her research? Is that individual amenable to working with residents? How fairly have residents been treated when working with faculty members on research projects in the past? (Have the residents done the work and been given secondary credit?)

Also find out about available facilities, funding, time, and support staff, such as statisticians, to do research. Does the department or institution provide these? Is research required, tolerated, or actively encouraged? In addition, if you do research and it is accepted for presentation at a national meeting, will the department pay your way there? Will they give you the necessary time off? Ask now to avoid disappointment later.

### 9. Is there administrative, bioethics, and legal training?

Although academicians have been slow to recognize it, medicine is also a business—sometimes a dangerous business. How much training in the administrative and legal aspects of medical practice will you get at this program? Will you have hands-on training dealing with insurance, billing, contracts, hiring, and similar problems? Or are you expected to learn it all at the "school of hard knocks" after you begin your own practice?

Will you receive in-depth training about the legal pitfalls now so common in medicine, or will this come only after your first malpractice suit? How about the ethical issues involved in your specialty?

Does the program offer a formal course of bioethics instruction? As medicine advances, practitioners must more frequently ask, "Just because I can do it, should I?" Bioethics helps answer this and other difficult clinical (and research) questions. Although the requirements for residency training now include the areas of law, ethics, and socioeconomics related to medicine, most training programs do not offer instruction in these areas. If you find one that does, it indicates that they have a dynamic and forward-looking residency director.

### 10. Is there a mentor/advisor system? How does it work?

Everyone expects to do well in his or her residency program. Problems can develop, however. The first may be simply learning the rules and the culture of a new institution. An experienced person who can guide you through this maze can work wonders. This may be a senior resident "buddied" with a new trainee, a faculty member at the program, or both. If this system exists, it suggests that the program is at least trying to ease your transition from medical student to resident. Later you may want to ask residents how well this mentoring system works.

Another recent innovation at some residencies is financial counseling. It's an excellent idea, since many residents carry an enormous debt burden and the repayment rules keep changing. Does this residency have such a program?

## 11. What type of resident evaluations are used? How often?

Interns struggle through their first year in one of two modes (sometimes alternating between them): they believe they are doing a dynamite job or, more frequently, they believe they are learning little and their performance is marginal. Neither extreme is usually the case. But in the strange world of neophyte medicine, it is hard to know where you stand without some feedback.

How often does the program supply this feedback? What mechanisms are used? In the past, many residents went through one or more years of training blissfully unaware that the faculty thought their performance was less than adequate, only to be suddenly dropped from the program. This was especially common in Surgical training programs. Residency programs must now demonstrate to reviewers their mechanisms for evaluation.

Many Internal Medicine programs now use not only periodic formal evaluations, but also "Early Warning Notes" and "Praise Cards," developed by the American Board of Internal Medicine, to deliver feedback between formal evaluations. Unfortunately, most faculty are not used to giving individual residents constructive feedback while they are working with them, so formal evaluations become very important in gauging how well you are doing.

Another evaluation method is the in-service examination given by many Boards. These measure "book knowledge," and are used to compare residents at the same level of training across the United States. Ask if such exams are available at the program. Will you be allowed time off to take the exams (including the night before so you won't fall asleep during the test)? How are the results used—to help the resident assess his or her strengths and weaknesses, or to eliminate "weak" residents? Does the program offer standardized evaluation examinations or other methods of self-assessment in addition to the national in-service tests? It is nice to know how you are doing compared not only to your peers locally, but also to all other residents with whom you will take your specialty board examination when you finish the program. These tests are one way of finding out.

**12. How has health care reform affected this program and institution?**

Far from an idle question, the 1990s saw the most devastating and grievous insult to medical student education in this century. Medicare rules and punitive actions (fining medical schools and residency faculties millions of dollars) have forced most teaching hospitals to seriously restrict many residents' clinical independence.

Medicare also has a demonstration project to pay 49 New York hospitals $400 million to decrease the number of residency positions by 20 to 25%. Their idea was that if this could be implemented nationwide, it would decrease the total number of U.S. physicians. As of 1999, at least 16 of these hospitals have dropped out of the project less than two years after it began, an indication of how much work residents do in hospitals.

In addition, the encroachment of managed care organizations has siphoned off many patients from hospitals' teaching services and clinics. Even when the patient census has remained stable, declining reimbursement has often decreased the number of ancillary staff, available services, and any amenities residents once had. How is this residency program and teaching institution responding to assure that trainees continue to get a quality clinical education? Are they financially stable? Have these changes adversely affected residents' and faculty's esprit de corps?

**13. Do you anticipate changes in the program's curriculum?**

This is another of those questions that you should ask the residency director. It is a safe inquiry and can be asked directly.

Are changes in the curriculum expected in the near future—if so, why? "Near future" is defined as your time in the program. Residency programs may anticipate changes based upon modifications of board requirements, alterations in the patient base, or new directions being taken by the specialty as a whole or the faculty in particular. These changes may make a difference in your evaluation of the program—either favorably or unfavorably.

In some cases, only general ideas about anticipated changes can be set forth. Usually the faculty is not dissembling, but rather demonstrating both their hopes for the program and the complexity involved in altering many training curricula. In any case, know that no matter what you are told, some changes most likely will take place during your training. No program's curriculum is chiseled in stone.

**14. What is the program's accreditation status?**

Another sensitive question. Does that specialty's Residency Review Committee accredit the program? (Actually it is the Accreditation Council for

Graduate Medical Education which accredits the programs, but let's not quibble.) This indicates that the program is certified to prepare residents for the specialty's board examination. There are four possible answers to this question.

The first answer is "No, the program is not accredited." If you go through such a program, which is not in the NRMP Match since it is not accredited, *you will not be eligible to take the specialty's board exam.* A negative answer to this question should, in virtually all cases, eliminate this program from your consideration.

The other possibilities all come under the "Yes" category. The simplest is "Yes, full accreditation." This means that the program has been accredited without restrictions for a number of years. This is as good as it gets.

Two other possibilities are "Yes, provisionally" and "Yes, on probation." The former indicates that the program either has not been in existence long enough to get a full accreditation or has had enough recent changes to warrant being considered a "new" program. The problems here, common to all new programs, revolve around the question of stability. The latter response, "Yes, on probation," indicates that the program is having major problems and is in danger of losing its accreditation. If that happens, any resident in the program may be left in the lurch, struggling to find another program to enter in mid-training. That is neither a pleasant possibility nor an easy thing to do.

Although you can indirectly look for information about accreditation in *FREIDA* (since non-accredited programs will not be listed) and some programs may mention their accreditation status in the material that they send to applicants, it is worthwhile confirming this at the interview; things do change. You should ask this question of the residency director. The most diplomatic way to do this might be, "You do have full accreditation?" This allows a complete answer. If the program does have full accreditation, there will be a simple answer. If not, the residency director will have an answer already prepared for you. Sit back and take it all in. It may "get a little deep" at this point and you may have to lift your feet off the floor part of the time.

### 15. Is this a pyramidal program?

Most often found in Surgery and Surgical specialties, a pyramidal training program is structured so that only a percentage, usually about half, of those starting in the PGY-1 year will be allowed to finish the entire program. This is usually because the program needs "bodies" to accomplish much of the clinical work, but only has enough significant procedures, such as major operations, to accommodate a few chief residents. If you plan to go into such a program, e.g., "Categorical" General Surgery, be prepared for intense competition with your peers. However, if you are applying only for a one- or two-year "Preliminary" position prior to entering a subspecialty such as Orthopedic Surgery, it might work in your favor. If you are accepted into the program, it will mean that fewer of the Categorical residents will have to be dropped from the pyramid. Make certain that you ask this question—the information, although very important to you, often will not be offered spontaneously.

Programs may no longer be pyramidal according to the ACGME's rules. Many residents, however, report that de facto pyramidal programs still exist.

### 16. Have any housestaff left the program?

Aside from being in pyramidal programs, residents leave training programs for many reasons. Most residencies have had residents leave, usually because of illness, family circumstances, or simply changing their minds about which specialty to enter. This information is not what you are after. You want to know whether any residents have left because they were discontented with the program, the faculty, or the training they were receiving.

A way to ferret out these individuals may be to ask, "Have any of the residents who have left this program gone into another program in the same specialty?" These are usually the folks who were discontented with the program. Simply ask why they left. Although you may not get specifics, the tenor of the answer may be enough to let you know if there is a potential problem for you.

### 17. Do you help your graduates find jobs?

This may be a new question to many residency faculty. In the past, there was little problem finding work once a resident finished training. Today, with a "doctor glut" in some specialties, there are fewer choice jobs to go around. So, you might need some help to find them, especially if you are interested in entering a difficult market, such as southern California. Ask if the program will help you.

If they say you are on your own, it indicates that they: (1) have little regard for your future welfare, and (2) have little understanding of what their job as teachers really entails. In either case, you are now forewarned.

If they do offer help to residents in finding employment after training, what have they done for recent graduates and current residents? Are there individual counseling sessions? Are faculty contacts used to get positions? Will the faculty review job offers with the residents?

These are but a few of the possible ways in which the program can assist residents in getting their first jobs. You are having a hard enough time getting into a residency. Ask this question now to avoid as many problems as you can when you finish your training.

### 18. Could you give me (show me) an example?

This is one of the most important questions you can ask during interviews. Ask it to supplement questions you ask of faculty and residents.

In the process of trying to ascertain whether you would fit into a program, you need to have some firm information, not unsubstantiated statements. "Our resident on-call schedule is very benign," says the chief resident. "Could you show me the current month's schedule?" you ask. After you see the schedule, you will know if it really is as easy as they claim it is. If it is just the resident's interpretation of what "benign" means, you will know that too.

Many questions lend themselves to confirmation or explanation. This is a safe, pleasant, and enlightening way to get further information about important points. You can never ask this question too often.

## The List—To Ask Residents

### 19. What contact will I have with the clinical faculty?

The material that the program sent to you listed 42 faculty members. Did they happen to specifically mention how often you will have contact with all of them? With *any* of them? The faculty only helps you if you have direct contact with them. If faculty members hide in their offices or labs rather than attend in the clinics, wards, emergency departments, or operating rooms, they might as well not be there.

So, the questions that you should ask the residents are, "How often are the faculty members present?" and "How often do you want faculty input but find that it is not available?" You might want to specifically ask "How available are they on nights and weekends?" Of course, as a resident, you want to be able to exercise some independent thought and judgment. But you need adequate guidance from knowledgeable faculty during residency training. Does this program really offer it?

### 20. Do residents regularly have an opportunity to formally evaluate faculty and the program? What changes have been made recently as a result of this feedback?

This question really asks, "How important is the educational mission?" Feedback on the faculty's performance is an essential part of all education.

If the residency is serious about education, it will have a good evaluation system. Virtually all residencies, however, will say that they have an evaluation system, since the residency review boards generally require it. What is really telling is if they can recite substantive changes that have been made based on these evaluations. That means that they not only have the system, but also value their residents' opinions.

When asking this question, you may also get information on the institution's or residency's grievance policy, such as that used for harassment. Listen closely. Is the resident telling you about problems they have had, or how they have used their system to avoid problems?

### 21. How much didactic time is there? Does it have priority?

If it is not in the material that you have already received, find out how much time is spent in lectures, seminars, journal clubs, and other didactic activities. If a current monthly schedule is available, ask for a copy to peruse at your leisure.

The more important question, which you need to ask of one or more residents (not the faculty), is "Which has a higher priority, attending conferences or performing clinical duties?" In most training programs, residents must, at least occasionally, attend to clinical duties while conferences are in progress. But if this is the norm rather than the exception, kiss any meaningful answers about the number of didactic sessions good-bye. If you cannot attend the teaching sessions, they don't exist. Remember that didactic sessions may have a significant impact on your learning, and on your passing in-service training exams and specialty board examinations.

### 22. What type of clinical experiences will I have?

Residencies are supposed to teach physicians to be excellent clinicians. For that, they must provide adequate clinical experience. How many clinical experiences will you have and how diverse will they be?

In surgical or procedural specialties, will you be performing procedures, or mostly watching? Is there a struggle between services or among residents on the same service for some procedures? At what level do residents graduate to more advanced procedures? In General Surgery, for example, if third- and fourth-year residents are still doing appendectomies, there is a definite problem. Similarly, if senior Pediatric, Family Practice, or Internal Medicine residents "hog" every tube and line placement, it suggests that they have not had enough experience doing these procedures. Have previous graduates really felt comfortable performing all necessary procedures by the time they graduated? If not, you should question whether such a marginal program is right for you.

A special situation exists in Obstetrics and Gynecology. Few programs now teach their residents how to perform elective abortions. If you plan (or think you might want) to do these procedures in your practice, ask specifically whether this training will be available to you.

Some programs offer unique learning opportunities, for example, new diagnostic or therapeutic techniques (such as neurohyperthermic therapy), older but rarely available methodologies (such as hyperbaric chambers), or special training in areas of faculty expertise. As a resident, will these opportunities be available to you?

### 23. *Tell me about the on-call rooms, cafeteria, library, computer access, and parking.*

You've already experienced a variety of call rooms during your clinical years. That was only a taste. When you seriously use these call rooms night after night, their ambiance (or lack thereof) can greatly affect your outlook on life and work. Not only should you be told about the call rooms, but, if possible, go see those at the institutions you visit during your interview trip. That way you can evaluate and compare them.

No resident has ever died from hospital food (at least I don't think so). But when you get a chance to eat, it's a lot better if the food is tasty, looks good, has some variety, is served in a setting with at least some semblance of quiet and pleasant décor, and is inexpensive (or free). More hospitals are finding that jazzing up their cafeterias improves their image with hospital staff, trainees, and patients' families. How do the cafeterias at the locations you will work measure up? Can you tolerate this food and setting (and cost) for the duration of your residency?

The library is the bellwether of an institution's educational commitment. Is it stocked with useful and up-to-date materials, staffed with knowledgeable and helpful people, and open long (or all) hours? Does the library have audiovisual and computer materials to supplement printed material? How about access to on-line databases? When you need to access material for tomorrow morning's grand rounds, are the library's facilities adequate?

Our new century is computerized, and the medical field, although currently lagging behind other segments of society, is no exception. Practitioners need to be computer literate, using the Web and local networks as readily as their stethoscopes. Does the residency provide access to computers and use them for teaching? Is Internet access available in the clinical areas? Are computer labs or specialists available to residents? How about special computer courses? It's no longer enough to know how to take a medical history and do a physical examination. You also need to know how to access computerized medical records, lab results, bedside nurses' notes, clinic schedules, library materials, databases, and, eventually, billing records.

Finally, how about parking at the hospital and clinics? Is it difficult to find or expensive? If you drive to your residency interview, you may get a taste of what the parking is like. Is this the norm for residents, or just for visitors?

## 24. Will I have time to read?

Your educational reading, of course, reflects a personal decision about what is important to you. However, if residents consistently answer that they are too tired to read, it suggests a deficiency in the program rather than in any individual. Education in any specialty depends on supplementing clinical experiences with reading. You cannot learn all you need to know on the wards, in the clinics, or in the OR. Reading will be important to you. Ask whether you will have time to do it from those who know—the residents. The answer to this question will also help to identify those departments that have residency programs primarily to fulfill their service commitments, rather than to educate.

Ask senior-level (PGY-2 and above) residents this question; nearly all interns will tell you that they are too tired to read. That is certainly understandable given their schedules.

## 25. What support staff is available? Are they helpful?

Residents commonly feel overworked because there are too few people to perform what are typically non-physician tasks. You owe it to yourself to find out how much "scut" work the residents at a program typically perform.

Who starts routine IV lines, draws blood, and does clerical work? Who pushes patients to x-ray or to radiation oncology for treatments?

Does the institution provide an adequate level of nursing and ancillary support? Is this staff supportive, or merely an obstacle to good patient care? Are there backup teams you can call when you are swamped with admissions?

Even if institutions have sufficient numbers of support staff, their quality and interest in helping you may vary based on personnel policy and tradition. What is it like at the institutions through which residents in this program rotate?

While faculty may be able to tell you about some of the available clinical support, ask the residents for the real answers. Don't complain after the fact. Find out in advance.

## 26. What is the call schedule?

There are two main things that directly affect your life during residency—and they both relate to the call schedule. The first is the amount of time you will actually work. The second is who arranges the schedule.

Ask the residents how much time they actually work at each level of training. Some states, such as New York, and all specialties have officially limited the number of hours their residents can work. Not everyone, however, plays by the rules. Being intelligent folks with ever-tighter budgets, many residency directors skirt the rules so the institution can avoid the cost of adding residents. Some of the worst offenders, at least in New York, have been the private hospitals. Surgical specialties and Obstetrics and Gynecology, due to the nature of their practices, continue to have the longest hours.

Not many years ago, an applicant got a Surgical internship after having, he thought, asked all the appropriate questions. He expected to work long hours, but was astonished when he found that in addition to taking call in-house on alternate nights, he had to take call from home when he was off duty! Ask in advance so you don't get any nasty surprises.

At many programs, the residency director, the secretary, a chief resident, or some unnamed individual in a back office makes the schedule. This leaves the residents feeling helpless and without control over their lives. Indeed, the lack of control over one's life is one of the biggest stressors among residents. Some programs allow the residents themselves to generate the call schedule (as well as conference, vacation, and off-service schedules). If a program offers this, your mental health will be much better.

Also find out if days off are built into the schedule. Although all residents are supposed to be allotted days off (a minimum number is usually four/month), many programs do not explicitly build them into the schedule, and then apply pressure on residents to work even on "free" days. This leads to rapid burnout, frustration, and disgust with practicing medicine and the specialty. Avoid this by asking whether days off are scheduled, and how many there are per month.

## 27. What is the patient population I will see?

Patients (their numbers and age distribution, the nature of their diseases, and who cares for them in what settings) are the basic element of all medical training programs. If the program lacks an adequate number of patient encounters, it doesn't matter what else it offers.

It is necessary to first ascertain how many patients residents care for. But aside from this, you also need to know how much time is spent and how much autonomy residents have when caring for private patients. While some programs have many patients coming through their offices or hospital beds, private practitioners often take care of the majority of them.

Find out about the patient population served and the distribution of disease processes. Some teaching hospitals have an overabundance of a few types of disease processes, such as penetrating trauma, tertiary oncology, or AIDS. A skewed distribution does not provide adequate training for clinicians who will eventually serve a more diverse population having more common diseases. Today, as more medical care is being delivered in outpatient settings, residents should see patients in the clinics and outpatient surgeries. Finally, ask if there are medical students on the service. If there are, ask if you will be responsible for teaching them. Whether this is a plus or minus for you, find out in advance what to expect.

### 28. Do the residents socialize as a group?

This is one element, or at least demonstrates one element, of esprit de corps. Are the social events program-wide or institution-wide? This may or may not be important to you. If it is, you may also want to ask about the ratio of married to single residents (in the program or institution), how many have children, and how often social events occur.

Does there seem to be any particular activity that is of special interest to the residents, or do their interests vary? Is socializing related to educational activities, such as journal clubs? Or are they separate events, such as volleyball games or picnics? Note that if the socialization is resident-organized, it may vary considerably from year to year.

## Confirm Questionable Points

A number of the questions that you raise may be critical. Which questions these are will depend upon your own "Must/Want" Analysis. However, you may not get straight answers to some of them. This may be because no one knows the answer at the moment. For example, in October no one may really know how many of the faculty will still be on-site next July. But you may be getting the runaround for other, more nefarious, reasons. If you ask the residency director about how much faculty interaction with residents there is, and the hemming and hawing begins, then you will need to get the real story. This is where the technique of cross-checking facts becomes useful.

Whenever you have some doubt about the answer to an important question, repeat the question to another interviewer. Or better yet, if it is appropriate, ask a resident in the program. In fact, if the issue is extremely important to you, ask everyone you talk to the same question. But be sure not to do so within earshot of others you have already asked (or will ask) that same question—it will be taken as a sign that you doubt their honesty, which, of course, you do. Remember that the program is trying to sell its product to you at the same time that you are selling yourself to it. Not all salesmen are honest. *Caveat emptor!*

# Things Not To Ask

There are specific questions that must not be asked during an interview, even though they are important to you. These questions basically involve four areas: salary, benefits, vacation, and competition. Let's discuss each one individually, so you will at least know what information to get from *appropriate* sources.

## Salary

The *salary* you will receive as a resident will, in large part, depend upon three factors.

1. The mean salaries of housestaff around the country in the previous year.

2. The type of institution in which the residency is located.

3. The region of the country in which the institution is situated.

Most institutions base their resident salaries upon a variation from the mean salary that residents are receiving nationally. The variations in many cases are based upon the cost of living in the region of the country where the institution is located. In addition, those programs that have a relatively difficult time attracting residents, such as community and non-university hospitals, will tend to have higher salaries. Those with very large numbers of applicants will generally offer lower salaries. But, of course, you would be more than happy to do the residency for free, wouldn't you? Probably not. However, this is the attitude to take during the interview process. Salary will keep you alive and pay your bills—but do not try to find out what it will be during the interview. What are you, money-hungry?

The only exception to this rule is if you have any hint that the position is unfunded. Despite rules to the contrary, these positions still exist. They are most commonly found in highly competitive fellowships (post-residency) and at some institutions whose residents are mostly international medical graduates. If this is the case, and you are still interested in the position, at least ask about the non-salary benefits offered.

## Benefits

*Benefit packages* are very important to you as a resident—as they will be for the rest of your career. Virtually all such packages include malpractice insurance and some type of medical insurance. Other benefits may be food or housing allowances, uniforms, cleaning expenses, disability insurance, moving expenses, parking, tuition fee waivers for the affiliated school, and childcare, to name some common ones (Figures 10.4 and 10.5).

Remember, if you can use the benefit, it counts as additional salary. However, if the program offers benefits that you cannot use, such as Obstetric care when you are not planning any children for now, the value of this benefit is lost to you. Do make certain that the medical insurance is comprehensive enough to cover serious illness or injury. You probably already are in debt up to your eyeballs and cannot afford steep medical bills.

Asking a faculty member about the benefit package, however, is generally like talking to your pet rock. He or she will normally have no idea what his or her own benefit package is, let alone yours. Don't make your interviewer look stupid. Avoid this topic during the interview.

## Vacation

If you don't think that *vacation* is important, wait until you have been up most of every night for a week. At that point, dreaming about an upcoming vacation may be all that keeps you going. Most interns have three weeks or less of vacation, while most residents in their second or higher years have at least three weeks of vacation (Figure 10.6) each year. In some programs, the vacation can all be taken at one time; in others, it must be taken as one-week blocks. The latter obviously doesn't allow much time for travel.

Asking an interviewer about vacation is akin to inquiring whether you would actually have to do any work during the residency. While everyone understands that vacation—even a resident's vacation—is important, interviewers assume that during the interview you will concentrate on the great educational experience that they offer, rather than your time off.

## Competition

Who is your *competition*? It doesn't matter! Asking about other applicants will serve no good purpose and only directs an interviewer's attention away from you. The key, as has been stressed throughout this book, is to put your own best efforts before the residency faculty and let them select you based upon what they see. Forget the others. Concentrate on selling yourself.

*Okay, so where do you find out about salary, benefits, and vacation?* First, look over the packet that the residency sent to you. Normally, you will discover most of the information there. If not, then three other excellent sources are *FREIDA* (which you have already accessed), the residency secretary, and the people in the institution's Graduate Education office. In fact, the latter site is the place where you can get the most up-to-date information. It is also the spot where you can obtain the data and still remain relatively anonymous. If all else fails, put your questions in writing when you get home and address them to the director of the institution's Housestaff or Graduate Education office. Even by mail, try to avoid querying the program directly about these non-educational areas.

# Things Not To Do

Just as there are certain questions that you should avoid, there are certain things that you should not do during the interview. The following are attitudes or actions that will evoke a negative response from an interviewer.

## Show Discouragement

Be upbeat! This is your time to shine. One poor interview should not influence the rest of your visit. Remember that the interviewer may not have thought it was a poor interview at all. Looking "down in the dumps" will destroy any positive effect that your interview could possibly have made.

Stand up straight. *SMILE*—it won't break your face. If you cannot find the courage to smile through some adversity now, you are really going to be in trouble when you get into your residency.

## Disparage Other Programs, Faculty, or Applicants

You might very well be asked about the other programs that you have visited. The question could be phrased as, "Tell me about the poorest programs that you have visited." Although this may be tempting—you may have interviewed at some really horrendous places—back up a minute to redirect the question. Say that you are not in a position to determine which programs are poor, but there may be some that do not seem to meet your needs. Then you can describe specific aspects of programs that you feel did not fully meet your expectations. But go easy. If you really berate a program that you have visited, the interviewer might wonder what you will say about his or her program when you go elsewhere.

Do not say anything derogatory about faculty at another institution. It should go without saying that you will not berate faculty at the institution at which you are interviewing. No matter what you think, academic medicine, especially within the confines of any one specialty, is rather close-knit. There is a good chance that the person you are describing is well-known to the interviewer.

## Falsify Background

Although it may appear that you could say almost anything about your background during the interview and get away with it, you do so only at great risk. The first danger is that you will immediately be discovered.

Not many years ago, a residency applicant was eloquently describing his activities in the Emergency Medical System. He stated that he responded to calls frequently even while in medical school. It was quite an impressive achievement. Yet, as he went on with his story, it became obvious to the interviewer that he was being less than honest. For, while he was describing activities in the opposite end of the country, it just so happened that the interviewer was also from that area and picked up on major factual errors in the story. These were confirmed by a call to his medical school.

The second danger is even worse. If information that you provide when you apply for any job, including a residency position, is later found to be false, it is grounds for immediate dismissal. Thus, giving fraudulent information puts you in jeopardy throughout your residency. Stick to the truth. Make it appear as favorable as possible, but stick to the truth.

## Inappropriate Humor

There is a place for humor in interviews. A good laugh can be enjoyed, but, unfortunately, rarely is during residency interviews. However, humor should not be offensive. Even if laughter ensues after you tell an off-color, sexist, or racist joke, you almost certainly will have lowered yourself in the eyes of the interviewer.

In fact, off-color or inappropriate humor is considered by a large number of administrators to be the major breach of etiquette in the workplace. If you have an uncontrollable urge to tell these types of jokes, at least keep them out of the interview.

## Drink Coffee, Smoke, Chew Gum, or Bite Nails

Four activities that you must not do during an interview are drink coffee, smoke, chew gum, or bite your nails. You may very well be offered coffee by each interviewer. They mean well. But do they also offer you a bathroom break in the middle of the interview? No! And if you are concentrating on a full bladder instead of the interviewer's questions, you could end up in deep trouble. Avoid diuretics.

There are four problems with smoking. The first is that it is unlikely that your interviewer smokes, since the habit is now relatively rare among physicians. The second is that smoking looks bad during an interview. So, even if you are addicted, hold out until the interview is over—or you have left the program for the day. The smell that lingers on your clothes and breath, if you smoke, will not endear you to non-smoking interviewers. Third, interviewers may be biased against hiring smokers. As of yet, no programs have gone public with an explicit ban on hiring smokers, but it is likely that it would be legal. There is no protection under current civil rights legislation for smokers. This makes it legal for an interviewer to inquire whether or not you are a smoker. Note, of course, that if they inquire, it can only be a (un-Lucky?) strike against you. About 25% of personnel directors admit that if offered two equivalent applicants, they would hire the non-smoker. Fourth, an old ploy, used to put an applicant in an awkward position, is to suggest that you smoke and then not have an ashtray available for you. You will avoid this (rare) problem by not smoking.

Chewing gum is absolutely out. It evokes a fatuous, sophomoric image which will destroy everything that you have worked so hard to achieve. If blowing bubbles is your "thing," hold out until you leave the hospital. No one is physiologically addicted to chewing gum (except, perhaps, nicotine gums—use patches during interviews). One stick of gum at the wrong time can cancel your chance for a residency slot that you really want.

Finally, even though you are nervous and your common response is to bite your nails, restrain yourself when at residency programs. It signals your neuroses to interviewers. For clinicians, it also demonstrates potentially dangerous, infection-producing behavior.

## Stressful Interviews

Stress interviews were very common at one time. Interviewers asked questions to purposely make applicants confused, fearful, and hostile. Employers believed they could weed out applicants who couldn't handle stress. The applicants they actually eliminated were individuals with enough self-esteem to determine that they didn't want to work for people who treated potential employees like dirt. While the business world long ago learned not to use this method, some residency programs still use the technique. Others treat applicants shabbily because that is how they treat their residents.

### Panel Interviews

The most common type of interview is the one-on-one serial interview, in which you go from interviewer to interviewer, with each asking his or her own questions. Occasionally, though, you will be faced with a rather unusual interview scenario—the panel or group interview, in which from two to twenty individuals will all be interviewing you at the same time. There is a reason business people call this the "gang bang." It is generally considered a rather poor interview technique, both from an employer's and from an applicant's perspective. However, it is still in use, primarily because it is thought to save the interviewers' time. Some people also believe this technique is useful for jobs that require sophisticated communication skills—such as that of a physician.

These interviews will generally be conducted using either a question or a scenario format. In the question format, each panel member asks his or her own questions. In the scenario format, you discuss one or more cases with the entire panel.

The best approach is to look at the individual who asked the question when you answer. In the case of the scenario, since it is a question from the entire group, look at all the members while answering. If an individual member asks you a follow-up question, look at that person when answering. Do not try to determine the most influential people on the panel and direct most of your attention to them. The others will feel slighted. When the panel members meet together later to discuss the candidates, your implied insult will damage your chance of getting a residency position.

A particularly nasty variation used at some residency programs is to sit the applicant between the wings of a V-shaped table facing the interviewers seated on both outside wings. They then pepper interviewees with questions, alternating sides to make candidates swivel their heads back and forth to answer each question. One applicant quickly adjusted by simply slowing down and completely turning to face each questioner when she answered. Her key was to avoid getting flustered. You could also get up and move your chair back so the angle to view the interviewers is not so acute.

Even worse is another technique employed (thankfully) by only a few Gestapo-like programs. At the end of an interview day, they bring two students at a time into a roomful of faculty. They then rapidly ask the students the same questions at the same time. This is really an abuse of power; my suggestion, if this happens to you, is to stand up, thank them for their time, and leave without participating.

If you are faced with any type of panel interview, remember that it will be as unnerving an experience for everyone else as it is for you. So, keep cool and knock their socks off!

## Non-Interview Visits

There is one type of program visit, still very rare, to which you may be invited. This is the non-interview visit, which is essentially the same as a traditional interview visit, but without the interviews. While it has the same implications as any other invitation to visit a residency, the programs handle it somewhat differently.

At present, only a few of the most highly selective programs use this type of visit. You are not rated on the basis of your performance during the visit (unless you act really obnoxious). Rather, the residency faculty screens applicants based on their performance in undergraduate or medical school, on the USMLE, and by using other written materials they feel are important.

They then assume that all of those they invite for a visit to their program would make acceptable residents.

Faculty use the non-interview visit primarily to show an applicant the program. During the visit, applicants normally have multiple opportunities to see the physical plant, didactic program, and social milieu of the residency. They are usually given many opportunities to interact with faculty and residents, and to have all their questions answered. Generally, they are given a better picture of the program than would be possible during a more traditional visit. Applicants invited for these visits get the maximum possible information; this assures that those ranking the program highly are doing so with a sound knowledge of what they are getting into.

There are several principles upon which this system is based. The first is that the interview system, especially when using physician-interviewers who are untrained in personnel selection, is as likely to give erroneous information as valid facts. A second is that creating a program with happy residents is best assured by giving applicants as much information as possible about it ahead of time. The last assumption is that if you have qualified applicants, those that are happy to come to a particular program for training make the best residents and, therefore, the best program.

This system is, at best, considered avant-garde. You probably will not be exposed to it. But if you are, do not be put off by it. You should still handle yourself in the same manner described elsewhere in this book.

## Silence

The most stressful time during any interview can be a period of silence. This is an occasion to reveal all of your twitches, nervousness, and insecurity. It is also an opportunity to show self-assurance. Be strong!

Silence occurs for several reasons. Rarely are physician-interviewers disciplined enough, or nasty enough, to impose a period of silence to simply test an applicant. Rather, they may remain quiet while they contemplate a question or your answer. They also may suddenly have remembered that they didn't turn off their headlights when they parked their car that morning. Don't feel that a period of silence is negatively directed at you.

Some people respond to silence during an interview by fidgeting. They brush their hair back, move around in their chairs, straighten their clothes, or mutter to themselves. Others try to break the silence by repeating (or worse, contradicting) what they just said. Don't do it; sit still, be calm, and be quiet—it too will end. One way experienced individuals combat periods of silence in interview-like situations is to simply begin counting the time to see how long the period lasts. It will seem like days, but it rarely lasts more than fifteen seconds.

You, too, can occasionally use silence to demonstrate your contemplative side. If an interviewer asks a particularly deep or thoughtful question, you don't have to jump in immediately with an answer, even if you are prepared for it. Wait a few seconds as you "think" it through. Rather than appearing impulsive, you now seem to be a deep thinker.

# Control The Interview—Gently

As you will see in the next chapter, it is often possible to steer the interview in a direction that is beneficial to you. You can mold your answers to interviewers' questions in such a way as to bring out some of your most favorable points. However, this must be done subtly. Some interviewers may see your pushing an interview in a specific direction as being impudent. This, of course, would be counterproductive. So, if you can, steer the interview in a beneficial direction—but do it so gently that the interviewer does not notice.

# Reasons Why Interviews Fail

## Inadequate Preparation

The first reason that interviews fail is due to inadequate preparation on the applicant's part. This book helps you to prepare for the residency interview. In the end, however, it is up to you to know about the specialty, the program, the faculty, your own ambitions and desires, and the questions that you will probably be asked during interviews. It takes hard work on your part to get ready for interviews, but in the end it is worth it.

## Not Listening To Questions

The second reason is because the applicant does not listen to the interviewer's questions. This results in discommunication, distorting the messages coming in and going out. This is what happens when you let your mind wander during an interview—and it spells disaster. Remember that an interview is a battle of wits. If your thoughts stray during this war game, you lose!

Even fast talkers listen faster than they talk. We usually speak only 100 to 150 words per minute, but process about 600 spoken words a minute. This provides a lot of time for our minds to wander—usually spent thinking about what we are going to say next rather than about what is being said. Since we can only listen or think, we may miss what the other person is saying. When we think and our eyes wander (even momentarily), the speaker knows that we are not listening. The epitome of ignoring the interviewer and the interview is the apocryphal candidate whose cellular phone rings during the interview, excuses herself, and proceeds to answer the phone.

Use "active listening." This involves briefly summarizing what you think the speaker has just said. It shows that you are carefully listening, allows the speaker to correct any misimpressions you may have gotten, and helps the conversation move forward. Don't wait until the end of the interview to do this, but rather intersperse it several times during the interview. For example, after the interviewer has described some attributes of their program, say "As I understand it, this residency's strengths are . . . ." You might then continue with, "How about . . . ?"

Since many residency interviews are conducted in busy offices, clinical settings, or even hallways, you may have to concentrate very hard on the interview to avoid the ever-present distractions, sometimes justifiably called "interview blockers" (Figure 17.1). This can be difficult, but your experiences working in noisy patient-care areas should help you to concentrate on the task at hand. And don't just listen to the question, listen to *how the question is asked.* Many times an interviewer will give the astute listener clues to the answer that he or she is looking for. Figure 19.2, "Guidelines for Effective Listening," should help you out.

When speaking, use your normal voice rather than the higher pitch that people often use when they are nervous. Avoid using "fillers" to pad a pause in the conversation, such as "um," "er," "ah," or "you know." Rather, simply pause or use "and," "or," or "but" to join your thoughts together.

Also, never robotically "give your presentation," downloading your spiel in a rote manner. Rather, keep in mind an outline of your "message" and interject it at appropriate points in the conversation.

---

### FIGURE 19.2
#### *Guidelines for Effective Listening*

1. Demonstrate attentiveness.
2. Listen for "what" and "why" questions.
3. Listen for key issues.
4. Mirror back the interviewer's messages.
5. Don't interrupt the interviewer.
6. Ask clarifying questions.
7. Identify feelings and attitudes in the interviewer.
8. Don't waste time evaluating the interviewer.

Occasionally your mind may go blank during an interview. It's okay. Just apologize to the interviewer and simply ask for a moment to think about the question or, second best, ask the interviewer to repeat the question. As Sam Donaldson, the television newsman, says, "Even the pros get tongue-tied."

**One caveat.** If you have carefully read the questions and answers in Chapter 20, you may be planning how to answer what you think will be the next question. Or, you may be analyzing how you might interact during your residency with the faculty and residents you have met. Stop! Turn off that mental audiotape and listen to the interviewer. By now you should be able to answer questions without rehearsing, and there will be plenty of time later to analyze your visit. Concentrate on what the interviewer is saying.

If you really listen, and you still can't understand what an interviewer is looking for, ask for clarification. This might also work (once) if you miss a question completely—but it would be unwise to count on using it repeatedly. Remember that the most ego-gratifying thing you can do for interviewers is to listen to them.

If you are asked a question you just don't know how to answer, be honest and say so. Perhaps you can say, "I'll have to think about that. Can we come back to that later?" Normally, the interviewer will oblige. It is then your responsibility to return to the question before the end of the interview. At that point, if you still cannot come up with an answer, say that you will continue to think about it and get back to the interviewer by letter. Then, in your thank-you letter, give that interviewer an answer to his or her question. In these cases, honesty (and thoughtfulness in later responding by letter), rather than bluffing your way through an answer, may be your key to success.

## Answering Questions Not Asked

A third reason for interview failures is that interviewers may get annoyed by having questions answered that were not asked. Many students, while attempting to highlight their strengths, routinely give answers that have no relation at all to the questions that were asked (much like politicians).

Here, you are treading the fine line between guiding the interview and destroying it. Answering a question about your spare-time activities with a description of your medical school awards makes no sense. Rather, talk about the rock band you organized or the Internet bulletin board you established. These both answer the question and highlight your initiative and talents.

Similar applicant behavior that interviewers detest includes answering questions with questions, telling jokes to change the subject, and answering with gibberish. Like reporters, good interviewers simply repeat their original question until they get a straight answer. Also, because interviewers are human, answers that might work one day may not on another. Many factors can influence an interviewer's behavior (Figure 19.3).

## Rambling

A fourth way to wreck your interview is to ramble, thus providing superfluous information. Interviewers are easily bored—not surprising given the number of applicants they must often see in one day.

If you have a lot of information to impart in answer to a specific question, tell the interviewer the main points, and then ask if he or she would like you to continue. For example, if you are asked to describe your medical school rotation in your chosen specialty, give the highlights in several sentences and then ask if the interviewer would like to know more. Since you are watching the interviewer while you answer, you may note nonverbal cues indicating that you have said enough. In general, keep your answers brief, to the point, and interesting.

## Giving Warning Signals

The fifth reason that interviews fail is that the applicant inadvertently gives warning signals to the interviewer that there may be an unstable personality lurking behind a deceptive smile. Trained interviewers seek specific warning signs (Figure 19.4).

Very few faculty interviewers are sophisticated enough in the techniques of employment interviewing to consciously recognize these signs. Being good clinicians, though, they unconsciously assimilate clues and will give the applicant a poor rating. It would be a good idea to review the warning signs and make certain that you do not demonstrate any unintentionally.

---

### FIGURE 19.3
#### *Factors Influencing an Interviewer's Behavior*

- Age and Stage in Life Cycle
- Cultural Background
- Interests
- Prior Experiences
- Goals/Aspirations
- Successes/Failures
- Mood
- Personality

---

### FIGURE 19.4
#### *Warning Signs for Interviewers*

- Inconsistent answers during the interview.
- Inconsistencies between what is said in the interview and past performance.
- Abrasiveness or any other personality quirk that makes the interviewer uncomfortable.
- Evasiveness.
- A pattern of unhappiness in former jobs.
- Blaming others for all the applicant's problems.
- Dullness when responding to questions.
- A pattern of taking advantage of, or of deceiving, other people.

---

Adapted from: Perham JC. Spotting bad apples: the warning signals. *Dun's Business Month*. October 1986, pp. 54-56.

## Interview Disasters

Life is often stranger than fiction, and so are some interviews. One national employment agency described some of the more unusual occurrences during interviews for professional positions:

- At the outset of the interview, the applicant sat down in the interviewer's chair and insisted that the interviewer sit elsewhere.
- When an applicant was asked about loyalty, he showed the interviewer a tattoo of his girlfriend's name.
- An applicant pulled out a tape recorder, saying that he taped all interviews.
- Another left the dry cleaning tag on his jacket, saying that he wanted to demonstrate just how neat and clean he was.
- When told to take his time answering questions, an applicant began writing out the answers before speaking.
- During the interview, an applicant received three cellular telephone calls.
- Another brought his five children and the family cat to the interview.
- At the end of the interview, the applicant asked if she could use the fax machine to send out some personal letters.

Hopefully, you won't make these types of errors. Just think, if this is how other applicants behave, you don't have much to worry about. Of course, most medical students are smart enough to avoid such crass behavior.

## Sell Yourself

The bottom line during an interview is that you must sell yourself. At the same time, you also need to elicit information. To have the best chance of being ranked highly by the programs, you must do a good job of showing your own wares. Interviewers are looking for specific attributes in applicants (Figure 19.5). When talking with the individuals at each program, remember that interviewers rate these elements in the applicants they interview. Although every program has a different rating form for interviewers to complete, the essential items will always be the same (Figure 19.6).

It is your job to point out how closely you resemble the interviewer's ideal candidate by exhibiting the sought-after traits. Remember, if you don't sell yourself, no one else will do it for you!

---

**FIGURE 19.5**
*Key Personality Traits Interviewers Seek*

**Personal**

- Enthusiasm
- Motivation/Initiative
- Communication skills
- Chemistry
- Energy
- Determination
- Confidence
- Humility
- Emotional control
- Common sense
- Good interpersonal skills
- Adaptability
- Intelligence

**Professional**

- Reliability
- Honesty/Integrity
- Pride
- Dedication
- Analytical skills
- Listening skills
- Ability to get things done
- Initiative
- Good work habits/work ethic
- Good judgment
- Motivation to achieve
- Problem-solving skills

FIGURE 19.6
### *Interviewer's Rating Form*

Applicant Name _____ Date _____

*Scale:* 1 = *Very Weak*    10 = *Very Strong*

**General**

_____ Physical appearance (dress, grooming)

_____ Character (reliability, honesty, integrity)

_____ Timeliness

_____ Knowledge about specialty

_____ Knowledge about program

_____ Computer literacy

_____ Energy

**Intellect**

_____ Mental ability          _____ Judgment

_____ Flexibility             _____ Communication ability

**Emotions**

_____ Work ethic           _____ Personality (fits program)

_____ Motivation           _____ Teachable

_____ Attitude              _____ Sense of humor

_____ Stability             _____ Outside interests

_____ Self-confidence

**Record**

_____ USMLE/COMLEX score      _____

_____ Class rank              _____

_____ Medical school         _____

_____ Quality of reference letters    _____

_____ Clinical performance (general)   _____

_____ Clinical performance (specialty)   _____

_____ Honors/Awards         _____

_____ Research              _____

_____ **Total**        _____ **Number of Scored Items**

_____ **Average of Scored Items**

# 20

# The Questions–The Answers

*Silence is the only good substitute for intelligence.*

– Folk Saying

*Judge a person not by his answers, but by his questions.*

– Voltaire

What must you remember in the process of preparing for the interview? And what must you remember during the interview? Only two things: *prepare in advance* and *sell yourself by showing your best qualities.*

Interviews generally start with some simple pleasantries and then move on to the skills/attitude evaluation (Figure 19.1). In this part of the interview, no matter what the format or the type of questions asked, most program directors look for three qualities in applicants: *intellectual strength, energy,* and *personal compatibility* with faculty, staff, and current residents.

Interviewers don't really want "the truth." They want "correct" answers. If you believe there is no such thing as the correct answer to a typical interview question, you are sadly mistaken. Good interviewers know exactly what they are looking for in a resident. They know how to extract the needed information in a way that is disarmingly benign. Their questions are simply tools with which to hammer out an impression of the applicant.

## Intellectual Strength

Program directors already know a great deal about your performance in this arena. Reference letters, USMLE/COMLEX scores, transcripts, and narratives of clinical performance have preceded you. That is what got you in the door for the interview. Now it is time to see if you can think on your feet. Can you apply what you know to new situations? Are you really interested in learning, or just in getting through a program so you can go into practice? Do you know about anything other than medicine? Was it your quick smile rather than a solid intellect that got you your good grades? Do you believe that you have very little left to learn? Basically, the interviewer is trying to determine what you know, how well you are able to use what you have learned, and if you really want to learn any more.

## Energy

Residents spend the majority of their time attending to patient care duties. No matter where a program is located or what the specialty is, fatigue, stress, and depression are pervasive. This is especially true during the PGY-1 year. The less this manifests itself in a program's residents, the fewer the problems with which the faculty must deal and, consequently, the happier they are. Make them happy. Demonstrate that you have the good humor, self-confidence, and stamina to go the distance. But don't just say the words—show them by your actions during the entire interview process.

## Personal Compatibility

Remember that you are being hired to join an established group of practicing physicians, albeit at a very junior level. You will be responsible for the care of the faculty's patients. You will be their representative to the medical and non-medical communities. They will have to live their professional lives with you for the duration of your training.

A "personality" already exists for the group, the residency, the department, and the institution. Will you fit in? Will they be comfortable with you? A little thought and a lot of care are necessary here. A hyper-aggressive image may work in some locales, but fail in others. Modify the image you project to meet the situation. But don't fool yourself. If you will not fit in with a group, it is better to find that out during the interview, rather than after you arrive for a several-year stint as a resident.

# Presenting Yourself

## Show Your Best Qualities

As you answer the interviewers' questions, remember to highlight your best qualities to *sell yourself!*

And do not sell yourself short! Know what your strengths are. Know what the residency is looking for. If you don't have an obvious opportunity to let the interviewers know how well you meet their needs, make an opportunity. This may come through answering questions—all questions—with different strength areas you want to demonstrate. Or it may come in the form of a "question" at the termination of the interview, e.g., "Is it true that many Orthopedic Surgeons have woodworking as a hobby? I have a workshop at home and have made prize-winning furniture." Remember, if you don't sell yourself, no one will do it for you.

## Prepare

When getting ready for the interview, it is absolutely essential to *prepare, prepare, prepare!* How many hours have you spent studying and preparing for exams? A thousand? Five thousand? The interview is, perhaps, the toughest exam of your life. Make sure that you spend enough time studying for it. The steps to preparing for an interview are very straightforward: learn to talk about yourself easily, and learn the types of questions interviewers ask and what they hope to learn from your answers. Then combine these and formulate your answers in advance.

### *Talking About Yourself*

Talking about yourself can be very difficult. Most people are loath to extol their own virtues. You must be ready to tell the interviewers your positive qualities so that they hear them loud and clear.

*First*, put yourself in the position of the residency faculty where you will be interviewing. What job skills and personal characteristics would you want in an individual applying to *your* program? You should be able to get a good idea from the material you have collected from the specialty societies, from the program's own information, and from talks with residents and specialists in the field. Write these characteristics down. Then write out questions you would ask an applicant to your program.

*Second*, list your strengths that match these characteristics. This step requires a good bit of objectivity. You may need some help from your adviser or a close friend. The following exercise will help you to get in the habit of thinking and talking positively about yourself.

### *Exercise*

List *three accomplishments* of which you are proud and what each accomplishment indicates about you:

1. _____

   _____

2. _____

   _____

3. _____

   _____

Next, list *three abilities* you have that will make you valuable as a resident in the specialty for which you are applying:

1. _____

_____

2. _____

_____

3. _____

_____

Now, can you use these accomplishments and abilities in a short narrative that describes you? If you can, you have made a good start toward a successful interview.

*Finally*, write some great answers to the questions you developed. Be sure to incorporate your accomplishments and abilities into your answers. But do not memorize them word for word—they will sound forced. Guests on television talk shows prepare by making a list of the ten questions they *don't* want to be asked—and then developing answers for each of them. Note that this process may change a bit as you gain interview experience. But the process gets easier each time you do it. And it is worth the effort.

It's said that the famous lawyer, F. Lee Bailey, doesn't believe that he has won so many difficult cases because he is any smarter than his opponents—it is just that he is more obsessive-compulsive. Preparation is his key to success. Your preparation will also be your key to getting a residency position.

## Types of Questions

Typical interviewers only use five types of interview questions, although they can be phrased in many different ways. Recognizing the type of question the interviewer asks helps you determine what information he or she is seeking.

### Closed Question

These questions ask for specific information and a simple, definitive answer. "How many years were you an undergraduate?" for example, deserves merely a simple answer, such as "four years." Nothing deep here. Interviewers use closed questions to elicit information seemingly absent from the application materials.

## Open-Ended, Informal Question

These questions also ask for specific information, but require more in-depth answers. Such a question might be, "What clinical experiences have you had in this specialty?" While the question requires specific information, it allows the applicant a chance to speak and become relaxed.

## Open-Ended, Attitudinal Question

These questions determine how well an applicant organizes his or her thoughts before speaking. An example is "What do you think of physician advertising?" Most interviewers want to see if the answer is concise and to the point.

## Probing Question

Interviewers ask probing questions as follow-ups to open-ended questions. They become especially useful after the applicant has given an answer expressing an opinion. An example of this type of question is "Why do you feel that way?" This forces applicants to defend and further explain their previous answer. It also allows an interviewer to control the direction of the interview.

Sometimes an interviewer will go back to an earlier answer, quote the applicant, and ask a question, such as "You said you felt this area of the country was more progressive medically than your medical school's area. Why is that?"

## Leading Question

Interviewers use leading questions to direct applicants' answers or to see if they have the gumption to express their own opinions. Unfortunately, it is not always easy to tell what is expected. Such a question might begin, "Residents in our specialty should go back to an every-other-night call schedule," and be followed by, "Don't you agree?" The interviewer may be serious or merely prodding the interviewee into an untenable position. If the intent is unclear, a way to find out before answering is simply to ask, "What makes you think that?"

# Interviewer Techniques

Interviewers have numerous methods to trap the unwary applicant. They may, for example, ask three questions together at the start of the interview. Are you cool enough to remember them without being prompted? One way to help remember them is to repeat them back "for clarification" after they are asked.

The interviewer may also give conflicting opinions about the same topic to see if the applicant will simply agree with both. Wrong move! Don't be a wimp! Suggest to the interviewer that the opinions "seem to conflict, if I understand you correctly."

Some interviewers treat the interview more like a psychological test by asking interviewees to complete sentences. Examples might be:

"If I were 10% more assertive, I would . . ."

"I sometimes act inappropriately when . . ."

"If I could say anything I wanted right now, I would say . . ."

As for psychological tests, about half of all U.S. companies use them, and about a fourth give formal personality tests to job applicants as part of the interview process. This has not yet caught on among residency programs. Prospective employers use these tests to measure "The Big Five"—emotional stability, extroversion, openness to new experiences, agreeableness, and conscientiousness. These test results (which can be faked by knowledgeable test takers) can then be validated in the interview. Residency faculty think that they can get the same information without using these tests.

Some savvy residency directors interview applicants twice—although one time may be during lunch or in a more informal setting. They may ask some of the same questions again. The second time they are interviewed, applicants are generally more relaxed and may give more complete information or even respond differently to the same questions.

Now, what are some of the specific questions you are likely to be asked?

## Questions & Answers

The following questions are those that residency applicants have been asked over the past several years. Following the prototypical question and a discussion of possible answers, I have listed similar questions that applicants have been asked. Some are much more thoughtful or original than the classic questions—such as "Why do you want to be a (fill in the specialty)?"—to which nearly all applicants tire of responding. Perhaps some interviewers will read this list and buff up their interviewing "act." However, it is impossible to prepare for or predict every possible question. If you prepare for the questions listed below, you will have the confidence to answer anything an interviewer asks.

These questions are often used in strange ways by interviewers. One residency applicant reported that she had been asked the (main) questions from this list *in the order in which they appear!* Don't count on this happening to you.

## 1. How are you today?

What a pleasant way for an interviewer to begin. A simple ice-breaker, you think. Wrong! Sophisticated interviewers use this and similar questions as rapid and effective screening tools. "Gee, it's raining outside and I got soaked coming here," said one applicant. "I'm really frustrated that my plane was late and that I had trouble getting a cab," whined another.

Interviewers look for individuals whose demeanor stays upbeat even under adversity. The travails on the interview circuit are insignificant compared to those during residency. Simple opening questions delivered in an off-hand manner often expose an applicant's true personality far better than the well-rehearsed "deep" questions that most applicants have come to expect.

Most people find the first three minutes of an interview to be the most difficult. Breaking the ice has tripped up many excellent candidates. You can ease this awkward moment—and make many interviewers grateful—by asking a question about a photograph, book, or other object in the office in which you are sitting. The interviewer then has the ball and must answer (giving you a little breathing space) and starts the interview on a warm, friendly note.

The point is, there are no innocent questions!

• Did you have any trouble finding us or getting here?
• You're looking a little flustered. What's wrong?

## 2. Do you have any questions?

This is the "behavioral" interviewer's classic opening. The interviewee is expected to take the initiative right from the start. Many applicants ask standard questions and, therefore, waste this opportunity. When the "any questions" opportunity begins an interview, ask questions that highlight your strengths and knowledge of the specialty. Get this information from reading recent "throwaway" journals or news magazines for this specialty, such as *Internal Medicine News*.

Use this question to show them the special expertise you can add to their program, and that you are achievement-oriented. An example might be, "I recently read in *Family Practice News* that Family Practice expects to be more involved in sports medicine. I have a real interest in this area based on my work as a football trainer in college, and I have taught new trainers. Do other people at this program also have an interest in sports medicine?"

Faculty members most commonly ask this question because they are poor employment interviewers. They often do not know what other questions to ask. Since many applicants report this is the most common question they are asked, make a long list of your own questions to use as answers. Never answer "No," since, no matter what the situation, a negative answer indicates that you have a less-than-serious interest in that program.

- Do you know much about our program?
- If you were in my (the interviewer's) seat, what would you ask? Okay, now answer those questions.

## 3. *Tell me about yourself.*

This is the granddaddy of open-ended questions (although, of course, it isn't really a question). You have the opportunity to say almost anything you want. You can put your best foot forward or stick it right in your mouth. This question gives you, by design, no hint of how to answer it. You can go off on almost any tangent. And if the interviewer is any good, you will be able to talk for as long as you want. The longer you talk, however, the less chance there is that you will score high on the interviewer's list of candidates.

To answer this question, and similar open-ended questions as well, first respond briefly and succinctly to the single question, "What motivates you?" For example, you might cite your most applicable qualities by stating, "I am a hard worker with a real interest in ENT. I like both the diagnostic and therapeutic aspects of the specialty and seem to be good at the technical procedures that I have been allowed to do."

Then stop. Ask the interviewer if you should continue. This demonstrates that you understand the interactive nature of interviews and that you have consideration for the other person's role. When you ask whether you should continue, many interviewers will direct you to other areas to discuss further. This will help both you and the interviewer a great deal by allowing you to answer the questions that the interviewer really wanted to ask.

- What three adjectives best describe you?
- Tell me a story about yourself that best describes you.
- If you were going to die in five minutes, what would you tell someone about yourself?
- If you died right now, what would you want on your tombstone?
- Of which accomplishments are you most proud?
- Do you have any hidden achievements or qualities of which you are secretly proud? What are they?
- What are your team-player/leadership qualities?
- What might give me a better picture of you than I can get from your résumé?
- Tell me about your adolescence.

- How have you changed since high school?
- What was the most important event in your life?
- What shaped you and got you to where you are today?
- What was the most difficult thing you have ever done?
- If you could be on the cover of any magazine next month, which one would it be? What would the caption say?
- What do you like to cook?
- How would your best-friend/roommates/relatives describe you? What negative things would they say?
- Why did you write . . . in your personal statement/essay?
- What do you recall about your day before you go to sleep at night?
- What one thing do you want conveyed to the residency committee?

## 4. What are your strengths and weaknesses?

This question represents the "Tell me about yourself" question phrased negatively. It asks, "Tell me what's wrong with you."

Would you want to answer that question? Of course not. And it is extremely unlikely that you will ever come up against it. But an inquiry about your strengths and weaknesses, essentially the same question, is very common. Basically, the interviewer asks you to jump off a cliff of your own design. All you need to do is to redesign the cliff so you can climb rather than jump.

First, answer the question about your strengths concisely. The only danger is talking too much. Then work on the other half of the question, the dangerous part.

Everyone has weaknesses. "Each and every one on you has something that makes you a jerk," says the Lt. Colonel briefing a group of officers about to be promoted to General. "Get in touch with your 'inner jerk' and work on losing that ugly part of your personality." Okay, so a little bit of you is a "jerk." How do you respond?

At this point, you must turn your "weaknesses" into more strengths. What character flaws would the faculty in this specialty approve of? Is your weakness that you are obsessive about completing your work in an exacting manner? Or is it an intolerance for those clinicians who do not perform their patient-related tasks with a professional attitude? Maybe it is an inability to go home at night unless all your work is completed. These are, undoubtedly, the types of "failings" that the faculty will be interested in encouraging rather than disparaging. But in relating these faults, show at least a little remorse about having them. Don't be glib.

- Tell me about your "secret identity," the part of your personality that you don't share with strangers.
- Are there any skeletons in your closet that you want to tell me about?
- How well do you take criticism?
- What is your pet peeve?
- If you could change one thing about your personality, what would it be?
- What are your three strongest qualities?
- What are your two worst qualities?
- Have you demonstrated leadership in any extracurricular activities?

### 5. If you could be any cell in the human body, which would you choose to be, and why?

This is not much different from the directive to "Tell me about yourself." It is, however, a bit more inventive and has been used by many interviewers, especially in Internal Medicine, ever since it found its way into *The New England Journal of Medicine* (1990;323:838). Unfortunately, you may have a hard time not being reminded of *Saturday Night Live's* Baba WaWa's similar question, "If you could be any kind of twee . . . ?"

The neuron was overwhelmingly favored by applicants for Internal Medicine internships, and for Gastroenterology and Geriatric fellowships. Most applicants said they wanted to be neurons "to be in control, to be stimulated and stimulating, and to be the center of all things." Since you are now prepared in advance for this question, try to be original. Don't be surprised if this question pops up along the interview route.

- Do you see yourself as more relaxed/casual/informal or as more serious/dedicated/committed?
- Which is more important, the ability to organize, structure and prioritize, or the ability to be flexible, modify, and make do as needed?
- Which is more important, knowledge or imagination?
- If you could be any kitchen object, what would you be?
- If you could sing any one song beautifully, which one would you choose?
- What is the strangest Halloween costume you ever wore?

## 6. If your house was burning, what three objects would you save?

Some residency interviewers really believe Freudian analysis will help them choose the best residents. While this may seem to be essentially the same type of question as the one above, think again. This question narrows the scope to a very concrete and personal level by asking, "What do you value in your own life?" How important are material objects to you? Are you "sensitive" enough to reach for your beloved's picture, or are you "sensible" enough to grab the car keys and credit cards?

There is no one correct answer to this question. The best answer depends upon the nature of the person asking the question. Sometimes the questioner actually wants to know whether you have planned ahead or can think quickly, since a fire is a real possibility in our lives—unlike turning into a tree or a cell.

An alternate form of this question is "If you had to repack your belongings, what wouldn't you have brought with you?" This question is even more concrete, at least for the majority of students traveling to interviews. The follow-up questions will certainly be "Why leave that behind?" and "Why did you bring it?" Pack carefully.

- If you had unlimited money and two free hours (one day, one week, one month) what would you do?
- If you had three wishes, what would they be? (Shades of Aladdin!)
- What in your life is most important to you?

## 7. What kinds of people are your friends?

"Know my friends, know me," goes an old expression. People attract similar folks as friends. Applicants' descriptions of their friends often gives interviewers deep insights into their personalities. These types of questions essentially ask you to talk about yourself in the third person.

Answer this type of question as if you were describing yourself. Interviewers often respond favorably when married applicants state that their spouse is their best friend. Describing a spouse's glowing personal attributes only serves to enhance the applicant, as long as these attributes are not used as a contrast to the candidate's own qualities.

- Describe your best friend/roommate/spouse and their life.
- How are you similar and dissimilar to your best friend?
- How would your friends or coworkers describe you?
- Has someone ever come to you for help with a major personal crisis? What have you done to alleviate their emotional pain?

## 8. Who are your heroes?

Related to the question "Tell me about yourself," this is a deep probe into your psyche. It evaluates your self-image, direction, and goals. How the interviewer interprets your answer may, to some degree, reflect his or her own personality, age, and background.

This is perhaps the most difficult interview question to answer. In an age without obvious heroes, your choice will, by necessity, be very personal There are several possible responses to this question.

One answer you may have already thought of is that you have no heroes. You have, however, just completed many years of schooling, during which you had many new experiences and met countless interesting people as teachers, friends, and patients. Viewed from that perspective, it would be an unusual, and perhaps very narrow-minded, individual who could not find someone to look up to as a role model.

Another possible answer is to cite a family member, friend, or personal acquaintance. The follow-up question, of course, will be "Why?" There should be some identifiable attribute this person demonstrates that justifies your distinguishing him or her as your hero. A parent, sibling, or spouse is usually a very good choice. It shows respect for your family and a firm commitment to your roots. If you choose a physician as your hero, be prepared to explain how you are trying, or will try, to emulate that person's attributes in your professional life.

Historic or public figures are perfectly acceptable answers. These heroes can be drawn from science, education, or many other fields. But tread lightly if your hero is a contemporary religious or political figure. An interviewer's bias may affect your evaluation if your choice of a hero exemplifies major philosophical differences between the two of you.

The worst answer is to name a contemporary star of television, the movies, or popular music. In that case, both you and your answer will probably be seen as very superficial.

- What is your favorite movie? Why?
- What is the last book you read?
- What do "success" and "failure" mean to you?
- If you could accomplish only one thing the rest of your life, what would that be?
- What do you believe?
- Do you have any Black, Hispanic, etc. role models in medicine?
- What physician characteristics do you admire most? least?
- If you could dine with anyone from the past, present or future, who would it be?

- Among the people at your school, whose work or life do you admire? Why?
- Tell me about your father/mother.

### 9. What do you do in your spare time?

The primary danger here is in giving too long an answer. Everyone likes to talk about him- or herself and this is an invitation to do just that. But keep it brief. If you collect rocks, for example, you might say, "I am an avid rock collector and have been for about ten years. I have had the opportunity to travel across the United States and Canada pursuing my hobby." Then stop. If the interviewer wants to know any more, he or she will ask.

Your answer should show that you are not a couch potato (although a computer aficionado is okay). Do not describe activities that may cause injuries resulting in prolonged sick leave. Also, pick a non-controversial topic; avoid discussing hunting, guns, or religion unless you are certain that you will not raise the interviewer's hackles. In general, speak about community-oriented and people-centered activities. The focus of the rock collector's description might be the people she meets at collector's conventions.

The questioner usually wants to learn three things from this query.

First, does the applicant have any interests outside medicine? An interviewee with no outside interests sends a serious danger signal. Residents who have no outlet for the anxieties, stresses, and frustrations of residency training may decompensate—and become a problem for the residency faculty. If you have no overriding outside interest, simply mention what you do in your spare time. Yes, spending lots of time with your spouse and children is certainly an outside interest.

Second, is the applicant more enthusiastic about his or her avocation than about the prospect of training for and practicing in this medical specialty? The key here is to show equal enthusiasm for both.

Third, the interviewer is screening out those applicants who are so wrapped up in themselves that they will not be able to pay any attention to their patients, peers, and faculty. How do they spot these individuals? They are the ones who go on and on and on about their other activities with no prompting—even after the interviewer gives negative cues, such as turning away from the applicant, coughing, or even standing up. Answer questions about your outside activities, as you have answered the other questions—fully, briefly, and with enthusiasm.

- What are your favorite games and sports? Why?
- Have you done any volunteer work?

- Why did you choose these outside activities?
- If you had a completely free day, what would you do?
- What is the most bizarre thing you have ever done (or did in high school or in college)?
- What was the most unusual occurrence in your life in the past month?
- Do you think you can remain intensely focused on learning this specialty for the length of the program? For the rest of your professional career?
- Would you work if you didn't have to? Why?
- Besides your future medical accomplishments, what do you wish to be known for by your peers, friends, and family?
- Where have you traveled? Why?
- What non-medical magazines do you regularly read?
- What have you contributed to groups and activities in which you participated?
- What have you learned from your volunteer work?

### 10. *It says on your résumé that . . .*

You wrote that you have a particular skill or learning experience. That may have been one reason you got this interview. Okay, show us how you would apply it.

This request is not made in the abstract. Rather, the interviewer gives you a specific situation, usually associated with medical practice, and possibly with the residency, and asks you to show your stuff. You wrote that you had experience working in a medical clinic for indigent patients. They ask you how you would obtain necessary medications for a child whose parents did not have the money to pay for them. Or you wrote that you served as the student on your hospital's bioethics committee. What elements do you look for when doing a bioethics consultation, asks the interviewer?

In some cases, the request can be even simpler. The interviewer starts speaking to you in Spanish or Russian. Well, you said you could speak it. Anything you put in your résumé is fair game for the interviewer, including your extracurricular activities, publications or research, ability in a foreign language, travel, etc. Don't embellish! You are certain to run across at least one interviewer who will want to speak to you in Serbo-Croatian if you said you speak it fluently. If you said you participated in a study of histamine in rats, an interviewer is sure to ask you to explain how you could study the chemical's role in headaches or toxic presentations during your residency.

Since you may be asked about them, bring any written materials, such as articles, book chapters, etc., listed in your résumé to the interview. Even if they haven't been published, bring a draft copy so you can show it to interviewers if asked.

This is called the "predictive interview technique." It is very effective when the interviewer can make a specific connection with something in the applicant's history. For interviewees, this can be a wonderful or a devastating experience. Be careful what you put in your application materials.

- What did you like about Kuala Lampur (to an applicant who said he had worked in a medical clinic there)?
- How would you design a study to test whether drug Z works in congestive heart failure (to an applicant who says she has done several drug-related studies)?

## 11. In what situations are you most efficient and effective?

Medicine, and especially residency, is best practiced by those who are time efficient. Residency directors know that those who can manage their time well will often make excellent residents. Part of managing time, however, is knowing what makes you efficient. Have you thought about how you optimize your use of time? Do you know the strategies that help you accomplish tasks faster, more successfully, and in a timely manner?

A particular interest in some specialties is whether you can multi-task. That is, can you walk and chew gum at the same time? Or more to the point, can you successfully handle multiple patient-related tasks for multiple patients at once? This is essential to function well in emergency departments, busy clinics, and on hectic ward services.

- When are you least efficient and effective?
- How do you handle interruptions when you are busy?
- When are you most creative?
- What makes you procrastinate?
- Do you see time as your ally or an enemy?

## 12. To which organizations do you belong?

People join organizations that further their own agendas, be they recreational, spiritual, political, or professional. The organizations you belong to reflect your goals, background, and interests. The question here is, how much do you want to reveal?

The groups you join often loudly signal your religion, political or sexual orientation, and cultural heritage. Since prejudice exists in many guises, it may be best to simply discuss the professional medical organizations to which you belong. These should include the student arm of the specialty's national organization, and might also include the AMA, AOA, or AMSA.

Most interviewers now understand that pressing you for information about other organizations might violate state and federal hiring rules. Note, however, that anything you included in your application materials is fair game during interviews. If you list an organization on your résumé, the interviewer may ask you about it.

- Your name sounds Hispanic (Arabic, Italian, Vietnamese, etc.). Is it?
- How did you learn to speak (non-English language)?
- When was the last time you went back to (country of origin or family's origin)?
- Why do you think you are a minority?
- Would you have any trouble working in this predominantly Catholic (LDS, Jewish, etc.) hospital?

### 13. *What are your plans for a family?*

You probably will be asked a variety of questions that are not only uncomfortable, but also patently illegal under state or federal statutes. These questions also provide ammunition for discrimination-in-hiring lawsuits. (These suits are rarely brought, however, because discrimination is hard to prove in court.)

The litmus test to see whether a question is illegal is to ask yourself, "Is it important to my job as a resident?" If it is relevant, then the question is probably legitimate. (The law, however, can be convoluted. See Figure 20.2.)

Questions about family, childcare, and birth control are most often directed at women applicants. Other candidates may hear inquiries about race, nationality, physical infirmities, religion, and other subjects which are illegal for employers to raise. (See also Chapter 13, "Marriage, Pregnancy, and Children," and "Illegal Questions" later in this chapter.")

How should you respond to such questions? This can be very tricky. There are several possible approaches. The most common one is to just answer the question in the most favorable manner possible. It is the most politic thing to do and will not eliminate you from the pool of potential candidates. For questions about family planning, you could simply state that you have no plans to interrupt your training to have a family at the present time. If you already have children, you might directly address the interviewer's concerns by stating that your past performance demonstrates that your family responsibilities will not detract from your work or affect your ability to show up on time. Directly answering such questions may be preferable to saying "I prefer not to answer." Just as when invoking your Fifth Amendment rights, the listener will often infer the most negative response.

You may not, however, want to answer such questions, either because of the answer that you would have to give or because your principles just will not allow it. You then have three choices.

The first choice, which will still permit you to remain a viable candidate, is to laughingly ask whether the answer to the question, or the question itself, is relevant to being a resident. If you do this lightly, the interviewer will be able to back off from the question without losing face.

If you derisively ask whether the question is relevant, or simply state that the question is illegal (your second choice), you will be on the interviewer's black list. Don't plan on getting into that residency program. But, if you do not get in and you still want to, you have the option of taking legal action against the program for violating your civil rights (your third choice). This has been done successfully in the business world many times. It is only a matter of (a short) time until these suits become frequent in the medical community. In fact, they may become commonplace enough that there will be much firmer control over the entire interview process in order to avoid legal entanglements.

Still, you should approach these illegal and uncomfortable questions in a relaxed manner. This will yield the best results.

A legal way to ask such questions might be "Is there anything about your personal life that may affect your performance in this demanding residency?" Your answer is "No."

- How important is your family to you?
- How do you propose to juggle marriage (relationship) and medical practice?
- What do your parents do for a living?

## 14. If you could no longer be a physician, what career would you choose?

Once again, let's see who is really hiding beneath the polished interview veneer. How deeply are you committed to medicine? Is it an interesting part of your life or is it the core of your existence? How easily can you come up with an answer that you find acceptable? How upset do you seem by such a prospect?

Very few people can fake a response to something this important. Interviewers, especially those who live and breathe medicine, use this question to find people who have the same level of commitment. Older interviewers may ask this more frequently, since many distrust the resolution of younger generations.

One other reason for asking this question is that some studies suggest that there is a high correlation between alternate career choices and certain specialties. Those going into Anesthesiology or Radiology, for example, usually select highly technical professional fields, such as engineering, research, the "hard" sciences, law, architecture, or finance-related business. Those entering Pediatrics tend to select teaching, other health-related professions, the humanities, the arts, or non-professional careers.

Variations of this question may also be used to test an applicant's grasp of reality. The interviewer may ask "What do you think you will do when you stop practicing medicine (at the end of a career)?" Others will probe even a strong answer to see whether applicants have considered any alternatives if they suddenly cannot practice medicine, at least in their specialty.

- Why did you choose to be a physician?
- If your brain was the only part of your body that worked, what would you do with your life?
- What will happen if you develop a debilitating disease while in residency?

## 15. *You seem really interested in research. How will you incorporate that interest into your residency and career?*

Are you sure you want to go to *this* residency? If you are interviewing at a program within a research institution, the interviewer may simply be assessing the strength of your interest in research and, perhaps, how strong a clinician-researcher you might be. However, if the interview is at a program that is primarily or solely clinical, the question may be asking how well you investigated the program before applying, whether your goals are consistent with those of the program, or if you will be happy going through this residency. This is a very legitimate faculty concern. If you have research as a possible career goal, be sure to apply to programs that share this interest.

- What are the most important traits for a clinician/researcher?
- How will the research you have done alter scientific thought? Help mankind?
- Let's discuss the details of the research you have done.
- How did the idea come to you for any research you initiated?
- How might acupuncture work? Do we know enough about physiology and biophysics to determine that?

## 16. In what subspecialty would you like to practice?

It is perfectly reasonable to say that you plan on practicing the primary specialty. But you may already have your heart set on becoming, for example, a cardiologist or neonatologist. Residency faculty know that a great many applicants, especially in the "primary care specialties" (General Internal Medicine, General Pediatrics, Family Practice, Obstetrics/Gynecology), plan to take subspecialty fellowships. Feel free to tell them that you are *considering* that course. Realize, though, that many residents change their minds about which specialty to enter once they get more clinical experience, so couch your answer with the reality that your future is not certain and you will make your decision at the appropriate time during your residency training.

If you do specify a subspecialty in which you are interested, be prepared for questions about that medical area. Also, you may be asked what you know about how well that subspecialty is represented at that residency's training institutions and program. Do you know who the subspecialists are? Do you know how much time you will spend with them during your residency? Given your interests, if that subspecialty is not well represented at their institutions why did you choose to interview at their program?

- In light of the bleak future for subspecialists, why would anyone go into cardiology or gastroenterology today?

## 17. How do you make important decisions?

As you discuss some very important life decisions you have made, the interviewer may wonder how you came to these decisions. Individuals vary in how they make important decisions. This reflects their personality and thought processes. Are they thoughtful, deliberate, and slow, or are they inattentive, impulsive, and quick? Or, does their decision-making method vary appropriately with the situation?

Be prepared to discuss your own decision-making strategies with interviewers. Think carefully before responding to this question, however. Remember, they may respond by asking if the method you describe matches the method you used to make your decisions to enter medicine and to apply for the specialty. Or they may inquire about how this process affects your ability to perform in specific clinical situations or to make other obvious life decisions, such as those revealed by your résumé.

If you use the Must/Want Analysis to help decide on the qualities you want in a residency, take a copy (without the program's ratings) to your interview and show it to any interviewer who asks you this question. They will probably be impressed with your logical and deliberate decision-making process.

- Are you a "risk-taker" or "safety-minded"?
- What made you choose your undergraduate major/minor?
- How did you select your undergraduate/medical school?
- What was the biggest obstacle in your life? How did you overcome it?
- What was the most difficult stand or position you ever defended? Why was it difficult?
- What was the most difficult decision you have had to make in your life? How did you make it?

## 18. *What were the major deficiencies in your medical school training?*

This is your opportunity to demonstrate some realistic insight into the past three-and-a-half years of your life. How well did your basic science courses prepare you for your clinical rotations? What were the strongest elements in your training? Where were the holes that you need to fill? No one believes that any medical school is perfect; residency faculty know this as well as anyone. However, avoid taking major swipes at your school. You will be an alumnus of the residency program at which you train no less than you will be an alumnus of your medical school. While a rah-rah response is not appropriate, neither is downgrading the training that you have received. Remember, your medical school training has gotten you as far as this interview.

While mentioning any deficiencies in your training you have the perfect opportunity to talk about your plans to remedy the deficit. These may include taking extra work or courses during the balance of your senior year and electives you plan to take while in residency.

- Why did you choose your medical school? How satisfied are you with your decision?
- What preclinical (clinical) medical school courses interested you the most?
- Did you enjoy your medical school classes? Why?

## 19. *How do you explain your . . . (low grades? leaves of absence? poor clinical narratives?)*

Not everyone who reads this book has an unblemished, stellar record. In fact, very few medical students do. Most have some areas of their records that require an explanation. Perhaps you failed a basic science course or a USMLE Step, and had to repeat it. Or maybe you had to take a leave of absence at some point in your training. You should expect to be asked about these deficiencies if the faculty members interviewing you are at all on the ball.

You already know what these issues are, and you need to be prepared to explain them. If there is a good justification for a questionable action, such as having to take time off due to a death in the family or a personal illness, explain. But if the poor grade or poor clinical performance on a rotation was, as is usual, due to your failure to put forth your best effort, just say so. Do not give excuses; they will sound lame to almost everyone except you. Your answer should be a variation of the terse military response, "No excuse, sir." Say that you did not give the course, rotation, etc. your best effort. If you think you can get away with it, blame it on immaturity, ignorance, or youth. This works best if the problem occurred during your first year in school, especially if you can demonstrate that you have expended more effort in subsequent years. If you have any questionable areas hanging over your application, be prepared in advance to answer for your aberrant behavior.

- If you could begin your schooling again, what would you change?
- Have you ever dropped a class? Why?
- Have you ever quit or been fired from a job? Why?
- With these grade(s) in (medical school subject[s]), how did you even get an interview here?
- Do you use drugs?
- Do you like to study? How do you study best? What motivates you to keep studying?
- What did you do during this (specified) period of time?

## 20. *Have you always done the best work of which you are capable?*

If you imagine that you can just answer yes or no to this question, you haven't gotten the drift of the interviewing business yet. The correct response to this question must not only show that you have put in a tremendous effort, but also demonstrate humility—by acknowledging that you could often have done a better job.

How to do this? Simply say that you have always striven to do the best possible job that you could, but the results did not always match your effort. This again stresses that you are a hard worker, you are humble, and you understand your limitations—all positive attributes. And this is all nicely wrapped up in that one-sentence answer. Very elegant.

- What have been your biggest failures in life?
- What have you done to ensure that these failures won't happen again?

## 21. *With which types of people do you have trouble working?*

This question asks, "Why won't you fit into the clinical team that exists at this residency?" In essence, what personality problems do you have? Will Rogers said, "I never met a man I didn't like." Maybe so, but most people have some difficulties with arbitrary, obnoxious, and loud individuals. This is not, however, what you want to say. The correct answer, if you cannot honestly state that you usually get along with everyone, is that you generally have problems with those individuals who do not pull their own weight.

This is also the answer to the parallel question, "What qualities drive you crazy in colleagues?" Again, this emphasizes your interest in, and ability to do, hard work. At the same time, it will normally hit a responsive chord in the interviewer, who also probably dislikes picking up the workload for slack colleagues. No one, of course, ever recognizes this problem in him- or herself.

Some interviewers will attempt to get the names of negative references by asking, "Who didn't you get along with in medical school or in past jobs?" Luckily, this is an unusual request, if only because programs are besieged with too many applicants to follow up on the information. If you are asked for such references, your willingness to provide them and your ability to explain why you didn't get along with certain individuals will say a lot about your self-confidence, honesty, and insight.

- Describe the best/worst attending or resident with whom you ever worked.
- Do you prefer to work under supervision or on your own?

## 22. *With which patients do you have trouble dealing?*

The interviewer in this case is trying to determine whether you will generate multiple patient complaints—a situation that faculty and administrators abhor.

No one expects you to be thrilled when you have to deal with whining, abusive, demanding, alcoholic, or drug-seeking patients. Most physicians do not like to treat such patients. You should state that while there are certain personalities that irritate you, you attempt to recognize these patients and then try even more than usual to act in a professional manner during interactions with them. This demonstrates professional maturity, survival skills, and common sense.

If you really dislike dealing with certain racial, ethnic, or age groups, or with people in general, you should probably reconsider your decision to pursue a medical career.

- What are patients most afraid of when they visit a doctor?
- If I called the last patient you took care of, what do you think they would say to me?
- What would you find most difficult to deal with if (when) you were a patient?

## 23. How do you normally handle conflict?

Hopefully, you can answer that your interactions with people rarely lead to conflict but, when there is conflict, you try to work the problem through to a reasonable and amicable settlement.

You may want to prepare an example of just such a situation that you faced and how it was resolved. Optimally, this example will demonstrate that the conflict was handled in a thoughtful and good-natured manner, with good will restored at the end. Your attitude, facial expressions, and body language when telling such a story will reveal much about your personality and your real ability to harmoniously work with others.

- How do you respond when you are having problems with a nurse, patient, another medical student, resident, or attending physician?
- What do you do if your senior resident or attending tells you to do something you know is absolutely wrong (medically or morally)?
- Have you ever challenged a teacher in class or a supervisor, resident, or attending physician at work? What were the circumstances?
- How do you handle disagreements with more senior colleagues, peers, nurses, and ancillary medical staff?
- How do you handle criticism, whether it's fair or unfair, from a superior, a subordinate, a peer, or a family member?
- What was the most useful criticism you ever received? Why?
- What was your most difficult/stressful life experience? How did you handle it?
- What frustrates you the most?

## 24. With what subject or rotation did you have the most difficulty?

Similar to the question concerning your strengths and weaknesses, this one asks you to incriminate yourself. You cannot plead the Fifth Amendment, so you need to know how to work through it. If you obviously had problems with a course, as evidenced by a poor grade or dismal narrative evaluations, you will have to address this. Do so in a direct manner.

Otherwise, use the same strategy you used for the strength and weakness question. Pick "difficulties" that will exhibit some of the strengths that you want the interviewer to see.

For example, by stating that your Internal Medicine rotation was difficult because of the vast amount of information you needed to assimilate through extensive reading and clinical time, you will impress the interviewer with both your insight and your hard work. Discussing the time it took you to master suturing techniques on your Surgery rotation suggests to the interviewer that you have gained a clinical skill that is a prerequisite to training in the specialty. In general, you should emphasize that any trouble that you have had was the result of the long hours you spent (explanation, not a complaint) in the learning process. However, if you really did poorly in a course or on a clinical rotation, you are probably being asked to explain why you did so poorly (Question 19).

Commonly, the interviewer will have already spotted your problem area and will also ask, "How will that affect your performance as a physician?" Of course, your answer is that it won't affect your performance, since you already have (or plan to) overcome any problems in this area through hard work or extra training.

- Tell me about your first day in anatomy. How did it change you?
- What has been your greatest challenge?

## 25. Why do you want to go into this specialty?

This is probably the question most often asked of residency applicants. The question poses two dangers. The first lies in not having a good answer. If you have gone through the steps in this book, you will have no trouble answering the question. You initially found out what aspects of medical practice you enjoyed and then matched them to the specialty that encompassed most of them. Then, you talked with multiple specialists working in the field, read as much as you could about the field, and tested your choice by spending volunteer time working in the specialty. With this background to support your answer, you should have little trouble convincing the interviewer that you have firm and valid reasons for entering the specialty.

The second danger is that interviewers will ask you this question so often—sometimes two or three times at each program—that you will become bored with your own answer. This will be obvious in your response and will reflect poorly upon your candidacy. Since each interviewer tends to ask applicants similar questions, your response will be compared with the answers from the other candidates they have seen. Be enthusiastic when replying to this question—every time. Try to take a new tack when answering the question with different interviewers. This way you will avoid repeating the same phrases, which will sound stale and trite not only to you but also to the interviewers. You have an excellent answer to this question; make certain that your delivery is just as good.

- What would you be willing to sacrifice to become a (specialist)?
- What is the greatest sacrifice you have already made to get where you are?
- If (this specialty) did not exist, what would you do?
- How much did lifestyle considerations fit into your choice of a specialty?

### 26. Why did you apply to this program?

No specialty has only one training program. So this question comes up quite often in interviews. Having based your program selections on your personal "Must/Want" Analysis, you have some excellent answers to this question. Maybe the program is particularly strong in research, which is an area you value highly. Or perhaps the faculty is outstanding. Your answer to this question should include whatever attracted you to the program. In addition, it never hurts to say that the program also got a strong recommendation from your specialty adviser.

Review all material you have about the program, as well as your personal evaluation of it, before beginning the day's interviews. If you remember to individualize your answer for each program, you should have no problem. Your knowledge about the program should include:

- Residency size
- Academic mission
- Key faculty names & specialties
- Research opportunities
- Number of key procedures performed

- Patient volume
- Clinical training sites
- Elective opportunities
- Patient population mix
- Percent women, minorities, or IMGs admitted

If you lack some of this information, that's okay. Make sure you ask for it at your first opportunity.

A more personal way of asking this question is, "Why are you willing to leave the West (or Northeast, Midwest, etc.) to come here to train?" Rather than obviously directing the question towards the program's educational elements, the question appears to be asking a more personal question. Without thinking, you may answer, "Well, I don't really want to live anywhere but the Boston area, but I heard this was a good program and I thought I'd take a look." Bad move! You have fallen into the interviewer's trap. It is not even worth considering you as an applicant now, since you said you would be unhappy away from Boston. The better answer is to say (hopefully with some truth) that you are willing to move anywhere there is a fine training program in this specialty. Then tell the interviewer what you consider to be the program's fine qualities.

- What qualities are you looking for in a program/residency?
- What interests you most about this program/residency?
- What have you heard about our program that you don't like?
- Are you applying here because it is a familiar environment?
- What do you think you will contribute to our specialty or to your community?
- How can you be sure that (specialty) is the right career for you?
- You said (a statement) in your application essay. What did you mean?
- What would you want your patients to say about you?
- What can be done to ensure that physicians are in (specialty) for the "right" reasons?
- Why do you want to leave (city or state where you live)?
- What do you think will be the most difficult aspect of living in this city, coming as you do from . . . ?
- Do you know what you are getting into? Have you talked with physicians about what a career in our specialty is really like?

### 27. What will be the toughest aspect of this specialty for you?

This is another way of asking you about your strengths and weaknesses. Only the most skilled interviewers usually ask this form of the question.

Every specialty has complex areas to master; each specialty has its onerous aspects. What do you foresee as difficult areas for you? Your answer may deal with your learning to master certain skills or with the vexing areas of the specialty's practice.

It would be unrealistic for you not to recognize some difficult areas of the specialty, and failure to cite some might indicate that you know little about the specialty, yourself, or both. A good way to answer this question is to note one or more small or commonly recognized difficult areas (such as physics training in Radiology) and describe how you intend to overcome any problems you might have. The fact that you envision only small problems will either placate the interviewer or lead to other questions to be certain that you haven't missed the big picture.

If the question is asked in the form of the "most enjoyable" part of the specialty for you, answer in the most specific terms you can. Cite examples of experiences you had while working in the specialty that excited you, stimulated you to read further, or suggested interesting research opportunities. The more specific you can be, the better your answer will be received, and the better the interviewer will remember you.

- How will you handle the least interesting or least pleasant parts of this specialty's practice?
- What qualities are most important in this specialty?
- What would you be willing to sacrifice to become a (specialist)?
- What is the greatest sacrifice you have already made to get where you are?
- Are you willing to work graveyard shifts and all weekends for a month or more at a time?
- How long have you stood on your feet at one time?
- Have you ever noticed negative aspects of (specialty) physicians with whom you have come in contact?
- What negative aspects do you see to pursuing a (specialty) career?

## 28. Why should we take you in preference to the other candidates?

Danger! This is one of those questions designed to quickly lead you down the garden path to disaster.

What is your first response? Most of you would attempt to defend yourself against attack, probably by trying to compare yourself favorably with other candidates whom you either know or imagine. Wrong move.

Start by acknowledging that you will not make the decision about who gets into the residency. State that you are not qualified to make that type of decision. In addition, acknowledge that there undoubtedly are many good candidates applying to the program. Then, state that you can really only describe your own qualities and ask the interviewer if he or she would like you to do just that. If the answer is yes, you have an excellent opportunity to tout your best qualities and finest achievements.

Obviously, to answer the interviewer's initial question, you will want to stress those qualities that distinguish you from other candidates. You should concentrate on some of the areas mentioned previously—*energy level*, the *desire to do and to learn*, and the *ability to get along with others* under all circumstances. Never disparage other candidates. Only stress your own excellence.

- What can you add to our program/residency class?
- What computer experience do you have?
- What are some of the qualities a good physician should possess? Do you possess them?
- How will your background in . . . be of any use in this specialty?
- If you were on our residency committee, what would you look for in an applicant?
- Why should I tell the residency committee to pick you?
- If we had one spot left in the residency class, what one of your attributes qualifies you more than any other candidate?
- What makes you unique?
- Give me your sales pitch.

## 29. I don't think you'd be right for this program/specialty.

Medicine has some pretty crass folks populating its ranks, but very few would actually invite you for an interview and really mean it when they tell you that you would not be right for their program, much less the specialty.

If you are told this, recognize it for the ploy that it is. It is meant to fluster and confuse an applicant. A rather nasty maneuver, used only by cruel interviewers, it can easily be sidestepped if you see it coming. This is a statement that can only be answered successfully with a question. That question is "Why do you say that?"

If you come out swinging to defend yourself, you lose. Put the interviewer on the defensive by asking the question in your nicest, most polite manner. This will throw him or her off guard, and you might even receive an apology.

- Describe your ideal residency program in this specialty.
- Montana . . . Hmm . . . Isn't that where the Unabomber lived?
- I see that neither of your parents graduated from high school. What does that say about your genetic background?
- How would you contribute to this residency's reputation?

## 30. What is your energy level like?

Although this may be an interviewer's standard question, watch out. Some only ask this of applicants who demonstrate less-than-adequate energy levels during their interviews. If you feel yourself fading, pump out a little more adrenaline and beef up your act. Now is the time to show your energy level. If you can't do it now, what will it be like at 3 A.M. while you are on call?

A question about your energy level must be answered with an enthusiastic "Very high." A very brief anecdote of just how high it is would be appropriate. An example might be, "I was able to make rounds on all my Medicine patients and write notes each morning before the residents even arrived." Try to make your anecdote appropriate to the specialty for which you are interviewing.

- When do you work harder than you ordinarily do?
- How many hours of sleep do you require each night?
- How well do you function without adequate sleep?

## 31. *How well do you function under pressure?*

Every physician, at one time or another, has been under pressure while practicing medicine. Some specialties have frequent stressors, and the physicians in them seem to thrive under this stress. Asking you about your performance under stress is, therefore, a natural question. The interviewer wants to know two things. First, have you thought about the pressures inherent in residency training, as well as those peculiar to this specialty? And second, are you up to them?

Assuming that you have gone through all the right steps to select this specialty, your answer should indicate that you operate at peak performance under the type of stressful conditions encountered in the specialty. Cite specific examples of your past performance under stress. Be sure that the examples, however, do not show that the stress resulted from your negligence, procrastination, or obstinacy. Assure the interviewer that you are up to the challenges this specialty has to offer.

A potential curve ball here may be a secondary question dealing with the administrative stressors brought on by government and third-party payer interference with medical practice. This question may be raised because it is constantly, and annoyingly, on many practitioners' minds. If this topic is raised, either state that you are certain that you will learn to handle these problems during residency, or respond by simply asking the interviewer "What are the biggest problems you are facing in this area?" In all likelihood, the interviewer will be pleased to speak about the subject at length. Be a good listener.

- How do you handle stress?
- Can you handle stress without the resources you are accustomed to relying on?
- When was the last time you cried?
- Have you ever faced death? How did you handle it?

## 32. *Tell me about the patient from whom you learned the most.*

This is a favorite question of elderly professors, as well as smarter young interviewers. It examines your medical knowledge, your insight into the patient's condition, your ability to think quickly, your attitude toward medicine and learning, and your compassion. If an interviewer asks this question, the balance of the interview remains on the same topic. How, then, should you approach it?

To be able to answer this question satisfactorily, you must prepare at least two patient cases in advance. Try to choose examples at least somewhat relevant to your chosen specialty. Select patients in whose care you were intimately involved. These should be people you helped treat for a prolonged period of time—either during many concentrated hours or periodically over time. If they had a specific disease or injury, read about it in depth. If they had a multisystem disease, be able to describe its effect on the various organs grossly and microscopically, as well as clinically.

What was it that you learned from these patients? Was it just the nature of the disease? Normally, this will not be enough. Did you learn something about your own limitations as a physician, the patient's fears and perceptions of the medical system, or the workings of the health care system itself? If you did, be prepared to say so. Also, know the follow-up information on the patients. If they were discharged, review their medical records to find out how they are doing now. If they died, did you attend the autopsy? (Attending your patients' autopsies is a good idea throughout your training—it reveals to you both what you missed and what you were powerless to change.) If you did not attend, obtain a copy of the autopsy report and read it. Following up on interesting patients demonstrates both a concern for them and your excitement in learning.

If you have prepared for this question and have begun to answer it appropriately, the interviewer may interrupt with a "war story" of his or her own. Sit back, listen, and enjoy. You did just fine.

Over the years, applicants throughout the country have consistently said that being prepared for this question was the best advance planning they did for their interviews.

- What were your most memorable experiences in medical school/ college?
- If you had to choose the single most valuable thing you have ever learned, what would it be?
- What was the (non-medical) situation in your life when you had the greatest responsibility?
- Tell me about the non-physician health care provider who most influenced you.

### 33. *What error have you made in patient care?*

This is very similar to the question above, concerning the patient from whom you learned the most. In fact, the case illustrating your biggest error may be the same as the one from which you learned the most. If it is, say so. This question is used to test your humility, to ascertain whether you were allowed to do enough on your own as a medical student so mistakes were possible, and to determine whether you can learn from your mistakes. Obviously, these are all significant issues. Make sure you have prepared your reply before you visit any programs.

- What is your greatest fear about practicing medicine?
- What is your greatest fear about entering this specialty?
- What was the worst thing that ever happened to you? Why?

### 34. *Where do you see yourself in five (ten) years?*

Some realism, as well as the ability to read what the program and the specialty desire, is required to accurately answer this question. The questioner is attempting to find out if you have some life goals—and if these are consistent with the training that the program has to offer.

Have you looked beyond your existence as a trainee? Are you realistic? Do you expect to be the Surgeon General of the United States within the decade following the completion of your residency? Or perhaps you propose to be a full professor and head of a department at a major medical school. Both expectations are, of course, not practical in the near future. On the other hand, applying to a high-powered academic residency program as preparation for working part-time at a small neighborhood clinic also may not demonstrate much realism.

The problem of incongruent goals stems from your evaluation either of your own abilities or of the program's goals for its residents. Residency faculties usually have at least a general vision of what they would like most of their graduates to do with their careers. They want your goals to be consistent with those of the program. This is beneficial to both you and them. For example, if a training program has been designed primarily to produce academic physicians, residents who hope to become community doctors will be very unhappy in it, and faculty may be very dissatisfied with residents as well.

To answer this question, you should have previously analyzed the program's written materials. Do they promote goals consistent with your personal goals? If the two widely diverge, perhaps you should consider looking elsewhere. Do not, however, be too certain about your final career direction. Many, if not most, residents significantly change their career orientation during or shortly after training. This should not upset you; it is a normal part of learning and maturation.

So, answer this question by giving a general response while listening to the interviewer. Try to understand the diversity of learning experiences that exist within the training program. Leave enough latitude in your reply, however, to allow for other possibilities in your future. Also, always phrase your answer in terms of a probability which may change with training, experience, and age.

- In ten years, in what specialty and under what circumstances will you be practicing? Who will be paying for your services?
- What are your life goals? What have you done to accomplish them?
- How would you describe "success"?
- Draw a picture of yourself in ten years.

## 35. How do you see the delivery of health care evolving in the twenty-first century?

This can be a very tricky question. It tests your knowledge of current events and politics, as well as your humility in recognizing that you do not have the ultimate answer. The interviewer, though, may think that he or she does. Only people who already have definite opinions about the trends in health care will ask this question. They actually may want to use it as a jumping-off point from which to expostulate on their pet theory. Since people like to hear themselves talk, give the interviewer a chance to say what is on his or her mind while appearing interested and you will do just fine.

The strategy for you is to give a broad answer to the initial question, such as "I expect that there will be numerous changes, not only in the way medicine is practiced, but also in the way it is paid for." You can go on to add that you do not have any definitive answers. This will give the interviewer a chance to jump in and give you either the lecture that was lying in wait, or at least some definite hints as to what he or she is thinking. You do not want to stick your neck out without some guidance.

This question is probably the closest that you will get to a direct inquiry about your political views, which is illegal in pre-employment questioning. Listen closely, nod your head a lot, and do not go out on a limb without some support. If you want some solid background, read the Institute of Medicine's *The Nation's Physician Workforce: Options for Balancing Supply and Requirements.* (Washington, DC: National Academy Press, 1996).

- Would you be willing to work under a single-payer (government-run) health care system?
- How little would your annual take-home pay have to be for you to leave medicine for another field?
- What are your thoughts about homeopaths, naturopaths, and herbal medicine?
- How do you think a socialized medical system will affect medical progress?
- If you were made King of the United States, what one thing would you change about health care delivery? Why?
- What is managed care? HMOs? PPOs? Capitation?
- What is the biggest challenge facing health care delivery?
- What does "a cross-cultural approach to healing" mean?
- What will you do as a physician to curb the rising costs of medicine?
- What is the nurse's role and how much responsibility should a nurse be given for patient care?
- Where does the money go in a prepaid medical system?
- What recent newsworthy medical event or announcement would you like to discuss?
- What is your least healthy personal habit?
- What is the solution to the health care crisis?

### 36. What problems will our specialty face over the next five (ten) years?

This question is an important variation on the question about health care in general. It provides an opportunity for you to take the broad concepts related to changes in health care and direct them towards the specific specialty to which you are applying. Have you given the specialty's future any thought? Have you given your own future enough thought? The information you obtained to answer the general question (above) about health care in the next century should give you plenty of ammunition to carry on a conversation about changes that might occur in this specialty. Of course, your wealth of knowledge about the specialty will also come in handy here.

As mentioned in the question relating to general changes in health care, give the interviewer an opportunity to sound off if it seems like that is what he or she wants to do. Listen actively. Be ready to jump in gently with an idea or two of your own, but don't argue. Some interviewers may bait you to see if they can make you angry or upset. No matter what they say, keep your cool. Remember that at least one of you has to remain professional.

- What do you think is the number one issue facing our specialty today?
- What would have to happen for you to leave (specialty) for another type of medical practice?
- Will new technological developments change our specialty? For better or for worse?

## 37. If a patient just stabbed your best friend . . . ?

A favorite question of many interviewers is the ethics scenario. In virtually all cases, it involves a situation in which there is no "correct" answer. However, as with all ethics questions, there are wrong answers.

The key to answering this question (the question itself is usually, "What would you do?") is to tell the interviewer that you need a moment to think about it. Then think through at least one answer that does not violate your personal values. Relate this to the interviewer. It is best if you do not give responses based upon your religion. Generalities, such as protecting patient autonomy or avoiding paternalism, work best.

Do not appear dogmatic; state that you are sure that there are other possible options. The interviewer may want to discuss the problem. If so, listen to the options presented and discuss them. Do not argue! Try to see the interviewer's point of view, but do not escalate the discussion into a religious debate or a shouting match. There's an old saying which suggests that one should never discuss religion or politics with friends, or you are bound to lose them. That applies just as well to residency interviewers.

- What would you do if the housestaff had a "job action" (strike)?
- What would you do if you saw another resident or physician snorting cocaine at a nightclub? On the job?
- What do you think about using animals in medical research and teaching?
- Should physicians be involved in assisted suicide or active euthanasia?
- What ethical questions will the health care delivery system face in the future?
- Should applicants who say they don't want to treat patients with (AIDS, hepatitis B, life-threatening plague, etc.) be admitted to our specialty?
- What would you do if you knew Dr. X was cheating on the in-service exam?

- Is health care rationing ethical?
- Would you treat a colleague and a patient, each coming to you with an unwanted pregnancy, differently?
- How would you respond if a resident or a colleague wanted to keep a therapeutic error a secret from a patient and the patient's family?
- What do you think of hospitals that refuse admission to patients without insurance?

## 38. What do you think of what is happening in the (economy, Eastern Europe, Congress)?

The interviewer is trying to find out if you have pulled your head out of your medical books in the past four years. It's wise to prepare for this question by reading weekly news magazines for a month or two prior to the interview season. It is also prudent to read the newspaper and, if possible, watch the morning news on the day of your interview.

As for the question itself, hope that it is on a relatively innocuous subject. If not, don't antagonize the interviewer by giving a polarized viewpoint. Try to take a balanced view—looking at both sides of the issue, e.g., "on the one hand . . . , but on the other hand . . ." This shows that you do not have your head in the sand and that you are a diplomat—both desirable qualities.

- What is the last non-medical book you read?
- Are physicians doing enough to improve public health policies?
- Are physicians doing enough for women's issues?
- What do you think is the largest problem facing American society on a statewide or a national basis?

## 39. Teach me something non-medical in five minutes.

This is now the question I use most often. It shows me a great deal about applicants, including how well many of them think on their feet. It is also more fun to start off an interview this way than with many of the routine questions most interviewers ask.

With this directive, applicants have a marvelous opportunity to discuss something in which they are an expert—and the interviewer has guaranteed that he or she will pay rapt attention. Pick a topic that you know really well and that you can explain a small piece of to a novice in five minutes.

But which topic is best? Is it something about your hobby, something unique you learned in childhood, something from a previous job, or something truly different, such as a lesson you learned through a difficult experience? The keys here are to pick a topic that will interest listeners, that fascinates you, and that can be successfully taught in the allotted time. Among the topics applicants have discussed are how to tie fishing lures, how to write a simple computer program, and how to select a melon. Not that I always understood them, but they were always interesting. Often this directive leads naturally to further questions about the topic.

Many applicants and interviewers find this the best, and most productive, interview question.

- Without using your hands, tell me how to tie a shoelace.
- How are art and medicine similar?
- What is "beauty"?
- Why are manhole covers round?
- Why is it called "the practice" of medicine?
- If you were the residency director for the next five minutes, how would you evaluate your performance halfway through your first year of residency.
- Give an example of a problem you solved and describe how you went about solving it.

## 40. *Does the reverse side have a reverse side?*

The comedian Steven Wright has made a career of asking unanswerable questions. Many of the questions attributed to him are actually from anonymous sources. This type of question can rattle, provoke, or amuse residency interviewees, depending on the intensity of the situation, their ability to understand spoken English, and the interviewer's attitude.

If you recognize that you are being asked this type of question—and most interviewees immediately will—laugh. Giving any other response is ridiculous.

- When the light goes out, where does it go?
- Why are there five syllables in the word "monosyllabic"?
- How come Superman could stop bullets with his chest, but always ducked when someone threw a gun at him?
- When I erase a word with a pencil, where does it go?
- Why do we wait until a pig is dead to "cure" it?
- Why do we put suits in a garment bag and put garments in a suitcase?
- How many ping pong balls fit in an airplane?

## 41. *Where else have you interviewed?*

This is many residency directors' favorite question. Don't become paranoid when you hear it. In most cases, they are not trying to test your interview choices. They are doing two things.

The first is determining whether you have selected programs in a reasonably sufficient quantity and of a quality to assure that you match with a program.

The second reason they ask is usually to find out current information about other training programs. Often, you are the best source of information that is available to them about other residency programs. Interviewers will be interested in pumping you for facts. Give them what they want. Tell them about what is going on in the places you visited. You may have to review all of your notes before each interview. If you just do not remember some of the specifics, be honest enough to say so. The interviewer will appreciate this. Be enthusiastic. But, as mentioned before, under no circumstances should you say anything derogatory about other programs or other faculty. If you say negative things about other programs to this interviewer, what will you say about this program when you go elsewhere? Negative comments are a sign of immaturity. Avoid them.

## 42. *What if you don't match?*

Okay. Now let's see you sweat a little. This question is most often asked during interviews for residency positions in the most-difficult-to-match-with specialties and programs. If you are not prepared for this question, you may internalize it and consider that it is a backhanded way of suggesting that you had better make other plans, since you won't be getting into a residency in this specialty. Keep cool. That is not why applicants are usually asked this question.

The interviewer is trying to determine whether you have had the foresight to plan for contingencies. Planning ahead says something about your personality. Not making alternative plans if you are applying to an Orthopedic Surgery or Emergency Medicine program is just plain foolish. And people who do foolish things with their lives are not the people these programs look for as residents. They also do not want applicants who are so uncommitted to the specialty that they say, unconcernedly, that they will simply train in another specialty if they do not match in this one. Interviewers would like you to mention alternative plans that include methods for getting into one of the specialty's training programs.

One such plan may be that you have also applied to some one-year programs, such as Preliminary Medicine or Surgery or some Transitional programs, so you will have a training slot for the coming year if you do not match in the specialty. However, you will still be in a position to re-apply to the specialty in the following year.

### 43. *Can you think of anything else you would like to add?*

The answer to this question should always be "Yes." If the interviewer has neglected any critical area that further explains your qualifications for a residency position, mention it now. Even if nothing was omitted, use this opportunity to give an abbreviated summary of your sales pitch.

This is an alternate form of the frequent query, "Do you have any (other) questions?" that can be positioned at either the beginning or the end of the interview. This question can be a disaster at the end of a long interview day when you are tired, hungry, and sleepy—just like an intern. The wimpy response, "No, I think all of my questions have been answered," is not likely to score very many points with an interviewer.

Even if prior interviewers have already answered all of your questions, ask one of them again. A very useful question, of course, is to ask for information that you wish to verify. Here you will have an opportunity to confirm or clarify the information. Another type of question to ask is one that will demonstrate your knowledge of the specialty's clinical or political activities. An example would be "What is your feeling about the new ultrasound treatment for cerebral tumors reported last month?" In any event, do not leave the interviewer in the lurch when you are given an opportunity to ask a final question.

• Is there anything else I should know about you?

### 44. *If we offered you a position today, would you accept?*

You are just finishing the last interview. Sitting with the residency director or department chief, you are suddenly faced with this question. Your first thought is "They can't ask me this. It's against Match rules."

Unfortunately, some programs disregard all rules, especially if they are desperate for good candidates. This question really puts you in a bind. If the program is clearly your top choice, no problem. If it isn't, or if you have not seen enough programs to know yet, what do you say? A perfectly reasonable response is, "I would love to accept a position in this program. I feel obligated, however, to keep the (six) other interview appointments I have made. I will be finished with these interviews in two weeks and could let you know then." Usually programs will accept this answer. Take care, though, to make sure you *really* do have a position guaranteed if you take them up on their offer (see Chapter 22, "Don't Believe Anything You Are Promised").

# Illegal Questions

Interviewers continue to ask many applicants, especially women, blatantly illegal questions (Figures 20.1 and 20.2). The most common of these are about marriage and family plans. Indeed, asking women about childbearing and childcare is the most common gaffe interviewers make. Besides implicitly asking whether a woman has children, this assumes that she must be the sole person responsible for making childcare arrangements. (Wrong!) Also, if a female applicant inquires about the provisions for maternity leave, she is often written off as not being a serious candidate.

---

### FIGURE 20.1

### *Illegal Questions–Sex Discrimination*

1. What was your maiden name?
2. Do you wish to be addressed as Miss? Mrs.? or Ms.?
3. Are you married? Single? Divorced? Separated? A single parent?
4. I notice that you are wearing an engagement ring. When are you going to be married?
5. What is your spouse's name? What does (s)he do for a living?
6. How does your spouse feel about your having a career?
7. Do you believe residents should use birth control?
8. Are you planning to have children? Anytime soon?
9. How will you take care of your children while at work?

---

### FIGURE 20.2

### *Other Questions–Legal & Illegal Forms*

| Legal Form | Illegal Form |
|---|---|
| • How well can you handle stress? | • Does stress ever affect your ability to be productive? |
| • Are you currently using illegal drugs? | • What medications do you currently use? |
| • Do you drink alcohol? | • How much alcohol do you drink per week? |
| • Do you have 20/20 corrected vision? | • What is your corrected vision? |
| • Can you perform as a resident with or without reasonable accommodations? | • Would you need reasonable accommodations to perform your job as a resident? |
| • How many days were you absent from school last year? | • How many days were you sick last year? |

---

Adapted from: Equal Employment Opportunity Commission. *Enforcement Guidance on Pre-Employment Disability-Related Inquiries.* Washington, DC:GPO, May 1994.

Another set of illegal questions relates to disabilities. According to the *Americans With Disabilities Act*, if an individual has a visible disability (for example, uses a wheelchair or guide dog), or discloses voluntarily that he or she has a disability, the interviewer may not ask about its nature, its severity, the condition causing the disability, the prognosis, or treatments. They may ask about the applicant's ability to satisfy essential functions or requirements of the position, as long as all applicants are asked the same questions.

Since illegal questions are apparently still being asked of all applicants (why this is allowed to continue is uncertain), it is important for you to be prepared for these questions.

## How Should You React To Illegal Questions?

If you are asked these questions, there are three possible ways to respond:

*Refuse to answer* the query, perhaps stating that it is illegal to ask such questions or that it is none of the interviewer's business. Such an answer, however, while it is perfectly correct and legitimate, is likely to ensure that you will not get a residency position at that site.

*Finesse the question.* One way to do this is to ask the interviewer whether such a question is really pertinent to obtaining a residency position. This gives the interviewer, who probably has been poorly prepared to do this type of interviewing, a chance to back off and save face at the same time. However, finessing a question must be handled with skill. Smile and be very pleasant while you parry these pointed questions. If you handle it correctly, you will still be a viable candidate for the program.

*Answer the question.* Most applicants take this tack, both in the medical field and in other employment situations. You can use either direct or indirect answers. For example, if asked about plans for a family and children, the direct answer might be "I plan to have children near the end of my residency." Since you might find this option distasteful, you could use an indirect answer, such as "My training comes first." These answers usually will not jeopardize your chance of obtaining a residency training position. Also, the interviewer probably does not even realize that he (or she) is being sexist and is violating both federal and state civil rights codes.

# 21

# Post-Visit Follow-Up

*We despise no source that can pay us a pleasing attention.*
– Mark Twain

Just because the interview is over does not mean you have finished your visit. You still have some work to do to maximize the effort you have already expended. This includes writing a thank-you letter, providing additional requested materials, and adjusting and completing your "Must/Want" Analysis for the program.

## Thank-You Letter

The key to using post-interview thank-you letters effectively is to remember that "out-of-sight is out-of-mind." Your letter reinforces the positive impression you left with the interviewers. Remember, you were not the only candidate interviewed that day. And by the time the faculty gets your letter, they may also have met more applicants.

Return yourself to the front of the interviewers' minds by sending them thank-you letters (see example, Figure 21.1). As with all aspects of the residency acquisition process, there are some rules to follow.

Send typed letters. Most of you would not want prospective employers to see your handwriting—even if you thought that they could read it. If your penmanship is particularly elegant, save it for a brief handwritten note at the bottom of a typewritten letter. That way you will achieve the maximum effect for each stamp you lick.

What should you include in the letter? First, direct the letter to the main interviewer—generally the residency director. In addition, mention all the interviewers. (Make sure that you save the list of names, with the correct spellings, of the people with whom you interview and tour the facilities.)

505

## FIGURE 21.1

### *Sample Follow-up Letter Format*

Use your personalized or laser-generated stationery, if possible.

Your Name
Your Current Address                    Date

Interviewer's Name
Interviewer's Position
Interviewer's Department
Interviewer's Address

Dear Dr. [Interviewer's Last Name]:

*Paragraph 1:* Thank the interviewer for the courtesy and consideration shown to you during your recent residency interview. Mention the date you interviewed.

*Paragraph 2:* Reaffirm your interest in the program. Mention anything you may not have mentioned in the interview that enhances yourself as a candidate for their program and for the specialty. (Make it brief.)

*Paragraph 3:* Provide any information you said you would send to this interviewer, including additional documentation or answers to questions deferred during the interview. If you write this immediately following the interviews and do not have this information with you, say that you will be sending the additional information subsequently. Also, always offer to provide any additional information the program or interviewer might need.

*Paragraph 4:* A simple, positive closing sentence, such as "I look forward to working with you in the future."

                              Sincerely yours,

                              [Sign your name]

                              Type your name

*P.S. Don't forget a handwritten note!*

Mention specific topics of mutual interest that were raised during your interview, e.g., "the exciting new neonatal transport program" or "the unique border-medicine experience." Include enough personal information to ensure that the reader will remember your interview from what you mention in the letter. Match the letter's formality to the tone of the interview you had. Don't go for wit or length in your letter; concentrate on making yourself memorable.

Don't forget the other interviewers. Many applicants who send thank-you letters ignore these folks, even though they often have a major say in deciding whether their program ranks candidates. Send each of them a copy of the letter you send to the residency director, but hand write (print if your penmanship is terrible) a personalized note to each of them. Again, you want them to remember you. Your note should mention a subject that you discussed with them during your interview. Try to make it something that only you, and not other applicants, may have discussed.

One tactic to enhance these letters is to quickly peruse each interviewer's office and bookshelves during your interview to try to ascertain his or her personal interests. Look for something unusual or unique you can mention during the interview. This will provide you with a subject to use as a good memory jogger later on. Of course, you will need to make notations on your Interview Notes form (Figure 17.2) to remind you of what to write to whom.

Also, with the new capability of computers and laser printers to produce quality photographs, it might be useful to have your picture on each of these letters, to better remind the interviewers who you are. Most local printing shops can quickly do this for you if you bring along a photograph.

Send the letters within 24 hours of the interview. You might not even be back home yet, and I know that trying to stop and produce these letters will be a major inconvenience. But it's worth the effort. Take materials with you on the road and get your thank-you letters out expeditiously. Some applicants now carry very small computers with them and stop by a local print-copy shop to print out their letters before they even leave the city where they interviewed.

## Telephone Follow-Ups

Although many job applicants often follow up their interviews with telephone calls, calling a residency director is usually counter-productive. Physicians are busy and do not like having their time wasted by sales pitches (from anyone). Unless you need to provide or obtain urgent information, or unless an interviewer specifically asked you to call, confine your follow-up messages to letters.

## Specific Information

Occasionally, you will receive requests for additional information, either during the interviews or from the residency secretary. This information can include anything from additional reference letters to a copy of an article that you quoted during the interview. State in your thank-you letter that you will send the requested material as soon as possible. And then send it. It will, again, reinforce the interviewer's positive image of you.

If you have signed up for a military scholarship program (HPSP), be sure that the programs to which you are applying have a written deferment on file, even if it was not requested. If a program does ask for this document, they will not seriously consider you unless you can supply it to them.

## Analyze Your Visit

There are two tasks to complete when analyzing your visit at each program. The first is to determine how well you performed. The second is to determine how well the program meets your needs. Let's discuss the personal analysis first.

The following questions will help you determine how well you did at the program, particularly in the interview setting. They are adapted from *The Robert Half Way to Get Hired in Today's Job Market* (Rawson, Wade Publishers, New York, 1981). Your analysis will also highlight problem areas to modify prior to visiting to the next residency program on your schedule.

1. Did I look as good as I am capable of looking?
2. Was I as informed about the program and the specialty as I should have been?
3. Was I relaxed and in control of myself?
4. Did I answer the questions in a way that stressed my ability, enthusiasm, and suitability for that program?
5. Did I listen closely to the interviewers?
6. Did I unobtrusively steer questions toward points I wanted to stress?
7. Did I tailor my answers to fit the type of interviewer I was with at the time?
8. Did I present an accurate and favorable picture of myself to all the program's personnel that I met?

The second task is to analyze how well the program did. Use your previously prepared "Must/Want" Analysis form (Figure 10.1) for the program. Fill it out immediately. Rate the program's strength for each factor you listed. Use the 1-to-10 rating scale, with "10" being perfect.

Once you have completed the score for each factor (for example, Faculty Availability), multiply its "Weight" by its "Score" to get a "Total" for that factor. Then add up the factor "Totals" to give the final Total ("Program Evaluation Score") for the program. You may now put this sheet away until you have completed a similar form for each program that you visit.

## Ranking The Programs For Success

### Using The "Must/Want" Analysis

Rather than relying on a *gestalt* or gut feeling of your impressions, you can use your completed "Must/Want" Analysis forms to give you an accurate picture of how well each program meets your needs. Once you have finished your interviews, you should have a file of completed "Must/Want" Analysis forms (Figure 10.1)—one for each program with which you have interviewed. Now you will see their true benefit.

Rank the programs that you have visited in order, based upon your own needs and wants, by using the "Program Evaluation Score" that you assigned to each program. Simply arrange the evaluation forms with the Program Evaluation Scores in numerical order to find out what your Rank-Order List for the Match should look like. Rank the program that received the highest Program Evaluation Score first and the one with the lowest score last, if at all.

One key point, however. You may be somewhat depressed after first ascertaining what you want in a program and then interviewing. You probably found that no program meets every one of your expectations. Hey, that is what life is all about. *There is no utopia.* In looking for a residency, as with any job search, some compromises are necessary. You should choose the program that best fits your own needs. The "Must/Want" analyses help you do this.

A conceptual way of how to look at your evaluation of residency programs is provided in Figure 21.2.

### List Enough Programs To Be Sure You Match

One of the keys to success in the Match is to rank enough programs. (It should go without saying that you must have interviewed at the programs that you list.) Several factors coincide to determine how many programs are "enough."

FIGURE 21.2

**How Applicants Evaluate Residency Programs**

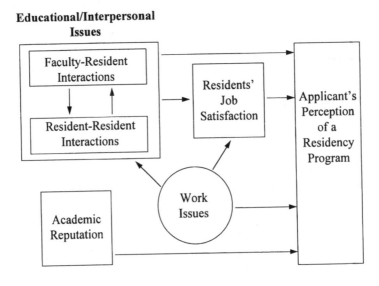

First, of course, is the specialty that you are trying to enter. The percentage of students who go unmatched in different specialties varies widely. There are tables that list the number of unmatched applicants in the *NRMP Data Book*, available from either your Dean of Students or your medical library. Note, however, that the numbers are incomplete, since many positions in Urology, Neurosurgery, Anesthesiology, Ophthalmology, Diagnostic Radiology, and Otolaryngology are filled outside the NRMP Match.

Nevertheless, by now you should know whether the specialty you have chosen is a "tough" or an "easy" match. If you still need some guidance, see the asterisk (*) ratings in Chapter 3. The tougher the specialty is to match in, the more programs you will have to interview with and rank. The number of applications graduates send to programs in their first choice of specialty is listed in Figure 11.1.

Geography also plays a part in the decision about how many programs to list. Some parts of the country are less desirable to medical school graduates than others. In some cases, this may have to do with the quality of programs located there. But it also is related to the ambiance of the surroundings. The deep South, Midwest, and large industrial or inner cities are locations that often have very good programs but have fewer applicants than elsewhere. It might be to your advantage to rank programs in one of these locales if you are not the strongest of candidates.

Program match rates also depend upon the type of institution in which they are located. If you are looking at mainly university and major-medical-center programs, be prepared for stiff competition. While not necessarily the best, these programs are where most students apply. Of course, you want to meet your own needs, not those of your peers. Therefore, consider carefully the type of program you want. If you want a program at a big center, be prepared to do a little more interviewing and make a longer Rank-Order List.

Your assessment of your competitiveness really determines how many programs you rank. The greatest danger is that you will overrate yourself, interview at and rank too few programs, and then be left without a position. If in doubt, do a little extra. It will pay off with a greater chance of success and provide more peace of mind until you receive those Match results.

## Hedge Your Bets As Necessary

Even if you have listed more programs than you think you will need to successfully match in the specialty of your choice, do not discard programs that you consider "sure bets" (weaker programs than those you have already ranked). Until you have a piece of paper in your hand stating that you have a residency position, nothing is certain.

Your best strategy (especially in the difficult-to-match-with specialties) is to list some "sure bets" at the bottom of your Rank-Order List, even if each of these is a slightly weaker program than others you have seen. Of course, if you think that the program is too weak, you may prefer not to match there. So, what should you do? Ask yourself, "Would I rather match at that program in the specialty of my choice, or not match in the specialty and take a chance on Unmatch Day?" If you can answer that question, you will know how to fill out the bottom of your Rank-Order List.

Plan ahead for all contingencies. That means interviewing at one or two less-competitive programs and, possibly, for a Transitional or Preliminary Surgery or Medicine slot. This will give you the "stoppers" on your list which will assure that you match. But it is your choice. If you are willing to "guts it out" and risk the Unmatch Day telephone scramble to find an open slot, then the best of luck to you.

## Go For The Gold

The preceding comments should not deter you from trying to secure the best residency position you can obtain.

As has already been mentioned, many of you will underestimate your own abilities and competitiveness. (Though a few of you will overestimate your chances.) Extend your sights and apply to the programs that you think will be the best for you. And, after you have applied and interviewed, make certain that you *rank your top choices first.*

Do not fill out your Rank-Order List in the order in which you think you will be selected by the programs. This will only decrease your chance of getting into the programs you really desire. Put your prime program choices at the top of the list. Then rank the others in descending order of preference. That way, when Match Day rolls around, you can be confident that you have matched with the best program possible.

# 22

# The NRMP & Other Matches

*It is good to hope, but bad to depend on it.*

– Folk Saying

The "Match" is officially known as the National Residency Matching Program (NRMP). It is how most medical students get their first-year (PGY-1, intern) training positions. Most of these positions are generally taken with the expectation on both the graduate's and the program's part that the entire training program will be completed.

In 2000, about 21,000 first-year positions were offered in the NRMP PGY-1 Match. This number must be compared with the total number of graduates enrolled in the Match from U.S. and Canadian medical schools (about 17,000), plus the total number of international medical graduates in the Match (about 10,000). This works out to about 0.8 positions offered per applicant (1.4 positions per U.S. senior student in the Match).

In 1999, 67% of the available NRMP first-year positions were filled by graduates of medical schools approved by the Liaison Committee on Medical Education (U.S., Puerto Rican, and Canadian medical schools), another 23% were filled by graduates of non-LCME-approved schools (IMGs), and 10% went unfilled through the Match. Usually, but not always, these unfilled positions were in the least desirable programs.

In the 1999 Match, nearly 94% of participating senior medical students from U.S. schools matched. About 60% of participating international medical graduates matched, with U.S.-citizen IMGs matching more often than non-U.S. citizens.

*Separate Matches exist for the specialties of Neurology, Ophthalmology, Neurosurgery, Otolaryngology, Plastic Surgery, and Urology.* See each specialty listing in Chapter 3 for details about these matching programs. There is negligible involvement in the NRMP Match by Nuclear Medicine, Medical Genetics, Child & Adolescent Psychiatry, and Preventive Medicine.

Osteopathic medical students match with American Osteopathic Association (AOA)-approved internships (other than those in the military) through the *Intern Registration Program*. This matching program is run under the AOA's auspices by National Matching Services (see description below). As of 1999, the AOA also runs a match for positions in their Orthopedic Surgery programs.

# The NRMP Match

In any competition, it is vitally important to know the rules *before* you play. This avoids having to learn through a process of trial and error. In as major an event in your life as the Match, learning as you go could be a disaster, so it behooves you to spend a few moments to become familiar with the way the system works. When you need more information or application materials, you can get them from your Dean of Students or the NRMP website (www.nrmp.aamc.org), 2501 M Street N.W., Suite 1, Washington, DC 20037-1307. The NRMP also maintains a 24-hour Voice Response System (VRS) at (202) 828-0566. You can quickly obtain assistance and specific materials through either the website or this telephone number.

## History of The Match

Prior to 1951, the matching of medical students to internship positions was a rather sordid affair. Appalling abuses of the system occurred, such as weak programs pressuring students to take less-than-optimal positions early rather than waiting for an offer from their top choice. And, while there was a purported uniform announcement date for several years, it proved to be unworkable.

As evidence of just how badly a new matching system was needed, in 1951, more than 98% of hospitals and 97% of students participated in the first Match. Organized by the National Student Internship Committee, the program was a huge success and led to the establishment of the National Intern Matching Program.

This organization has changed its name and membership several times over the years. Currently, it is organized as the National Resident Matching Program (NRMP). Its board of directors consists of representatives from the Association of American Medical Colleges, American Hospital Association, American Medical Association, American Board of Medical Specialties, American Medical Student Association, AAMC Organization of Student Representatives, Council of Medical Specialty Societies, AMA Medical Student Section, and the Consortium of Medical Student Organizations.

The original matching program used a card-sorting system which was state-of-the-art in the early 1950s. This method, though it became antiquated, was not changed until 1970, when electronic data-processing techniques were introduced. But it was not until 1974 that the entire system was fully computerized. Currently, the entire computer program for the Match takes about six minutes to run. While the Match process has many flaws, as Winston Churchill said of democracy, it is "the worst [system] except all those other forms that have been tried from time to time."

## NRMP Match Algorithm

The key element in the Match is the "algorithm" (see "NRMP Algorithm," pg. 522). The algorithm favors applicants, although how many residency programs this adversely affects is debatable. Due to complaints, the NRMP changed their matching algorithm in 1998 from one that favored programs (program-optimal) to one that favors applicants (student-optimal).

No matter what the truth is, of those students matched through the NRMP in 1999, 57% matched with their first choice, 15% with their second choice, 8% with their third choice, 5% with their fourth choice, and 9% with their fifth or lower choice of program. The others did not find a position in the Match.

The matching process has developed to the point where it can now accommodate all programs in all specialties that offer positions to senior medical students, regardless of the postgraduate level at which the program begins. However, many programs still do not offer their positions through the NRMP Match.

The San Francisco Matching Program for Ophthalmology, Otolaryngology, Neurology, Neurological Surgery, Plastic Surgery, and a number of subspecialties in these areas, changed their matching algorithm in 1997 so that applicant preferences would always prevail.

## Participating Specialties

Most PGY-1 positions are offered through the NRMP Match. The majority of those not offered are in military internships. However, PGY-2 positions in many specialties are either not offered through any Match (so you will have to negotiate directly with programs) or offered through the specialty's own Matching program. The number of specialties and programs participating in, and how many positions in each of these specialties are offered through the NRMP Match changes from year to year. The best sources for current information on your chosen specialty are listed in the "Specialty Descriptions" in Chapter 3.

## Intern Positions

Some PGY-1 positions for medical students are classified as "*Categorical (C)*." These are in the broad specialties and do not require preliminary graduate training. They are designed for individuals who want to remain in the same program throughout their residency. Categorical positions are found in Family Practice, Internal Medicine, Pediatrics, Emergency Medicine, Obstetrics and Gynecology, General Surgery, and Pathology. In addition, other specialties whose boards require a preliminary broad clinical experience can also offer Categorical positions if the individual program has made arrangements for this experience.

"*Preliminary (P)*" programs are designed for students seeking one or two years of broad prerequisite clinical experience prior to entering another specialty. They are available in Internal Medicine, General Surgery, and Transitional programs. They are not designed to act as entry points for a full residency in either Internal Medicine or General Surgery, but can occasionally be used as just such a pathway.

## Advanced Positions

There are also positions available through the NRMP's Matches beyond the PGY-1 year. These are "*Advanced*" residency positions (designated by an "S" in the *NRMP Directory*) and "*Fellowships*." (Also see "Matching in Advance [PGY-2 and Above]," below.) Advanced residency positions are those positions above the PGY-1 level that are available for senior students. The presumption is that students will complete preliminary training before entering these programs. Fellowships are for individuals who have completed, or are about to complete, residencies in a primary specialty and desire more specialized training.

### Advanced ("S")

"*Advanced (S)*" programs offer positions *beginning at the PGY-2 or higher level* to senior medical students (Figures 14.2 and 22.2). The problem is that many programs offering such positions do not go through the NRMP PGY-1 Match. Applicants to these programs need to apply for the Advanced Position and also to the NRMP PGY-1 Match to fulfill their initial training requirement. This is especially true in Otolaryngology, Ophthalmology, Neurosurgery, and Radiology. The prerequisite internships acceptable for further training in other specialties are listed in Figure 22.1. The numbers and types of training programs and positions available, as of 2000, are listed in Figures 22.2 and 22.8.

All graduates of Osteopathic medical schools must complete an AOA-approved rotating internship before beginning Osteopathic specialty training (Figure 3.2), although *specialty track* internships in Internal Medicine, Obstetrics and Gynecology, Otolaryngology/Facial Plastic Surgery, Pediatrics, and Urological Surgery essentially eliminate the requirement in these specialties.

## Fellowships

Some specialty fellowship programs have positions available through the NRMP and other matching programs (Figure 22.8). Participation in these Matches is limited to individuals who have completed or are about to complete programs in the prerequisite specialties.

The largest of these matching programs is the NRMP Medical Specialties Matching Program run by the NRMP. It currently includes Internal Medicine subspecialty programs in Cardiovascular Disease, Gastroenterology, Infectious Disease, and Pulmonary Diseases (including Pulmonary Diseases-Critical Care). This program requires applicants to return their Applicant Agreement and fee by mid-March and to submit their Rank Order List by mid-May. Match results are announced in late June.

Most fellowships in the medical subspecialties other than the four listed above are arranged directly with the individual programs. Fellowships that use an NRMP Combined Musculoskeletal Match are Foot and Ankle Surgery, Hand Surgery, Orthopedic Sports Medicine, and Pediatric Orthopedic Surgery.

The San Francisco Matching Program runs fellowship matches in Craniofacial Surgery, Facial Plastic Surgery, Head & Neck Oncologic Surgery, Mohs Micrographic Surgery, Otology/Neurolotology, Pediatric Otolaryngology, and all Neurological Surgery and Ophthalmology fellowships.

Nearly all fellowships require completion of the basic residency before beginning the program. See also the Fellowship descriptions in Chapter 3, listed either under the parent specialty or separately (designated by an "F" following their names).

FIGURE 22.1

PGY-1 Training Acceptable to Various M.D. Specialties*

| Specialty | — Training — | | | | | | | | |
|---|---|---|---|---|---|---|---|---|---|
| | Internal Medicine | Pediatrics | Surgery | Family Practice | OB/Gyn | Transitional | Neurology | Emergency Medicine |
| Anesthesiology | X | X | X | X | X | ** | X | X |
| Dermatology*** | X | X | X | X | — | X | — | X |
| Neurology | X | — | — | — | — | — | — | — |
| Nuclear Medicine | X | X | X | X | X | X | X | X |
| Ophthalmology | X | X | X | X | ** | X | X | X |
| Orthopedic Surgery | X | X | X | ** | — | ** | — | ** |
| Physical Med & Rehab | X | X | X | X | — | ** | ** | ** |
| Psychiatry | X | X | ** | X | ** | ** | ** | ** |
| Diagnostic Radiology | X | X | X | X | X | X | X | X |
| Radiation Oncology | X | X | X | X | — | X | — | — |

*The traditional PGY-1 (intern) year for Osteopathic (D.O.) physicians is acceptable to all AOA-approved specialties; Few M.D. programs give credit for that year.
**Must be approved by program director.
***Broad-based clinical training year.

FIGURE 22.2

## ACGME-Approved Specialties, Programs, & Entry-Level Positions Offered

**Column 1** lists the specialties. **Column 2** lists the number of programs in NRMP PGY-1 or Advanced Match (as of January 3, 2000) and, in parentheses "( )," the total number of approved programs. **Column 3** lists the total number of positions available to medical students through the NRMP Match. **Column 4** lists total number of entry-level specialty positions.

| 1 | 2# | 3* | 4+ |
|---|---|---|---|
| Addiction Psychiatry | 0 (24) | 0 | 56 |
| Adolescent Medicine | 0 (0) | 0 | 15 |
| Adult Reconstructive Orthopedics | 0 (12) | 0 | 18 |
| Allergy & Immunology | 0 (79) | 0 | 127 |
| Anesthesiology | 186 (192) | 381 | 1,075 |
| Blood Banking/Transfusion Med | 0 (48) | 0 | 56 |
| Cardiology | 0 (199) | 0 | 656 |
| Child and Adolescent Psychiatry | 4 (116) | 8 | 387 |
| Child Neurology | 0 (71) | 0 | 84 |
| Clinical Cardiac Electrophysiology | 0 (69) | 0 | 107 |
| Clinical & Laboratory Immunology | 0 (12) | 0 | 12 |
| Clinical Neurophysiology | 0 (63) | 0 | 163 |
| Colon & Rectal Surgery | 0 (30) | 0 | 55 |
| Critical Care (all adult) | 0 (164) | 0 | 486 |
| Cytopathology | 0 (70) | 0 | 100 |
| Dermatology | 99 (101) | 41 | 291 |
| Dermatopathology | 0 (41) | 0 | 50 |
| Emergency Medicine | 121 (121) | 1,131 | 1,131 |
| Emergency Med-Internal Med | 8 (11) | 19 | 21 |
| Endocrinology | 0 (130) | 0 | 213 |
| Family Practice | 516 (516) | 3,365 | 3,365 |
| Family Practice-Internal Med | 2 (2) | 8 | 8 |
| Family Practice-Psychiatry | 10 (12) | 17 | 19 |
| Forensic Pathology | 0 (42) | 0 | 72 |
| Forensic Psychiatry | 0 (19) | 0 | 44 |
| Gastroenterology | 11 (170) | 0 | 329 |
| Geriatrics (IM, FP) | 0 (107) | 0 | 262 |
| Geriatric Psychiatry | 0 (47) | 0 | 107 |
| Hand Surgery (all) | 60 (72) | 0 | 135 |
| Hematology (all) | 0 (98) | 0 | 147 |

FIGURE 22.2 (continued)

| 1 | 2# | 3* | 4+ |
|---|---|---|---|
| Hematology & Oncology (IM) | 0 (105) | 0 | 289 |
| Infectious Diseases | 0 (142) | 0 | 307 |
| Immunopathology | 0 (9) | 0 | 9 |
| Internal Medicine | 375 (406) | 5,312 | 5,629 |
| Internal Med-Neurology | 4 (16) | 6 | 19 |
| Internal Med-Pediatrics | 104 (108) | 454 | 463 |
| Internal Med-Physical Med/Rehab | 6 (15) | 9 | 16 |
| Internal Med-Preliminary | 261 (261) | 1,556 | 1,556 |
| Internal Med-Preventive Med | 0 (3) | 0 | 3 |
| Internal Med-Primary | 90 (90) | 649 | 649 |
| Internal Med-Psychiatry | 23 (28) | 49 | 52 |
| Medical Genetics | 0 (35) | 0 | 44 |
| Medical Microbiology | 0 (9) | 0 | 11 |
| Medical Toxicology | 0 (28) | 0 | 42 |
| Musculoskeletal Oncology | 0 (8) | 0 | 9 |
| Neonatology | 0 (100) | 0 | 181 |
| Nephrology | 0 (135) | 0 | 321 |
| Neurological Surgery | 24 (99) | 34 | 136 |
| Neurology | 21 (122) | 56 | 487 |
| Neurology-Psychiatry | 4 (9) | 5 | 12 |
| Neuropathology | 0 (46) | 0 | 39 |
| Neuroradiology | 0 (90) | 0 | 160 |
| Nuclear Medicine | 5 (76) | 7 | 113 |
| Nuclear Radiology | 0 (34) | 0 | 54 |
| Obstetrics & Gynecology | 252 (264) | 1,135 | 1,246 |
| Oncology | 0 (45) | 0 | 133 |
| Ophthalmology | 4 (132) | 9 | 467 |
| Orthopedic Surgery | 154 (157) | 560 | 601 |
| Orthopedic Surgery of the Spine | 0 (14) | 0 | 21 |
| Otolaryngology | 20 (105) | 44 | 277 |
| Pain Management | 0 (95) | 0 | 250 |
| Pathology (Anatomic & Clinical) | 143 (174) | 452 | 549 |
| Pediatric Anesthesiology | 0 (0) | 0 | 45 |
| Pediatric Cardiology | 0 (48) | 0 | 101 |
| Pediatric Critical Care | 0 (63) | 0 | 94 |
| Pediatric Emergency Medicine | 2 (59) | 4 | 95 |
| Pediatric Endocrinology | 0 (63) | 0 | 67 |
| Pediatric Gastroenterology | 0 (46) | 0 | 47 |
| Pediatric Hematology/Oncology | 0 (65) | 0 | 99 |
| Pediatric Infectious Diseases | 0 (0) | 0 | 49 |

FIGURE 22.2 (continued)

| 1 | 2# | 3* | 4+ |
|---|---|---|---|
| Pediatric Nephrology | 0 (45) | 0 | 46 |
| Pediatric Orthopedic | 0 (27) | 0 | 43 |
| Pediatric Pathology | 0 (25) | 0 | 28 |
| Pediatric Pulmonary | 0 (45) | 0 | 43 |
| Pediatric Radiology | 0 (49) | 0 | 64 |
| Pediatric Rheumatology | 0 (16) | 0 | 17 |
| Pediatric Surgery | 0 (32) | 0 | 28 |
| Pediatrics | 203 (216) | 2,314 | 2,515 |
| Pediatrics/Psychiatry/Child Psych | 10 (10) | 20 | 20 |
| Physical Med & Rehabilitation | 96 (98) | 76 | 330 |
| Plastic Surgery (All) | 43 (98) | 67 | 331 |
| Preventive Med/Public Health | 7 (43) | 15 | 179 |
| Aerospace Medicine | 0 (4) | 0 | 42 |
| Occupational Medicine | 0 (29) | 0 | 78 |
| Psychiatry | 197 (197) | 1,080 | 1,080 |
| Pulmonary Diseases | 15 (62) | 0 | 111 |
| Pulmonary Diseases/Critical Care | 100 (100) | 0 | 269 |
| Radiation Oncology | 62 (82) | 100 | 128 |
| Radiology-Diagnostic | 213 (213) | 161 | 884 |
| Rheumatology | 0 (107) | 0 | 167 |
| Selective Pathology | 0 (9) | 0 | 44 |
| Sports Medicine-Orthopedics | 0 (58) | 0 | 121 |
| Sports Medicine-Primary Care | 0 (33) | 0 | 44 |
| Surgery-General | 243 (246) | 1,035 | 1,040 |
| Surgery-General–Preliminary | 200 (201) | 998 | 1,000 |
| Thoracic Surgery | 0 (91) | 0 | 149 |
| Transitional | 129 (161) | 1,046 | 1,360 |
| Trauma Surgery | 0 (25**) | 0 | 44 |
| Urology | 30 (121) | 62 | 249 |
| Vascular Surgery | 0 (80) | 0 | 89 |
| Vascular/Interventional Radiology | 0 (83) | 0 | 183 |

#These are the numbers of institutions participating. Some institutions separate their applicants into two or more "programs" based on whether they are applying as Categorical, Preliminary, Advanced, or Physician candidates.

*These positions may be at either the PGY-1 level or at the PGY-2 level (Advanced). All of these are available for medical student matching. Not included are the few positions in some specialties, labeled "R," that are open only to physicians.

**Programs complying with guidelines from the American Association for the Surgery of Trauma; this subspecialty is not recognized by the ACGME.

+These numbers are an approximation of all entry-level positions available in accredited programs in the specialty. The positions occur at various years of training. Some are not available to medical students, but must be matched with during internship or residency. Others are available only through the military's matching program.

Numbers derived from: Appendix II, Table 10. *JAMA.* 1999;282(9):904-6; AMA-*FREIDA*; and Waldo Wentz at the National Resident Matching Program (January 2000).

# The NRMP Match Rules—General

## NRMP Algorithm

The NRMP Match algorithm is somewhat complex. While it is described in the *NRMP Handbook for Students*, this is a brief summary:

1. The Match handles each applicant in sequence.
2. An attempt is first made to place an applicant into his or her most-preferred program.
3. If this is unsuccessful, an attempt is then made to place the applicant into the second, third, etc., choices on his or her Rank-Order List.
4. This process continues until there is a (tentative) match or until the applicant's listed programs have been exhausted.
5. When subsequent applicants go through the process, an attempt is first made to place them into their most-preferred program.
6. If a program they ranked highly has ranked them higher than applicants already tentatively matched, the new applicants get the spot and the previously matched applicants go back through the algorithm.
7. When applicants are "bumped" from a spot and go back through the Match, the process again begins with their first choice program.
8. The Match is complete when all applicants have either been matched with one of their choices or all the programs listed by applicants have filled their positions.

One element of this algorithm generally goes unsaid. The NRMP allows several hundred hospitals each year to designate positions in one program that, if unfilled in the Match, can be transferred to positions in another program that can be filled.

## Rank-Order Lists

The order in which you list the programs is called your Rank-Order List (ROL). The programs complete a similar list of candidates. After you complete the worksheets from the NRMP website, your ROL is entered into the NRMP's computer system from any terminal with Netscape 4.0 or higher, Microsoft Internet Explorer 4.0 or higher, or another Web browser compatible with these browsers.

The ROL can be entered in one or more sessions and can be modified as often as necessary until the posted deadline, usually in mid-February. It is best to finish using ROLIC a few days before the deadline, since the system becomes very slow (due to use by procrastinators) during the last

24 hours before the deadline. Applicants are responsible for the correctness of their individual Rank-Order Lists. You can print a copy of your personal ROL at any time during the process by clicking on the Display/Print button and using your Web Browser's print button. The NRMP only accepts ROLs via computer. Do not mail or fax them your list.

Security is guaranteed by granting access to the system only to individuals with both an Applicant Code and a PIN (Personal Identification Number). The unique six-digit NRMP Applicant Code and the unique five-digit PIN are assigned during enrollment in the Match and listed on the Confirmation. The PIN should be kept strictly confidential, (do not share it with anyone else) and in a safe place.

Upon completing your ROL, "certify" the list by clicking on the "List Complete" button and reenter your PIN/Password. If you reenter your ROL after this, you will invalidate the certification and will need to recertify the list in order for the NRMP to accept it.

IMGs can participate in the NRMP Match even without an ECFMG Certificate *if the ECFMG notifies the NRMP that all requirements for Certification have been met* before the Match is run.

In 2000, the basic NRMP Match registration cost for students in LCME-approved schools was $40.00. It was $90.00 for independent applicants. This fee allows the applicant, without additional charge, to rank up to fifteen different programs on the ROL, as well as a total of fifteen different PGY-1 programs on one or more Supplemental ROLs. Each couple's partner pays the individual fee and there is a $15 fee for submitting as a couple. This allows them to rank fifteen different programs (plus "unmatched") in up to 300 combinations without additional charge. Each additional program pair listed costs $15. Each additional listed program for individuals or for couples costs $30.

For each program you list, you will include the program's "Rank Order" (number 1 through as many as you choose to list); "Hospital Name/City, State"; "Program Description" (specialty and type of program, e.g., Surgery-Categorical); and "NRMP Program Code" (from the current *NRMP Directory* listing). The form you use depends upon whether you are applying as an individual, which includes those applying for shared-schedule positions, or as a couple.

The Supplemental ROLs are used by students applying to one or more Advanced Programs for Students (listed as "S" on the *NRMP Directory* website). The Advanced programs are initially listed on the primary ROL. For each Advanced program or group of programs listed, acceptable associated PGY-1 programs should be listed on the Supplemental ROL. If, for example, you list five Advanced programs, all in widely dispersed locations, then you will probably have five Supplemental ROLs, each with one or more associated PGY-1 positions listed. For each additional PGY-1 program listed over a total of fifteen, there is a charge of $30.00.

Although there is no limit to the number of specialties (or programs) you can include on your list, it has been demonstrated that the individuals with the greatest success in the Match are those who rank only one specialty. However, if you are attempting to get into a relatively difficult specialty, such as Emergency Medicine, this does not preclude you from listing some Transitional or Preliminary (Medicine, Surgery) programs at the bottom of your list.

## Optimizing Your Rank-Order List

What techniques can you use to achieve the best possible outcome in the Match? There are two things to remember: *list your first-choice program first* and carefully *consider how many programs you should list.*

*Applicants consistently do best if they list their top choice first.* After listing the top choice, applicants might theoretically get better results if they listed programs based on knowing how all other applicants rate programs—information which is unavailable. Therefore, *rank programs in the order of their acceptability to you*—not in the order in which you think you are acceptable to the programs. This gives you the best chance of matching at a site you think is optimal for you.

How long should your ROL be? If you apply to a highly competitive specialty (see ratings in Chapter 3), or to programs in an area of the country where matching is difficult, it's probably better to have a long ROL. If, however, you apply to programs that are easier to match with, you may want to have a relatively short list.

The key to success is to consider, for each program you list, whether you would rather go to that program or whether you would prefer to be unmatched and take your chances in the scramble of unmatched candidates for positions. The higher the number of programs applicants list on their ROLs, the better their chance of matching (Figure 22.3).

No matter how competitive (or non-competitive) the specialty, list all the programs with which you would like to match. If this isn't a long list, or if you are applying to a specialty that generally has many positions open after the Match, a reasonable strategy may be to list fewer programs (only those with which you *really* want to match). See Figure 22.4 for a decision tree to help you decide whether to rank a program.

## Confidentiality

Match rules do not allow programs or applicants to ask each other how they will be ranked. The Rank-Order Lists from both parties are considered

FIGURE 22.3

*Average Number of Programs on Applicants' ROLs*

| Year | Matched Applicants | Unmatched Applicants |
|------|--------------------|----------------------|
| 1996 | 6.4 Programs | 5.4 Programs |
| 1997 | 6.9 Programs | 5.2 Programs |
| 1998 | 7.3 Programs | 5.0 Programs |
| 1999 | 7.4 Programs | 5.1 Programs |

Adapted from NRMP information, January 2000.

confidential. Either party can, if they so desire, release this information to the other. What is said, however, is not binding. Many students have been grossly misled by a program's faculty member who told them that they would be "ranked high enough to match." Of course, many did not match with those programs although the students listed them first.

Programs are not supposed to offer contracts for appointment to applicants prior to the general announcement of NRMP Match results. To enforce this, applicants are expected to report any such offers to the NRMP, who will presumably take punitive action. In fact, in recent years, eight percent of students have reported that they were asked to make a commitment before a Match result, either NRMP or specialty, was announced. So much for the ethics of academic physicians.

## Match Results

Match results are released stepwise over the course of "Match Week" (Figure 22.5). All information is available to applicants simultaneously through postings on the NRMP website and the NRMP Voice Response System (202-828-0566). Access to either one requires an applicant's NRMP code and PIN.

Match Day is now in mid-March. Applicants can discover whether they matched at noon Eastern Standard Time (EST) three days prior to Match Day. The locations of filled and unfilled positions are posted at noon (EST) two days before Match Day. Unmatched applicants are then free to contact programs to try to acquire unfilled residency positions. This is commonly referred to as "The Scramble." Matched applicants can discover to which programs they will be going at 1:00 P.M. on Match Day. Both applicants and programs are, by the NRMP rules, bound by the Match results just as if they had already signed the official appointment documents.

FIGURE 22.4

*NRMP Rank-Order List Decision Tree*

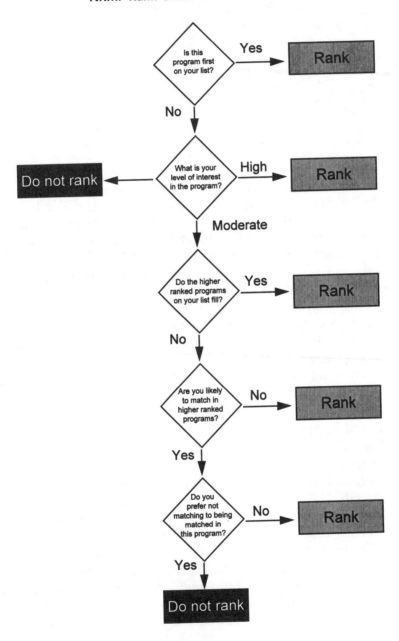

Adapted from a similar algorithm produced by Christopher Leadem, Ph.D., Dean of Students, University of Arizona College of Medicine, Tucson.

## Employment Requirements

Even after you match with a program, you may need to successfully complete specific pre-employment requirements, such as drug testing, to get the position. If applicants must fulfill such requirements, they should be informed of this before they submit their Rank-Order List, preferably in the material provided by the institution.

## Illegal Behavior

The NRMP considers two actions illegal for an applicant or a program. The first is supplying forged credentials or letters of recommendation to programs. This is not only illegal in terms of the Match, but also may be either a misdemeanor or a felony in some states. It certainly could prevent you from ever getting a license to practice medicine.

The second is for a program to refuse to accept an applicant who has matched into that program (program illegality) or for an applicant who has matched to refuse to accept a position (applicant illegality). While in the past the NRMP took action if it received "credible evidence" that such activities had occurred, the NRMP now expects that the individuals and programs will settle any disagreements themselves.

## Schedule of Events

Beginning in 1987, a uniform national date for *releasing the Dean's letters was set at November 1*. Although not all Deans play strictly by the rules (some offer to essentially read the letter to program directors over the telephone), most Dean's letters go out on that date.

The dates for both the NRMP and "early" (Ophthalmology, Neurology, Urology, Neurosurgery, Otolaryngology) Specialty Matches were also pushed back. This generally gives students an additional six weeks to complete the decision and application process. For the NRMP PGY-1 Match, the Rank-Order Lists are due in mid-February and Match results are released in mid-March. Although it varies by specialty, "early" Matches require their Rank-Order Lists in early to mid-January, with Match results released in mid- to late January.

The exact dates for the events in the Matching program change from year to year. Figure 22.5 gives a list of the *approximate dates* for each of the mileposts in the process. For the exact dates each year, check the back cover of the current *NRMP Directory*.

## FIGURE 22.5
### Important Dates in the NRMP Application Process

**March-November:** Students request residency application materials from individual programs.

**April:** Application materials are sent to medical school Deans.

**May:** Application materials are sent to the hospitals and programs.

**June:** Application materials are sent to Independent Applicants.

**Mid- to late July:** Students and institutions sign and return NRMP agreements.

**Summer to Fall:** Students apply to individual programs. Applicants can also register with ERAS (separate from the NRMP).

**Mid-September:** *NRMP Directory of Programs* posted on the NRMP website (www.nrmp.aamc.org) and updated weekly thereafter.

**Mid-November:** NRMP must receive *Sponsored Graduate Agreements* (from M.D. graduates being "sponsored" by an LCME-accredited school), *Independent Applicant Agreements*, and *Shared-Residency Pair Forms*.

**Early January:** Programs must submit their final program information on the number of available positions.

**Early January to Mid-February:** Applicants and programs enter their *Rank Order Lists* using the *Rank Order List Input Confirmation System (ROLIC)* via the World Wide Web.

**Mid-February:** *Rank Order List Input Confirmation System (ROLIC)* closes. NRMP must have received both applicants' and programs' *Rank Order Lists* by this time.

**Mid-March:**

**Three Days Prior to Match Day** – Applicants find out if they matched at 12:00 noon (EST) via the NRMP website or Voice Response System (VRS). The Dean of Students finds out at 11:30 A.M. (EST).

**Two Days Prior to Match Day** – Filled and unfilled positions are posted by specialty and program on the NRMP's website at 11:30 A.M. (EST). Locations of all unfilled positions are released to applicants at 12:00 noon (EST). Unmatched students and programs can begin filling at this time.

**One Day Prior to Match Day** – Confidential list of applicants matched with each residency program posted to the NRMP website at 2:00 P.M. (EST).

**Match Day** – Match results posted on the NRMP website at 1:00 P.M. (EST).

**Mid-March to Mid-April:** Programs/applicants mail and receive letters of appointment.

## Institution

*All* programs at a participating institution are required to offer *all* available PGY-1 positions to student applicants through the NRMP Match. Unfortunately, the same does not hold true for the institution's Advanced (PGY-2 and above) positions. Therefore, some Advanced positions may be offered through the Match, while others are matched in other ways. This practice leads to a considerable amount of confusion.

## Name & Address Changes

The NRMP keeps only the addresses of Independent Applicants on file. Individual schools keep the addresses for students. If Independent Applicants have address changes, these must be forwarded to the NRMP in writing. They are due on the same date as the ROL.

If any applicant has a name change after mid-November but before the Match, the applicant must supply the following to each program to which he or she is applying: their old name, their new name, and their NRMP Applicant Code. The NRMP will not change names on their records after mid-November. Entering a new E-mail address in the ROLIC system will not decertify an applicant's Rank-Order List.

## Withdrawal From Matching Program

By signing the NRMP contract to participate in their Match, you agree to withdraw from the Match only if you:

1. Accept an appointment from the military.
2. Decide not to pursue a PGY-1 training position in that year.
3. Otherwise obtain a residency position that begins in the current year.

In this last case, the program director must send a letter to the NRMP. (Matching through the Canadian Resident Matching Service [CaRMS] is not considered a withdrawal.)

To withdraw from the Match, permission from your Dean is required. Some students think they can easily withdraw from the Match either by not turning in their ROL or by turning in a blank ROL. This is not true, because a list of all NRMP Match participants who have not turned in Rank-Order Lists, or who have turned in blank lists, is sent to their medical school Dean.

The NRMP automatically withdraws candidates who cannot verify their medical school attendance or graduation, candidates who do not pay the required fees, IMGs who have not completed the ECFMG requirements, and Fifth-Pathway students or graduates who have not completed USMLE Steps 1 and 2.

# Student Candidates

## Schools

Although the majority of participants in the NRMP Match are graduates of U.S. schools granting M.D. degrees, you can participate even if you do not fall into this category. However, the rules change slightly depending upon the category into which you fall.

### LCME-Accredited Schools

Students from schools accredited by the Liaison Committee on Medical Education (LCME), which includes virtually all M.D.-granting institutions in the United States, Puerto Rico, and Canada, enter the Match by permission of their Dean. For students in U.S. schools, the medical school's Dean decides upon each student's eligibility to participate. The question the Dean must answer is, "Will the student graduate this year?" Materials for the Match are sent to the Dean's office and from there are distributed to individual students. Confirmation notices from the NRMP with student information and a form on which to make any corrections are also distributed through the school.

Canadian medical students need to contact the NRMP directly and apply as "Independent Applicants." They must show proof of enrollment in medical school. Physicians who have already graduated but who are, nevertheless, applying for positions through the Match have the option of going either through their medical school (as Sponsored Graduates) or directly through the NRMP (as Independent Applicants). The NRMP mails Agreement Confirmations to Independent Applicants, who must make any necessary corrections, sign, date, and return a copy to the NRMP.

### Canadian Resident Matching Service (CaRMS)

Canada has its own matching program. Individuals may, if they wish, enter both matching programs. However, since the CaRMS completes its Match before the NRMP does, candidates entering both programs essentially rank all Canadian programs on their list higher than U.S. programs. If an individual matches through the CaRMS (www.carms.ca), the NRMP automatically removes that applicant's name from the NRMP lists.

### AOA-Approved Schools

Students from medical schools approved by the American Osteopathic Association may also participate in the NRMP Match. However, PGY-1 programs available through the NRMP Match do not fulfill the requirements for licensure of Osteopaths in many states (Figure 7.9). It is important that you check with the state *before* you decide to enter the Match.

If you want to participate in the Match, you do so as an Independent Applicant and communicate directly with the NRMP. You will have to furnish proof of enrollment in or graduation from your medical school.

### Non-LCME-Approved Schools
Students at or graduates of medical schools not approved by the LCME, which includes virtually all medical schools outside the United States, Puerto Rico, and Canada and a very few within these jurisdictions (you already know if you are in this group), can apply to the Match only as Independent Applicants. This includes International Medical Graduates (FNIMGs and EVIMGs), U.S. citizens graduating from non-LCME approved schools (USIMGs), and Fifth-Pathway students.

To participate in the Match, each applicant must furnish proof that he or she has either passed the examinations for the Examination Council for Foreign Medical Graduates (ECFMG) certification, or obtained a full and unrestricted license to practice medicine in the United States. While you can sign up for the NRMP Match and submit a ROL without being certified by the ECFMG, you must have passed all examinations necessary for this certification by the time the ROL is due (mid- to late February). The NRMP will check with the ECFMG at that time. If you do not meet the requirements, you will not be allowed to proceed in the Match.

## Couples Match
With the understanding that physician-physician couples were becoming more common, the NRMP instituted a Couples Match several years ago to assist couples in matching in the same geographic location. In recent years, couples' match rates have been comparable to those of students matching as individuals. The Couples Match is *not* only for those who are married or engaged. Any pair can use this Match, including those who are dating, gay/lesbians, or even close friends. Independent applicants, such as Osteo-pathic students, graduate physicians, and international medical graduates can also use the Couples Match.

There are, however, significant differences between going through the Match alone and going through as a couple. The initial step in entering the Couples Match is simply for each member of the couple to enroll in the Match and indicate in the ROLIC system that they want to be in the Match as part of a couple. A final decision about whether to match as a couple need not be made until the Rank-Order Lists are entered.

Unlike those in a shared-schedule position (described in the next section), couples apply to and interview at programs separately. They should, of course, try to select programs in corresponding geographic areas.

For example, if one partner applies only in Washington, DC and the other only in San Francisco, there would certainly be no way to find programs where they could live together while they complete their residencies. However, if they both apply to programs in each city, there should be some compatible matches (see Figures 22.6 and 22.7).

The special worksheet and instructions for the Couples Match can be found on the NRMP's website. After the partners apply to and interview at programs, each needs to evaluate the programs just as if he or she were matching as an individual. They then must work together to develop the combinations of programs to put on their Couples Rank-Order List Worksheet. Figure 22.7 is an example of one couple's list. Up to 300 pairs of programs can be listed without extra charge. The programs are matched by rank order and any combination of specialties and locations can be used. Note that PGY-1 choices on a Supplemental ROL are not paired in the Match. Therefore, any PGY-1 spots listed to accompany Advanced Programs should be geographically compatible with the partner's paired choices.

In many cases, programs will be listed more than once. This may be especially true for the higher-ranked programs. It is also possible for one partner to elect to be unmatched against the other partner's selection. This option is normally reserved for the bottom of the Rank-Order List, where it is used as a "stopper" to attempt to prevent both partners from going unmatched.

When entering the ROL on the ROLIC system, each partner enters his or her choices independently. Be careful that the numbers of the choices for both partners' lists match. One safeguard is that the partners are required to have the same number of listings, even though some of those listings may be "unmatched." Both applicants need to know their partner's NRMP Applicant Code, not their ROLIC password, to enter an ROL in the Couples Match.

---

### FIGURE 22.6
#### *Example of a Couple's Worksheet*

| Partner 1 | Partner 2 |
|---|---|
| Washington, DC–Prog A | San Francisco–Prog 1 |
| Washington, DC–Prog B | Washington, DC–Prog 1 |
| San Francisco–Prog A | San Francisco–Prog 2 |
| | Washington, DC–Prog 2 |

This is the way each partner independently ranked the programs at which they interviewed. They now need to work together to form combinations of these selections within each geographic area for their Couples ROL. (This is shown in Figure 22.7.)

---

FIGURE 22.7

### *Example of a Couple's Rank-Order List*

| Partner 1 | Partner 2 |
|---|---|
| Washington, DC–Prog A | Washington, DC–Prog 1 |
| San Francisco–Prog A | San Francisco–Prog 1 |
| Washington, DC–Prog B | Washington, DC–Prog 1 |
| Washington, DC–Prog A | Washington, DC–Prog 2 |
| San Francisco–Prog A | San Francisco–Prog 2 |
| Washington, DC–Prog B | Washington, DC–Prog 2 |
| Unmatched | Any Program Listed Above |

(Based on the individual preferences in Figure 22.6.)

---

Three important things to note: First, if one partner withdraws from the Match, the other partner will be ranked as a single candidate using the ROL he or she submitted. Second, couples are treated only as a single unit, meaning that if they do not obtain a match using any of their pairs of programs, the NRMP will not run their lists independently to find a match. Finally, the NRMP is not your mother. It does not inquire how or why a couple is trying to match together. However, your Dean of Students will know that you are using the Couples Match. If you wish this information to be kept confidential, you may want to make a special appointment to talk to your Dean.

Even more complicated for some couples are the problems that occur when both partners are not going through the NRMP PGY-1 Match. For example, if one partner is interested in Otolaryngology and the other in Internal Medicine, major problems can develop. Since Otolaryngology is one of the specialties that sponsors its own Match, there is no way the NRMP's Couples Match will work for them.

The best solution in this case would be for the pair to make up a tentative list similar in nature to that made up by those going through the Couples Match. Then each partner should explain the situation to the program and department directors during their interviews. If you find yourself in this situation, ask them to make a commitment to you. If one residency position can be secured in advance, the partner can then attempt to match only with geographically compatible programs.

It is perfectly legal for program directors to make a commitment to you in advance. But programs participating in the NRMP PGY-1 Match are not allowed to offer you a contract. You, of course, have to place a great deal of trust in the program unless you are offered a contract to sign. Program directors, however, cannot bind you to a commitment if they participate in the NRMP Match, and so they also need to trust you. Remember, if you do not deal honestly with the programs, the next couple coming through will have a much more difficult time.

### Shared-Schedule/Part-Time Position Match

A shared-schedule position, unlike the Couples Match, is one residency position held by two individuals. As explained in Chapter 13, the individuals involved want to do their training on a part-time basis, over a longer period of time than is normal. Programs that offer part-time (shared-schedule) positions are most frequently found in Family Practice, Pediatrics, Preventive Medicine, Internal Medicine, Psychiatry, and Child and Adolescent Psychiatry. There is a separate listing of all programs offering shared-schedule positions in the AMA's *Graduate Medical Education Directory Supplement*, published annually and available at most medical school libraries. This information is also available in each program's description on *FREIDA*.

To participate in the NRMP Match for a shared-schedule position, it is necessary for the pair to submit a "Shared-Residency Pair Form," found on the NRMP website, by late October. The NRMP then issues the pair a single NRMP Applicant Code to be used in the Match. In addition, a single combined name is used on the candidate list sent to the residency programs. For example, applicants Robert Smith and Mary Jones would be the candidate "Smith/Jones" for purposes of the Match. They would submit only one Rank-Order List, and could only be matched as a pair.

## Physician Candidates

Physicians already in training or who have completed a training program can apply to enter the NRMP Match either as Independent Candidates or, if they are graduates of a U.S. LCME-approved school, as Sponsored Graduates. Sponsored Graduates apply to the Match through their Dean's office, similarly to applicants who are currently students. Non-LCME graduates must furnish proof either of ECFMG certification or of a full and unrestricted license to practice medicine in the United States. About 32 positions in 15 programs, labeled "R" in the *NRMP Directory*, are open only to physician candidates.

## Military Appointments

Military medical training programs usually will accept only those individuals already obligated to do military service due to training at the medical school of the Uniform Services University of the Health Sciences, participation in the Health Professions Scholarship Program, or another type of prior commitment. There are usually too few military positions available for the number of individuals who apply.

In order to have the best chance of obtaining a position, you will have to participate in both the military and NRMP PGY-1 Matches. The military selects their residents before the NRMP PGY-1 Match (except for the Army and Navy PGY-1 slots in the NRMP Match), so those individuals who do not get military positions outside the Match will still be able to get a residency position through the NRMP Match. *Those students who do match with the military outside the NRMP Match are obligated to notify the NRMP or the American Osteopathic Association that they have withdrawn from the Match.* The military does not notify the NRMP.

## Don't Believe Anything You Are Promised

Several years ago, an applicant, whom our program had ranked highly, called to say that she had not matched. That was rather surprising, since she was a very competitive applicant. Looking for a position, somewhat desperate, she admitted that she had listed only one program on her Rank-Order List. Why had she done this? Not for any of the common reasons related to family or other personal commitments. Instead, she had relied upon a promise from the residency director of a particular program, which was her first choice, that she would be ranked high enough to guarantee her a position. But that did not happen and she was left out in the cold. I have seen similar scenarios play out numerous times—often involving excellent students who have reason to believe that they will match with a particular program, only to find that they are either unmatched with any program or psychologically unprepared to go to their second-choice program.

The moral of such stories is that you should be extremely wary of any faculty member's promise to match you at a program. This holds true up until the point that either you get your Match results or you actually get a *firm and specific offer, in writing, from an individual authorized to make it.* (One student wrote saying he got just such a verbal offer and showed them this section of the book to demonstrate that he really did need a legitimate written offer. He got it.) If you fall for a specious promise, your dream of matching with the ideal residency may prove to be ephemeral.

According to surveys, residency programs contacted about two-thirds of applicants to inform them that they were being ranked highly. About one-third felt that programs lied to them, and one-quarter felt that programs made at least informal commitments to them. This doesn't seem to portray medical educators as excellent role models.

As mentioned previously, couples with one or both partners applying to specialties outside the NRMP PGY-1 Match must take a calculated risk by asking for just such a commitment. In these cases, obtain the commitment from both the residency director and department chairman, if possible. And make it clear that you are willing to sign a contract if it is offered.

Be aware, however, that *even a written contract for a position offered in the NRMP Match may not be valid.* The NRMP Match rules say that any contract for a position offered in the NRMP Match which is signed before the Match results are released is superseded by the results of the Match. Some specialties and programs, however, do not offer positions through the Match. If these programs offer you a position, they should simultaneously offer you a contract.

## What To Do If You Don't Match

If, for some reason, you do not match, you will be notified during "The Unmatch" or "The Scramble," the two days before Match Day. This does *not* mean that you have failed; *matching is not the final measure of your worth.* If you are currently enrolled in an LCME-approved medical school, there will be, in all probability, a formal mechanism in place to help you find a residency position. You will certainly not be the first individual in the school's history who did not match. And you will probably find some of your classmates in the same situation. By going through the steps in this book, you are less likely to find yourself unmatched than some of your classmates. In addition, the preparation you have already done will not be wasted. It will give you an edge, even if you do end up without a position. The first rule is: DON'T PANIC!

You may first want to consider whether the specialty you chose is still what you want. Many students have second thoughts after making their initial commitment. You now have a chance to reconsider—but you must reconsider quickly. As soon as you hear that you haven't matched, you must be on the telephone with residency programs. If you aren't sure about a specialty, one option is to pick one of the many Preliminary Surgery or Medicine slots that go unmatched. These may act as stepping-stones to PGY-2 openings in the new specialty of your choice.

If you decide that you still want to go into the specialty you initially selected, you will need to be geographically flexible. Training in the urban ghetto or the rural hinterlands (sites with many unmatched positions) may not be so bad after all; you will get a chance to expand your horizons, and you may even grow to like it. If you are flexible, you are almost sure to get a reasonable position in most specialties. (A few specialties, like Orthopedic Surgery, rarely have spots open after the Match.)

## Telephone Match

If you find yourself unmatched, listen to the advice from your Dean of Students and proceed in an orderly manner to find a position. This search, unlike the deliberate steps you took to locate a residency slot before the Match, will be more like the harried and frenetic activity of a commodities broker with telephones to both ears at once.

If you are not currently a student at an LCME school, the process is the same. The only difference is that you will not have as much moral support behind you.

Three days before Match Day, if you learn that you have not matched, contact both your advisor and the Dean of Students to find out what procedures and resources they have to help you. Two days before Match Day, the first day of "The Scramble," unmatched applicants and unfilled programs are free to search each other out and to contract for positions. Print out the relevant lists of available residency positions from the NRMP website. When printing your lists, remember that some programs and specialties that would not initially consider you may be happy to seriously consider you now. After all, they also need to fill their slots. Make a list of their telephone numbers, E-mail addresses, and websites before you begin by looking them up in *FREIDA*. If you want more information about a program than *FREIDA* supplies, look at their website.

List the programs in the order they interest you. Then, beginning at 12:00 noon (EST), call them in that order. If their line is busy, send the residency director an E-mail expressing your interest and detailing how best to contact you. Are you carrying a beeper or cell phone?

Have a copy of your Dean's letter, transcript, personal statement, NBME transcript, and reference letters available. You will probably be asked to immediately fax copies of these documents to the programs that are interested in you. If you have a copy of your ERAS packet, that would be optimal. If possible, have your specialty advisor available to make some personal calls to verify that you are an excellent candidate.

If the folks on the other end of the line appear somewhat curt, understand that they also feel oppressed by having to scramble to fill their residency position with the best available person. In addition, unlike you, their program is listed on the "Unmatched" website. This announces to the world that their program did not fill. They are not having a good day either, so be tolerant.

Be wary of programs that request that you go for an interview before being considered. At this stage of the game, *you need to conclude negotiations for a position by telephone.* If you take the time to interview for a position and do not get it, your chances of getting any reasonable PGY-1 slot are almost non-existent. At this point, both applicants and programs should be willing to interview and make decisions over the telephone. If they are not, they may not really be making a serious offer. You need a position, they need a resident—and you both need them *now.*

Finally, remember that many "scramblers" enter excellent residencies, some get into difficult-to-enter specialties, and despite this very temporary setback, most go on to become excellent clinicians.

## A Scrambled Future?
The NRMP has a plan to unscramble "The Scramble." According to a white paper presented at the October 1999 NRMP meeting, one possibility for the future will be, rather than a "scramble" of unmatched candidates and programs, a mandatory "amble" through a second Match. The plan is similar to one used in the Canadian Resident Matching Service.

It would mean that once the first (now only) Match was completed, all unmatched candidates would be required to resubmit electronic applications for open program slots. They would then undergo telephone interviews. Both applicants and programs would then resubmit Rank-Order Lists and these would be run through the matching algorithm. The results would be as binding as the primary Match.

The earliest that this can be implemented will be for the Spring 2002 Match. Political resistance from both applicants and programs will probably delay, if not eliminate, using this system.

## Other Training Opportunities
If you haven't matched, there is another avenue to consider. That is post-poning your training at the PGY-1 level to pursue parallel training. You may have an interest in pursuing a graduate degree (for example, an M.P.H. or M.S.) or in doing research. This is a perfect opportunity. It gives you a chance to regroup and rethink both your decision about a specialty choice and your method of pursuing it. In addition, success in this year, if it is used to advantage, may even bolster your chance of getting the position you want. The bottom line is, don't waste this year, even if you decide not to do an internship immediately.

## Matching In Advance (PGY-2 & Above)

One of the most confusing and frustrating aspects of the Match is that not all specialties participate. And some of those that do, do so only incompletely. Although listed in the *NRMP Directory*, Neurology, Neurosurgery, Ophthalmology, Otolaryngology, Plastic Surgery, and Urology essentially do not participate in the NRMP Match.

Most of these specialties use separate Matches, sponsored by one of their academic societies, to fill their PGY-2 positions. (See Figure 22.8.) The positions are predominantly filled one or two years ahead of time by senior medical students who will enter these programs after finishing preliminary training. These specialty Matches require that Rank-Order Lists be submitted by early January and they release their Match results in mid- to late January. The cost for these Matches is $35 (2000 Match).

Information and applications for Neurology, Neurosurgery, Otolaryngology, Ophthalmology, and Plastic Surgery can be obtained by writing (designate which specialty) the Matching Program, P.O. Box 7999, San Francisco, CA 94120; www.sfmatch.org. Telephone numbers for each specialty's "vacancy line," which offers information about positions that have become available, will also be included. Information about the Urology Match can be obtained by writing the American Urological Association Residency Matching Program, P.O. Box 201820, Houston, TX 77216-1820; www.auanet.org. The Urology Match cost $50 in 2000.

Orthopedic Surgery, Anesthesiology, Emergency Medicine, and Psychiatry offer both PGY-1 and PGY-2 (Advanced [S]) positions through the NRMP PGY-1 Match. Nearly all programs in these specialties participate in the NRMP Match. Diagnostic Radiology has both PGY-1 and PGY-2 (Advanced [S]) positions available through the NRMP Match. Other positions are available as advanced placements (PGY-2 and above) outside the Match.

The NRMP also runs the Combined Musculoskeletal Specialty Match the Medical Specialties Matching Program, and selected Obstetric-Gynecology fellowship matches.

## Not Using A Match

Some residents get their positions without going through the NRMP or any specialty Matches. In recent years, nearly one-fifth of the residents in training programs had not gone through the NRMP Match to obtain their positions. Just how many of these individuals went through the specialty Matches, and exactly which positions (and their quality) were obtained, is unknown. There are opportunities outside of the Match, though. And it is important to know about these options.

FIGURE 22.8

### Positions Available through Other (Non-NRMP-PGY-1) Matches

| Specialty Match | Total Programs (Programs in Match) | Total Positions (Positions in Match)[+] |
|---|---|---|
| Anterior Segment Surgery[#] | 0 (13) | 0 (15) |
| Cardiovascular Disease* | 199 (149) | 656 (465) |
| Cornea/External Disease[#] | 58 (53) | 64 (76) |
| Foot and Ankle Surgery* | 20 (19) | 24 (23) |
| Gastroenterology* | 170 (11) | 329 (14) |
| Glaucoma[#] | 46 (39) | 52 (49) |
| Hand Surgery* | 72 (61) | 135 (119) |
| Infectious Diseases* | 142 (105) | 307 (223) |
| Maternal-Fetal Medicine* | 60 (47) | 84 (60) |
| Neurological Surgery[#] | 99 (92) | 136 (144) |
| Neurology[#] | 122 (119) | 487 (452) |
| Neuro-Ophthalmology[#] | 19 (8) | 13 (8) |
| Ophthalmology[#] | 132 (122) | 467 (437) |
| Ophthalmology Plastic/Recon Surg* | 23 (23) | 21 (21) |
| Otolaryngology[#] | 105 (104) | 277 (257) |
| Pediatric Ophthalmology[#] | 35 (29) | 42 (38) |
| Pediatric Orthopedic Surgery* | 27 (18) | 42 (26) |
| Plastic Surgery (PGY-4)[#] | 98 (66) | 331 (117) |
| Pulmonary Diseases (all Int Med)* | 162 (116) | 380 (303) |
| Retina-Vitreous Surgery[#] | 71 (58) | 65 (78) |
| Sports Medicine-Orthopedic* | 58 (52) | 121 (115) |
| Urology** | 112 (121) | 232 (223) |

*Match run by NRMP (Information from NRMP, January 2000).
[#]Match run by the San Francisco Match (Information from Douglas Perry, January 2000).
**Match run by the American Urological Assn.
[+]Many of the positions not in the matches are offered through the U.S. military.

## Early Graduation

The NRMP PGY-1 Match is only for residency positions beginning in July. While not generally advertised, many programs have or can make positions available at other times. These are open for several reasons. For example, the program may not have been fully matched in previous years, it could be expanding, or a resident may have left voluntarily or been dropped from the program. Some programs have actually designed one or more positions to begin at midyear. Residency positions beginning in January, February, or March are not normally listed by the NRMP. However, there are not many of these positions (see "Programs offering multiple start dates" in each specialty's listing).

The best way to find positions that begin at times other than July is to write to the programs and inquire. (A list of programs that claim to offer multiple start dates can be found in the American Medical Association's *Graduate Medical Education Directory—Supplement* for the current year.) Your inquiry should be specific. Tell them when you want to start and whether you will have officially graduated. Also, indicate whether you will have a letter from your school certifying that you have completed all the requirements for graduation if your diploma will not be granted early.

If you go outside the Match, there are some additional rules. These revolve around actually obtaining the position. Unlike using the Match, you will need to decipher when you are actually being offered a position and how firm the offer really is. Most programs do not have as rigid a structure for interviewing or selecting applicants for midyear positions as they have for those that are available in July. The selection process, in fact, may be a little sloppy.

Aside from the other rules listed for optimal interviewing, you must also nail down exactly when and how you will be notified of the program's decision. It is perfectly reasonable to let the interviewers know that you are applying to more than one program for a midyear slot and, though you would *really* like to go to their program, you will, of necessity, have to accept the first available position. This, of course, is not completely true. If your second-choice program offers you a position, get at least a 24-hour delay to consider the offer. Virtually all programs will give you that long. Then contact your first choice and press them for a decision. But don't bluff. While this may get you a position at your first-choice program, it might also leave you out in the cold if you force an early decision without having been offered a slot at another program.

Specifically, ask the residency director when you can expect to hear back from the program. Emphasize that an early decision is crucial. They will, undoubtedly, understand this. If you are a competitive candidate for the position, you will be seen as being even stronger at midyear. The program is not likely to wait for someone just a little bit better—that individual might not show up. So, be assertive. The day after you were supposed to hear a decision, assuming that you haven't, call the residency director's office and find out what is going on. In many cases, the program just will not have "gotten it together" enough to decide yet. Your demonstration of enthusiasm will be very effective. *For midyear matching, being assertive is the key to success.*

## New Programs

New programs, specifically those that have just recently been approved to offer training but are not yet in the NRMP Match, are potential gold mines for those with initiative. Not only will there be less competition for slots, but you have the potential of matching early—avoiding the hassle of sweating it out until March.

In addition, these programs offer you the unique opportunity to help shape a training program. The first residents through any program, though they encounter a lot of rough spots and often have no senior residents to act as role models, inevitably have closer contacts with the faculty than subsequent classes. They are frequently given more responsibility and obtain more intense training.

But how do you find out about these programs? There are a number of sources. Your mentor and the Dean of Students are the sources closest to home. Prominent individuals, especially other program directors and notable teachers in that specialty, often receive advance notification about new programs that have been approved to begin training residents.

The specialty society is another source of information. Call and ask to talk to their Director of Educational Programs. New programs will often place advertisements in their specialty journals. Advertisements can also be found in general readership journals such as the *New England Journal of Medicine* and the *Journal of the American Medical Association*. Finally, search the Internet. Many new programs list themselves so that potential applicants can find out about them before they are listed either on *FREIDA* or in the "Green Book."

Once again, the student who puts forth a little extra effort will reap gold from these opportunities. Also remember that new programs have fewer applicants. This is true not only for their first year, but also in the next few years. If you are not the most stellar of candidates, this source of training opportunities may be one of your best bets.

## Following Other Training

Some people suggest that you might have better luck getting into a highly competitive specialty such as Neurosurgery, Dermatology, or Orthopedic Surgery, if you first complete specialty training in another area, such as Internal Medicine. The theory is that with the greater emphasis on patient care in teaching centers, any trainee who is already competent in basic patient care will be prized. In some cases, this might be true, but experience suggests otherwise.

Program directors ask the following questions: Why is someone who could go out and practice medicine applying for another training program?

Are they unsure of themselves or their goals? Are they planning to become perpetual students? Are they even educable at this stage of their training? In addition, some recent federal rules restrict a program's reimbursement to training residents for their first completed specialty. So they ask, Do I want this applicant badly enough to reduce the Medicare payments we get for residents? Obviously, this is a risky road to follow—not to mention a long one. Think hard before you take this path.

### Specialties Without Matching Programs

Preventive Medicine, Medical Genetics, and Nuclear Medicine do not have matching programs and do not, for all intents and purposes, participate in the NRMP Match. Other than Orthopedic Surgery, Osteopathic residencies also do not participate in a match. If you are interested in these specialties, you must apply to the individual programs and make individual contracts. Most programs in Aerospace Medicine, a section of Preventive Medicine, are in the military match.

### Non-Approved Programs

Of all the non-Match methods for getting a residency training position, this definitely has the most risk. "Non-approved" means that the Residency Review Committee for that specialty has not certified a program. These committees send out surveyors to assess training programs using preset criteria. A program that does not gain approval was probably deficient in more than one area that was felt to be essential for an adequate training program. *Training at a non-approved program may leave you unqualified to take the specialty's board examination.*

You should be aware of some other terms used to describe the accreditation of programs. Some programs have "provisional" approval. This only means that a program is relatively new or has undergone significant changes. However, if the program is on "probation," assess it carefully. It is in danger of falling into the "non-approved" category. And, while provisions are usually made to accredit the training of the most senior residents in such programs, those in subsequent classes may be in trouble.

## Osteopathic Matching Program

Osteopathic medical students match with American Osteopathic Association (AOA)-approved internships (other than those in the military) through the *Intern Registration Program*. This program is run under the AOA's auspices through National Matching Services (NMS), 595 Bay St.,

Suite 301, Box 29, Toronto, Ontario M5G 2C2, Canada; telephone (416) 977-3431 or (716) 282-4013; fax (416) 977-5020 or (716) 282-0611; www.natmatch.com. The algorithm they use for the Match is applicant-optimal, i.e., it gives applicants' choices of programs a slight edge over programs' applicant choices.

Osteopathic medical students automatically receive an information-application packet, including Agreement forms, by the end of June in their junior year (Figure 22.10). Other applicants must contact the NMS directly. Agreement forms must be returned to the NMS by mid-September; the NMS then sends students confirmation of their participation. In October of their senior year, the NMS sends participants a personalized Rank-Order List on which to submit their preferences, as well as the codes for individual programs. All students and programs must submit their ROLs in early January.

A vital piece of information, which all Match participants should access through the AOA website (www.am-osteo-assn.org), is the AOA's *Opportunities—[Annual] Directory of Osteopathic Postdoctoral Education Programs*. This lists all available Osteopathic training positions. However, not all listed programs or positions really exist. Within each listing, look for the number of "funded positions"; you can only match into a funded position. Disregard any programs or positions that are only listed as "approved positions." (See Figure 22.9 for the number of funded programs and positions in each specialty.)

The Intern Registration Program includes traditional Osteopathic internships, as well as "*specialty-track*" internships for Internal Medicine, Obstetrics/Gynecology, Otolaryngology/Facial Plastic Surgery, Pediatrics, and Urological Surgery. (Specialty-track internships usually shorten specialty training by one year.) The Program also includes "*special-emphasis*" internships in Anesthesiology, Emergency Medicine, Family Practice, Psychiatry, and Radiology. Although these internships follow the specialty's curriculum, they do not reduce the number of subsequent training years.

Participants can access their Match results on the AOA website at noon (EST) on "AOA Intern Registration Day," usually at the end of January. Individuals who don't match can also access a list of programs with available positions. Since relatively few participants don't match and quite a few positions don't fill, students should have no problem finding a spot at which to train.

Match results are binding. If a matched participant does not sign a contract with that program within 30 days, he is banned from entering any other AOA-approved training program for one year. The only exception is if both the program and the applicant agree, in writing, to release each other from this obligation. Osteopaths with military commitments participate in the military matching program. If they fail to obtain a military residency position (announced prior to the Intern Registration Program), they may participate in the Osteopathic match. Fewer than three-fourths of Osteopathic graduates take Osteopathic internships. With the numbers varying widely, Osteopathic schools have from 3% to 47% of their new graduates opting for ACGME-approved (M.D.) programs.

FIGURE 22.9

### Osteopathic Specialties with Annual Number of Funded Entry-Level Positions*

| Specialty | Number of Programs | Number of Entry-Level Positions |
|---|---|---|
| Anesthesiology | 13 | 10 |
| Cardiology | 8 | 15 |
| Child Psychiatry | 1 | 0 |
| Critical Care | 4 | 1 |
| Dermatology | 11 | 8 |
| Diagnostic Radiology | 14 | 20 |
| Emergency Medicine | 28 | 96 |
| Emergency Med–Fam Practice | 4 | 4 |
| Emergency Med–Internal Med | 12 | 17 |
| Family Practice | 117 | 373 |
| Fam Prac–Osteo Manipul Med | 4 | 2 |
| Gastroenterology | 5 | 3 |
| Geriatrics (All) | 6 | 2 |
| Hematology/Oncology | 1 | 1 |
| Infectious Diseases | 2 | 2 |
| Internal Medicine** | 50 | 198 |
| Internal Medicine–Pediatrics** | 1 | <1 |
| Maternal-Fetal Medicine | 1 | <1 |
| Nephrology | 1 | <1 |
| Neurological Surgery | 8 | 4 |
| Neurology | 5 | 5 |
| Obstetrics/Gynecology** | 35 | 60 |
| Occupational Medicine | 1 | <1 |
| Ophthalmology | 10 | 8 |
| Orthopedic Surgery | 29 | 46 |
| Osteopathic Manipulative Med | 13 | 15 |
| Otolaryngology | 2 | 1 |
| Otolaryngology/Facial Plastic Surg** | 20 | 17 |
| Pediatrics** | 13 | 28 |
| Pediatric Emergency Medicine | 1 | <1 |

FIGURE 22.9 (continued)

| Specialty | Number of Programs | Number of Entry-Level Positions |
|---|---|---|
| Physical Med & Rehabilitation | 1 | 1 |
| Plastic & Reconstructive Surg | 3 | 1 |
| Proctology | 1 | 1 |
| Preventive Medicine | 1 | 1 |
| Psychiatry | 4 | 11 |
| Pulmonary Medicine | 3 | 2 |
| Pulmonary Med–Critical Care | 1 | 1 |
| Radiation Oncology | 1 | 0 |
| Sports Medicine | 7 | 2 |
| Surgery (General) | 38 | 64 |
| Thoracic Surgery | 2 | 2 |
| Urological Surgery** | 13 | 5 |
| Vascular Surgery (General) | 8 | 3 |
| Internships** | 296 | 1,949 |

*Many programs list positions for which they do not have funding. This chart lists only funded (real) positions available for Osteopaths going through the Match.

**An internship is required before any Osteopathic residency training can be started. Taking a *specialty track* internship in Internal Medicine, Obstetrics and Gynecology, Otolaryngology/Facial Plastic Surgery, Pediatrics, and Urological Surgery can shorten the total residency length by one year.

Information from: American Osteopathic Association, December 1999.

---

FIGURE 22.10

### Osteopathic Intern Registration Program Schedule

**June:** Schools distribute Intern Registration Program materials to students completing their junior year.

**June-October:** Students gather program information and apply directly to programs.

**Early September:** Students return completed Agreement Form and fees to National Matching Service (NMS).

**Mid-September:** NMS sends confirmation to applicants.

**By late October:** NMS sends Rank-Order List forms and a list of participating programs to applicants.

**October-December:** Students interview with residency programs.

**Early January:** NMS must receive Rank-Order Lists or Statement of Military Obligation.

**Late January:** Match results released. Unmatched students receive a list of unfilled positions.

**By late February:** Hospitals send contracts to matched applicants.

**By late March:** Student must sign and return contract to the institution within 30 days of its receipt.

# 23

# You've Matched–Now What?

*Eureka! Eureka!*

– Archimedes

Congratulations! You have gotten a residency position. You have matched! But you are still not through. As they say in tennis, it's the follow-through that makes winners. (I can't even hit the ball, but I know the rules.)

You will be firmly attached to this residency training program for the next several years. What you do in the next few hours and days will make a lasting impression on your new employers.

## Telephone Follow-Up To Program

As soon as you find out where you have matched and can calm down to a reasonable level of intelligibility, make a telephone call to your new residency director. The call should be brief and enthusiastic, even if the program was not your first choice. Tell him or her how glad you are to have matched with the program and how much you are looking forward to starting your residency training.

This also is a good time to ask if the program needs any additional information from you, their new resident. During this *short* telephone call, keep in mind that you want to establish a positive image of yourself in the residency director's mind. Now that you have an employer-employee relationship, doesn't that seem wise?

## Letter Follow-Up

Now that you have matched, you also have some letters to write.

The first is to the program with which you have matched. Repeat your enthusiastic response to matching with them and starting your residency training. Ask again if they need any additional information. Also, of prime importance, *give them sufficient addresses and telephone numbers for the next*

547

*several months* so they can send you any materials you might need. Every year some new interns fail to get their first few paychecks on time because they could not be reached in advance to fill out the necessary paperwork.

Your second letter should be to your adviser or mentor. This is the individual who has probably done the most to help get you the position that you wanted. Of course, it is most appropriate to tell your adviser about your Match results in person, as soon as possible. But also send a note of thanks, saying how much you appreciate all his or her efforts on your behalf. It is also proper, if you so desire, to give a small gift as a token of your thanks. This, however, is purely optional and will depend upon the relationship you have developed.

The final letters you should send are to those individuals who wrote you reference letters. Thank them for writing the letters and tell them where you will be going for training. They will appreciate your thoughtfulness and this will, hopefully, help you to continue these valuable professional ties that you have established.

## Post-Purchase Dissonance

Have you ever thought long and hard before buying a car, a home, or a stereo—only to finally buy it and be fraught with uncertainty over whether you made the correct decision? Of course you have. It is normal human behavior. This behavior is called post-purchase dissonance.

You have just spent the past six months, and probably much longer, investigating specialties and residency programs before you "bought." You might now feel similarly uncertain about that choice. You may, from some source, receive additional information about your program (no matter whether it is correct or not) or about your specialty (significant or not), and you suddenly are unsure about the life decision that you have made. Don't worry! This happens to almost everyone. If you have gone through the steps outlined in this book, you will be just fine. Now is the time to relax and enjoy yourself—you've earned it.

You might also wonder if the program's faculty does not also feel some post-purchase dissonance. They often do. But if you have contacted them as outlined above, their dissonance, if they have any, will not be directed toward you.

## Contracting With The Program

After matching, you should soon receive a contract to sign from the program. The contract and accompanying information a program sends you should specify

- the length of the residency program
- the duration of your appointment
- the conditions for your reappointment
- your responsibilities in the program
- the amount of your salary
- the amount of other stipends (meals, uniforms, laundry)
- liability, health, and disability insurance coverage
- other benefits
- vacation and leave policies (including sick and professional leave)
- disciplinary and grievance procedures
- policies on sexual harassment
- policies on moonlighting

While no residency contract is perfect, programs should supply as much information as possible, in writing, before you start the residency. This will eliminate confusion later on.

Occasionally, the information in a residency contract will vary from that provided when you were interviewing. It is not unusual for programs to slightly alter the benefit programs as the sponsoring institution changes its benefits. If, however, there are important differences between this material and what you were initially told, immediately contact the program director to clarify the situation.

You might also want to look carefully for any pre-employment screening requirements, such as drug tests or infectious disease screens. The NRMP now takes the position that matching with the program is only part of the agreement, and that a prospective resident must pass any required screening before being hired. This is information that you should (ideally) know before you rank any program. Be certain that you look for it now, in case the program has a requirement you cannot pass.

## Debt Management

As you embark on your new career, you may not want to think about the medical school debt that hangs heavy over most graduates' heads; but now is the time to do it. Before you leave your school, it may be wise to have a final meeting with the financial aid officer. He or she may be able to give you some advice about how to best handle your debt burden.

Several other valuable tools exist to help residents manage their debts. The Association of American Medical Colleges (AAMC) runs a listserver called MONEYMATTERS for debt-ridden residents. They also have a "Layman's Guide to Educational Debt Management for Residents and Graduate Medical Education Staff," an excellent on-line publication. It discusses eight strategies for residents to use to manage their debt.

1. Know your portfolio.
2. Know the "relative cost" of your loans.
3. Know your grace, deferment, and forbearance options.
4. Know your decision points and keep a calendar.
5. "Run the numbers" before choosing any repayment plan or consolidation option.
6. Keep good records.
7. Know when you need outside professional help.
8. Know and use your support systems.

Both resources can be accessed through the AAMC website (www.aamc.org). Click on "Student and Applicant Information." The listserver can be accessed using a password that you get via the E-mail address at the site. Additionally, the AAMC runs "Debt Management Workshops" periodically for residents. Check their website for dates and locations. A video of this conference can be accessed through their website using a password available from your medical school's financial aid officer.

The American Medical Association's "Student Loan Manager" (free to resident members) contains additional information. For information about consolidating loans, contact: U.S. Department of Education (www.hrsa. dhhs.gov/newsroom/releases/HEALrefinance.htm), Federal Direct Consolidation Loan Information Center (www.ed.gov/offices/OPE/ Direct Loan), Direct Student Loan Consolidation (www.pueblo.gsa.gov), and Sallie Mae (www.salliemae.com).

## Your New Home

A number of websites now exist to help you choose a new residence. Some that seem to be good are:

- www.hypervigilance.com/househunt.htm
- www.homepath.com
- www.homefair/mortcalc.htm (helps calculate mortgage payments)
- realestate.yahoo.com/realestate/schools
  (find areas with the best schools )

More sites are popping up all the time. Use your search engine to find them and you can eliminate a lot of hassle.

# Moving

If you have gotten a position far from where you now live, or you have just decided it is time to live in nicer quarters now that you will be getting paid (a little) for what you do, you need to move. Since this may be a new experience for you, and because many students have told me that they got "burned" when using movers, here are some helpful tips for hiring professional movers.

**Call your local Better Business Bureau** before contacting any mover, to find out if they have had any complaints lodged against them.

**Contact and get estimates from at least three movers.**

**Get a written estimate.** Estimates come in three forms: *Binding*, where the price remains fixed once the estimate is signed by both parties; *Non-binding*, where you can be charged almost any price; and *Not-to-exceed $X*, which sets an upper limit on cost.

**Get details about charges not covered by the estimate.** These may include packing, unpacking, surcharges for long distances from the house or apartment to the truck or for stairs (on either end of the trip), packing materials, and insurance.

**Carry irreplaceable items with you.** Do not entrust diplomas, other legal documents, heirlooms, family photographs, jewelry, safe-deposit-box contents, or other highly valued or easily breakable items to the movers. Take them with you.

**Get adequate insurance for the possessions you will move.** Check to see if your homeowners' insurance policy covers your possessions while the mover has them. *Basic (interstate) moving insurance* only covers about 50 cents for each pound of material lost. The other options are *full-replacement-value insurance*, which costs about 85 cents per $100 of declared value of your goods; *depreciated-value-of-goods insurance* (what the goods are worth today), which costs about 25 cents per $100 of declared value of your goods; or a *full-replacement-less-a-deductible insurance* policy. This latter is relatively inexpensive, but you must pay the deductible before the insurance company pays anything.

**Make a detailed list of all goods moved**, including a list of everything in each box. The mover will make his own list of items and note whether furniture is "scratched," "dented," etc. Go over this list with the mover and be certain the items' conditions are correctly stated on his list. Number the boxes so you quickly know if any are missing. (While it may be a pain, be sure to account for each box or item at the end of the move—before the movers leave.)

**Take photographs** of any large or expensive items you must entrust to the movers, such as electronic equipment. Carry these photographs with you.

**Carry contact numbers** for your mover's dispatcher so you can locate your truck when it is delayed. (The frequent-mover's law: Never expect the truck to arrive when scheduled.)

## Conclusion

Now you are ready to begin residency training. Let me welcome you to what will undoubtedly be one of the most stimulating and exciting periods of your professional life. You have planned well and have used your own wants and needs to guide your selection of both a specialty and a training program. *Good luck in all your future endeavors. You deserve it!*

### A New Beginning

To an intern, personal time is always reckoned in minuses. It is the time remaining when work-ups, conferences, dictations, and clinic sessions are taken away or it equals the time left over after work, sleep and errand running are subtracted from a day. Figured by whatever means, personal time often seems like a sum that is unaccounted for, the small amount that balances the ledger of hours. And in the tallying of hourly expenditures that every intern makes, it always lies on the debit side. Personal time is time still owed . . .

Having spent the last two years of medical school rotating disaffectedly from one clinical service to another—with hardly any involvement in patient care and hardly any sense of continuity—I gladly forfeited any claim to private time in order to have greater responsibility for patients and a more permanent station in life.

Stephen A. Hoffmann. *Under the Ether Dome: A Physician's Apprenticeship at Massachusetts General Hospital.* New York: Scribner, 1986, p. 209.

# Glossary

AAMC—*see* Association of American Medical Colleges.

Advanced Positions—Residency positions obtained through a matching program at least eighteen months before the slot opens.

Adviser—One of a number of faculty members who give you information about medical school, rotations, courses, specialties, and residency programs. This individual may also be your mentor.

AHA—*see* American Hospital Association.

Allopathic Physicians—*Not* M.D.s, but rather a therapeutic tradition believing that diseases are treated by producing a second condition that is incompatible with or antagonistic to the first.

AMA—*see* American Medical Association.

AMA-Fellowship and Residency Electronic Interactive Database Access—This AMA-produced computer program, popularly known as *FREIDA*, has in-depth information about nearly all residencies and many fellowship programs.

American Hospital Association—A professional organization of U.S. hospitals. It lobbies for and monitors hospitals, and has a large say (through the JCAHO) in the setting and enforcement of hospital standards.

American Medical Association—An association of physician members which establishes standards of care, monitors legal issues, and lobbies members of the U.S. Congress on issues important to physicians and their patients. It has special sections for IMGs, residents, students, and young physicians. The AMA publishes the *Journal of the American Medical Association* (*JAMA*) and other specialty journals, as well as reliable resources on many health-related issues.

American Medical Women's Association—An independent organization representing the interests of women physicians and medical students.

American Osteopathic Association—An association of Osteopathic physicians which establishes standards of care, monitors legal issues, and lobbies members of the U.S. Congress on issues important to physicians and their patients. It also sponsors its own Intern Registration Program. All Osteopathic medical students must be AOA members.

AMWA—*see* American Medical Women's Association.

AOA—*see* American Osteopathic Association.

AOA (award)—Alpha Omega Alpha, the best-known and most prestigious medical student honorary society.

Association of American Medical Colleges—An association of U.S. and Canadian Medical schools, the AAMC accredits schools in the United States, Canada, and Puerto Rico. The AAMC also conducts an annual meeting, provides consultation, and publishes useful directories and educational materials.

Audition Electives—Senior clerkships taken to demonstrate your abilities to the faculty at residencies you wish to attend.

Canadian Resident Matching Service—The Canadian equivalent of the NRMP Match. Formerly called the Canadian Intern Matching Service (CIMS).

**CaRMS**—*see* Canadian Resident Matching Service.

**Categorical Intern**—A first-year residency position in Internal Medicine or General Surgery designed for those who plan to complete a residency in that field.

**Clerkship**—Structured clinical education provided to medical students.

**Clinical Research Fellow**—Designates either a U.S. physician or an IMG engaged primarily in research associated with patient care. Physicians in this category need full medical licensure if significant patient contact is involved, but no license if there is minimal patient contact under the supervision of a licensed physician.

**Clinical Skills Assessment**—An examination given by the Educational Commission for Foreign Medical Graduates (ECFMG) to test both clinical skills and facility with spoken English.

**Clinical years**—The period of medical school when students "rotate" through the various clinical services. In a traditional four-year school, these are the third (junior) and fourth (senior) years.

**Combined Musculoskeletal Match**—NRMP-run matching program for selected Orthopedic Surgery fellowships.

**COMLEX**—*see* Comprehensive Osteopathic Medical Licensing Examination.

**Comprehensive Osteopathic Medical Licensing Examination**—A method of licensure available only to Osteopathic Physicians. It is a three-part written exam.

**COTH**—The Council of Teaching Hospitals, which publishes several useful references for residency applicants.

**Couples Match**—A method by which couples can rank their residency choices in program pairs in the NRMP Match so that they can stay in geographic proximity to one another.

**CSA**—*see* Clinical Skills Assessment.

**Curriculum Vitae (C.V.)**—A résumé.

**Dean of Students**—The key individual to ask for information about, and for assistance during, specialty selection and the matching process.

**ECFMG**—*see* Educational Commission for Foreign Medical Graduates.

**Educational Commission for Foreign Medical Graduates**—A nonprofit foundation sponsored by standard-setting associations and agencies to monitor competency of graduates of foreign medical schools.

**Electronic Residency Application Service**—A method for residency applicants to submit their applications through their Dean's office via the Internet. Most M.D. specialties now use the system.

**ERAS**—see Electronic Residency Application Service.

**EVIMG**—*see* Exchange-Visitor International Medical Graduate.

**Exchange-Visitor International Medical Graduate**—The largest subset of FNIMGs applying for residency slots, these individuals are in the United States only temporarily as Exchange Visitors (with J-1 visas) to study, teach, or do research.

**Externship**—A clinical rotation taken at a location away from your primary teaching institutions.

**Federation Licensing Examination**—A medical licensing examination which is no longer given. However, if it was previously passed, it still may be used for licensure.

**Federation of State Medical Boards of the United States**—This organization maintains contact information for individual medical licensing authorities and responds to inquiries regarding medical licensure.

**Fellow**—An academic term used to designate one engaged in postgraduate training after completing a residency program. Also used for experienced scholars engaged in research, writing, or teaching.

**FLEX**—*see* Federation Licensing Examination.

**FMG**—A term used by some organizations to indicate foreign-national physicians who are IMGs.

**FMGEMS**—*see* Foreign Medical Graduate Examination.

**FNIMG**—*see* Foreign-National International Medical Graduate.

**Foreign Medical Graduate Examination**—An examination once used to obtain an ECFMG Certificate, but not a medical license. It is no longer given.

**Foreign-National International Medical Graduate**—A non-U.S. citizen whose basic medical degree or qualification was conferred by a medical school not approved by the LCME, usually located outside the United States, Canada, and Puerto Rico.

**FREIDA**—*see* AMA-Fellowship and Residency Electronic Interactive Database Access.

**FSMB**—*see* Federation of State Medical Boards of the United States.

**Green Book**—The AMA-produced *Graduate Medical Education Directory*. This book lists most residency and fellowship programs. It also contains listings of the standards residency programs must meet and the requirements to take the specialty board examinations.

**Health Maintenance Organization**—A managed care plan under which medical treatment is prepaid through monthly premiums. HMO physicians are paid set salaries rather than collecting patient fees. Patients have a limited choice of physicians and, except in emergencies, must be admitted to HMO-designated hospitals.

**Health Professions Scholarship Program**—Military-sponsored scholarships for medical students.

**HMO**—*see* Health Maintenance Organization.

**HPSP**—*see* Health Professions Scholarship Program.

**IAP-66**—Visa document issued to a J-1 visa holder.

**IMG**—*see* International Medical Graduate.

**Independent Applicants**—Anyone in the NRMP Match who is neither a current student at nor a Sponsored Graduate of an LCME-approved medical school.

**Individual Provider Association**—The group contracting with independent physicians to provide services to an HMO's patients.

**Intern**—The historical term for individuals in their first year of training after medical school. While not officially used except to designate specific positions (Transitional, Preliminary, and Categorical internships), clinicians still commonly use the term.

**Intern Registration Program**—A matching program for obtaining AOA-approved internships.

**International Medical Graduate**—A foreign national educated at a U.S., Canadian, or an accredited Puerto Rican medical school (EVIMG); a foreign national who trains outside the U.S., Canada, or an accredited Puerto Rican medical school (FNIMG); or a U.S. or Canadian citizen who trains in a foreign medical school and then returns to the United States or Puerto Rico (USIMG).

**IPA**—*see* Individual Provider Association.

**LCME**—*see* Liaison Committee on Medical Education.

**Liaison Committee on Medical Education**—This organization accredits U.S., Canadian, and some Puerto Rican medical schools. Foreign-national graduates of these schools do not have to obtain an ECFMG Certificate to continue training in the United States.

**License**—A state's permission to practice medicine. Each state has its own licensure requirements.

**Managed Care**—Any type of health insurance that uses only specified physicians to see their patients. Examples include HMOs, IPAs, and PPOs.

**Match Day**—The day on which residency applicants participating in the NRMP or AOA Matches find out with which program they have matched.

**Matching Programs**—One of the various methods by which students or physicians obtain a position in a residency or fellowship training program.

**Medical Matching Program**—NRMP-run matching program for selected Internal Medicine fellowships.

**Mentor**—The faculty member who helps guide you through medical school and through the residency-application process.

**Moonlighting**—Extra clinical work done for pay, usually away from the institution where one is a resident.

**Must/Want Analysis**—The best method to determine what you want in a residency program and which programs meet those needs.

**National Board of Medical Examiners**—The organization that produces national physician licensing examinations, including the USMLE.

**National Board of Osteopathic Examiners**—An organization which gives an alternative licensing examination for Osteopathic physicians. This examination is not widely accepted by licensing bodies.

**National Residency Matching Program**—A national program to match applicants with accredited U.S. residency programs.

**NBOE**—*see* National Board of Osteopathic Examiners.

**NRMP**—*see* National Residency Matching Program.

**Objective Structured Clinical Examination**—A patient-simulation examination used to test medical students and similar to the CSA test given to international medical graduates.

**OSCE**—*see* Objective Structured Clinical Examination.

**Participating Institution**—One part of a multi-institutional graduate education program.

**Part-Time Positions**—*see* Shared-Schedule Positions.

**PGY-1**—Postgraduate Year-1. The internship year, otherwise known as the first year of residency.

**PPO**—*see* Preferred Provider Organization.

**Preclinical years**—The period of medical school preceding clinical rotations, usually the first two years.

**Preferred Provider Organization**—A group of hospitals or physicians that contracts to provide comprehensive health coverage at a competitive rate. These networks combine aspects of a traditional health care system and an HMO.

**Preliminary Intern**—First-year positions in Internal Medicine or General Surgery designed for those who do not necessarily plan to complete a residency in that specialty. Many students who take these positions either are undecided about their career plans or plan to go into another field that requires prior clinical training.

**Program**—The designation for both a place and a curriculum to train residents.

**Rank-Order List**—The program rankings each applicant submits and the applicant ranking each residency program submits to matching programs.

**Rank-Order List Input Code**—The code needed for each applicant to enter a Rank-Order List in the computer system for the NRMP Match.

**Research Scholar**—Term used to designate an individual holding a Ph.D., M.D., or equivalent degree who is in a research training program. The term implies that no patient contact is involved in the training.

**Résumé**—Also called a curriculum vitae or C.V., it briefly summarizes a person's accomplishments.

**ROL**—*see* Rank-Order List.

**ROLIC**—*see* Rank-Order List Input Code.

**San Francisco Matching Program**—The program running many of the "early" matches for specialties such as Neurology, Neurosurgery, Otolaryngology, and Ophthalmology.

**Scramble**—*see* Unmatch Days.

**Shared-Schedule Position**—One residency position shared by two individuals.

**Special Purpose Examination**—A one-day examination to test the knowledge base of physicians who seek licensure in a new state or relicensure in the same state at least five years after graduation from medical school.

**Special-Emphasis Internship**—Available for Osteopathic Physicians in Anesthesiology, Emergency Medicine, Family Practice, Psychiatry, and Radiology. Although these internships follow the curriculum of the specialty, they *do not* reduce the number of subsequent training years.

**Specialty-Track Internship**—Available for Osteopathic Physicians in Internal Medicine, Obstetrics/Gynecology, Otolaryngology/Facial Plastic Surgery, Pediatrics, and Urological Surgery. These internships usually shorten specialty training by one year.

**SPEX**—*see* Special Purpose Examination.

**Sponsoring Institution**—The main hospital or clinic responsible for a residency training program. Often it is also the primary training site.

**Subinternship**—A clinical rotation that gives a senior medical student added responsibility.

**TOEFL**—An examination called *Toward English as a Foreign Language*. Currently used as the ECFMG English examination.

**Transitional Internship**—Also called a "rotating internship," it allows interns to rotate through a variety of clinical services, usually in most of the same specialties they went through during their third-year clerkships.

**Unmatch Days**—The two days before Match Day when those who fail to match with a residency program begin to "scramble" for a residency position.

**USIMG**—A U.S. citizen whose basic medical degree or qualification was conferred by a medical school not approved by the LCME, usually located outside the United States, Canada, or Puerto Rico.

**United States Medical Licensing Examination**—The examination required to practice medicine in the U.S. Implemented in 1994 as the only licensing examination for physicians (M.D.s or equivalents) without regard to their nationalities or medical schools.

**USMLE**— *see* United States Medical Licensing Examination.

**Voice Response System**—The NRMP's automated telephone system that gives applicants information and match results.

# Annotated Bibliography*

*Knowledge is power.*

– Hobbes, Leviathan

## Medicine—The Big Picture

Drayer J. *The Cost-Effective Use of Leeches and Other Musings of a Medical School Survivor.* Tucson, AZ: Galen Press, Ltd., 1998. Hilarious stories, cartoons, and poems (based on Dr. Seuss), describing one medical student's trials and tribulations as he wended his way through medical school. A must read—if you don't take yourself too seriously. ★

Lewis S. *Arrowsmith.* New York: Penguin Books, 1924. An inspiring classic that led many people to medicine as a career. It shows what physicians can do, as well as their limitations, in medical practice and in the laboratory. Although written in the pre-antibiotic era, the story remains as current today as it was then. ★

London O. *Kill as Few Patients as Possible: and Fifty-Six Other Essays on How to be the World's Best Doctor.* Berkeley, CA: Ten-Speed Press, 1987. Funny, short essays illustrate this practicing physician's rules about how to be a successful (and humane and compassionate) physician. While the essays are tongue-in-cheek, much of the underlying advice really will make you an excellent physician. ★

Polk SR. *The Medical Student's Survival Guide.* 4th ed. Denver, CO: MedinCom, 1995. The strategies you need to know for medical school, internship, residency, and medical practice. Written in an easy and often humorous style familiar to most medical students, this book should give you a start on navigating through the dangers inherent in medical education. ★

Reynolds R, Stone J. *On Doctoring: Stories, Poems, Essays.* 2nd ed. New York: Simon & Schuster, 1995. Classic and pithy descriptions of physicians, medical practice, diseases, and patients. Contributors include physicians (Sir Arthur Conan Doyle, William Carlos Williams, Richard Selzer, and others) and noted writers (Anton Chekhov, Ernest Hemingway, Kurt Vonnegut, and Alice Walker). A book to be repeatedly read through an entire medical career. ★

Schiedermayer DL. *House Calls, Rounds, and Healings.* Tucson, AZ: Galen Press, Ltd., 1996. Revealing the human vulnerabilities in doctor-patient relationships, this small book of verses provides powerful insight into how excellent clinicians bond with the great variety of patients they encounter. Written by a practicing internist with diverse experiences. It brings the humanity back into medical practice—something we all occasionally miss. ★

---

*\*Code:*
- See Chapter 9 for a more detailed description.
- ■ Address at end of Bibliography.
- ★ Reference can be obtained through *The Galen Press Catalog*, P.O. Box 64400, Tucson, AZ 85728-4400; telephone (800) 442-5369.

## The Specialties

American Academy of Family Physicians. *Can I Afford to Be a Family Physician? The Medical Student's Guide to Considering Financial Aspects of Specialty Choice.* 1998. AAFP, 11400 Tomahawk Creek Parkway, Leawood, KS 66211-2672. Well, can you afford it? Can you afford not to become an FP if that's what you really want? Obviously, a somewhat skewed perspective, but worth a look.

American Academy of Pediatrics. *Pediatrics: What's It Really Like?* AAP, 141 Northwest Point Blvd., Elk Grove Village, IL 60007-1098. A compilation of eleven articles from several sources, with various publication dates, detailing aspects of Pediatrics. Urban, rural, small town, academic, and alternative Pediatric practices are discussed in a positive way by practicing Pediatricians.

American Association for the Surgery of Trauma. Guidelines for trauma care fellowships. *J Trauma.* 1992;33(4):491-4. This document lays out the requirements for Trauma Surgery fellowships in a manner similar to that used by the "Green Book" for primary residencies. Well worth a look for those interested in pursuing this specialty.

American Board of Medical Specialties. *Annual Report & Reference Handbook.* Evanston, IL: ABMS, published annually. This lists the currently approved specialties and subspecialties for M.D.s.

American College of Surgeons. *Socio-Economic Factbook for Surgery.* ACS, 633 North St. Clair Street, Chicago, IL 60611-3211. Published in alternate years. A wealth of statistics compiled into tables, giving an up-to-date picture of Surgery. Sections on surgical manpower, surgical education, and utilization of surgeons. There are also statements by the American College of Surgeons on ambulatory surgery, trauma systems, prepaid health plans, and unnecessary surgery.

American Medical Association. *JAMA's* "Contempo Issue" (published annually). A review of the newest scientific advances and future perspectives in the clinical practice of most specialties. Written by noted individuals in each field. ∎

Berry AJ, Hall JR. Work hours of residents in seven anesthesiology training programs. *Anesth Analg.* 1993;76(1):96-101. This article describes residents' work hours and activities at seven university-based residency training programs.

Biro FM, Siegel DM, Parker RM, Gillman MW. A comparison of self-perceived clinical competencies in primary care residency graduates. *Ped Resrch.* 1993;34(5):555-9. This paper describes how comfortable Family Practice, Pediatric, Internal Medicine, and Internal Medicine-Pediatric residency graduates feel when taking care of different types of primary care patients. This may be something to consider when deciding between various primary care residencies.

Colen BD. *O.R.: The True Story of 24 Hours in a Hospital Operating Room.* New York: Signet (Penguin), 1994. A Pulitzer-Prize-winning author's gripping, minute-by-minute account of the operating room, as seen from several perspectives. From extraordinary surgical feats to the mundane. After reading this, you will either be a confirmed surgeon or know why you don't want to enter this world. ★

Committee on Strengthening the Geriatric Content of Medical Training. Strengthening training in geriatrics for physicians. *J Am Geriat Soc.* 1994;42(5):559-65. A good description of the specialty, including the use of non-physician practitioners. It contains descriptions of what current Geriatricians do in practice and their estimate for future need.

Delbridge TR. *Emergency Medicine in Focus: A Handbook for Medical Students & Prospective Residents.* 1991. Emergency Medicine Residents Association, P.O. Box 619911, Dallas, TX 75261-9911. Everything you wanted to know about Emergency Medicine, albeit with a very personal and sometimes biased slant. Topics include the history of the specialty, career options within Emergency Medicine, the future of the specialty, how Emergency Medicine residencies and fellowships function, and how to apply.

DeLisa JA, Jain SS, Campagnolo DI. Factors used by physical medicine and rehabilitation residency training directors to select their residents. *Am J Phys Med Rehab.* 1994;73(3): 152-6. The title says it all. What does it take to get into a PM & R program?

DeLisa JA, Leonard JA, Smith BS, Kirshblum S. Common questions asked by medical students about physiatry. *Am J Phys Med Rehab.* 1995;74(2):145-54. The authors answer all common questions and correct the misunderstandings about Physical Medicine and Rehabilitation. Well worth reading.

Gabram SGA, Allen LW, Deckers PJ. Surgical residents in the 1990s: issues and concerns for men and women. *Arch Surg.* 1995;130(1):24-8. If you plan on going through all or part of a Surgical residency, read this article to learn the frustrations and concerns you will face.

International Medicine Centre to Advance Research and Education. *Internal Medicine Data Book.* IMCARE, 2011 Pennsylvania Avenue N.W., #800, Washington, DC 20006-1808. First published in December 1992, this booklet contains nearly every statistic anyone could want to know about internists and Internal Medicine. Much of the data is drawn from the AMA's data, but the items are broken out to compare Internal Medicine with other specialties. The booklet's information is divided into sections on medical education, specialty distribution and characteristics, patient information, practice characteristics, and medical economics. Definitely worth looking over if you are considering Internal Medicine or one of its subspecialties.

Lull RJ, Littlefield JL. Work force problems in nuclear medicine and possible solutions. *Seminars Nuclear Med.* 1993;23(1):31-45. An excellent review of who practices Nuclear Medicine and how they practice. It also gives some predictions for the specialty.

Miller RH. Otolaryngology residency and fellowship training. *Arch Otolaryngol.* 1994; 120(10):1057-61. This article clearly describes the positive and negative aspects of different ENT residency and fellowship training programs.

Pawluch D. *The New Pediatrics: A Profession In Transition.* Hawthorne, NY: Aldine de Gruyter, 1996. Written by a sociologist, this book highlights the negative aspects of Pediatric practice, especially the "dissatisfied Pediatrician syndrome." Since it is always best to know the negatives about a potential specialty as well as the positives, it is definitely worth a look for those contemplating Pediatrics.

Senf JH, Campos-Outcalt D, Watkins AJ, Bastacky S, Killian C. A systematic analysis of how medical school characteristics relate to graduates' choices of primary care specialties. *Acad Med.* 1997;72(6):524-33. What makes you think you want to enter a primary care specialty? Is it one of the factors described in this excellent study?

Wachter RM, Goldman L. The emerging role of "hospitalists" in the American healthcare system. *N Engl J Med.* 1996;335(7):514-7. This is the article that first brought the idea of hospitalists to the forefront. It describes the concept and its possible future.

Weissman S. American psychiatry in the 21st century: the discipline, its practice, and its work force. *Bull Menninger Clin.* 1994;58(4):502-18. A review of the current state of Psychiatry and where it may go in the early part of the next millennia.

Zussman R. *Intensive Care.* Chicago: Univ Chicago Press, 1992. Excellent book for anyone considering a specialty where you may spend time in the ICU. This well-written book gives the real scoop on what happens and what practitioners do there, rather than what they want you to think they do. ★

## Selecting a Specialty

American Medical Association. *Specialty Profiles*. Chicago: AMA, published annually. A weighty volume containing all the recognized specialties, plus a few more such as Legal Medicine and Clinical Pharmacology. Each chapter has a brief history and a current perspective on the specialty. A large section is devoted to the demographics of current practitioners in the specialty, with lots of charts, graphs, and tables. ▪

Burack JH, Irby DM, Carline JD, et al. A study of medical students' specialty-choice pathways: trying on possible selves. *Acad Med*. 1997;72(6):534-41. Are you thinking about a primary care specialty? This paper describes factors that previous students considered important when either entering or rejecting a primary care career. No doubt you will recognize yourself in some of these vignettes.

Ducatman BS. Be careful what you wish for. *JAMA* 1997;278(14):1130. An insightful and beautifully written one-page piece on a student's experience with the consummate rural family practitioners—and reasons to rethink what seem to be idyllic career choices.

*Glaxo Welcome Medical Specialties Survey*. Glaxo Welcome Pharmaceuticals, Inc. 1999. Contains some of the most complete descriptions of most of the medical specialties and major subspecialties. It includes a background of each specialty, profiles of individual practitioners, and anecdotes about why individuals entered the fields. It then goes on to detail and rate, on a linear scale, how important seventeen different aspects of practice are to physicians in that specialty. These factors include continuity of care, schedule, diversity, autonomy, manual activities, security, and income. It also contains an exercise by which you can rate your interests against the typical profile in each of the specialty areas. This material is on a CD-ROM, which, along with many other materials, is *free* to participants in the Glaxo Welcome Pathway Evaluation Program. If you haven't already gone through it, ask your Dean to set it up for your class.

Iserson KV. *Non-Standard Medical Electives in the U.S. and Canada*. Tucson, AZ: Galen Press, Ltd., 1998. This is the way to find out about unusual specialties and the out-of-the-way corners of medicine. Only for those interested in something other than the humdrum electives normally offered to medical students, this book gives the information necessary to take really special away rotations. There are hundreds of listings, including Aviation Psychiatry, Wilderness Medicine, Medical Ignorance, Aging Brain, Spiritual Care of Patients, and NIH Research Electives. ★

Kassebaum DG, Szenas PL. Medical students' career indecision and specialty rejection: roads not taken. *Acad Med*. 1995;70(10):937-43. So you think you know what specialty you want to enter? Think again—as did many of your cohorts. This article reviews the alternative decisions students made about their career choices as they proceeded through medical school.

Taylor AD. *How to Choose a Medical Specialty*, 3rd ed. Philadephia, PA: WB Saunders, 1999. A correlate to the Glaxo Welcome Pathway Evaluation Program and Chapter 4 in this book, it provides an additional way to see if you are heading toward the right specialty.

## The USMLE, Other Exams, and Licensure

American Medical Association. *State Medical Licensure Requirements and Statistics*. Chicago: AMA, published annually. This is where to find the nitty gritty details about state licensure, both for U.S. and international medical graduates. It contains all the basic information about licensure requirements in every state and territory of the United States. All the permutations and combinations of licensing are included in easy-to-read charts. It includes a way to contact individual state boards for answers to additional questions and updates, as well as hard-to-get information on IMG licensure requirements. ▪

Asta LM. Board games: a no-nonsense guide to acing the national medical licensing exams. *New Phys.* 1995;44(9):15-8. A short, excellent summary on how to prepare for the USMLE. It includes specifics about some of the review courses and materials, as well as some good hints about how to prepare for and take the examinations.

The Federation of State Medical Boards of the U.S., Inc. *Exchange–Section 1: USMLE and M.D. Licensing Requirements.* Euless, TX: FSMB, published biannually. Contains the USMLE Step 3 eligibility requirements and administrative rules. Also has the requirements for initial licensure, licensure by endorsement, reregistration of one's license, licenses for postgraduate education, and special licenses. ▪

——*Exchange–Section 2: USMLE and D.O. Licensing Requirements.* Euless, TX: FSMB, published biannually. Contains the USMLE Step 3 eligibility requirements and administrative rules. Also has the requirements for initial licensure, licensure by endorsement, reregistration of one's license, licenses for postgraduate education, and special licenses. ▪

——*Exchange–Section 3: Licensing Boards, Structure and Disciplinary Functions.* Euless, TX: FSMB, published biannually. Contains the basic structure and operation of each state medical board, their review and disciplinary functions, and contacts for both of these functions. ▪

National Board of Medical Examiners and The Federation of State Medical Boards of the U.S., Inc. *USMLE Step 1 (or 2, or 3) General Instructions, Content Outline, and Sample Items.* (published annually). These valuable booklets list the current examination dates and eligibility requirements for the three Steps, as well as certification and registration procedures. Most important, there are subject/content outlines for all three Steps of the exam. The Step 3 booklet can be obtained from the state licensing board through which you will take the examination. ▪

Reteguiz J. *Mastering the OSCE/CSA.* New York: McGraw-Hill, 1999. This book helps examinees improve their performance on the OSCE (Objective Structured Clinical Examination) and the CSA (Clinical Skills Assessment). In each case, it helps you develop a checklist so you can better interact with SPs.

## The Paperwork

Hunt DD, MacLaren CF, Scott CS, Chu J, Leiden LI. Characteristics of dean's letters in 1981 and 1992. *Acad Med.* 1993;68(12):905-11. An excellent review of what is contained in Dean's letters. It should give you a good idea of what information might be included but that is not in yours, or what information you may want to suggest *not* be included in your own letter.

Taylor CA, Weinstein L, Mayhew HE. The process of resident selection: a view from the residency director's desk. *Obstet Gynecol.* 1995;85(2):299-303. This article contains the results of a survey of Family Practice and Obstetrics & Gynecology residency directors. The results seem to reflect the decision-making processes residency directors use in Internal Medicine, Pediatrics, Psychiatry, and surgical specialties.

Tysinger J: *Résumés and Personal Statements for Health Professionals*, 2nd ed. Tucson, AZ: Galen Press, 1998. A classic, this book guides you through the arduous process of describing your accomplishments in the best possible way to develop unique résumés and personal statements that reflect who you really are. Describes how to develop a personal inventory, and then how to apply the inventory items to a professional-looking document that will impress residency directors. Lots of examples to help. Also discusses cover and thank-you letters. A must for all applicants. Written by an educator with years of experience showing health professionals how to get a position by describing themselves in the best possible way. ★

Venolia J. *Write Right! A Desktop Digest of Punctuation, Grammar, and Style.* 3rd ed. Berkeley, CA: Ten-Speed Press, 1995. A powerful and easy-to-understand pocket guide on how to avoid making mistakes on résumés, personal statements, and other important documents. ★

## Selecting a Residency Program

American Academy of Family Physicians. *Directory of Family Practice Residency Programs.* Kansas City, MO: AAFP, published annually. This substantial volume lists all the currently approved Family Practice residencies. Information includes: How many positions exist at each level of training and what type of graduate (U.S. or IMG) is filling them; salaries; benefits; whether moonlighting is permitted; night-call frequency; number of hospitals and Family Practice centers in the program; faculty to resident ratio; number and type (M.D., Ph.D., etc.) of full-time-equivalent faculty/staff; time spent working in Family Practice center; number of Family Practice conferences; level of resident responsibility by postgraduate year; and resident research encouragement.

American Medical Association. *Fellowship and Residency Electronic Interactive Database Access (AMA-FREIDA®).* For most residency applicants, this system has replaced the "Green Book." Hundreds of items of information are available on-line about training programs and their parent institutions. The information the programs provide is not validated by any outside source; verify that the information is correct. Applicants can access the system through any on-line computer. • ■

——*Graduate Medical Education Directory.* Chicago: AMA, published annually. Known as "The Green Book," the Directory includes information on nearly all ACGME-accredited and combined specialty programs. Also included are Institutional and Program Requirements for all approved M.D. specialties/subspecialties and the requirements for medical specialty board certification. The *FREIDA* system has mostly replaced this book. • ■

——*Graduate Medical Education Directory Supplement.* Chicago: AMA, published annually. Contains a listing of those residency programs that begin in January, Quarterly, and at negotiable times. It also lists programs that offer part-time/shared residency positions. ■

American Medical Student Association. *AMSA's Student Guide to the Appraisal and Selection of House Staff Training Programs.* Reston, VA: AMSA, 1997. This short text briefly describes many aspects of the residency selection process. It has a brief section on the questions you may want to ask during the residency interview. ■

American Osteopathic Association. *Opportunities–Directory of Osteopathic Postdoctoral Educational Programs.* Chicago: AOA, published annually. A current listing of all AOA-approved internships and residency programs. It also includes policies and procedures for entering the Intern Registration Program (Match), and requirements for getting the AOA to approve non-AOA training. An absolute necessity for all Osteopathic students, it can be obtained free from the AOA or your Dean of Students. ■

American Psychiatric Association. *Directory of Psychiatry Residency Training Programs.* (Published annually.) American Psychiatric Press, 1400 K Street, N.W., Washington, DC 20005. A complete listing of accredited Psychiatry and Child/Adolescent Psychiatry residencies, with extensive information about each program. Also has a short introductory chapter on what psychiatric training includes and about some of the functional (official and not official) subspecialties in Psychiatry. It also explains how to use the APA clearinghouse of available residency positions. Two pages for each program list the number of available NRMP and non-NRMP positions, and positions filled and whether women, minorities or IMGs filled them; the facilities used and their demographics; the number and type of faculty; salary and benefits; patient load; frequency of night call; required rotations and electives; and available fellowships or combined training programs (e.g., Psychiatry-Internal Medicine). Each Child/Adolescent Psychiatry program has a similar separate listing. An appendix lists the available training programs combined with other specialties; all post-residency fellowships in Psychiatry; and the requirements United States and Canadian residency programs in Psychiatry and Child/Adolescent Psychiatry must follow. Essential for anyone applying to Psychiatry residencies.

American Urological Association. *Accredited Urology Training Programs*. (Published in odd-numbered years.) AUA, 6750 W. Loop South, Suite 900, Bellaire, TX 77401-4114. This book gives a brief description of all accredited Urology residencies. While the book duplicates much of the information in *FREIDA*, it does state how many applicants each program interviews each year, whether the two-year "pre-Urology training must be at the same institution as the residency, and how much time is devoted solely to research.

Association for Hospital Medical Education. *Transitional Year Program Directory* (formerly called *The Purple Book*). (Published annually.) AHME, 1200 19th Street N.W., #300, Washington, DC 20036-2412. This book lists most of the available transitional programs, contact information, months of required and elective rotations, presence of other training programs, type of individuals who match with the program, difficulty of getting a slot, night-call frequency, and opportunities for a PGY-2 year at the same institution. Despite *FREIDA*, this book remains an excellent source of hard-to-come-by information. •

Association of Academic Physiatrists. *Directory of Physical Medicine & Rehabilitation Residency Training Programs*. (Published annually.) AAP, 5987 E. 71st St., Suite 112, Indianapolis, IN 46220. This book gives a good picture of residency training programs available in Physical Medicine and Rehabilitation. Information about specific programs includes: academic affiliation and status; number of residents at each level; number and type of faculty; elective and conference time; required research and teaching; on-call frequency; hospitals used and their demographics; evaluation methods; salary and benefits; and whether moonlighting is permitted. Some information may not be current, so recheck specific information with the programs. Also contains the special requirements for Physiatry residencies and general guidelines for applicants to the specialty.

Council of Teaching Hospitals. *COTH Directory*. Washington, DC: Association of American Medical Colleges, published annually. Lists all the hospitals that are members of COTH, with a description of each institution. • ■

——*COTH Survey of Housestaff Stipends, Benefits, and Funding*. Washington, DC: Association of American Medical Colleges, published annually. An extensive description of salaries and benefits provided to residents. The information is broken down by the type of institution and region of the country. It is also available at the AAMC website. • ■

Raff MJ, Schwartz IS. An applicant's evaluation of a medical house-officership. *N Engl J Med.* 1974;291(12):601-5. A very extensive list of questions that can be used to supplement the "Must/Want" Analysis list. Although the paper is nearly three decades old, virtually all the questions are still pertinent.

Simmonds AC, Robbins JM, Brinker MR, Rice JC, Kerstein MD. Factors important to students in selecting a residency program. *Acad Med.* 1990(10);65:640-43. What is important to students when making the big decision? This study suggests some answers.

Society of Critical Care Medicine. *Directory of Critical Care Medicine Programs in the United States and Canada*. Published annually in *Critical Care Medicine*. A list of identified programs in adult and pediatric Critical Care. The programs are described in detail. The listing, however, does not imply that the programs are either approved or sanctioned, only that they exist.

Society of General Internal Medicine. *SGIM Directory of General Internal Medicine Fellowship Programs.* (Periodically updated.) A national list of Internal Medicine fellowship programs in General Internal Medicine. Can be searched by geographic area and contains information similar to that contained in *FREIDA* for residencies. It can be found at: www.sgim.org/fellowship/fellowshipwelcome.htm

——*SGIM Directory of Primary Care Internal Medicine Residency Programs.* (Periodically updated.) A national list of Internal Medicine residency programs with primary care orientations. It contains information not in *FREIDA*. It can be found at: www.sgim.org/residency/residencywelcome.htm

## International Medical Graduates

Ball LB: *The International Medical Graduate's Guide to U.S. Medicine: Negotiating the Maze.* Tucson, AZ: Galen Press, 1995. Excellent descriptions of the process and pitfalls of obtaining visas, ECFMG certification, and U.S. medical training. Designed for U.S. citizens, U.S. permanent residents, and foreign nationals with foreign medical training; Canadians; and foreign nationals in U.S. medical schools. It also covers physicians applying for Research Scholar positions and families accompanying physicians to the United States. ★

James D. Coming to America. *New Phys.* 1998;October:25-30. A good overview of the current status of international medical graduates attempting to enter U.S. residency programs. It only briefly discusses the CSA exam, since there was little experience with it at the time this was written.

Riley JD, Hannis M, Rice KG. Are international medial graduates a factor in residency program selection? A survey of fourth-year medical students. *Acad Med.* 1996;71(4):381-6. Does the presence of IMGs dissuade U.S. graduates from applying to certain residency programs. This study suggests that it does.

Sutnick AI, Stillman PL, Norcini JJ, et al. Pilot study of the use of the ECFMG clinical competence assessment to provide profiles of clinical competencies of graduates of foreign medical schools for residency directors. *Acad Med.* 1994;69(1):65-7. This article provides a glimpse of the Clinical Competence Assessment (CCA) examination that is being used as part of the testing for ECFMG Certificates.

World Health Organization. *World Directory of Medical Schools.* (Published intermittently.) WHO, 49 Sheridan Ave., Albany, NY 12210. Graduates of the listed medical schools are allowed to obtain ECFMG certification. If your school is not listed, you cannot attempt to practice medicine in the United States.

## Women in Medicine

Association of American Medical Colleges. *Women in Medicine Update.* (Published quarterly.) A newsletter that describes new studies and recent events affecting women in medicine and women's health. Available on the AAMC website. ▪

Asta LM. Halting harassment. *New Phys.* 1995;44:30-8. A good review of sexual harassment in the medical education environment, including some valuable resources to use if necessary.

Bickel J, Ruffin A. Gender-associated differences in matriculating and graduating medical students. *Acad Med.* 1995;70(6):552-9. An overview of the differences in how male and female medical students envision their career paths at the time of graduation.

Carr P, Ash AS; Friedman RH; et al. Relation of family responsibilities and gender to the productivity and career satisfaction of medical faculty. *Ann Int Med.* 1998;129(7):532-8. A large study showing that women faculty with children did not do as well as did men or women without children.

Conley FK. *Walking Out On the Boys*. New York: Farrar, Strauss & Giroux, 1998. A very interesting book written by a female tenured neurosurgery professor at Stanford University School of Medicine who resigned her position to protest sexual harassment and gender-based discrimination. She has since regained her position and continues to be active in the movement against gender-based discrimination.

Durso C. The long and winding road. *New Phys.* 1995;44:24-9. An excellent review of the tortuous path women's medical training has taken in the United States. A sidebar to the article looks at how women are faring in medicine around the globe.

Frank E, Brogan D, Schiffman M. Prevalence and correlates of harassment. *Arch Int Med.* 1998;158:352-8. This large study shows that while their experiences of and sensitivity to harassment differ, women physicians commonly perceive that they have been harassed.

Frank E, McMurray JE, Linzer M. Career satisfaction of U.S. women physicians. *Arch Internal Med.* 1999;159(13):1417-26. Are women who entered medicine pleased with their decisions? What do they like about medicine and what do they want changed?

Langelan MJ. *Back Off! How to Confront and Stop Sexual Harassment and Harassers*. New York: Simon & Schuster, 1993. The title pretty much says it, and the book delivers this message. ★

Nora LM. Sexual harassment in medical education: a review of the literature with comments from the law. *Acad Med.* 1996;71(1):S113-8. An excellent, comprehensive review of the prevalence of sexual harassment in medical education, including a balanced and insightful view of the legal status of claims of harassment.

Wiebe C. From here to maternity. *New Phys.* 1995;44:40-4. A good description of some problems pregnant women physicians faced during medical school and residency. They also have some helpful suggestions.

## Parenting

American Academy of Pediatrics. *Child Care: What's Best for Your Family?* A Web-based update of their excellent guide to childcare services, it gives detailed instructions on the different types of childcare services, what to look for, what questions to ask, and the different childcare needs of children as they grow and when they are ill. Available on the AAP website: www.aap.org/family/childcare.htm

Bickel J. *Medicine and Parenting*. Washington, DC: AAMC, 1991. Although dated, still an excellent source of information about the problems of physicians as parents—with some excellent solutions. ▪

Potee RA, Gerber AJ, Ickovics JR. Medicine and motherhood: shifting trends among female physicians from 1922 to 1999. *Acad Med.* 1999;74(8):911-19. How have things changed over the years? Is it better, or only different?

## Disabled Students

Essex-Sorlie D. The Americans with Disabilities Act: I. History, summary, and key components. *Acad Med.* 1994;69(7):519-24. An excellent overview of the Americans with Disabilities Act and how it relates to medical schools. While it does not address questions of residency application directly, it gives enough information from which to extrapolate. Clear, concise, and not filled with legal mumbo-jumbo.

Helms LB, Helms CM. Medical education and disability discrimination: the law and future implications. *Acad Med.* 1994;69(7):535-43. A bit more about the legal background, relevant court findings, and possible directions of Americans with Disabilities Act implementation.

## Special Situations

Baldwin DC, Daugherty SR, Rowley BD. Racial and ethnic discrimination during residency: results of a national survey. *Acad Med.* 1994;69(10 Supp):S19-21. How commonly does racial and ethnic discrimination appear during residency training? This is one of the few papers that help assess the problem.

Carling PC, Hayward K, Coakley EH, Wolf AMD. Part-time residency training in internal medicine: analysis of a ten-year experience. *Acad Med.* 1999;74(3):282-4. If you are considering doing a part-time/shared-schedule residency, see what others have experienced.

Humphrey D. You say you want a revolution. Part 1 (Sept, pp. 14-20) and When worlds collide. Part 2 (Nov, pp. 15-21). *New Phys,* 1997. Excellent two-part article describing the Indian Health Service, part of the U.S. Public Health Service.

Mullan F. The journey back: a physician retrains. *JAMA.* 1997;278(4):281-3. An excellent description of an experienced (older) physician-administrator retraining to enter clinical practice.

Ramos MM, Téllez CM, Palley TB, Umland BE, Skipper BJ. Attitudes of physicians practicing in New Mexico toward gay men and lesbians in the profession. *Acad Med.* 1998;73(4): 436-8. Things have changed for the better, but not as much as you might suppose.

## Osteopathic Medicine

American Osteopathic Association. *[Annual] Yearbook and Directory of Osteopathic Physicians.* Chicago: AOA. Contains current information on Osteopathic residency programs, medical schools, and state-by-state and international licensure requirements. ▪

——Division of Postdoctoral Training. Osteopathic graduate medical education. *JAOA.* (November). This annual article gives an overview of the number of available AOA-approved and funded residency positions, the number of graduates, how many D.O.s are taking ACGME-approved training, and new rules for specialty certification. ▪

Cummings M, Lemon M. Combined allopathic and osteopathic GME programs: a good thing, but will they continue? *Acad Med.* 1999;74(9):948-50. Some residency programs are combined. Will they last? One perspective on this ever more common arrangement.

Gevitz N. *The D.O.'s–Osteopathic Medicine in America.* Baltimore, MD: Johns Hopkins Univ Press, 1982. An entertaining and enlightening look at the development of Osteopathy in the United States. Unfortunately, it only takes the history up to 1981. It is, nevertheless, required reading for all D.O.s and anyone else interested in Osteopathy. ★

Meyer CT, Price A. Osteopathic medicine: a call for reform. *JAOA.* 1993;93(4):473-85. A plea to move away from conflict with M.D.s and to further integrate Osteopathic and M.D. graduate medical education. It also suggests that the two branches of medicine work together to help forge a national health policy.

Ross-Lee B, Weiser MA, Kiss L. The outlook for Osteopathic medical specialists within a reformed healthcare system. *JAOA.* 1994;94(7):558-67. An excellent overview of what may occur within Osteopathy with the changing health care environment.

## Selecting Candidates and Interviewing

Biegeleisen JI. *Make Your Job Interview a Success.* 4th ed. New York: Prentice-Hall, 1994. The chapter, "63 Guaranteed Ways to Muff a Job Interview," is enlightening reading. It is also funny. Well worth the time; it may prevent you from making a serious faux pas. ★

Krogh C. Residency interviews. *New Phys.* 1986;35(7):33-6. A discussion of the feedback from his previous article on residency interviews. The comments, based on students' experiences, are both interesting and enlightening.

Krogh C, Vorhes C, Abbott G. The residency interview: advice from the interviewers. *New Phys.* 1984;33(5):8-11, 34. The inside scoop from some experienced interviewers of residency applicants. Old, but still valuable information; interviewing has not changed much over the years.

Molidor JB, Campe JL. It's show time: mastering the art of being interviewed. *The Advisor.* 1997;18:21-6. An excellent mnemonic to use when faced with a stressful interview.

Molidor JB, Duff JL. Whatcha gonna do when they come for you? Preparing your responses for your interview. *The Advisor.* 1998;18:45-9. Another in this author's series on how to approach the high-stakes interview.

Wagoner NE, Suriano JR. Program directors' response to a survey on variables used to select residents in a time of change. *Acad Med.* 1999;74(1):51-8. What are program directors in various specialties actually searching for in residency applicants? This article gives some clues.

## The Match

*Academic Medicine.* Association of American Medical Colleges. Available at all medical school libraries or through your Dean's office. The June or July issue each year contains the results of the prior year's NRMP Match. ▪

Hirthler MA, Glick PL, Hassett JM. Evaluation of the pediatric surgical matching program by the directors of pediatric surgical training programs. *J Ped Surg.* 1994;29(10):1370-4. An evaluation highlighting the elements that fellowship directors seek in successful candidates.

National Resident Matching Program. *NRMP Data.* Washington, DC: NRMP, published annually. An annual description in words and charts of the results, both in general and by specialty, of the prior year's NRMP Match. You can see a copy by asking your Dean of Students. Much of this information used to be in the *NRMP Directory*, and was of enormous interest to applicants. Unfortunately, it is now a little more difficult to come by, but is worth seeking out. ● ▪

——*NRMP Directory.* Washington, DC: NRMP, published annually. The annual listing of programs participating in the NRMP Match. Available to registered applicants on the NRMP website. ● ▪

——*NRMP Handbook for Students.* Washington, DC: NRMP, published annually. This is a supplement to the *NRMP Directory*, available on the NRMP website. It contains special information about the Couples Match, Shared-Schedule positions, matching into Advanced positions, and getting your Match results. ▪

——*Results [Annual]: Number of Candidates Sought and Number Matched for Each Participating Hospital and Unfilled Programs by Specialty.* Washington, DC: NRMP. Known as the "Results Book," this is a listing of the outcome of the annual NRMP Match, listed by specialty and institution. ● ▪

Pevehouse BC, Colenbrander A. The United States Neurological Surgery Residency Matching Program. *Neurosurg.* 1994;35(6):1172-82. This article describes the specialty match in Neurosurgery, including a description of the algorithm and a summary of how well different applicant classes have done.

## Medical Practice

American Hospital Association. *Guide to the Health Care Field.* Chicago: AHA, published annually. Contains a detailed listing and description of over 7000 teaching hospitals in the United States. • ■

American Medical Association. *Physician Characteristics and Distribution in the United States.* Chicago: AMA, published annually. This book contains an extensive breakdown of the characteristics of physicians practicing in each specialty in the United States. It goes into the specifics of who, what, and where the physicians are. The descriptions are broken down both by specialty and by county. ■

——*Physician Marketplace Statistics: Profile for Detailed Specialties, Selected States and Practice Arrangements.* Chicago: AMA, published annually. This book provides detailed information on a variety of physician practice characteristics, including fees for selected procedures, measures of Medicare utilization, and deferred physician income statistics. It is intended to compliment *Physician Socioeconomic Statistics.* ■

——*Physician Socioeconomic Statistics.* Chicago: AMA, published annually. Extensive description of the hours worked, patient contact, costs of practice, and income of most major specialists in the United States. ■

——*U.S. Medical Licensure Statistics and Current Licensure Requirements.* Chicago: AMA, published annually. This book contains the in-depth requirements, by state, for medical licensure. This is a particularly helpful book for international medical graduates and those seeking licenses in more than one state. ■

Council on Graduate Medical Education. *Managed Health Care: Implications for the Physician Workforce and Medical Education.* Washington, DC: Health Resources & Services Administration, U.S. Dept. of Health & Human Services, 1995. This comprehensive document reviews the changing health care environment. It also specifically analyzes the impact of managed care on the need for physicians and on medical education.

Pathman DE, Konrad TR, Ricketts TC III. The National Health Service Corps experience for rural physicians in the late 1980s. *JAMA.* 1994;272(17):1341-8. A disheartening picture of the NHSC, demonstrating low morale and poor retention. Much of this is caused by disregarding the needs and preferences of the NHSC physicians and their families.

*Resident and Staff Physician.* "Board Review Issue." (annually in May.) Details the current utilization and rules for the various licensing examinations, as well as the licensing requirements for each state (M.D. and D.O.). It also usually includes information on specialty societies and current Board requirements in most specialties.

Tschida M. Corps or less. *New Phys.* 1995;44:12-6. An overview of the state of the National Health Service Corps. Although it tries to be upbeat, it's not a pretty picture.

Villanueva AM, Kaye D, Abdelhak SS, Morahan PS. Comparing selection criteria of residency directors and physicians' employers. *Acad Med.* 1995;70(4):261-71. This article lays out what residency directors in Pediatrics, Surgery, Family Practice, and Internal Medicine seek in residency candidates' applications. It then compares the personal qualities they desire in residents with the qualities that academic medical centers, private practices, managed care organizations, hospitals, and other health care systems look for when hiring new physicians.

## General Information

*The New Physician.* American Medical Student Association. Published monthly and free with membership in AMSA. Has frequent articles about medical specialties, interviewing, the Match, international medical graduates, medical practice, and other topics of vital interest to medical students. ■

# Contact Information

American Hospital Association, 325 7th Street N.W., Suite 700, Washington, DC 20004-2802; (202) 626-4631; www.aha.org

American Medical Association, 515 N. State Street, Chicago, IL 60610; (312) 464-5000; www.ama-assn.org

AMA-FREIDA: www.ama-assn.org/cgi-bin/freida/freida.cgi
E-mail: freida@ama-assn.org

American Medical Student Association (AMSA), 1902 Association Drive, Reston, VA 20191; (703) 620-6600; fax (703) 620-5873; www.amsa.org; E-mail: amsa@amsa.org

American Medical Women's Association, 801 N. Fairfax Street, Suite 400, Alexandria, VA 22314; (703) 838-0500; fax (703) 549-3864; www.amwa-doc.org

American Osteopathic Association, 142 E. Ontario Street, Chicago, IL 60611; www. am-osteo-assn.org

American Urological Association Residency Matching Program, P.O. Box 201820, Houston, TX 77216-1820; fax (713) 622-2898; www.auanet.org; E-mail: www.resmatch@auanet.org

Association of American Medical Colleges, 2450 N Street N.W., Washington, DC 20037-1127; (202) 828-0400; www.aamc.org

AAMC-ERAS, www.aamc.org/eras; Help desk E-mail: swshelp@aamc.org

Canadian Resident Matching Service (CaRMS), 151 Slater Street, Suite 802, Ottawa, Ontario K1P-5H3, Canada; (613) 237-0075; www.carms.ca; E-mail: carmsmail@carms.ca

Council of Medical Specialty Societies, 51 Sherwood Terrace, Suite M, Lake Bluff, IL 60044-2232; (847) 295-3456; www.cmss.org

Council of Teaching Hospitals, Association of American Medical Colleges, 2450 N Street N.W., Washington, DC 20037-1126; www.aamc.org/hlthcare/teach

Most recent survey of housestaff stipends and benefits: www.aamc.org/hlthcare/coth-hss/

Educational Commission for Foreign Medical Graduates (ECFMG)/ERAS, P.O. Box 13467, Philadelphia, PA 19104-3467; (215) 387-9963, fax (215) 222-5641; www.ecfmg.org; Help desk E-mail: erashelp@ecfmg.org

Applicant Document Tracking System (ADTS)
Website: eraspo3.aamc.org/adts/ or www.aamc.org/eras

*For completed diskettes without payment or with payment by credit card,* ERAS Program, P.O. Box 13467, Philadelphia, PA 19101-3467.

*For completed diskettes with payment,* ERAS Diskettes at PNC, P.O. Box 820010, Philadelphia, PA 19182-0010.

*For completed diskettes by courier delivery,* ERAS Program, 3624 Market Street, Philadelphia, PA 19104.

**ECFMG/USMLE Information,** 3624 Market Street, 4th Floor, Philadelphia, PA 19104-2685; (215) 386-5900

**Federation of State Medical Boards of the U.S., Inc.,** 400 Fuller Wiser Rd., Suite 300, Euless, TX 76039-3855; (817) 868-4000; fax (817) 868-4099; www.fsmb.org

**National Board of Medical Examiners,** 3750 Market Street, Philadelphia, PA 19104-3190; (215) 590-9500; www.nbme.org

**National Board of Osteopathic Medical Examiners,** 8765 W. Higgins Rd., Suite 200, Chicago, IL 60631-4101; (773) 714-0622; fax (773) 714-0631; www.nbome.org

**National Health Service Corps, Bureau of Primary Health Care,** 4350 East West Highway, 8th Floor West, Bethesda, MD 20814; (301) 594-4130, (800) 221-9393, (800) 638-0824; www.bphc.hrsa.dhhs.gov/nhsc/pages/toc.htm

**National Medical Association,** 1012 10th Street N.W., Washington, DC 20001; (202) 347-1895; fax (202) 842-3293; www.nmanet.org/menu.html

**National Resident Matching Program,** 2501 M Street N.W., Suite 1, Washington, DC 20037-1307; www.nrmp.aamc.org/nrmp

**San Francisco Matching Programs. (Specialty) Matching Program,** P.O. Box 7584, San Francisco, CA 94120-7584; (414) 447-0350 [including Vacancy Line]; fax (415) 561-8535; Overnight Mail address: 655 Beach Street, San Francisco, CA 94109; www.sfmatch.org

# Index

# – M –

## – Q –

# About the Author

**Kenneth V. Iserson, M.D., M.B.A., FACEP**, is a noted medical teacher, clinician, and researcher. A past president of the Society of Teachers of Emergency Medicine and a Professor of Surgery, he directed the Residency Program in Emergency Medicine at the University of Arizona College of Medicine in Tucson for a decade. He frequently speaks to medical students, advisers, and residency directors throughout the country on the complex process of selecting a medical specialty; choosing a residency program; and applying to, interviewing for, and obtaining a desired residency position.

Dr. Iserson is also the author of the following books, all published by Galen Press, Tucson, Arizona:

- *Death to Dust: What Happens to Dead Bodies?, 2nd ed.* (2000)
- *Ethics in Emergency Medicine, 2nd ed.* (1995)
- *Get Into Medical School! A Guide for the Perplexed* (1997)
- *Grave Words: Notifying Survivors About Sudden, Unexpected Deaths* (1999)
- *Pocket Protocols: Notifying Survivors About Sudden, Unexpected Deaths* (1999)
- *Non-Standard Medical Electives in the U.S. and Canada* (1998)
- *Dying to Know: A Compendium of the Morbid, Mortal, & Macabre* (October, 2000)

## *Galen*

*Galen of Pergamum* (A.D. 130-201), the Greek physician whose writings guided medicine for more than a millennium after his death, inspired the name, Galen Press. As the father of modern anatomy and physiology, Galen wrote more than 100 treatises while attempting to change medicine from an art form into a science. As a practicing physician, Galen first ministered to gladiators and then to Roman Emperor Marcus Aurelius. Far more than Hippocrates, Galen's work influenced Western physicians, and was the "truth" until the late Middle Ages when physicians and scientists challenged his teachings.

Galen Press, which publishes non-clinical, health-related books, follows Galen's advice that "the chief merit of language is clearness . . . nothing detracts so much from this as unfamiliar terms."

## Also by Galen Press, LTD.

*After-Death Planning Guide*
by Kenneth V. Iserson, M.D.

*Civil War Medicine\**
by Alfred Jay Bollet, M. D.

*The Cost-Effective Use of Leeches
and Other Musings of a Medical School Survivor*
by Jeffrey A. Drayer, M.D.

*Death Investigation: The Basics*
by Brad Randall, M.D.

*Death To Dust: What Happens To Dead Bodies?*
by Kenneth V. Iserson, M.D.

*Ethics in Emergency Medicine, 2nd ed.*
Edited by Kenneth V. Iserson, M.D. Arthur B. Sanders, M.D.,
and Deborah Mathieu, Ph.D.

*Get Into Medical School! A Guide for the Perplexed*
by Kenneth V. Iserson, M.D.

*Getting Into A Residency Companion Disks*
DOS and Windows™ versions

*Grave Words: Notifying Survivors about Sudden, Unexpected Deaths*
by Kenneth V. Iserson, M.D.

*House Calls, Rounds, and Healings: A Poetry Casebook*
by David Schiedermayer, M.D.

*Non-Standard Medical Electives in the U.S. & Canada, 2nd ed.*
by Kenneth V. Iserson, M.D.

*The International Medical Graduate's Guide to U.S. Medicine, 2nd ed.\**
by Gloria A. Goldman, J.D.

*Resumes and Personal Statements for Health Professionals, 2nd ed.*
by James W. Tysinger, Ph.D.

---

*For more information, please contact:*
**Customer Service, Galen Press, LTD.**
P.O. Box 64400, Tucson, AZ 85728-4400 USA
Internet: Http://www.galenpress.com
Tel: (520) 577-8363     Fax: (520) 529-6459

*call for information

## Pocket Protocols
### for Notifying Survivors about Sudden, Unexpected Deaths
Pocket-sized booklet containing the protocols from *Grave Words*

ISBN: 1-883620-05-8                    $ 6.95 (Bulk discounts available.)

---

## Slides for Grave Words

- Slide Sets of the Protocols & other tables from Grave Words
- Build your own Death Notification and Death & Dying Course using the specialized slide sets

| Slide Set | Number of Slides |
|---|---|
| A. Main Protocol for Death Notification | 66 |
| B. General Set: Sudden Death/Nurse Interactions/ Grief/Communication/Survivors' Questions | 49 |
| C. Chaplains/Religions | 41 |
| D. Emergency Medicine/Trauma | 35 |
| E. Phrases: Helping and Hurtful | 23 |
| F. Telephone Notification Protocol | 20 |
| G. Students' Deaths | 17 |
| H. Emergency Medical Services | 16 |
| I. Telling Friends | 16 |
| J. Children: Telling & Grieving | 13 |
| K. Obstetrics | 14 |
| L. Disaster Survivors' Protocol | 10 |
| M. Organ Donation | 10 |

*Prices:*  **Item 1:** Complete set of 330 slides:           $ 395.00
**Item 2:** Main Protocol + Any three other sets:     $ 345.00
**Item 3:** Main Protocol + Any two other sets:      $ 295.00
**Item 4:** Main Protocol + Any one other set:       $ 250.00
**Item 5:** Individual set:                 $3.00/slide

**Items 1-4:** Includes one copy each of *Grave Words & Pocket Protocols*. **Free shipping.**

**Item 5: Add shipping** of $7 for first set and $3 for each additional set. (Priority mail.)

---

### To order, and for more information, please contact Galen Press, LTD., at:
P.O. Box 64400   Tucson, AZ 85728-4400  USA
Internet: Http://www.galenpress.com
Tel: (520) 577-8363    Fax: (520) 529-6459

**Previews:** We keep our prices low by not offering previews. See our 30-Day Guarantee.

**Thirty Day Money Back Guarantee:** You may return your purchase *within thirty days* for a refund of the purchase price. (Shipping costs not refundable.)

# Order Form     Order Form     Order Form

*Yes! . . . Please send me:*

\_\_\_\_\_ copies of **Getting Into A Residency: A Guide For Medical Students, 5th ed.** @ $36.95 each          $ _____

\_\_\_\_\_ copies of **The Companion Disk** @ $12.00
❑ DOS version      ❑ Windows® version          $ _____

\_\_\_\_\_ copies of **Grave Words: Notifying Survivors about Sudden, Unexpected Deaths** @ $38.95 each          $ _____

\_\_\_\_\_ copies of **Pocket Protocols** @ $6.95 each          $ _____

\_\_\_\_\_ copies of **Death to Dust: What Happens to Dead Bodies?** @ $44.95 each          $ _____

\_\_\_\_\_ copies of **After-Death Planning Guide** @ $3.00 each          $ _____

\_\_\_\_\_ copies of **Ethics In Emergency Medicine, 2nd ed.** @ $39.95 each          $ _____

\_\_\_\_\_ copies of **Résumés and Personal Statements for Health Professionals, 2nd ed.** @ $18.95 each          $ _____

\_\_\_\_\_ copies of **Death Investigation: The Basics** @ $24.95 each     $ _____

\_\_\_\_\_ copies of **Non-Standard Medical Electives in the U.S. & Canada, 2nd ed.** @ $31.95 each          $ _____

\_\_\_\_\_ copies of **Get Into Medical School! A Guide for the Perplexed** @ $34.95 each          $ _____

\_\_\_\_\_ copies of **The International Medical Graduates' Guide to U.S. Medicine** @ $31.95 each          $ _____

\_\_\_\_\_ copies of **House Calls, Rounds, and Healings: A Poetry Casebook** @ $12.95 each          $ _____

\_\_\_\_\_ copies of **The Cost-Effective Use of Leeches and Other Musings of a Medical School Survivor** @ $14.95 each          $ _____

AZ Residents – Add 7% sales tax          $ _____

**Shipping: $3.00 for 1st Book, $1.00 / each additional**          $ _____

Priority Mail: **ADD** $3.00 for 1st Book, $2.00 / each additional     $ _____

**TOTAL ENCLOSED (U.S. Funds Only)**          $ _____

❑ Check  ❑ VISA  ❑ MasterCard  ❑ Institutional Purchase Order

SHIP TO: Name _____

Address _____

_____

City/State/Zip _____

Phone **(required)** _____

**CREDIT CARD** Number: _____

Expiration date: _____  Signature: _____

**Send completed form and payment to:**

Galen Press, Ltd.                                        Tel (520) 577-8363
PO Box 64400-R5                                      Fax (520) 529-6459
Tucson, AZ 85728-4400 USA          Orders: 1-800-442-5369 (US/Canada)

**Visit our Home Page at http://www.galenpress.com**

*Also available through your local bookstore.*

## Pocket Protocols
### for Notifying Survivors about Sudden, Unexpected Deaths
Pocket-sized booklet containing the protocols from *Grave Words*

ISBN: 1-883620-05-8 $ 6.95 (Bulk discounts available.)

---

# Slides for Grave Words

- Slide Sets of the Protocols & other tables from Grave Words
- Build your own Death Notification and Death & Dying Course using the specialized slide sets

| Slide Set | Number of Slides |
| --- | --- |
| A. Main Protocol for Death Notification | 66 |
| B. General Set: Sudden Death/Nurse Interactions/ Grief/Communication/Survivors' Questions | 49 |
| C. Chaplains/Religions | 41 |
| D. Emergency Medicine/Trauma | 35 |
| E. Phrases: Helping and Hurtful | 23 |
| F. Telephone Notification Protocol | 20 |
| G. Students' Deaths | 17 |
| H. Emergency Medical Services | 16 |
| I. Telling Friends | 16 |
| J. Children: Telling & Grieving | 13 |
| K. Obstetrics | 14 |
| L. Disaster Survivors' Protocol | 10 |
| M. Organ Donation | 10 |

*Prices:*
**Item 1:** Complete set of 330 slides: $ 395.00
**Item 2:** Main Protocol + Any three other sets: $ 345.00
**Item 3:** Main Protocol + Any two other sets: $ 295.00
**Item 4:** Main Protocol + Any one other set: $ 250.00
**Item 5:** Individual set: $3.00/slide

**Items 1-4:** Includes one copy each of ***Grave Words & Pocket Protocols***. **Free shipping.**
**Item 5: Add shipping** of $7 for first set and $3 for each additional set. (Priority mail.)

---

**To order, and for more information, please contact Galen Press, LTD., at:**
P.O. Box 64400 Tucson, AZ 85728-4400 USA
Internet: Http://www.galenpress.com
Tel: (520) 577-8363 Fax: (520) 529-6459

**Previews:** We keep our prices low by not offering previews. See our 30-Day Guarantee.

**Thirty Day Money Back Guarantee:** You may return your purchase *within thirty days* for a refund of the purchase price. (Shipping costs not refundable.)

# Order Form  Order Form  Order Form

*Yes! . . . Please send me:*

_____ copies of **Getting Into A Residency: A Guide For Medical Students, 5th ed.** @ $36.95 each      $ _____

_____ copies of **The Companion Disk** @ $12.00
    ❑ DOS version     ❑ Windows® version      $ _____

_____ copies of **Grave Words: Notifying Survivors about Sudden, Unexpected Deaths** @ $38.95 each      $ _____

_____ copies of **Pocket Protocols** @ $6.95 each      $ _____

_____ copies of **Death to Dust: What Happens to Dead Bodies?** @ $44.95 each      $ _____

_____ copies of **After-Death Planning Guide** @ $3.00 each      $ _____

_____ copies of **Ethics In Emergency Medicine, 2nd ed.** @ $39.95 each      $ _____

_____ copies of **Résumés and Personal Statements for Health Professionals, 2nd ed.** @ $18.95 each      $ _____

_____ copies of **Death Investigation: The Basics** @ $24.95 each      $ _____

_____ copies of **Non-Standard Medical Electives in the U.S. & Canada, 2nd ed.** @ $31.95 each      $ _____

_____ copies of **Get Into Medical School! A Guide for the Perplexed** @ $34.95 each      $ _____

_____ copies of **The International Medical Graduates' Guide to U.S. Medicine** @ $31.95 each      $ _____

_____ copies of **House Calls, Rounds, and Healings: A Poetry Casebook** @ $12.95 each      $ _____

_____ copies of **The Cost-Effective Use of Leeches and Other Musings of a Medical School Survivor** @ $14.95 each      $ _____

AZ Residents – Add 7% sales tax      $ _____

**Shipping: $3.00 for 1st Book, $1.00 / each additional**      $ _____

Priority Mail: **ADD** $3.00 for 1st Book, $2.00 / each additional      $ _____

**TOTAL ENCLOSED (U.S. Funds Only)**      $ _____

❑ Check   ❑ VISA   ❑ MasterCard   ❑ Institutional Purchase Order

SHIP TO: Name _____

  Address _____

_____

  City/State/Zip _____

  Phone **(required)** _____

**CREDIT CARD** Number: _____

Expiration date: _____ Signature: _____

**Send completed form and payment to:**

Galen Press, Ltd.        Tel (520) 577-8363
PO Box 64400-R5        Fax (520) 529-6459
Tucson, AZ 85728-4400 USA      Orders: 1-800-442-5369 (US/Canada)

**Visit our Home Page at http://www.galenpress.com**

*Also available through your local bookstore.*

# Pocket Protocols
### for Notifying Survivors about Sudden, Unexpected Deaths
Pocket-sized booklet containing the protocols from *Grave Words*

ISBN: 1-883620-05-8                    $ 6.95  (Bulk discounts available.)

---

# Slides for Grave Words

- Slide Sets of the Protocols & other tables from Grave Words
- Build your own Death Notification and Death & Dying Course using the specialized slide sets

| Slide Set | Number of Slides |
|---|---|
| A. Main Protocol for Death Notification | 66 |
| B. General Set: Sudden Death/Nurse Interactions/ Grief/Communication/Survivors' Questions | 49 |
| C. Chaplains/Religions | 41 |
| D. Emergency Medicine/Trauma | 35 |
| E. Phrases: Helping and Hurtful | 23 |
| F. Telephone Notification Protocol | 20 |
| G. Students' Deaths | 17 |
| H. Emergency Medical Services | 16 |
| I. Telling Friends | 16 |
| J. Children: Telling & Grieving | 13 |
| K. Obstetrics | 14 |
| L. Disaster Survivors' Protocol | 10 |
| M. Organ Donation | 10 |

**Prices:**
| | | |
|---|---|---|
| **Item 1:** Complete set of 330 slides: | $ 395.00 |
| **Item 2:** Main Protocol + Any three other sets: | $ 345.00 |
| **Item 3:** Main Protocol + Any two other sets: | $ 295.00 |
| **Item 4:** Main Protocol + Any one other set: | $ 250.00 |
| **Item 5:** Individual set: | $3.00/slide |

**Items 1-4:** Includes one copy each of *Grave Words & Pocket Protocols*. **Free shipping.**

**Item 5: Add shipping** of $7 for first set and $3 for each additional set. (Priority mail.)

---

### To order, and for more information, please contact Galen Press, LTD., at:
P.O. Box 64400    Tucson, AZ  85728-4400  USA
Internet: Http://www.galenpress.com
Tel: (520) 577-8363    Fax: (520) 529-6459

**Previews:** We keep our prices low by not offering previews. See our 30-Day Guarantee.

**Thirty Day Money Back Guarantee:** You may return your purchase *within thirty days* for a refund of the purchase price. (Shipping costs not refundable.)

# Order Form    Order Form    Order Form

*Yes! . . . Please send me:*

_____ copies of **Getting Into A Residency: A Guide For
Medical Students, 5th ed.** @ $36.95 each                    $ _____

_____ copies of **The Companion Disk** @ $12.00
❏ DOS version    ❏ Windows® version                    $ _____

_____ copies of **Grave Words: Notifying Survivors about
Sudden, Unexpected Deaths** @ $38.95 each                    $ _____

_____ copies of **Pocket Protocols** @ $6.95 each                    $ _____

_____ copies of **Death to Dust: What Happens to
Dead Bodies?** @ $44.95 each                    $ _____

_____ copies of **After-Death Planning Guide** @ $3.00 each          $ _____

_____ copies of **Ethics In Emergency Medicine, 2nd ed.**
@ $39.95 each                    $ _____

_____ copies of **Résumés and Personal Statements for Health
Professionals, 2nd ed.** @ $18.95 each                    $ _____

_____ copies of **Death Investigation: The Basics** @ $24.95 each   $ _____

_____ copies of **Non-Standard Medical Electives in the
U.S. & Canada, 2nd ed.** @ $31.95 each                    $ _____

_____ copies of **Get Into Medical School! A Guide for the
Perplexed** @ $34.95 each                    $ _____

_____ copies of **The International Medical Graduates' Guide
to U.S. Medicine** @ $31.95 each                    $ _____

_____ copies of **House Calls, Rounds, and Healings:
A Poetry Casebook** @ $12.95 each                    $ _____

_____ copies of **The Cost-Effective Use of Leeches and Other
Musings of a Medical School Survivor** @ $14.95 each          $ _____

AZ Residents – Add 7% sales tax                    $ _____

**Shipping: $3.00 for 1st Book, $1.00 / each additional**          $ _____

Priority Mail: **ADD** $3.00 for 1st Book, $2.00 / each additional   $ _____

**TOTAL ENCLOSED (U.S. Funds Only)**                    $ _____

❏ Check   ❏ VISA   ❏ MasterCard   ❏ Institutional Purchase Order

SHIP TO: Name _____

Address _____

_____

City/State/Zip _____

Phone **(required)** _____

**CREDIT CARD** Number: _____

Expiration date: _____    Signature: _____

**Send completed form and payment to:**

Galen Press, Ltd.                                        Tel (520) 577-8363
PO Box 64400-R5                                        Fax (520) 529-6459
Tucson, AZ 85728-4400 USA              Orders: 1-800-442-5369 (US/Canada)

**Visit our Home Page at http://www.galenpress.com**

*Also available through your local bookstore.*

## Pocket Protocols
### for Notifying Survivors about Sudden, Unexpected Deaths

Pocket-sized booklet containing the protocols from *Grave Words*

ISBN: 1-883620-05-8                    $ 6.95  (Bulk discounts available.)

## Slides for Grave Words

- Slide Sets of the Protocols & other tables from Grave Words
- Build your own Death Notification and Death & Dying Course using the specialized slide sets

| Slide Set | Number of Slides |
|---|---|
| A. Main Protocol for Death Notification | 66 |
| B. General Set: Sudden Death/Nurse Interactions/ Grief/Communication/Survivors' Questions | 49 |
| C. Chaplains/Religions | 41 |
| D. Emergency Medicine/Trauma | 35 |
| E. Phrases: Helping and Hurtful | 23 |
| F. Telephone Notification Protocol | 20 |
| G. Students' Deaths | 17 |
| H. Emergency Medical Services | 16 |
| I. Telling Friends | 16 |
| J. Children: Telling & Grieving | 13 |
| K. Obstetrics | 14 |
| L. Disaster Survivors' Protocol | 10 |
| M. Organ Donation | 10 |

**Prices:**

| | | |
|---|---|---|
| **Item 1:** Complete set of 330 slides: | | $ 395.00 |
| **Item 2:** Main Protocol + Any three other sets: | | $ 345.00 |
| **Item 3:** Main Protocol + Any two other sets: | | $ 295.00 |
| **Item 4:** Main Protocol + Any one other set: | | $ 250.00 |
| **Item 5:** Individual set: | | $3.00/slide |

**Items 1-4:** Includes one copy each of *Grave Words & Pocket Protocols*. **Free shipping.**

**Item 5: Add shipping** of $7 for first set and $3 for each additional set. (Priority mail.)

### *To order, and for more information, please contact Galen Press, LTD., at:*

P.O. Box 64400    Tucson, AZ  85728-4400  USA

Internet: Http://www.galenpress.com

Tel: (520) 577-8363    Fax: (520) 529-6459

**Previews:** We keep our prices low by not offering previews. See our 30-Day Guarantee.

**Thirty Day Money Back Guarantee:** You may return your purchase *within thirty days* for a refund of the purchase price. (Shipping costs not refundable.)

# Order Form     Order Form     Order Form

*Yes! . . . Please send me:*

_____ copies of **Getting Into A Residency: A Guide For Medical Students, 5th ed.** @ $36.95 each $ _____

_____ copies of **The Companion Disk** @ $12.00
　　　　❏ DOS version 　　❏ Windows® version $ _____

_____ copies of **Grave Words: Notifying Survivors about Sudden, Unexpected Deaths** @ $38.95 each $ _____

_____ copies of **Pocket Protocols** @ $6.95 each $ _____

_____ copies of **Death to Dust: What Happens to Dead Bodies?** @ $44.95 each $ _____

_____ copies of **After-Death Planning Guide** @ $3.00 each $ _____

_____ copies of **Ethics In Emergency Medicine, 2nd ed.** @ $39.95 each $ _____

_____ copies of **Résumés and Personal Statements for Health Professionals, 2nd ed.** @ $18.95 each $ _____

_____ copies of **Death Investigation: The Basics** @ $24.95 each $ _____

_____ copies of **Non-Standard Medical Electives in the U.S. & Canada, 2nd ed.** @ $31.95 each $ _____

_____ copies of **Get Into Medical School! A Guide for the Perplexed** @ $34.95 each $ _____

_____ copies of **The International Medical Graduates' Guide to U.S. Medicine** @ $31.95 each $ _____

_____ copies of **House Calls, Rounds, and Healings: A Poetry Casebook** @ $12.95 each $ _____

_____ copies of **The Cost-Effective Use of Leeches and Other Musings of a Medical School Survivor** @ $14.95 each $ _____

AZ Residents – Add 7% sales tax $ _____

**Shipping: $3.00 for 1st Book, $1.00 / each additional** $ _____

Priority Mail: **ADD** $3.00 for 1st Book, $2.00 / each additional $ _____

**TOTAL ENCLOSED (U.S. Funds Only)** $ _____

❏ Check 　❏ VISA 　❏ MasterCard 　❏ Institutional Purchase Order

SHIP TO:　Name _____

　Address _____

　_____

　City/State/Zip _____

　Phone **(required)** _____

**CREDIT CARD** Number: _____

Expiration date: _____　Signature: _____

**Send completed form and payment to:**

Galen Press, Ltd.
PO Box 64400-R5
Tucson, AZ 85728-4400 USA

Tel (520) 577-8363
Fax (520) 529-6459
Orders: 1-800-442-5369 (US/Canada)

**Visit our Home Page at http://www.galenpress.com**

*Also available through your local bookstore.*